Unexplained Infertility

Glenn L. Schattman • Sandro C. Esteves
Ashok Agarwal
Editors

Unexplained Infertility

Pathophysiology, Evaluation and Treatment

Springer

Editors
Glenn L. Schattman
Ronald O. Perelman and Claudia Cohen Center for Reproductive Medicine
Weill Cornell Medical College
New York, NY, USA

Sandro C. Esteves
ANDROFERT, Andrology and Human Reproduction Clinic
Referral Center for Male Reproduction
Campinas, São Paulo, Brazil

Ashok Agarwal
Lerner College of Medicine
Case Western Reserve University
Andrology Center &
Center for Reproductive Medicine
Cleveland Clinic
Cleveland, OH, USA

ISBN 978-1-4939-2139-3 ISBN 978-1-4939-2140-9 (eBook)
DOI 10.1007/978-1-4939-2140-9

Library of Congress Control Number: 2014955347

Springer New York Heidelberg Dordrecht London

Printed on acid-free paper

Springer is part of Springer Science+Business Media (www.springer.com)

Preface

Infertility, or involuntary childlessness, is customarily defined as the failure of a couple to conceive after 12 months of unprotected regular intercourse. It has been estimated that 10–15 % of couples seek medical assistance for fertility evaluation, and the problem is apparently equally shared between male and female partners. However, after extensive evaluation of both partners by routinely used tests and without physical or endocrine abnormalities, up to 30 % of infertile couples remain childless devoid of identifiable causes—leading to a diagnosis of unexplained infertility.

Potential etiologies of unexplained infertility include couples' miscomprehension of the concept of the female fertile window, improper coital techniques, erectile dysfunction, and molecular and functional causes of male and female infertility. Interestingly, contemporary advanced technologies have demonstrated various ultrastructural, molecular and genetic etiologies in male or female partners with unexplained infertility. Men with unexplained infertility typically have normal semen parameters with no demonstrable abnormalities in their history, physical or endocrinological examination. Possible underlying causes of unexplained male infertility include mainly immune, humoral or cellular sensitization against sperm, genetic defects, sperm dysfunction and fertilization incompetence.

Even more interestingly, highly intricate testing methods provide a great deal of information about the potential contribution of female factors in UI. Cervical hostility, endometrial receptivity problems, fallopian tube dysfunction and oocyte quality may all weaken female fertility potential. Further, immunity against sperm, genetic causes, oxidative stress and subtle foci of endometriosis are some of the conditions that need to be evaluated in a patient with unexplained infertility, in order to understand the underlying cause(s) of unexplained infertility. These conditions may serve as a guide in any future research plans to solve the infertility dilemma.

This book introduces unexplained infertility, its definition and incidence in both males and females. The current use of the 2010 WHO guidelines in semen analysis has an impact on the diagnosis of unexplained infertility. The pathophysiological factors of this type of infertility include physical, immunological and genetic abnormalities. Factors that cause the development of oxidative stress and a variety of environmental factors have a role in the etiology of unexplained infertility. The management of unexplained infertility is complex, as its diagnosis was likely made by exclusion of various potential causes of infertility. Unexplained infertility may be managed through medications that may help normalize the endocrine profile or soothe immunological imbalances. Active interventions and the outcomes of each treatment modality are also considered. Couples dealing with a diagnosis of either male or female factor unexplained infertility very often resort to assisted reproductive technology to achieve conception, and the outcomes of these interventions will be discussed.

This textbook, the first of its kind, is intended to provide the reader with a thoughtful and comprehensive review of the clinical and scientific significance of unexplained infertility. We had invited leading, internationally recognized clinicians and basic scientists with expertise in male and female infertility to contribute their thoughts on these various aspects of unexplained infertility. The experts from the various sub-specialties have contributed for this textbook. This book puts together information that serves as an invaluable tool both for the basic scientists with an interest in reproductive medicine and for clinicians working in the field of infertility (e.g., urologists, andrologists, gynaecologists and reproductive endocrinologists and embryologists). It is hoped that the topics discussed in this book serves to enlighten the readers regarding unexplained infertility and provide an in-depth perspective of this form of infertility.

Glenn L. Schattman
Sandro C. Esteves
Ashok Agarwal

Contents

Contributors

Yapo Guillaume Aboua Division of Medical Physiology, Department of Biomedical Sciences, Stellenbosch University, Cape Town, South Africa

Ashok Agarwal Center for Reproductive Medicine, Cleveland Clinic, Cleveland, OH, USA

Alfredo Guillén Antón Department of Reproductive Medicine IVI Madrid, Rey Juan Carlos University, Madrid, Spain

Michael S. Bloom Obstetrics, Gynecology and Reproductive Sciences, University of California at San Francisco, San Francisco, CA, USA

Jamin Brahmbhatt Department of Urology, University of Florida & Winter Haven Hospital, Winter Haven, FL, USA

Spyridon Chouliaras Reproductive Medicine and Gynecology, Gynehealth, Manchester, UK

Marcello Cocuzza Department of Urology, University of Sao Paulo (USP), Sao Paulo, SP, Brazil

Ali A. Dabaja Department of Urology, Weill Cornell Medical College, New York-Presbyterian Hospital, New York, NY, USA

Anderson Sanches de Melo Department of Obstetrics and Gynecology, University of São Paulo, Ribeirão Preto, São Paulo, Brazil

Marcello Desgro Department of Gynecology and Division of Gynecology and Reproductive Medicine, IRCCS Istituto Clinico Humanitas, Rozzano (Milano), Italy

Richard P Dickey The Fertility Institute, Mandeville, LA, USA

Sejal B. Doshi Center for Reproductive Medicine, Cleveland Clinic, Cleveland, OH, USA

Stefan S. du Plessis Division of Medical Physiology, Department of Biomedical Sciences, Stellenbosch University, Parow, Western Cape, South Africa

Damayanthi Durairajanayagam Center for Reproductive Medicine, Cleveland Clinic, Cleveland, OH, USA

Sandro C. Esteves ANDROFERT, Andrology and Human Reproduction Clinic, Referral Center for Male Reproduction, Campinas, Sao Paulo, Brazil

Fathy Ezzeldin Department of Obstetrics and Gynaecology, Alexandria University, Alexandria, Egypt

Rogério de Barros Ferreira Leão ANDROFERT, Andrology and Human Reproduction Clinic, Referral Center for Male Reproduction, Campinas, SP, Brazil

Rui Alberto Ferriani Department of Obstetrics and Gynecology, University of São Paulo, Ribeirão Preto, São Paulo, Brazil

Victor Y. Fujimoto Obstetrics, Gynecology and Reproductive Sciences, University of California at San Francisco, San Francisco, CA, USA

Daniela Galliano Department of Reproduction, Instituto Valenciano Iinfertilidad (IVI), Barcelona, Spain

Bhushan K. Gangrade Center for Reproductive Medicine, Orlando, FL, USA

Juan Antonio García Velasco Department of Reproductive Medicine IVI Madrid, Rey Juan Carlos University, Madrid, Spain

Jaime Gosálvez Biology Department, Genetics Unit, Universidad Autónoma de Madrid, Madrid, Spain

Lawrence Grunfeld Department of Obstetrics, Gynecology, & Reproductive Medicine, Icahn School of Medicine at Mount Sinai, New York, NY, USA

Ahmet Gudeloglu Department of Urology, University of Florida & Winter Haven Hospital, Winter Haven, FL, USA

Brent M Hardin Division of Urology, Department of Surgery, University of Tennessee Graduate School of Medicine, Knoxville, TN, USA

Avner Hershlag Department of Obstetrics, Gynecology and Reproductive Medicine, North Shore-Long Island Jewish Hospital of Hofstra University School of Medicine, Manhasset, NY, USA

Roy Homburg Fertility Centre, Homerton University Hospitals NHS Trust, Homerton, London, UK

Edward D Kim Division of Urology, Department of Surgery, University of Tennessee Graduate School of Medicine, Knoxville, TN, USA

Walter K.H. Krause Deptartment of Dermatology and Allergology, University Hospital, Philipp University, Marburg, Germany

Pieter Johann Maartens Division of Medical Physiology, Department of Biomedical Sciences, Stellenbosch University, Cape Town, South Africa

Avinash Maganty Department of Urology, New York—Presbyterian Hospital, Weill Cornell Medical College, New York, NY, New York, USA

Ricardo Miyaoka ANDROFERT, Andrology and Human Reproduction Clinic, Referral Center for Male Reproduction, Campinas, SP, Brazil

Ben Willem Mol Department Gynecology/Obstetrics, Academic Medical Center at the University of Amsterdam, Amsterdam, The Netherlands

Fabiana Y. Nakano Androfert, Campinas, SP, Brazil

Anupa Nandi Fertility Centre, Homerton University Hospitals NHS Trust, Homerton, London, UK

Luciano G. Nardo Reproductive Medicine and Gynecology, Gynehealth, Manchester, UK

Paula Andrea de Albuquerque de Salles Navarro Department of Obstetrics and Gynecology, University of São Paulo, Ribeirão Preto, São Paulo, Brazil

Rajesh K. Naz Department of Obstetrics and Gynecology, West Virginia University School of Medicine, Morgantown, WV, USA

Darius Paduch Department of Urology, Weill Cornell Medical College, New York-Presbyterian Hospital, New York, NY, USA

Sijo Parekattil Department of Urology, University of Florida & Winter Haven Hospital, Winter Haven, FL, USA

Sejal Dhana Patel Center for Reproductive Medicine, Orlando, FL, USA

Zamip Patel Center for Reproductive Medicine, Orlando, FL, USA

Pasquale Patrizio Department of Gynecology and Division of Gynecology and Reproductive Medicine, IRCCS Istituto Clinico Humanitas, Rozzano (Milano), Italy

Antonio Pellicer Department of Reproduction, Instituto Valenciano Iinfertilidad (IVI), Barcelona, Spain

Ranjith Ramasamy Department of Urology, New York—Presbyterian Hospital, Weill Cornell Medical College, New York, NY, New York, USA

Patricia Rekawek Department of Obstetrics, Gynecology, & Reproductive Medicine, Icahn School of Medicine at Mount Sinai, New York, NY, USA

A. K. Rengan Center for Reproductive Medicine, Cleveland Clinic, Cleveland, OH, USA

Edmund S. Sabanegh Department of Urology, The Cleveland Clinic, Cleveland, OH, USA

Hassan Sallam Department of Obstetrics and Gynaecology, Alexandria University, Alexandria, Egypt

Nooman Sallam Department of Obstetrics and Gynaecology, Alexandria University, Alexandria, Egypt

Glenn L. Schattman Ronald O. Perelman and Claudia Cohen Center for Reproductive Medicine, Weill Cornell Medical College, New York, NY, USA

Peter N. Schlegel Department of Urology, New York—Presbyterian Hospital, Weill Cornell Medical College, New York, NY, New York, USA

Thalia R. Segal Department of Obstetrics, Gynecology and Reproductive Medicine, North Shore-Long Island Jewish Hospital of Hofstra University School of Medicine, Manhasset, NY, USA

Lucky H. Sekhon Department of Obstetrics, Gynecology, & Reproductive Medicine, Icahn School of Medicine at Mount Sinai, New York, NY, USA

Paolo Emanuele Levi Setti Department of Gynecology and Division of Gynecology and Reproductive Medicine, IRCCS Istituto Clinico Humanitas, Rozzano (Milano), Italy

Rakesh K. Sharma Center for Reproductive Medicine, Cleveland Clinic, Cleveland, OH, USA

Christopher L. Starks The Urology Group of Virginia, Glickman Urologic and Kidney Institute, The Cleveland Clinic Foundation, Cleveland, Suite 112 Leesburg, USA

Bruno Camargo Tiseo Department of Urology, University of Sao Paulo (USP), Sao Paulo, SP, Brazil

Alberto Vaiarelli Department of Gynecology and Division of Gynecology and Reproductive Medicine, IRCCS Istituto Clinico Humanitas, Rozzano (Milano), Italy

N. M. van den Boogaard Gynaecology and Obstetrics and Reproductive medicine, VU medical centre and AMC medical centre, Amsterdam, Pieter Lodewijk Takstraat 31, The Netherlands

Michelle van der Linde Division of Medical Physiology, Department of Biomedical Sciences, Stellenbosch University, Parow, Western Cape, South Africa

Fulco van der Veen Department of Gynecology, Academic Medical Center, Amsterdam, The Netherlands

Fatma Ferda Verit Department of Obstetrics & Gynecology, Infertility Research & Treatment Center, Suleymaniye Maternity, Research &Training Hospital, Istanbul, Turkey

Sidney Verza Jr. ANDROFERT, Referral Center for Male Reproduction, Andrology and Human Reproduction Clinic, Campinas, Sao Paulo, Brazil

Irene Zerbetto Department of Gynecology and Division of Gynecology and Reproductive Medicine, IRCCS Istituto Clinico Humanitas, Rozzano (Milano), Italy

About the Editors

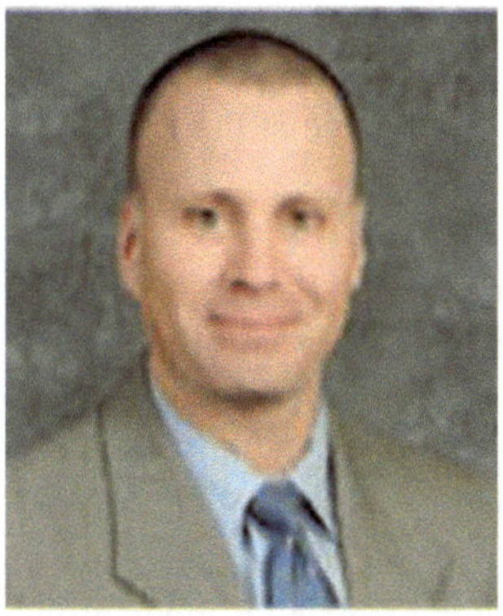

Dr. Glenn L. Schattman MD is an Associate Professor of Clinical Obstetrics and Gynecology and Clinical Reproductive Medicine at the Ronald O. Perelman and Claudia Cohen Center for Reproductive Medicine (CRM) of Weill Cornell Medical College. Dr. Schattman is board certified in Obstetrics and Gynecology and Reproductive Endocrinology and Infertility. He is a noted specialist in in vitro fertilization (IVF), fertility preservation, minimally invasive reproductive surgery and problems of sexual development in girls and young women.

Dr. Schattman is a leading minimally invasive surgeon. He was one of the first gynecologic surgeons to perform robotic surgery for reversal of tubal ligation and excision of uterine fibroids.

Dr. Schattman earned a Bachelor of Science from St. Lawrence University in Canton, New York, in 1983 and his medical degree from the State University of New York, Downstate Medical Center, in Brooklyn, New York, in 1987. He completed his residency training in Obstetrics and Gynecology at The George Washington University Medical Center in 1991. He finished his training with a fellowship in Reproductive Endocrinology and Infertility at the Center for Reproductive Medicine and became a CRM faculty member in 1993.

He was the 2011–2012 President of the Society for Assisted Reproductive Technology (SART), the leading association of in vitro fertilization-specialized physicians. Dr. Schattman was the Chair of SART's Practice Committee from 2004 to 2009 and is a member or fellow of numerous medical associations, including the American Society for Reproductive Medicine and the American Association of Gynecologic Laparoscopists.

Dr. Schattman has authored numerous articles and textbook chapters and lectures both nationally and internationally on a wide range of topics in reproductive medicine.

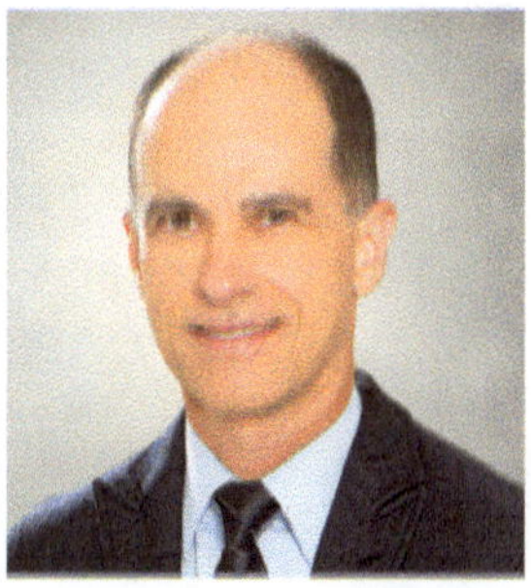

Sandro C. Esteves MD, PhD is Director of ANDROFERT—Andrology and Human Reproduction Clinic in Campinas, Brazil.

Sandro Esteves graduated in 1990 at the University of Campinas Medical School (UNICAMP), Brazil, where he accomplished a residency program in General Surgery and Urology (1991–1995). He received his Master Degree in Surgery in 1996 from UNICAMP, and a PhD in Medicine in 1998 from the Federal University of São Paulo (UNIFESP). He did his post-residency training in Andrology and Male Infertility under a fellowship from the Cleveland Clinic Foundation International Center at the Center for Reproductive Medicine of the Glickman Urological & Kidney Institute in Cleveland, Ohio (1995–1996). Dr. Esteves is a board-certified Urologist by the Brazilian Society of Urology, and member or office bearer of several professional societies, including the Brazilian Society of Urology (SBU), Brazilian Society of Human Reproduction (SBRH), Brazilian Society for Assisted Reproduction (SBRA), American Society for Reproductive Medicine (ASRM), Society for the Study of Male Reproduction and Urology (SMRU). He is an 'ad hoc' consultant in the area of germinative tissues at the Brazilian National Agency of Sanitary Surveillance.

Dr. Esteves is the founder of ANDROFERT, the first Center dedicated to male reproduction in Brazil. ANDROFERT has become a Referral Center for Male Infertility, and was the first Brazilian Human Reproduction Clinic to obtain full ISO 9001:2008 certification.

Dr. Esteves has authored and edited medical textbooks on human reproduction and published over 200 peer-reviewed articles and book chapters over the past 20 years (http://www.researchgate.net/profile/Sandro_Esteves/publications/). He serves as Associate Editor of the International Brazilian Journal of Urology and Area Editor of Clinics (Sao Paulo), International Urology and Nephrology, and MedicalExpress. Dr. Esteves' major interest areas are clinical male infertility, reproductive endocrinology, microsurgery, cryobiology, andrology and IVF laboratory technique, and quality management applied to Fertility Centers.

Dr. Esteves is a Research Collaborator and External Faculty at the Cleveland Clinic's Center for Reproductive Medicine, a Clinical Tutor in the College of Medicine at the University of Edinburgh.

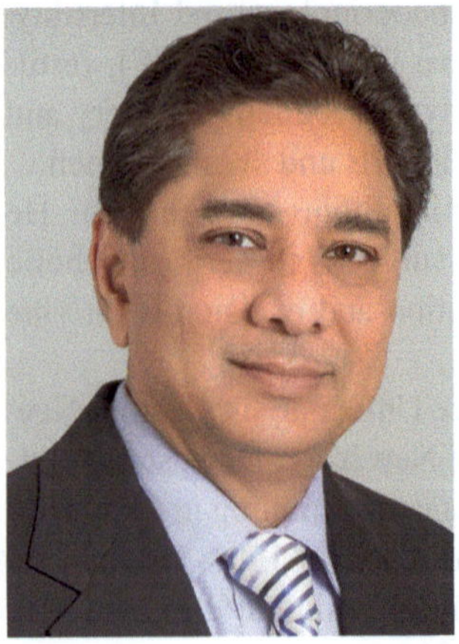

Ashok Agarwal PhD is a Professor at Lerner College of Medicine, Case Western Reserve University and the head of the Andrology Center. He is the Director of Research at the Center for Reproductive Medicine, Cleveland Clinic, USA. He has researched extensively on oxidative stress and its implications on human fertility and his group has published over 500 research articles. Ashok is an editor of over 26 medical text books/ manuals related to male infertility, ART, fertility preservation, DNA damage and antioxidants. Dr. Agarwal serves on the editorial boards of several key journals in human reproduction. His current research interests are the study of molecular markers of oxidative stress, DNA fragmentation and apoptosis using proteomics and bioinformatics tools, as well as fertility preservation in patients with cancer, and the efficacy of certain antioxidants in improving male fertility.

Part I

Definitions and Epidemiology

Definitions and Relevance of Unexplained Infertility in Reproductive Medicine

1

Sandro C. Esteves, Glenn L. Schattman and Ashok Agarwal

Infertility is customarily defined as the inability of a sexually active couple with no contraception to achieve natural pregnancy within one year [1]. The American Society for Reproductive Medicine (ASRM) considers infertility as a disease, which by definition is "any deviation from or interruption of the normal structure or function of any part, organ, or system of the body as manifested by characteristic symptoms and signs; the etiology, pathology, and prognosis may be known or unknown" [2, 3].

It has been estimated that 15% of couples seek medical assistance for infertility, and the origins of the problem seem to be equally distributed between male and female partners [1]. Taking into account a global perspective and a world population of 7 billion people, these figures indicate that approximately 140 million people (2.2%) face infertility [4, 5].

Infertility depends at large on the age of the female partner. As such, the ASRM states that an early evaluation and treatment is warranted after 6 months for women aged 35 years or older [3].

In men, about 8% seek medical assistance for fertility-related problems [6]. In its most updated version (2010) on "the optimal evaluation of the infertile male," the American Urological Association (AUA) recommends that the initial screening should be done if pregnancy has not occurred within one year of unprotected intercourse, or earlier in cases of known male or female infertility risk factors [7]. Male infertility can result from congenital or acquired urogenital abnormalities, urogenital tract infections, increased scrotal temperature such as a consequence of varicocele, endocrine disturbances, genetic abnormalities, immunological factors, lifestyle habits (e.g., obesity, smoking, and use of gonadotoxins), systemic diseases, erectile dysfunction, and incorrect coital habitus. Unfortunately, owed to limitations in our understanding of the events that take place during natural conception, and in view of the crude diagnostic tests available to identify potential abnormalities, the cause of infertility is not determined in nearly half of the cases. Moreover, approximately 5% of couples remain unwillingly childless despite multiple interventions [1, 8, 9].

Infertility of unknown origin comprises both idiopathic and unexplained infertility. Men presenting with idiopathic infertility have no obvious history of fertility problems, and both physical examination and endocrine laboratory testing are normal. However, semen analysis as routinely performed reveals sperm abnormalities that come alone or in combination. The reported prevalence of men with unexplained reduction of semen quality ranges from 30 to 40% [1, 10].

In contrast to idiopathic infertility, the term "unexplained infertility" is reserved for couples in whom routine semen analysis is within the reference values, and a definitive female infertility factor has not been identified [11]. In females with unexplained infertility, no definitive abnormality can be identified, but a reduced fecundity potential may be suspected in ovulatory woman with evidence of diminished ovarian reserve testing, including elevated follicle stimulating hormone (FSH) or low anti-Mullerian hormone (AMH) levels. In addition, direct evidence of diminished ovarian reserve can be determined by low antral follicle counts or lack of response to exogenous gonadotropins despite normal ovarian reserve testing. This category of 'poor ovarian response (POR)' or 'diminished ovarian response (DOR)' is difficult to define and the leading experts in the field were still unable to arrive at a conclusive definition [12].

The reported prevalence of unexplained infertility ranges from 6 to 30% [1, 8, 9, 11, 13], and this highly variable

S. C. Esteves (✉)
ANDROFERT, Andrology and Human Reproduction Clinic, Referral Center for Male Reproduction, Avenida Dr. Heitor Penteado, Campinas 1464, Sao Paulo, Brazil
e-mail: s.esteves@androfert.com.br

G. L. Schattman
Center for Reproductive Medicine, Weill Cornell Medical College, 1305 York Avenue, 10021 New York, NY, USA
e-mail: glschatt@med.cornell.edu

A. Agarwal
Center for Reproductive Medicine, Cleveland Clinic, 10681 Carnegie Avenue, Desk X-11, Cleveland, OH, 44195 USA
e-mail: agarwaa@ccf.org

G. L. Schattman et al. (eds.), *Unexplained Infertility*, DOI 10.1007/978-1-4939-2140-9_1,

prevalence strongly depends on the criteria used for diagnosis. In countries with limited resources for testing, it is likely that the prevalence of unexplained or unexplored infertility is increased [14]. Also, its prevalence is related to national or societies' guidelines and infertility centers' policies toward infertility evaluation. In a group of 2383 subfertile males attending one of the editors' (SE) tertiary center for male reproduction, in which all male partners underwent a systematic workup regardless of semen analyses results, 12.1% of the individuals were categorized as having infertility of unknown origin [9]. Depending on the method and criteria used for semen analysis, the percentage of men defined as "normal" will be variable. The AUA guidelines state that the initial evaluation for male infertility should include a reproductive history and two properly performed semen analyses, and that a full evaluation (which includes a throughout physical examination and additional testing) is warranted in the following cases: (i) presence of abnormalities in the initial evaluation; (ii) presence of unexplained infertility; and (iii) presence of persistent infertility despite proper treatment of identified female factors.

In contrast, the European Association of Urology (EAU) recommends that the male examination should be undertaken in individuals with abnormal semen analysis results [10]. According to the EAU guidelines on male infertility, a single seminal evaluation is sufficient if the semen analysis results are within the reference limits according to the World Health Organization (WHO) criteria. The EAU recommendations pose potential problems since semen analyses results, as routinely performed, are limited in their validity as surrogates for the assessment of male fertility status [15, 16]. First, the prognostic value of semen characteristics, such as sperm concentration, percent motility, and morphology, as surrogate markers for male fertility is confounded in several ways; a man's fertility potential is influenced by sexual activity, function of accessory sex glands, and other conditions. Second, routine semen analysis has its own limitations, and it does not account for sperm dysfunctions such as immature chromatin or DNA damage. It is known that about 30% of men misdiagnosed as having unexplained male infertility have sperm deficiencies that can be solely identified using sperm functional tests, including DNA integrity, oxidative stress, and antisperm antibodies testing [17–19]. Third, it is erroneous to assume that a single ejaculate represents the seminal profile owed to the large variability of semen parameters from the same individuals over different time periods. Results from at least two, preferably three, seminal analyses must be obtained before any statement is made regarding sperm production [20]. Finally, the criteria for normalcy, especially concerning sperm morphology, vary according to the edition of the WHO laboratory manual for the examination and processing of human semen [21–24].

These considerations highlight the shortcomings of the routine semen analysis. The male evaluation regarding fertility must go far beyond counting spermatozoa and assessing motility and morphology. It has to be complemented with a proper clinical examination, a comprehensive history-taking, and relevant endocrine, genetic as well as other investigations. The goals of an andrological investigation are to identify potential life-threatening diseases and to treat reversible conditions, including poor lifestyle habits, subclinical infections, hormone disorders, and clinical varicocele, to cite a few. Nevertheless, it is still a matter of debate not only what is considered a thorough evaluation, but also which tests are useful in the evaluation of couples with unexplained infertility.

Potential etiologies of unexplained infertility (UI) encompass a couple's miscomprehension of the concept of the female fertile window, improper coital techniques, erectile dysfunction, and molecular and functional causes of male and female infertility.

Altogether, these considerations form the backbone of this book, intended to unravel the mysteries of unexplained infertility. Modern insights on reproductive function are provided, including a detailed appraisal of the conditions that affect reproductive health in both males and females. Further insight is contemplated into the treatment options, including expectant management as well as active interventions. The benefits of each intervention and its inherent risk are discussed in detail, thus allowing appropriate patient counseling. Our readers will find this book as the ultimate resource to unexplained infertility, and we recommend it not only to clinicians working in the field of infertility but also to everyone with an interest in reproductive medicine.

References

1. World Health Organization. WHO Manual for the standardised investigation and diagnosis of the infertile couple. Cambridge: Cambridge University Press; 2000.
2. Practice Committee of the American Society for Reproductive Medicine. Definitions of infertility and recurrent pregnancy loss (Committee opinion). Fertil Steril. 2008;90:60.
3. Dorland WAN, editor. Dorland's illustrated medical dictionary, 31st ed. New York: Elsevier; 2007. p. 53.
4. US Census Bureau. Population estimates. U.S. Census Bureau, Methodology and Standards Council: (updated: 17th August 2011; cited 24th December 2011). http://www.census.gov. Accessed 21 June 2014.
5. Right Diagnosis.com. Statistics by country for infertility. Health Grades Inc.: (updated: 23rd August 2011; cited: 24th December 2011). http://www.rightdiagnosis.com/i/infertility/stats-country.htm. Accessed 21 June 2014.
6. CDC. Vital and Health Statistics, series 23, no. 26. http://www.cdc.gov (cited: 24th Dec 2011). Accessed 21 June 2014.
7. American Urological Association. Best practice statement on the optimal evaluation of the infertile male (revised 2010). http://www.auanet.org/content/media/optimalevaluation2010.pdf. Accessed 21 June 2014.

8. Moghissi KS, Wallach EE. Unexplained infertility. Fertil Steril. 1983;39:5–21.
9. Hamada A, Esteves SC, Agarwal A. Unexplained male infertility: potential causes and management. Hum Androl. 2011;1:2–16.
10. European Association of Urology. Guidelines on Male Infertility 2010. http://www.uroweb.org/gls/pdf/Male%20Infertility%20 2010.pdf. Accessed 21 June 2014.
11. Sigman M, Lipshultz L, Howard S. Office evaluation of the subfertile male. In: Lipshultz LI, Howards SS, Craig S, Niederberger CS, editors. Infertility in the male. 4th ed. Cambridge: Cambridge University Press; 2009, pp. 153–76.
12. Ferraretti AP, La Marca A, Fauser BCJM, Tarlatzis B, Nargund G, Gianaroli L. On behalf of the ESHRE working group on Poor Ovarian Response Definition. ESHRE consensus on the definition of 'poor response' to ovarian stimulation for in vitro fertilization: the Bologna criteria. Hum Reprod. 2011;26:1616–24.
13. Esteves SC, Miyaoka R, Agarwal A. An update on the clinical assessment of the infertile male. Clinics. 2011; 66:691–700.
14. Cates W, Farley TM, Rowe PJ. Worldwide patterns of infertility: is Africa different? Lancet. 1985;2:596–598.
15. Cooper TG, Noonan E, von Eckardstein S, et al. World Health Organization reference values for human semen characteristics. Hum Reprod Update. 2010;16:231–245.
16. Esteves SC, Zini A, Aziz N, Alvarez JG, Sabanegh ES Jr, Agarwal A. Critical appraisal of World Health Organization's new reference values for human semen characteristics and effect on diagnosis and treatment of subfertile men. Urology. 2012;79:16–22.
17. Bungum M, Bungum L, Giwercman A. Sperm chromatin structure assay (SCSA): a tool in diagnosis and treatment of infertility. AJA. 2010;13:69–75.
18. Agarwal A, Makker K, Sharma R. Clinical relevance of oxidative stress in male factor infertility: an update. Am J Reprod Immunol. 2008;59:2–11.
19. Esteves SC, Sharma RK, Gosálvez J, Agarwal A. A translational medicine appraisal of specialized andrology testing in unexplained male infertility. Int Urol Nephrol. 2014;46(6):1037–52.
20. Esteves SC. Clinical relevance of routine semen analysis and controversies surrounding the 2010 World Health Organization criteria for semen examination. Int Braz J Urol. 2014. (Epub ahead of print).
21. World Health Organization. WHO Laboratory Manual for the examination of human semen and sperm-cervical mucus interaction, 2nd ed. Cambridge: Cambridge University Press; 1987.
22. World Health Organization. WHO Laboratory Manual for the examination of human semen and sperm-cervical mucus interaction, 3rd ed. Cambridge: Cambridge University Press; 1992.
23. World Health Organization. WHO Laboratory Manual for the examination of human semen and sperm-cervical mucus interaction, 4th ed. Cambridge: Cambridge University Press; 1999.
24. World Health Organization. WHO Laboratory Manual for the examination and processing of human semen, 5th ed. Geneva: WHO press; 2010.

Definitions and Epidemiology of Unexplained Male Infertility

2

Ahmet Gudeloglu, Jamin Brahmbhatt and Sijo Parekattil

Introduction

Infertility is defined as the inability to achieve a successful pregnancy after 12 months of unprotected intercourse or therapeutic donor insemination [1]. An estimated 15 % of the world population including 6 million couples in the USA are affected by infertility [2, 3]. A male factor is responsible in about 50 % of infertility cases; it is the sole reason in about 20 % of the cases, and is a contributory factor in 30–40 % of the cases [4].

After a thorough workup including history, physical examination, semen analysis, and laboratory testing a clear cause for the infertility can be identified in only half the patients [5]. Table 2.1 lists the most commonly identified causes of male factor infertility [6]. When there is no identifiable cause, the patients are categorized as having male infertility of unknown origin. This classification is further divided into idiopathic (IMI) versus unexplained (UMI). The prevalence of IMI is three times higher than UMI (33 % versus 11 %). Patients with IMI generally have normal physical examination and endocrine testing with a decrease in semen quality [7]. In contrast, patients with UMI will have a normal semen analysis.

Beyond these basic tests the evaluation for UMI may include postcoital testing, motility assessment, and sperm function tests, including fertilization potential, reactive oxygen testing, and chromatin defects [7]. Based on the findings from these studies treatments can be recommended. In this chapter, we will continue to define and discuss the epidemiology and potential etiologies of UMI.

S. Parekattil (✉) · A. Gudeloglu · J. Brahmbhatt
Department of Urology, University of Florida & Winter Haven Hospital, 199 Ave B NW Suite 310, Winter Haven, FL 33881, USA
e-mail: sijo.parekattil@winterhavenhospital.org

Table 2.1 Male infertility associated factors and percentage in 10,469 patients. (Reprinted from Jungwirth A, Giwercman A, Tournaye H et al. European Association of Urology Guidelines on Male Infertility: The 2012 Update. European Urology 2012; 62(2):324–32. With permission from Elsevier)

Male infertility associated factor	Percentage
Idiopathic	31
Maldescended testis	7.8
Infection	8
Disorders of semen deposition and sexual factors	5.9
Systemic disease	3.1
Varicocele	15.6
Endocrine	8.9
Immunologic	4.5
Obstructions	1.7
Other	5.5

Semen Analysis

Semen analysis is standard for the evaluation of male factor infertility. Approximately 40 % of infertile men have normal semen analysis parameters [8]. The test is generally repeated if the first sample is abnormal. Tested parameters include semen volume, sperm concentration, total count, motility, and morphology [5]. All these parameters can reveal significant information about testicular and auxiliary gland function and reproductive anatomy. In 2010, the World Health Organization (WHO) changed the standard values where the reference values were lowered based on a population study of fertile men from seven countries [9, 10]. It is recommended to use the WHO guidelines with caution for men who have normal semen quality because men can be infertile even though their sperm counts are above the lower limit of WHO criteria [11].

Low sperm concentrations are associated with low likelihood of pregnancy but in contrast higher sperm concentrations are not associated with increased likelihood of pregnancy [11]. Although semen analysis is critical in the evaluation of male factor infertility it rarely provides a diagnosis [12]. Semen analysis can provide reasonably precise

G. L. Schattman et al. (eds.), *Unexplained Infertility*, DOI 10.1007/978-1-4939-2140-9_2,

prognosis only if the parameters are at extreme levels [12]. Spontaneous pregnancy rates in couples where the male had normal and abnormal sperm parameters have been 24 and 23 %, respectively [8].

In UMI, the semen analysis is generally normal and given the recent changes in the WHO classification more men are now placed into this category. In these men, specialized testing is undertaken since standard semen analysis does not take into account several steps of the fertilization process such as sperm transport, sperm interaction with the cervical mucus, and/or oocyte. In a small number of patients, these tests may assist in deciding treatment options. These tests can focus on immune disorders, sperm genetic defects, environmental factors, and fertilization defects.

Immune Disorders

Since sperm are produced after puberty they are at risk for an autoimmune response from the developed immune system. They remain protected by the testicular blood-testis barrier and secretion of immunosuppressive agents by macrophages and/or sertoli cells [13]. The barrier protects postmeiotic spermatocytes and mature germ cells in the adluminal compartment [14]. However, spermatogonia and early spermatocytes are not protected because they develop below this layer and depend on the secretion of immunosuppressive agents. These barriers can be destroyed after trauma, vasectomy, orchitis and/or epididymitis, varicocele, and spinal cord injury [15–21]. This then allows the formation of antisperm antibodies (ASA), which can be found outside the sperm on seminal plasma, cervical mucus, and follicular fluid. Sperm antibodies are polyclonal and can bind multiple sperm antigens. The presence of antibodies does not always lead to functional sperm impairment.

Direct (detecting ASA on the sperm surface) and indirect (detecting ASA in the female genital tract or partners serum) testing can help identify ASA [22]. Both direct immunobead (D-IBT) and mixed antiglobulin reaction (MAR) tests show sperm bound ASA. Sperm immobilization test (SIT), tray agglutination test (TAT), gel agglutination test (GAT), enzyme-linked immunosorbent assay (ELISA), flow cytometry, and radioimmunoassay tests can indirectly measure ASA within seminal fluid, sperm extract, cervical mucus, and/or sera. Each of these tests has its advantages and disadvantages in terms of sensitivity, specificity, providing quantitative information, requirement of skilled staff, and cost [23].

The actual ASA prevalence is limited by the test utilized for detection. Analysis of serum (indirect) from 698 infertile couples revealed 31.1 % of couples (16.5 % of the men and 21.6 % of the women) possessed at least one positive result for ASA [24]. In another study, serum from 186 men and 194 women and cervical mucus of 155 women and semen of 202 men were evaluated with direct and indirect immunobead binding tests. ASA positivity was seen 11.1 % (7 % males and 4.1 % females). Overall, 3.2 % of cervical mucus and 10.4 % of semen samples were also ASA positive [25]. In a study evaluating 471 couples with direct testing using D-IBT, TAT, and GAT, 8.1 % of males and 3.1 % of females were found to be ASA positive [26]. Busacca et al. demonstrated that 16.2 % of the men and 7.3 % of the women in infertile couples had antibodies for sperm antigens [27].

Menge et al. found that the incidence of pregnancy was influenced significantly by the presence of circulating ASA in an infertile couple [24]. Prefertilization effects from ASA include sperm agglutination, sperm cytotoxicity, poor cervical penetration, acrosome reaction, and poor oocyte binding [28, 29]. Sperm agglutination can impair motility and cervical penetration and is higher in patients with the presence of ASA [30, 31]. ASA can also activate complement-mediated cellular lysis of the sperm [32]. A study comparing fertile nonautoimmune and infertile autoimmune men showed that sperm counts and motility were significantly lower in autoimmune infertile men than their fertile controls [33]. The presence of autologous cytotoxic antibodies lowers motility and leads to decreased sperm survival [34]. ASA also leads to decreased sperm penetration into cervical mucosa [27, 35] and decreased capacitation by inhibiting the fluidity of the plasma membranes of human spermatozoa [36]. Acrosome reaction is another important phase of fertilization process and Bandoh et al. found the inhibition of this reaction by ASA [37]. Furthermore, inhibited sperm-zona pellucida binding has been suggested by Liu et al [38].

Postfertilization antibodies can affect the viability of the embryo. ASA against sperm-derived protein CS-1 may play a role in postfertilization embryo defects [39]. Witkin and David demonstrated ASA on female sera and ejaculated sperm can cause unsuccessful conception and first trimester abortion [40]. In another study, Mandelbaum et al. found significant levels of ASA in women with unexplained infertility who had undergone in vitro fertilization/embryo transfer (IVF/ET) than women who had only tubal infertility [41]. All these studies suggest that ASA can cause infertility blocking different phases of fertility in the presence of normal semen parameters.

Genetic Disorders

Genetic disorders can lead to infertility by altering spermatogenesis and/or sperm function. These disorders include karyotype abnormalities (both autosomal and/or sex chromosomal) and deletions or mutations of specific genes within various chromosomal loci. In a review of 9766 infertile men with azoospermia and/or oligozoospermia the incidence of chromosomal abnormalities was 5.8 % (autosomal anomalies 1.5 % and sex chromosome anomalies 4.2 %) [42]. This incidence was significantly higher compared to the 0.38 % (0.14 % sex chromosomal and 0.25 % autosomal) reported in routine newborn screens [43]. The incidence of karyotype anomalies is inversely proportional to sperm concentration and is therefore less than 1 % in patients with normal sperm count [44].

Polymerase gamma (POLG) is a key enzyme involved in the elongation and repair of mitochondrial DNA strands that encode for the POLG gene. Studies have shown an association between POLG gene polymorphisms and UMI [45, 46]. It has been demonstrated that polymorphism of this gene can decrease sperm oocyte penetration and fertilization when sperm parameters are normal [45, 46]. This information may prove beneficial when recommending infertile couples for assisted reproduction.

Previous studies have shown that sperm DNA integrity has predictive value for both normal physiologic and assisted reproduction [47–49]. Protamine deficiency, oxidative stress, unrepaired DNA breaks during chromatin remodeling, abortive apoptosis during spermatogenesis, endogenous endonucleases, caspases, exogenous gonadotoxic agents, and the reactive oxygen species can cause DNA damage [50]. It has also been found that a negative correlation exists between semen parameters and sperm with fragmented DNA [48]. In comparison, infertile men who have normal semen analysis may also have higher percentage of sperm DNA fragmentation. Saleh et al. demonstrated that 43 % of infertile men who have normal sperm parameters have higher DNA fragmentation index then fertile counterparts [51]. Avendano et al. have demonstrated that the DNA fragmentation in morphologically normal spermatozoa has a statistically significant negative effect on embryo quality and pregnancy outcome in intracytoplasmic sperm injection (ICSI) patients [49]. Therefore, the sperm DNA damage can be another responsible factor for UMI. Terminal deoxynucleotidyl transferase-mediated deoxyuridine triphosphate nick end labeling (TUNEL), sperm chromatin structure assays (SCSA), and sperm chromatin dispersion (SCD) have been utilized to measure sperm DNA fragmentation.

Environmental Factors

Oxygen is essential in maintaining the lifecycle and is vital to several biochemical reactions. Reactive oxygen species (ROS) are free radicals that are derived from the metabolism of oxygen. Approximately 30 to 80 % of infertile patients may have high levels of seminal ROS [52]. The term free radical is used to define molecules that contain an unpaired electron in their outer layer. These molecules are highly unstable and include superoxide (O_2^-), hydrogen peroxide (H_2O_2), and hydroxyl (OH^-) radicals [52]. These molecules have an important role in the phagocytosis of microorganisms by neutrophils and macrophages. In order to protect the harmful effects of ROS, there are a variety of defense mechanisms, including enzymes (superoxide dismutase and catalase) and small molecules called antioxidants (vitamin E, C, and uric acid). Total antioxidant capacity (TAC) can be measured with enhanced chemiluminescence techniques [53]. Normally there is a balance between ROS and antioxidant system; distortion of this balance can cause excessive accumulation of ROS. Oxidative stress is used to describe this state of excess generation of ROS and diminished capacity of free radical scavenging by antioxidants [52].

Oxidative stress is a potential source for DNA fragmentation as well as abortive apoptosis and deficiencies in DNA recombination and chromatin packing [54]. ROS-induced DNA damage can lead to apoptosis and resultant decrease in sperm counts. The significance of sperm DNA integrity in both physiologic and assisted reproduction has been demonstrated [47–50]. Host et al. demonstrated the negative correlation between disrupted DNA integrity and fertilization rates in men with UMI undergoing IVF treatment [55]. They suggest the measurement of DNA strand breaks in spermatozoa in patients undergoing IVF with a history of unexplained infertility.

It has been shown that ROS-mediated damage to the sperm plasma membrane can change the membrane fluidity through lipid peroxidation, which adversely affects sperm-zona interactions [56]. De Lamirande et al. also found that ROS can decrease sperm motility reducing ATP levels [57]. All these are factors that can affect potential fertility.

Normal physiologic levels of ROS are needed for maturation, capacitation hyperactivation, acrosome reaction, and sperm–oocyte fusion [58]. Excessive levels of ROS are detrimental through lipid peroxidation, DNA damage, and apoptosis. It has been established that endogenous sources of ROS are leucocytes and immature or abnormal morphologic sperm [59, 60]. Henkel et al. found that leucocyte-derived (extrinsic) ROS negatively correlates with sperm concentration and motile sperm count. They also found another negative correlation between sperm-derived (intrinsic) ROS and motility and motile sperm count [61]. Increased ROS has been linked to smoking, alcohol, varicocele, and environmental factors such as radiation, heavy metals, and biological hazards [51, 62–65]. Therefore, a detailed patient history is essential when evaluating UMI.

The association between oxidative stress and idiopathic male infertility is well demonstrated by Pasqualotto et al. They found higher ROS levels as well as lower TAC levels in idiopathic infertile men compared to the control group [66]. Oxidative stress is clearly associated with male factor infertility by altering sperm quantity and quality, sperm function, and sperm–oocyte interaction [58, 66, 67]. It has also been verified that higher ROS levels can reduce fertility capacity without altering sperm parameters [68]. Pasqualotto et al. reported higher level of ROS in normospermic infertile patients than normal healthy man. They also concluded that oxidative stress may explain previously unexplained infertility in men [68]. Shekarriz et al. showed 40 % increased ROS formation in suspected subfertile men who had at least 60×10^6/ml sperm count [69]. In another study, 28 UMI patients with normal semen parameters compared with 30 normal fertile controls had significantly higher ROS and fragmented DNA levels (79 and 89 %) [70]. These studies suggest that ROS is one of the possible causes for UMI.

Fertilization Defect

Hyperactivation of the human spermatozoa during capacitation is associated with infertility [71–74]. Defects in capacitation and sperm mobility in males who have UMI are related to lower IVF rates [75]. Increased flagellar Ca^{+2} through plasma membrane CatSper channels triggers sperm hyperactivation [76]. Mutations in the CatSper channel genes can be considered another potential cause in UMI [7, 77].

Another important process of fertilization is sperm–oocyte interaction and acrosome reaction in sperm after this interaction. Defective sperm-zona pellucida binding is found in 13 % of infertile men with normal semen parameters. This study also showed that 27 % of these men have defective zona pellucida-induced acrosome reaction [78].

Conclusion

Approximately half of infertility is secondary to a male factor. Males with UMI have normal examination and semen parameters. The causes of UMI can be immunologic, genetic, structural, or environmental. A high index of suspicion needs to be present for these disorders to trigger further testing.

References

1. Practice Committee of the American Society for Reproductive Medicine. Definitions of infertility and recurrent pregnancy loss: a committee opinion. Fertil Steril. 2013;99(1):63.
2. Brugh VM, 3rd, Lipshultz LI. Male factor infertility: evaluation and management. Med Clin North Am. 2004;88:367–85.
3. Rowe PJ, Comhaire FH, Hargreave TB, Mahmoud AMA. WHO manual for the standardized investigation, diagnosis and management of the infertile male. Cambridge:Cambridge University Press; 2000.
4. Thonneau P, Marchand S, Tallec A, et al. Incidence and main causes of infertility in a resident population (1,850,000) of three French regions (1988–1989). Hum Reprod. 1991;6:811–6.
5. American Urological Association Education and Research, Inc. The optimal evaluation of the infertile male: AUA best practice statement. Linthicum (MD); 2010:38 p. https://www.auanet.org/common/pdf/education/clinical-guidance/Male-Infertility-d.pdf.
6. Jungwirth A, Giwercman A, Tournaye H, et al. European association of urology guidelines on male infertility: the 2012 update. Eur Urol. 2012;62(2):324–32.
7. Hamada A, Esteves SC, Nizza M, Agarwal A. Unexplained male infertility: diagnosis and management. Int Braz J Urol. 2012;38:576–94.
8. van der Steeg JW, Steures P, Eijkemans MJ, et al. Role of semen analysis in subfertile couples. Fertil Steril. 2011;95:1013–9.
9. World Health Organization (WHO). WHO laboratory manual for the examination and processing of human semen. 5th ed. Geneva: World Health Organization; 2010.
10. Esteves SC, Zini A, Aziz N, Alvarez JG, Sabanegh ES Jr, Agarwal A. Critical appraisal of World Health Organization's new reference values for human semen characteristics and effect on diagnosis and treatment of subfertile men. Urology. 2012;79:16–22.
11. Bonde JP, Ernst E, Jensen TK, et al. Relation between semen quality and fertility: a population-based study of 430 first-pregnancy planners. The Lancet. 1998;352:1172–7.
12. Jequier AM. Is quality assurance in semen analysis still really necessary? A clinician's viewpoint. Hum Reprod. 2005;20:2039–42.
13. Jacobo P, Guazzone VA, Theas MS, Lustig L. Testicular autoimmunity. Autoimmun Rev. 2011;10:201–4.
14. Ohl DA, Naz RK. Infertility due to antisperm antibodies. Urology. 1995;46:591–602.
15. Iqbal PK, Adeghe AJ, Hughes Y, Samra JS, Obhari MS, Cuthbert J. Clinical characteristics of subfertile men with antisperm antibodies. Br J Obstet Gynaecol. 1989;96:107–10.
16. Mulhall BP, Fieldhouse S, Clark S, et al. Anti-sperm antibodies in homosexual men: prevalence and correlation with sexual behaviour. Genitourin Med. 1990;66:5–7.
17. Awsare NS, Krishnan J, Boustead GB, Hanbury DC, McNicholas TA. Complications of vasectomy. Ann R Coll Surg Engl. 2005;87:406–10.
18. Lekili M, Tekgul S, Ergen A, Tasar C, Hascelik G. Acute experimental unilateral orchitis in the rabbit and its effect on fertility. Int Urol Nephrol. 1992;24:291–7.
19. Heidenreich A, Bonfig R, Wilbert DM, Strohmaier WL, Engelmann UH. Risk factors for antisperm antibodies in infertile men. Am J Reprod Immunol. 1994;31:69–76.
20. Knudson G, Ross L, Stuhldreher D, Houlihan D, Bruns E, Prins G. Prevalence of sperm bound antibodies in infertile men with varicocele: the effect of varicocele ligation on antibody levels and semen response. J Urol. 1994;151:1260–2.
21. Hirsch IH, Sedor J, Callahan HJ, Staas WE. Antisperm antibodies in seminal plasma of spinal cord-injured men. Urology. 1992;39:243–7.
22. Shibahara H, Koriyama J. Methods for direct and indirect antisperm antibody testing. Methods Mol Biol. 2013;927:51–60.
23. Mazumdar S, Levine AS. Antisperm antibodies: etiology, pathogenesis, diagnosis, and treatment. Fertil Steril. 1998;70:799–810.
24. Menge AC, Medley NE, Mangione CM, Dietrich JW. The incidence and influence of antisperm antibodies in infertile human couples on sperm-cervical mucus interactions and subsequent fertility. Fertil Steril. 1982;38:439–46.
25. Kamieniczna M, Domagala A, Kurpisz M. The frequency of antisperm antibodies in infertile couples—a Polish pilot study. Med Sci Monit. 2003;9:CR142–9.
26. Collins JA, Burrows EA, Yeo J, YoungLai EV. Frequency and predictive value of antisperm antibodies among infertile couples. Hum Reprod. 1993;8:592–8.
27. Busacca M, Fusi F, Brigante C, Doldi N, Smid M, Vigano P. Evaluation of antisperm antibodies in infertile couples with immunobead test: prevalence and prognostic value. Acta Eur Fertil. 1989;20:77–82.

28. Shibahara H, Shiraishi Y, Suzuki M. Diagnosis and treatment of immunologically infertile males with antisperm antibodies. Reprod Med and Biol. 2005;4:133–41.
29. Shibahara H, Koriyama J, Shiraishi Y, Hirano Y, Suzuki M, Koyama K. Diagnosis and treatment of immunologically infertile women with sperm-immobilizing antibodies in their sera. J Reprod Immunol. 2009;83:139–44.
30. Clarke GN, Elliott PJ, Smaila C. Detection of sperm antibodies in semen using the immunobead test: a survey of 813 consecutive patients. Am J Reprod Immunol Microbiol. 1985;7:118–23.
31. Moulik S, Gopalkrishnan K, Hinduja I, Shahani SK. Presence of sperm antibodies and association with viscosity of semen. Hum Reprod. 1989;4:290–1.
32. D'Cruz OJ, Haas GG Jr, Wang BL, DeBault LE. Activation of human complement by IgG antisperm antibody and the demonstration of C3 and C5b-9-mediated immune injury to human sperm. J Immunol. 1991;146:611–20.
33. Mathur S, Barber M, Carlton M, Zeigler J, Williamson HO. Motion characteristics of spermatozoa from men with cytotoxic sperm antibodies. Am J Reprod Immunol Microbiol. 1986;12:87–90.
34. Mathur S, Rosenlund C, Carlton M, et al. Studies on sperm survival and motility in the presence of cytotoxic sperm antibodies. Am J Reprod Immunol Microbiol. 1988;17:41–7.
35. Menge AC, Beitner O. Interrelationships among semen characteristics, antisperm antibodies, and cervical mucus penetration assays in infertile human couples. Fertil Steril. 1989;51:486–92.
36. Nakagawa K, Yamano S, Kamada M, et al. Sperm-immobilizing antibodies suppress an increase in the plasma membrane fluidity of human spermatozoa. Fertil Steril. 2004;82(Suppl 3):1054–8.
37. Bandoh R, Yamano S, Kamada M, Daitoh T, Aono T. Effect of sperm-immobilizing antibodies on the acrosome reaction of human spermatozoa. Fertil Steril. 1992;57:387–92.
38. Liu DY, Clarke GN, Baker HW. Inhibition of human sperm-zona pellucida and sperm-oolemma binding by antisperm antibodies. Fertil Steril. 1991;55:440–2.
39. Naz RK. Effects of antisperm antibodies on early cleavage of fertilized ova. Biol Reprod. 1992;46:130–9.
40. Witkin SS, David SS. Effect of sperm antibodies on pregnancy outcome in a subfertile population. Am J Obstet Gynecol. 1988;158:59–62.
41. Mandelbaum SL, Diamond MP, DeCherney AH. Relationship of antibodies to sperm head to etiology of infertility in patients undergoing in vitro fertilization/embryo transfer. Am J Reprod Immunol. 1989;19:3–5.
42. Johnson MD. Genetic risks of intracytoplasmic sperm injection in the treatment of male infertility: recommendations for genetic counseling and screening. Fertil Steril. 1998;70:397–411.
43. Van Assche E, Bonduelle M, Tournaye H, et al. Cytogenetics of infertile men. Hum Reprod. 1996;11(Suppl 4):1–24 (discussion 5–6).
44. De Braekeleer M, Dao TN. Cytogenetic studies in male infertility: a review. Hum Reprod. 1991;6:245–50.
45. Rovio AT, Marchington DR, Donat S, et al. Mutations at the mitochondrial DNA polymerase (POLG) locus associated with male infertility. Nat Genet. 2001;29:261–2.
46. Jensen M, Leffers H, Petersen JH, et al. Frequent polymorphism of the mitochondrial DNA polymerase gamma gene (POLG) in patients with normal spermiograms and unexplained subfertility. Hum Reprod. 2004;19:65–70.
47. Spano M, Bonde JP, Hjollund HI, Kolstad HA, Cordelli E, Leter G. Sperm chromatin damage impairs human fertility. The Danish first pregnancy planner study team. Fertil Steril. 2000;73:43–50.
48. Sun JG, Jurisicova A, Casper RF. Detection of deoxyribonucleic acid fragmentation in human sperm: correlation with fertilization in vitro. Biol Reprod. 1997;56:602–7.
49. Avendano C, Franchi A, Duran H, Oehninger S. DNA fragmentation of normal spermatozoa negatively impacts embryo quality and intracytoplasmic sperm injection outcome. Fertil Steril. 2010;94:549–57.
50. Beshay VE, Bukulmez O. Sperm DNA damage: how relevant is it clinically? Curr Opin Obstet Gynecol. 2012;24:172–9.
51. Saleh RA, Agarwal A, Sharma RK, Nelson DR, Thomas AJ, Jr. Effect of cigarette smoking on levels of seminal oxidative stress in infertile men: a prospective study. Fertil Steril. 2002;78:491–9.
52. Agarwal A, Prabakaran S, Allamaneni S. What an andrologist/urologist should know about free radicals and why. Urology. 2006;67:2–8.
53. Whitehead T, Thorpe G, Maxwell S. Enhanced chemiluminescent assay for antioxidant capacity in biological fluids. Anal Chim Acta. 1992;266:265–77.
54. Aitken RJ, Krausz C. Oxidative stress, DNA damage and the Y chromosome. Reproduction. 2001;122:497–506.
55. Host E, Lindenberg S, Smidt-Jensen S. DNA strand breaks in human spermatozoa: correlation with fertilization in vitro in oligozoospermic men and in men with unexplained infertility. Acta Obstet Gynecol Scand. 2000;79:189–93.
56. Aitken RJ, Clarkson JS, Fishel S. Generation of reactive oxygen species, lipid peroxidation, and human sperm function. Biol Reprod. 1989;41:183–97.
57. de Lamirande E, Gagnon C. Reactive oxygen species and human spermatozoa. II. Depletion of adenosine triphosphate plays an important role in the inhibition of sperm motility. J Androl. 1992;13:379–86.
58. Kothari S, Thompson A, Agarwal A, du Plessis SS. Free radicals: their beneficial and detrimental effects on sperm function. Indian J Exp Biol. 2010;48:425–35.
59. Aitken RJ, West KM. Analysis of the relationship between reactive oxygen species production and leucocyte infiltration in fractions of human semen separated on Percoll gradients. Int J Androl. 1990;13:433–51.
60. Gomez E, Irvine DS, Aitken RJ. Evaluation of a spectrophotometric assay for the measurement of malondialdehyde and 4-hydroxyalkenals in human spermatozoa: relationships with semen quality and sperm function. Int J Androl. 1998;21:81–94.
61. Henkel R, Kierspel E, Stalf T, et al. Effect of reactive oxygen species produced by spermatozoa and leukocytes on sperm functions in non-leukocytospermic patients. Fertil Steril. 2005;83:635–42.
62. Adedara IA, Farombi EO. Induction of oxidative damage in the testes and spermatozoa and hematotoxicity in rats exposed to multiple doses of ethylene glycol monoethyl ether. Hum Exp Toxicol. 2010;29:801–12.
63. Agarwal A, Hamada A, Esteves SC. Insight into oxidative stress in varicocele-associated male infertility: part 1. Nature reviews. Urology. 2012;9:678–90.
64. Mathur PP, D'Cruz SC. The effect of environmental contaminants on testicular function. Asian J Androl. 2011;13:585–91.
65. Lavranos G, Balla M, Tzortzopoulou A, Syriou V, Angelopoulou R. Investigating ROS sources in male infertility: a common end for numerous pathways. Reprod Toxicol. 2012;34:298–307.
66. Pasqualotto FF, Sharma RK, Pasqualotto EB, Agarwal A. Poor semen quality and ROS-TAC scores in patients with idiopathic infertility. Urol Int. 2008;81:263–70.
67. Pasqualotto FF, Sharma RK, Nelson DR, Thomas AJ, Agarwal A. Relationship between oxidative stress, semen characteristics, and clinical diagnosis in men undergoing infertility investigation. Fertil Steril. 2000;73:459–64.
68. Pasqualotto FF, Sharma RK, Kobayashi H, Nelson DR, Thomas AJ Jr, Agarwal A. Oxidative stress in normospermic men undergoing infertility evaluation. J Androl. 2001;22:316–22.
69. Shekarriz M, Thomas AJ Jr, Agarwal A. Incidence and level of seminal reactive oxygen species in normal men. Urology. 1995;45:103–7.

70. Venkatesh S, Shamsi MB, Deka D, Saxena V, Kumar R, Dada R. Clinical implications of oxidative stress & sperm DNA damage in normozoospermic infertile men. Indian J Med Res. 2011;134: 396–8.
71. Burkman LJ. Characterization of hyperactivated motility by human spermatozoa during capacitation: comparison of fertile and oligozoospermic sperm populations. Arch Androl. 1984;13: 153–65.
72. Suarez SS, Ho HC. Hyperactivation of mammalian sperm. Cell Mol Biol (Noisy-le-grand). 2003;49:351–6.
73. Luconi M, Forti G, Baldi E. Pathophysiology of sperm motility. Front Biosci. 2006;11:1433–47.
74. Kay VJ, Robertson L. Hyperactivated motility of human spermatozoa: a review of physiological function and application in assisted reproduction. Hum Reprod Update. 1998;4:776–86.
75. Mackenna A. Contribution of the male factor to unexplained infertility: a review. Int J Androl. 1995;18(Suppl 1):58–61.
76. Suarez SS. Control of hyperactivation in sperm. Hum Reprod Update. 2008;14:647–57.
77. Hildebrand MS, Avenarius MR, Fellous M, et al. Genetic male infertility and mutation of CATSPER ion channels. Eur J Hum Genet. 2010;18:1178–84.
78. Liu de Y, Liu ML, Garrett C, Baker HW. Comparison of the frequency of defective sperm-zona pellucida (ZP) binding and the ZP-induced acrosome reaction between subfertile men with normal and abnormal semen. Hum Reprod. 2007;22:1878–84.

Controversies Surrounding the 2010 World Health Organization Cutoff Values for Human Semen Characteristics and Its Impact on Unexplained Infertility

3

Sandro C. Esteves

Introduction

The World Health Organization (WHO) periodically releases manuals for the laboratory examination and processing of human semen. While laboratories use these manuals as a practical guide of standardized methods for performing semen analyses, clinicians rely on the reference of normal limits for interpreting semen analysis results. The first manual, published in 1980, summarized the clinical experience and research from the previous 80 years. In its subsequent updates in 1987, 1992, 1999, and 2010, the WHO manuals provided substantial improvements on how to assess the seminal parameters. The reference values that were thought to be compatible with normal male fertility have also changed (Table 3.1) [1–4].

In its latest fifth edition (WHO 2010), the semen analysis reference values are markedly lower than those of previous editions. Much debate has taken place thereafter, and a series of reports has questioned the validity of the newly released reference values [5–9].

In this chapter, I discuss the controversy surrounding the new 2010 WHO criteria for semen analyses. First, I point out the importance and limitations of the routine semen analysis in the workup of male infertility. Then, I present the 2010 WHO cutoff values for human semen characteristics and how they compare with previous references. Third, I critically discuss the methods used for generating these new limits and present our hypotheses to explain these lowered limits. Subsequently, I analyze the likely effect of the 2010 WHO cutoff values on the clinical management of men with unexplained infertility. Finally, I propose a practical approach to report semen analysis results for those contemplating adopting the 2010 WHO cutoff values for semen characteristics.

Importance and Limitations of Semen Analysis for Male Infertility Evaluation

Semen analysis is the most widely used biomarker to predict the male fertility potential [10]. It provides information on the functional status of the seminiferous tubules, epididymis and accessory sex glands, and its results are often taken as a surrogate measure of a man's ability to father a pregnancy. Routine semen analyses include: (a) physical characteristics of semen, including liquefaction, viscosity, pH, color, and odor; (b) specimen volume; (c) sperm concentration; (d) sperm motility and progression; (e) sperm morphology; (f) leukocyte quantification; and (g) fructose detection in cases where no spermatozoa are found and ejaculate volume is low [11].

Owed to its widespread availability, health care providers usually use semen analysis alone as the main marker to determine male partner referral for further investigation. However, semen characteristics that discriminate between infertile and fertile men are not well defined and results are normal in up to 40 % of those suffering from infertility [12–14]. Not only sperm production varies widely in same men but also conventional semen analysis neither tests for the diverse array of biological properties spermatozoa express as an eminently specialized cell nor accounts for putative sperm dysfunctions such as immature chromatin or fragmented DNA. In addition, there is a wide variation on how laboratories perform semen analysis. In this section, I will continue to discuss the major drawbacks of semen analysis for male infertility evaluation.

S. C. Esteves (✉)
ANDROFERT, Andrology and Human Reproduction Clinic, Referral Center for Male Reproduction, Avenida Dr. Heitor Penteado 1464, Campinas, São Paulo, Brazil
e-mail: s.esteves@androfert.com.br

G. L. Schattman et al. (eds.), *Unexplained Infertility,* DOI 10.1007/978-1-4939-2140-9_3,

Table 3.1 Cutoff reference values for semen characteristics as published in consecutive WHO manuals. (Esteves et al. [6], with permission from Excerpta Medica, Inc.)

Semen characteristics	WHO 1980	WHO 1987	WHO 1992	WHO 1999	WHO 2010[a]
Volume (mL)	ND	≥2	≥2	≥2	1.5
Sperm count (106/mL)	20–200	≥20	≥20	≥20	15
Total sperm count (10^6)	ND	≥40	≥40	≥40	39
Total motility (% motile)	≥60	≥50	≥50	≥50	40
Progressive motility[b]	≥2[c]	≥25%	≥25% (grade a)	≥25% (grade a)	32% (a+b)
Vitality (% alive)	ND	≥50	≥75	≥75	58
Morphology (% normal forms)	80.5	≥50	≥30[d]	(14)[e]	4[f]
Leukocyte count (10^6/mL)	<4.7	<1.0	<1.0	<1.0	<1.0

ND not defined
[a] Lower reference limits generated from the lower fifth centile value
[b] Grade a=rapid progressive motility (>25 μm/s); grade b=slow/sluggish progressive motility (5–25 μm/s); normal=50% motility (grades a+b) or 25% progressive motility (grade a) within 60 min of ejaculation
[c] Forward progression (scale 0–3)
[d] Arbitrary value
[e] Value not defined but strict criterion is suggested
[f] Strict (Tygerberg) criterion

Biological Intraindividual Variability of Semen Parameters

The semen parameters from same individuals are highly variable. Many conditions including the duration of ejaculatory abstinence, activity of the accessory sex glands, analytical errors, and inherent biological variability account for such discrepancies [15–18]. In one study, the within-subject variability of 20 healthy subjects assessed over a 10-week follow-up ranged from 10.3 to 26.8% [15]. Sperm concentration showed the highest within-subject variation (26.8%), followed by morphology (19.6%) and progressive motility (15.2%) whereas vitality had the lowest variation (10.3%). The utility of population-based reference values is related to the individual variability of a particular analyte. Reference values of analytes with attributable individuality, including the ones routinely assessed in the semen, are generally of limited utility. It means that individual subjects could present results that were very unusual for them, and such results might have been accounted when establishing the reference thresholds. For the aforesaid reasons and other uncontrolled factors such as the regression toward the mean, it is impossible to take the results of a single-semen specimen as a surrogate for a man's ability to father a child unless when at extreme low levels [19]. Regression toward the mean is the phenomenon in which a variable would tend to be closer to the average on a second measurement if it was extreme in its first measurement. This uncontrolled factor should be contemplated when designing studies involving semen analysis because following an extreme random event the next random event is less likely to be extreme. It has been shown that sperm concentration and motility were significantly higher in the second test in men with previous abnormal semen analyses results [20]. Regression toward the mean can be reduced in its magnitude by using means of multiple samples (two or three in the case of semen analysis). Hence, it is prudent that clinicians request at least two semen specimens following 2–5 days of ejaculatory abstinence to allow a better understanding of the baseline semen quality status of a given individual [21–23].

Sperm Dysfunctions Not Tested in the Routine Semen Analysis

Up to 30% of men with difficulties to father a child have no demonstrable abnormalities after an initial male infertility workup. Additional tests have been developed to unravel functional disorders and other sperm abnormalities that cannot be identified by conventional semen analysis [11, 24]. Some of these tests include the hypo-osmotic swelling test, computer-assisted sperm analysis, antisperm antibody test, sperm penetration assay, hemizona assay, reactive oxygen species (ROS) tests, and sperm chromatin integrity test [25]. Despite being available, there are inherent difficulties to set up these tests including cost of equipment and technical complexity. In addition, their predictive value in assessing the male fertility status is either variable or unknown [26]. Not surprisingly, many couples with unexplained infertility choose assisted reproduction techniques (ART) because of their widespread availability and overall success irrespective of the male infertility cause [27]. Yet, the assessment of sperm oxidative stress (OS) and DNA integrity has gained clinical importance in recent years. OS, which is present anywhere from 30 to 80 % in infertile men, is a result of the generation of ROS from contaminating leukocytes, defective sperm, and antioxidant depletion [28, 29]. ROS target sperm DNA molecules and ultimately affect the quality of the genetic material transmitted from the parents to the offspring. Damage to sperm DNA integrity can also result from apoptosis during spermiogenesis, alterations in chromatin remodeling during spermiogenesis, as well as exposure to environmental toxicants and gonadotoxins such as chemotherapy and radiotherapy [30]. Abnormal levels of DNA damage are observed in approximately 5 and 25 % of infertile men with normal and abnormal semen analysis, respectively [31–33]. Therefore, some authors propose that the assessment of both conditions might be included to the male infertility workup algorithm [34, 35].

Evidence of Poor Standardization in Semen Analysis Among Laboratories

Accuracy, the degree to which the measurement reflects the true value, and precision, the reproducibility of the results, are vitally important for clinicians who rely upon the values provided by the laboratory to direct the further work-up, diagnosis and counseling of the infertile male [36]. When both accuracy and precision are assured, the clinician is able to rely upon the semen analysis results to provide adequate counseling to the infertile couple. However, data from surveys of laboratory practice in the USA and the UK indicate that semen analysis techniques are still poorly standardized.

Among 536 clinical laboratories in the USA only about 60 % reported abstinence and indicated the criteria adopted for sperm morphology assessments. Moreover, fewer than half of them performed quality control for commonly assessed parameters such as sperm counts, motility, and morphology [37]. A survey involving 37 laboratories in the UK about the methods used to assess sperm morphology revealed that only 5 % complied with all WHO guidelines [38]. In the aforementioned study, participating laboratories had high interobserver variability when evaluating the same specimen. This data were corroborated by another study in which interlaboratory coefficient of variation was as high as 34 % for sperm concentration, 20 % for total sperm motility, 40 % for sperm vitality, and 70 % for sperm morphology (strict criterion) [39]. Discrepancies were also seen in laboratories enrolled in quality control programs, thus indicating that there is a need of global standardization among the laboratories and the providers of external quality control [40].

Owed to its complex nature, semen analysis should ideally be carried out in a dedicated andrology laboratory attired with experienced technicians, internal and external quality control, validation of test systems, quality assurance during all testing processes, and proper in place communication with clinicians and patients [41]. Despite being nonspecific for identifying male factor infertility etiologies, semen analysis is often the gateway test from which multiple expensive and often invasive treatments are based. Therefore, the importance of a reliable andrology laboratory cannot be underestimated.

The 2010 WHO Criteria for Semen Analysis

The WHO department of reproductive health and research workgroup made important changes in the 2010 laboratory manual for the examination of human semen and sperm-cervical mucus interaction [4]. While the WHO workgroup reviewed and updated in great detail all the methods delineated in previous manuals, it incorporated new protocols and tests. One of its main features was the inclusion of new references ranges and limits that were markedly lower than those reported in previous manuals.

Data characterizing the semen quality of fertile men provided the reference ranges for the manual [42]. For the first time, semen analysis results from recent fathers with known time-to-pregnancy (TTP), defined as months (or cycles) from stopping contraception to achieving a pregnancy, were analyzed. Raw data obtained from five studies of seven countries on three continents were pooled then assessed [43–48]. Approximately 1900 men who had fathered a child within 1 year of trying to initiate a pregnancy provided each one semen sample for sperm counts, motility, and volume assessments. Data on sperm morphology were extracted from four studies comprising approximately 1800 men whereas sperm vitality, assessed by the eosin–nigrosin method, was obtained from approximately 400 men of two countries [43, 45, 47, 48]. The mean ($\pm$SD) male age was 31 ($\pm$5) years (range 18–53) and only ten men were over 45 years old. Participating laboratories practiced internal and external quality control and used standardized methods for semen analysis according to the WHO manual for the examination of human semen current at the time of the original studies [42].

The 95 % interval for sperm volume, count, motility, vitality, and morphology were generated and the one-sided lower reference limits (the fifth centile) proposed as the lower cutoff limits for normality [42]. It was then assumed that values below these limits would come from a different population. Of note, assessment of progressive motility according to grades, as recommended by the previous WHO manuals, was replaced by categorizing motile sperm as being "progressive" or "nonprogressive." In addition, the strict criterion for morphology assessment was incorporated at last as the standard method. The lower limits of these distributions were lower than the values presented in previous editions except for the total sperm number per ejaculate (Table 3.1) [1–4]. Leukocyte reference values ($<1\times10^6$/mL) were not determined and remained the same as in previous manuals.

Controversies Surrounding the Validity of the 2010 WHO Thresholds

The lower reference limits in the 2010 WHO manual aimed to provide evidence-based thresholds that may aid clinicians in estimating the relative fertility of a given patient. Besides the aforesaid limitations of routine semen analysis in evaluating the male reproductive potential, methodological concerns arise from a careful examination of the studies that generated the current reference values. In a recent review, we critically analyzed these issues and concluded that it was unsound to assume that the 2010 reference standards represented the distribution of fertile men across the globe [6]. The group of studied men represented a limited population of individuals who live in large cities in the North hemisphere but for a small subset of men from Australia. Of note it was the absence of men from densely populated areas in Asia, Middle East, Latin America, and Africa, which represent the areas where most men live nowadays. This fact precludes the examination of regional and racial discrepancies that could account for semen quality variability. The selection criteria were arbitrary as stated by Cooper et al. "laboratories and data were identified through the known literature and personal communication with investigators and the editorial group of the fifth edition of the WHO laboratory manual" [42]. Not surprisingly, there was a significant overlap of authorship in the included studies. In addition, a single-semen specimen of each man was included for the pooled analysis, thus limiting the appraisal of the already discussed large intraindividual biological variability [6].

Some authors have claimed that the lowered 2010 WHO thresholds resulted from the declines in sperm count caused by endocrine disruptors and other environmental pollutants, such as insecticides and pesticides [49–51]. I, otherwise, conjecture that the observed discrepancies are likely to be associated with the patient selection criteria, the higher laboratory quality control standards and the methods used for semen assessment, such as the strict criterion for morphology determination. It means that methodology issues related to data generation might explain the discrepancies in the reference thresholds among WHO guidelines.

Collectively, these findings cast to doubt on the validity of the proposed reference range and cutoff limits about universally represent the distribution of semen results of fertile men.

Effects of the 2010 WHO Criteria for Semen Analysis in the Management of Male Infertility

Clinicians involved in the care of infertile couples still rely on the semen analyses results to determine a management plan. Abnormal semen parameters are taken into account not only to define male infertility but also to recommend further evaluation and treatment. One example is unexplained infertility which is based on the absence of female infertility, and the presence of at least two normal semen analyses and no identifiable causes after a thorough work-up including history, physical examination, and endocrine laboratory testing [24]. The adoption of the new WHO reference values will likely lead to more men being classified as "fertile", which is of particular importance for gynecologists who rely on semen analysis alone as a surrogate measure for male fertility. In a recent study, up to 15 % of men with at least one parameter below the 1999 WHO reference values were reclassified as "normal" by having all parameters at or above the 2010 WHO thresholds [8]. We have also contemplated our own data involving 982 men seeking evaluation for infertility that had abnormal semen analysis results based on the 1990 WHO criteria. We found that approximately 39 % of these men would be reclassified as "normal" by the new 2010 criteria. Morphology itself accounted for over 50 % of the reclassifications (unpublished data). Patient referral for evaluation could then be postponed or not undertaken if fertility status would be based on semen analyses alone. Albeit it is ambiguous yet whether this reclassification will lead to a more cost-effective evaluation, it is also possible that it could delay the definitive diagnosis and management of the infertile couple and lead to a more pronounced infertility condition with ageing.

The current guidelines for male infertility evaluation also rely on the concept of semen abnormality for patient management. The American Urological Association (AUA) defines that the initial male evaluation should include a reproductive history and two properly performed semen analyses, and that an extended evaluation is warranted in the presence of semen abnormalities in the initial evaluation [52]. In contrast, the European Association of Urology (EAU) recommends undertaking a male examination in individuals with abnormal semen analysis results [53]. Surprisingly, a single seminal evaluation would then be sufficient if the semen analysis results were normal according to the EAU. These recommendations understate the limitations of the semen analysis results and do not discuss the paradigm shift that is likely to occur in referrals and management on the face of the recent changes in the WHO reference thresholds.

Similarly, the recommendation for treatment has also been based on the results of routine semen analysis. Current guidelines for varicocele propose that treatment should be offered to men with clinical varicoceles in the presence of abnormal semen analyses [54–57]. Application of the new WHO reference values might lead to patients earlier deemed to be candidates for varicocele repair now be considered ineligible for treatment if their semen parameters are above the fifth centile. This may create a situation where health care providers might not reimburse treatment if semen parameters were above the new thresholds. As stated by Esteves et al. "the concern is that by denying these men a varicocele repair we may prevent them from achieving a substantial improvement in semen parameters and a greater chance of spontaneous pregnancy." Of note, the most recent Practice Committee report on varicocele by the American Society for Reproductive Medicine (ASRM) has withdrawn the presence of an abnormal sperm function test as an indication for varicocele treatment that had been listed in their document published in 2008 [57]. Yet, another example is sperm morphology results in which infertility specialists have relied on to recommend treatment modalities owed to their relationship with in vivo and in vitro fertilization [58]. The thresholds of sperm morphology (strict criteria; Tygerberg method) were lowered to 4 % in the 2010 WHO criteria compared with 14 % in the previous 1999 standards [3, 4].Infertility specialists recommend intracytoplasmic sperm injection (ICSI) instead of conventional IVF or intrauterine insemination (IUI) on the face of morphology results of below 4 % owed to the markedly lower pregnancy outcomes of these two treatment methods when using semen with low proportion of normal sperm [59, 60]. Interestingly, the distribution of semen analysis results of fertile men in centiles, as shown by the new WHO standards, clearly shows that though 5 % of the studied men had morphology values below the 4 % cutoff point they still could initiate an unassisted pregnancy within 12 months of unprotected intercourse [6, 42].

In summary, these considerations raise the question on how the 2010 WHO references thresholds would affect the current male infertility practice. It should be noted, however, that reference values, as proposed by the WHO, merely represent the distribution of semen parameters of a limited group of recent fathers. Physicians treating infertile couples should exercise circumspection when interpreting the results of routine semen analysis. Semen analysis alone is only a tool among several others for determining clinical care. The male infertility evaluation must go far beyond a simple semen analysis, as it has to be complemented with a proper physical examination, a comprehensive history taking, and relevant endocrine, genetic, and other investigations [10, 11].

A Modified Semen Analysis Report

Semen analysis reports usually present the specimen data and include the cutoff limits as a reference for interpretation [61]. Despite having updated to the 2010 WHO criteria, our andrology laboratory has changed the way results are reported. We have included the 95 % reference interval of the semen characteristics from recent fathers, as generated by the WHO workgroup, instead of only providing the lower reference limits.

It might be clinically useful to determine in which centile the patient specimen fits in comparison with the reference standards instead of simply classify the specimen as "normal" or "abnormal." This approach is more realistic and clinicians would have a better understanding of the patient's seminal profile by comparing the specimen results with the reference group. I propose that laboratories willing to adopt the 2010 WHO references include the full reference interval and I therefore offer my own andrology laboratory report as a template (Fig. 3.1).

Conclusions

The 2010 WHO semen analysis criteria are likely to have a significant effect on the management of male infertility, including reclassification of "normal" and "abnormal" semen analyses reports, deferment of patient referral for proper evaluation, and recommendation for treatment. These new reference limits were derived from a limited number of semen samples used to initiate natural conceptions. Albeit values below the thresholds may indicate a need for infertility treatment they cannot be used to determine the nature of that treatment. Several methodological shortcomings are associated with the new references standards that might explain why references were lowered in comparison with previous WHO guidelines. Semen parameters within the reference interval do not guarantee fertility nor do values outside those limits necessarily imply male infertility or pathology. Physicians treating infertile couples should exercise circumspection when interpreting the results of routine semen analysis. Semen analysis alone is usually insufficient for the diagnosis because it does not account for sperm dysfunction, such as immature chromatin, OS and DNA damage. Semen quality must be interpreted within the context of the patient's clinical information. The male infertility evaluation must go far beyond a simple semen analysis, as it has to be complemented with a proper physical examination, a comprehensive history taking, and relevant endocrine, genetic, and other investigations.

ANDROFERT

CENTRO DE REFERÊNCIA PARA REPRODUÇÃO MASCULINA

Semen Analysis Report

Patient Information

Report#	ID#	Patient Name:	Age (years):
1028/12	02815	xxxxxxxxxxxxxxxxxxxxxxxxxxxxxxxxxx	35

Physician:	Reason:	Date (dd/mm/yy):
Dr. Sandro Esteves	Postoperative folow-up: varicocele repair	16/10/2012

Ejaculate:	Collection Method:	Collection Site:
Total	Masturbation	Laboratory

Medication in use:	Difficulties in collection:	Complete Sample?: Yes No
None	Not Reported	Yes

Macroscopic Examination

Appearance:	Viscosity:	Liquefaction:	pH:	Agglutination:
Normal	Abnormal	Normal	8.0	1

Abstinence (days):	Collection Time:	Specimen Examination (minutes after collection):
02	08:50 am	25

Microscopic Examination

	Patient results	Reference Values: WHO 2010*		
		Lower limit (5th percentile)	Median (50th percentile)	Upper limit (95th percentile)
Volume (mL)	1.9	1.5	3.7	6.8
Sperm concentration/mL ($\times 10^6$)	15.50	15.00	73.00	213.00
Total sperm number ($\times 10^6$/ejaculate)	29.45	39.00	255.00	802.00
Total motility (%)	65	40%	61%	78%
Progressive motility (%)	51	32%	55%	72%
Normal forms (%)	04	04%	15%	44%
Vitality (%)	59	58%	79%	91%

* Reference values obtained from a population of approximately 2,000 recent fathers from five countries (time to pregnancy from stopping contraception to obtaining natural conception ≤12 months). Values may not be representative of the Brazilian population. Values outside the reference limits do not necessarily imply infertility; they should be interpreted in conjunction with clinical information. Semen analysis performed in accordance to the World Health Organization laboratory manual for the examination and processing of human semen, fifth edition, 2010.

Fig. 3.1 Modified semen analysis report template. The main difference from the routinely used templates is the inclusion of the "centile" distribution of semen characteristics from the reference population rather than solely the lower thresholds. The patient values (*left* column) are then compared with the reference limits thus aiding the clinician to appreciate how a given patient seminal profile fit within the "centile" distribution

References

1. World Health Organization. WHO laboratory manual for the examination of human semen and sperm-cervical mucus interaction, 2nd ed. Cambridge: Cambridge University Press; 1987. p. 80.
2. World Health Organization. WHO laboratory manual for the examination of human semen and sperm-cervical mucus interaction, 3rd ed. Cambridge: Cambridge University Press; 1992. p. 107.
3. World Health Organization. WHO laboratory manual for the examination of human semen and sperm-cervical mucus interaction, 4th ed. Cambridge: Cambridge University Press; 1999. p. 128.
4. World Health Organization. WHO laboratory manual for the examination and processing of human semen, 5th ed. Geneva: World Health Organization; 2010. p. 271.
5. Christopher LR, Barratt CLR, Mansell S, Beaton C, Tardif S, Oxenham SK. Diagnostic tools in male infertility—the question of sperm dysfunction. Asian J Androl. 2011;13:53–8.
6. Esteves SC, Zini A, Aziz N, Alvarez JG, Sabanegh ES Jr, Agarwal A. Critical appraisal of World Health Organization's new reference values for human semen characteristics and effect on diagnosis and treatment of subfertile men. Urology. 2012;79(1):16–22.
7. Haidl G. New WHO-reference limits-revolution or storm in a teapot? Asian J Androl. 2011;13(2):208–11.
8. Murray KS, James A, McGeady JB, Reed ML, Kuang WW, Nangia AK. The effect of the new 2010 World Health Organization criteria for semen analyses on male infertility. Fertil Steril. 2012;98(6):1428–31.
9. Yerram N, Sandlow JI, Brannigan RE. Clinical implications of the new 2010 WHO reference ranges for human semen characteristics. J Androl. 2012;33(3):289–90.
10. Esteves SC, Hamada A, Kondray V, Pitchika A, Agarwal A. What every gynecologist should know about male infertility: an update. Arch Gynecol Obstet. 2012;286(1):217–29.
11. Esteves SC, Miyaoka R, Agarwal A. An update on the clinical assessment of the infertile male. [corrected]. Clinics (Sao Paulo). 2011;66:691–700. (Erratum in: Clinics (Sao Paulo). 2012;67:203).
12. Guzick DS, Overstreet JW, Factor-Litvak P, Brazil CK, Nakajima ST, Coutifaris C, Carson SA, Cisneros P, Steinkampf MP, Hill JA, Xu D, Vogel DL, National Cooperative Reproductive Medicine Network. Sperm morphology, motility, and concentration in fertile and infertile men. N Engl J Med. 2001;345(19):1388–93.
13. Moghissi KS, Wallach EE. Unexplained infertility. Fertil Steril 1983; 39: 5–21.
14. van der Steeg JW, Steures P, Eijkemans MJ, F Habbema JD, Hompes PG, Kremer JA, et al. Role of semen analysis in subfertile couples. Fertil Steril. 2011;95:1013–9.
15. Álvarez C, Castilla JA, Martínez L, Ramírez JP, Vergara F, Gaforio JJ. Biological variation of seminal parameters in healthy subjects. Hum Reprod. 2003;18(10):2082–8.
16. Castilla JA, Alvarez C, Aguilar J, González-Varea C, Gonzalvo MC, Martínez L. Influence of analytical and biological variation on the clinical interpretation of seminal parameters. Hum Reprod. 2006;21(4):847–51.
17. Keel BA. Within- and between-subject variation in semen parameters in infertile men and normal semen donors. Fertil Steril. 2006;85(1):128–34.
18. Poland ML, Moghissi KS, Giblin PT, Ager JW, Olson JM. Variation of semen measures within normal men. Fertil Steril. 1985;44(3):396–400.
19. Jequier AM. Is quality assurance in semen analysis still really necessary? A clinician's viewpoint. Hum Reprod. 2005;20:2039–42.
20. Baker HW, Kovacs GT. Spontaneous improvement in semen quality: regression towards the mean. Int J Androl. 1985;8(6):421–6.
21. Berman NG, Wang C, Paulsen CA. Methodological issues in the analysis of human sperm concentration data. J Androl. 1996;17(1):68–73.
22. Carlsen E, Petersen JH, Andersson AM, Skakkebaek NE. Effects of ejaculatory frequency and season on variations in semen quality. Fertil Steril. 2004;82(2):358–66.
23. Sánchez-Pozo MC, Mendiola J, Serrano M, Mozas J, Björndahl L, Menkveld R, Lewis SEM, Mortimer D, Jørgensen N, Barratt CLR, Fernández MF, Castilla JA. Proposal of guidelines for the appraisal of SEMen QUAlity studies (SEMQUA). Hum Reprod. 2013;28(1):10–21.
24. Hamada A, Esteves SC, Nizza M, Agarwal A. Unexplained male infertility: diagnosis and management. Int Braz J Urol. 2012;38:576–94.
25. Samplaski MK, Agarwal A, Sharma R, Sabanegh E. New generation of diagnostic tests for infertility: review of specialized semen tests. Int J Urol. 2010;17:839–47.
26. Kovac JR, Pastuszak AW, Lamb DJ. The use of genomics, proteomics, and metabolomics in identifying biomarkers of male infertility. Fertil Steril. 2013;99:998–1007.
27. Sullivan EA, Zegers-Hochschild F, Mansour R, Ishihara O, de Mouzon J, Nygren KG, Adamson GD. International Committee for Monitoring Assisted Reproductive Technologies (ICMART) world report: assisted reproductive technology 2004. Hum Reprod. 2013;28:1375–90.
28. Agarwal A, Makker K, Sharma R. Clinical relevance of oxidative stress in male factor infertility: an update. Am J Reprod Immunol. 2008;59(1):2–11.
29. Esteves SC, Agarwal A. Novel concepts in male infertility. Int Braz J Urol. 2011;37(1):5–15.
30. Ashwood-Smith MJ, Edwards RG. DNA repair by oocytes. Mol Hum Reprod. 1996;2:46–51.
31. Kodama H, Yamaguchi R, Fukuda J, Kasai H, Tanaka T. Increased oxidative deoxyribonucleic acid damage in the spermatozoa of infertile male patients. Fertil Steril. 1997;68(3):519–24.
32. Spano M, Bonde JP, Hjollund HI, Kolstad HA, Cordelli E, Leter G. Sperm chromatin damage impairs human fertility. The Danish first pregnancy planner study team. Fertil Steril. 2000;73(1):43–50.
33. Zini A, Bielecki R, Phang D, Zenzes MT. Correlations between two markers of sperm DNA integrity, DNA denaturation and DNA fragmentation, in fertile and infertile men. Fertil Steril. 2001;75(4):674–77.
34. Agarwal A, Sigman M. Is sperm DNA integrity assessment useful? Opposing views. J Urol. 2013;90:1645–7.
35. Zini A, Sigman M. Are tests of sperm DNA damage clinically useful? Pros and cons. J Androl. 2009;30(3):219–29.
36. Snow-Lisy D, Sabanegh E Jr. What does the clinician need from an andrology laboratory? Front Biosci (Elite Ed). 2013;5:289–304.
37. Keel BA, Sternbridge TW, Pineda G, Serafy NT. Lack of standardisation in performance of the semen analysis among laboratories in the United States. Fertil Steril. 2002;78:603–8.
38. Riddell D, Pacey A, Whittington K. Lack of compliance in UK andrology laboratories to World Health Organisation recommendations for sperm morphology assessment. Hum Reprod. 2005;20:3441–5.
39. Alvarez C, Castilla JA, Ramírez JP, et al. External quality control program for semen analysis: Spanish experience. J Assist Reprod Genet. 2005;22:379–87.
40. Cooper TG, Björndahl L, Vreeburg J, et al. Semen analysis and external quality control schemes for semen analysis need global standardization. Int J Androl. 2002;25:(3)6–11.
41. Esteves SC, Agarwal A. Ensuring that reproductive laboratories provide high-quality services. In: Bento FC, Esteves SC, Agarwal A. Quality management in ART clinics: a practical guide, 1st ed. New York: Springer US 2013;129–46.
42. Cooper TG, Noonan E, von Eckardstein S, Auger J, Baker HW, Behre HM, et al. World Health Organization reference values for human semen characteristics. Hum Reprod Update. 2010;16:231–245.

43. Stewart TM, Liu DY, Garrett C, Jørgensen N, Brown EH, Baker HW. Associations between andrological measures, hormones and semen quality in fertile Australian men: inverse relationship between obesity and sperm output. Hum Reprod. 2009;24(7):1561–8.
44. Slama R, Eustache F, Ducot B, Jensen TK, Jørgensen N, Horte A, et al. Time to pregnancy and semen parameters: a cross-sectional study among fertile couples from four European cities. Hum Reprod. 2002;17(2):503–15.
45. Swan SH, Brazil C, Drobnis EZ, Liu F, Kruse RL, Hatch M, Redmon JB, Wang C, Overstreet JW, Study for Future Families Research Group. Geographic differences in semen quality of fertile U.S. males. Environ Health Perspect. 2003;111(4):414–20.
46. Jensen TK, Slama R, Ducot B, Suominen J, Cawood EH, Andersen AG, et al. Regional differences in waiting time to pregnancy among fertile couples from four European cities. Hum Reprod. 2001;16(12):2697–704.
47. Haugen TB, Egeland T, Magnus O. Semen parameters in Norwegian fertile men. J Androl. 2006:27:66–71.
48. Auger J, Eustache F, Andersen AG, Irvine DS, Jørgensen N, Skakkebaek NE. Sperm morphological defects related to environment, lifestyle and medical history of 1001 male partners of pregnant women from four European cities. Hum Reprod. 2001;16(12):2710–7.
49. Handelsman DJ. Estrogens and falling sperm counts. Reprod Fertil Dev. 2001;13:317–24.
50. Sadeu JC, Hughes CL, Agarwal S, Foster WG. Alcohol, drugs, caffeine, tobacco, and environmental contaminant exposure: reproductive health consequences and clinical implications. Crit Rev Toxicol. 2010;40(7):633–52.
51. Carlsen E, Giwercman A, Keiding N, et al. Evidence for decreasing quality of semen during past 50 years. BMJ. 1992;305:609–13.
52. American Urological Association. Best practice statement on the optimal evaluation of the infertile male (revised 2010). http://www.auanet.org/content/media/optimalevaluation2010.pdf. Accessed 5 Oct 2013.
53. Dohle GR, Diemer T, Giwercman A, et al. Chapter 2: Investigations. In: Dohle GR, Diemer T, Giwercman A, et al. Guidelines on male infertility. European Association of Urology. 2010. http://www.uroweb.org/gls/pdf/Male%20Infertility%202010.pdf. Accessed 5 Oct 2013.
54. The Male Infertility Best Practice Policy Committee of the American Urological Association. Practice Committee of the American Society for Reproductive Medicine. Report on varicocele and infertility. Fertil Steril. 2004;82:S142–5.
55. Dohle GR, Diemer T, Giwercman A, et al. Chapter 6: Varicocele. In: Dohle GR, Diemer T, Giwercman A, et al. (eds). Guidelines on male infertility. European Association of Urology; 2010. http://www.uroweb.org/gls/pdf/Male%20Infertility%202010.pdf. Accessed 5 Oct 2013.
56. Sociedade Brasileira de Urologia & Colégio Brasileiro de Radiologia; Projeto Diretrizes da Associação Médica Brasileira: Varicocele. http://www.projetodiretrizes.org.br/8_volume/40-Varicocele.pdf. Accessed: 5 Oct 2013.
57. Practice Committee of the American Society for Reproductive Medicine: Report on varicocele and infertility: a committee opinion. Fertil Steril. 2014;102:1556-60.
58. Kruger TF, Acosta AA, Simmons KF, Swanson RJ, Matta JF, Oehninger S, et al. Predictive value of abnormal sperm morphology in in vitro fertilization. Fertil Steril. 1988;49:112–7.
59. Coetzee K, Kruge TF, Lombard CJ. Predictive value of normal sperm morphology: a structured literature review. Hum Reprod Update. 1998;4:73–82.
60. Van Waart J, Kruger TF, Lombard CJ, Ombelet W. Predictive value of normal sperm morphology in intrauterine insemination (IUI): a structured literature review. Hum Reprod Update. 2001;7:495–500.
61. World Health Organization. WHO laboratory manual for the examination and processing of human semen, 5th ed. Geneva: World Health Organization; 2010. Appendix 6, p. 252.

Definitions and Epidemiology of Unexplained Female Infertility

4

Luciano G. Nardo and Spyridon Chouliaras

Introduction

Infertility causes, according to the current consensus include anovulation, male factor, tubal factor, cervical factor, endometriosis and unexplained infertility (UI). UI is a diagnosis of exclusion [1]. Traditionally, the term has been used when the basic investigations such as tests for tubal patency, ovulation and semen analysis are all normal [2].

Moreover, there are two distinct categories of infertility:

- Primary infertility, which is defined as infertility in a woman who has never had any pregnancies.
- Secondary infertility, which is the inability to conceive after at least one pregnancy (regardless of whether this has resulted in a live birth or not).

Therefore, UI should also be classified into unexplained primary or secondary infertility. Unexplained female infertility should be a term used when the female reproductive system has been evaluated according to current agreed standards, and no abnormalities are detected. Male factor infertility should have been ruled out with at least two normal semen analyses and with no demonstrable physical or endocrine abnormalities [3].

The latest opinion paper by the Practice Committee of the American Society for Reproductive Medicine (ASRM) published in 2012 [4] on the diagnostic evaluation of the infertile female, which replaces the 2006 document titled "Optimal evaluation of the infertile female" is a step forward towards understanding female infertility.

Evaluation according to this document should include:

1. Detailed history and clinical examination
2. Assessment of ovulatory function
3. Measuring the ovarian reserve
4. Exclusion of abnormalities of uterine anatomy
5. Confirmation of tubal patency
6. Consideration of peritoneal factors (such as endometriosis).

The post coital test for excluding cervical factor infertility is no longer recommended. This does not necessarily exclude a potential cervical factor such as aetiology for the infertility. It merely implies that our diagnostic ability to identify subtle defects in sperm–cervical mucousinteraction is limited.

All the above investigations will be discussed in more detail in this book. This document though clearly demonstrates a shift away from the concept of using the term UI as an 'umbrella' term for all women with normal ovulation and tubal patency tests, to a more elaborate assessment of the female and the couple. The potential for creation of new infertility categories arises.

Definition

The necessity for an accurate and globally accepted definition of UI, in both male and female, is undisputable. It is paramount for clinicians and healthcare providers alike in an era of increasing cost consciousness, to be able to monitor the incidence and prevalence of this condition in order to best understand how to investigate and treat the infertility efficiently.

Defining UI is far from straightforward. One of the reasons is that there is an inherent disparity between the clinical, the epidemiological and the demographic version of the definitions of infertility.

The differences correspond to:

1. The measured endpoint: conception, clinical pregnancy or live birth. Demographers measured endpoint is live birth. Clinicians on the other hand are interested in all outcomes and the data presented in different studies can vary significantly making comparisons between them difficult.

L. G. Nardo (✉) · S. Chouliaras
Reproductive Medicine and Gynecology, Gynehealth, 3-5 St. John Street, Manchester M34DN, UK
e-mail: lnardo@gyne-health.co.uk

G. L. Schattman et al. (eds.), *Unexplained Infertility,* DOI 10.1007/978-1-4939-2140-9_4,

2. The time to endpoint: lack of conception for 12–24 months is what is usually reported in most clinical and epidemiological definitions.

   In demographic studies of infertility, the data used are primarily based on Demographic Health Surveys (DHS) that contain complete birth reports but often scarce or poor data about miscarriages, terminations of pregnancies, intrauterine deaths and no data on the female's desire for pregnancy. Due to the inherent difficulty of assessing such data, longer periods of exposure are used (up to 7 years).

There are therefore numerous definitions of infertility in textbooks and other publications, and this fact on its own proves that it is an area where controversies still exist. This necessity for a generally accepted definition, and a consensus in that matter has been extensively argued [5–8]. One widely used definition of infertility is 1 year of unwanted non-conception with unprotected intercourse in the fertile phase of the menstrual cycles [9].

Another definition by Gnoth et al. describes infertility as failure to conceive after six cycles of unprotected intercourse irrespective of age [10].

The ASRM in 2008 also published a definition of infertility [11]. The document states that infertility is a disease, defined by the failure to achieve a successful pregnancy after 12 months or more of regular unprotected intercourse. The female age at presentation is also taken into account, distinguishing between those above and below the age of 35. The former category according to the ASRM warrants investigations and treatment after 6 months of failure to conceive. The same may apply for younger women, when indicated by history and clinical examination.

In 2009, the International Committee for Monitoring Assisted Reproductive Technology and the World Health Organization, produced a similar definition [12].

The shift towards taking into account the female age when defining infertility was also advocated by Bhattacharya et al. [8], who suggested defining infertility based on the length of trying (or exposure to pregnancy) adjusted for female age. This, according to the authors, is a more clinically meaningful definition and is already used in everyday practice.

The most up-to-date definition (2013) is a revised one by the ASRM [13], which replaced their 2008 definition:

> Infertility is a disease, defined by the failure to achieve a successful pregnancy after 12 months or more of appropriate, timed unprotected intercourse or therapeutic donor insemination. Earlier evaluation and treatment may be justified based on medical history and physical findings and is warranted after 6 months for women over age 35 years.

It is an elaborate definition that has the potential to replace all the others.

On the other hand, it is debatable whether a universal definition of infertility is pragmatic. A global consensus between fertility physicians may remain a utopia.

When attempting to define UI, it is appropriate to define fecundity and childlessness in humans:

- Fecundity is defined as the capacity of the female to produce a live birth.
- Childlessness is the condition of being without offspring, and can be the result of infertility, infecundity, and/or infant mortality.

Once infertility has been ascertained, regardless of which definition one uses, the 'diagnosis' of unexplained female infertility is made when tubal patency and normal ovulatory function are established in the presence of a normal semen analysis. By definition this would mean that all the appropriate tests have been performed. The interpretation of some of the diagnostic tests though is operator-dependant such as the tests for tubal patency. It is well known that the sensitivity of many diagnostics tests (i.e., contrast infusion ultrasound (Hycosy) and Hysterosalpingogram) is far from 100 %, and the diagnosis of UI may vary depending on the individual performing or interpreting the results.

Most importantly, there could be causes accounting for female infertility that are not recognised, either due to lack or omission of appropriate and accurate testing, or even due to investigating a clinician's beliefs and personal experience. In addition, an aetiology may also be assigned by some physicians with a bias towards specific diagnoses in the absence of objective evidence.

Below is a brief list of potential causes of female infertility that are generally thought to be associated with the "diagnosis" of UI and frequently unexplored.

1. Endometriosis
   Visible and non-visible or microscopic: even if a laparoscopy has been performed, the ability to identify the disease remains operator-dependant. Moreover, the presence of disease may not be macroscopically visible even to the most experienced surgeons.
2. Adenomyosis
   With the progress in imaging techniques and the non-invasive diagnosis of adenomyosis, new links between this condition and infertility are currently proposed and being investigated [14].
3. Congenital uterine abnormalities
   There is an increasing trend to investigate and treat such abnormalities like the septate uterus. They are thought to be associated with recurrent miscarriage and infertility. Three dimensional ultrasound scanning with or without contrast and MRI are currently the only non-invasive methods to diagnose congenital uterine abnormalities [15].

4. Leiomyomata (fibroids)
   The presence of certain types of uterine leiomyomata (submucous, large intramural fibroids distorting anatomy, etc.) has been demonstrated to affect fertility, and surgical management is accepted as treatment of choice at least for submucous and possibly for large intramural fibroids close to or distorting the uterine cavity [16, 17].
5. Reduced ovarian reserve and advanced female age.
6. Immunological factors
   Considerable controversy surrounds the significance of immunological factors and their impact on fertility, and there is significant interest in pursuing further research in this diagnosis by both physicians and patients. Future research may reveal novel links, which may be used to identify and treat certain infertile couples.
7. Tubal factor
   Although tubal patency may be confirmed by standard tests, tubal function is more difficult to evaluate and may be compromised leading to reduced oocyte recovery from the ovary during ovulation or defective sperm/oocyte transport.
8. Dietary and lifestyle causes [18].
9. Cervical factors.

As already discussed, there is an ongoing debate regarding the potential role of cervical factors in "so called" UI.

To conclude, the female partner of a couple suffering from UI should be extensively investigated according to the most up-to-date information with state-of-the-art testing. Only after such an evaluation has been performed and there has been no suggestion of pathology contributing to infertility should the "diagnosis" of UI be used. Some have even proposed that the term should be abandoned altogether as there is no place for such a diagnostic entity [19]. On the other hand, it has been suggested that the term is useful, both, from a clinical and practical perspective. The argument is that it may not be in the best interests of patients to undergo extensive testing, which may also not be cost effective if the information is not going to alter the proposed treatment or affect the outcome [20].

The authors' opinion is that the terminology should be preserved not only in an effort to provide clinical explanations for pathology, but also to provide focus for treatment regimens for individual patients.

The healthcare provider should equally take into account the patients' understanding and background as well as their emotions and psychological well-being. It can be extremely frustrating for the patient to be told that the reason for the infertility cannot be explained or the physician has failed to identify a diagnosis. Even where no specific targeted treatment is available, we believe that there is an advantage in providing the patient with a potential explanation to their problem.

A change in terminology will not only reduce the incidence of "UI" as a diagnosis, but will instigate more research into developing focused interventions driven forward by patients' demand.

Suggested terms that have been widely advocated are idiopathic infertility and undiagnosed infertility [19] in cases where after a "complete" evaluation, based on currently accepted diagnostic tests and interpretations, there is still no diagnosis.

Epidemiology

Establishing that the prevalence of infertility has significant demographic as well as health implications.

The incidence of truly unexplained female infertility is particularly difficult to elicit. One of the reasons and perhaps the most significant is that our current understanding of normal reproduction remains limited, and much of our understanding relies on animal research, the results of which may not be consistent with human reproduction. New information from both basic and clinical research is identified at a rapid pace and sometimes conflicts with our current thinking. Another reason is the disagreement between researchers in the definition of the term itself leading to significant differences in study populations between studies. There is very little published data regarding the prevalence of unexplained female infertility as such, so we will approach the subject by mainly looking at epidemiological studies of UI in couples.

When discussing the epidemiology of infertility, one would think that the prevalence would be different between the developed and the developing world. However, in the largest published review of its kind, the authors concluded that the prevalence of infertility is similar between more- and less-developed nations [21]. As the majority the world's population lives in the developing world, we can presume that this is where most of the infertile couples live as well. It was also reported that there is little change in the global rates of infertility over the last 20 years [22].

The similarities in prevalence of infertility between the developed and developing world may be true, but the aetiology contributing to infertility may not be the same. It is obvious that the percentage of couples suffering with UI will depend on the extent to which they have been investigated. For a couple to be diagnosed with UI by definition, they need to first seek evaluation by a reproductive specialist. In the Western world, it is estimated that between 44 and 73 % of infertile couples will present to a specialist for an evaluation [23–27]. In the study mentioned above by Boivin et al., the proportion of infertile couples living in the developed world who see a specialist varies between 27 and 74 %.

The difference in the percentages of couples seeing a reproductive specialist and the factors that could affect the reported prevalence of UI are as follows:

A. Economical
   Worldwide, there are extreme discrepancies in access to health care. Even in developed countries where state-of-the-art hospitals and treatment centres exist; access to these centres and the economic means of couples to undergo potentially expensive investigations can vary. Infertility investigations may be government funded in some countries, as for example in the UK. Therefore, women who present are investigated, irrespective of whether funding for any potential fertility treatment is secured. However, the extent of the tests that the clinician can order may vary in different areas across this country.
B. Religious
   Beliefs could direct whether the couple presents for investigations, whether certain tests are acceptable and can affect frequency or timing of coitus.
C. Social
   Society's perception of subfertility, expectations from relatives, sexual education, socially acceptable age and pattern of fecundability are all relevant.
D. Geographical
   Limitations to the size of the family as is the practice in China, or the prevalence of STIs (sexually transmitted infections), which are more common in Africa, could be important factors affecting reproductive potential.

UI accounts for 40 % of female infertility [28] and 25 [1] to 30 % [29] of infertility overall. Different studies report different findings depending on the selection criteria used [30, 31]. The limitations of all these studies are more or less due to their retrospective design. The differences in diagnostic methods to evaluate the infertile couples and variable means of data collection make them very inhomogeneous. Women suffering from unexplained subfertility have both delayed and decreased fecundity with an average cycle fecundity reported between 2 and 4 % per menstrual cycle [32, 33].

When discussing the prevalence of unexplained female infertility, stratification according to age groups should be discussed. A recent interesting study showed that the prevalence of UI in women aged less than 35 years was 21 %. However, in women over 35 years, this percentage rose to 26 % [34].

This concept of the parallel increase in UI with increasing chronological age of the female is widely recognised. Until now, though there is no such category as infertility due to "ovarian ageing" or "reproductive ageing". With the increasing use of ovarian reserve tests, such as anti-Mullerian hormone (AMH) and antral follicle count (AFC), it is likely that in the future a new category of women will be characterised as suffering from infertility related to decreased ovarian reserve and diminished oocyte quality.

Conclusions

Investigating and treating couples who suffer from UI has been described as putting a "jig-saw" puzzle together [35]. Out of the clues of this puzzle, the ones relating to the female partner appear to be more complex to investigate, and at the same time attract increased interest and opportunities for research into developing diagnostic tests and treatment options. The mystery of unexplained male infertility is starting to be unravelled and the factors that contribute to sperm dysfunction are being better understood [3]. It is our opinion that there will be some overlap between unexplained female and male infertility as new data and scientific discoveries come to light. Shedding light on these aetiologies will lead to better, more cost effective and less invasive treatments.

References

1. NICE clinical guideline 156. Fertility assessment and treatment for people with fertility problems, February 2013. Available: guidance.nice.org.uk/cg156. Accessed 20 May 2014.
2. Crosignani PG, Collins J, Cooke ID, Diczfalusy E, Rubin B. Recommendations of the ESHRE workshop on 'Unexplained Infertility'. Anacapri, 28–9 August 1992. Hum Reprod. 1993 Jun;8(6):977–80.
3. Hamada A, Esteves SC, Agarwal A. The role of contemporary andrology in unraveling the mystery of unexplained male infertility. Open Reprod Sci J. 2011;4:27–41.
4. Practice Committee of American Society for Reproductive Medicine. Diagnostic evaluation of the infertile female: a committee opinion. Fertil Steril. 2012 Aug;98(2):302–7.
5. Habbema JD, Collins J, Leridon H, Evers JL, Lunenfeld B, te Velde ER. Towards less confusing terminology in reproductive medicine: a proposal. Hum Reprod. 2004 Jul;19(7):1497–501.
6. Gnoth C, Godehardt E, Frank-Herrmann P, Friol K, Tigges J, Freundl G. Definition and prevalence of subfertility and infertility. Hum Reprod. 2005;20:1144–7.
7. Larsen U. Research on infertility: which definition should we use? Fertil Steril. 2005;83:846–852
8. Gurunath S, Pandian Z, Anderson RA, Bhattacharya S. Defining infertility-a systematic review of prevalence studies. Hum Reprod Update. 2011 Sep–Oct;17(5):575–88.
9. Evers JL. Female subfertility. Lancet. 2002 Jul 13;360(9327):151–9.
10. Gnoth C, Godehardt D, Godehardt E, Frank-Herrmann P, Freundl G. Time to pregnancy: results of the German prospective study and impact on the management of infertility. Hum Reprod. 2003 Sep;18(9):1959–66.
11. Practice Committee of American Society for Reproductive Medicine. Definitions of infertility and recurrent pregnancy loss. Fertil Steril. 2008 Nov;90(5 Suppl):S60.
12. Zegers-Hochschild F, Adamson GD, de Mouzon J, Ishihara O, Mansour R, Nygren K et al. International Committee for Monitoring Assisted Reproductive Technology (ICMART) and the World Health Organization (WHO) revised glossary of ART terminology, 2009. Fertil Steril. 2009 Nov;92(5):1520–4.
13. Practice Committee of American Society for Reproductive Medicine. Definitions of infertility and recurrent pregnancy loss: a committee opinion. Fertil Steril. 2013 Jan;99(1):63.
14. Campo S, Campo V, Benagiano G. Adenomyosis and infertility. Reprod Biomed Online. 2012 Jan;24(1):35–46.
15. Saravelos SH, Cocksedge KA, Li TC. Prevalence and diagnosis of congenital uterine anomalies in women with reproductive failure:

a critical appraisal. Hum Reprod Update. 2008 Sep–Oct;14(5): 415–29.
16. Pritts EA. Fibroids and infertility: a systematic review of the evidence. Obstet Gynecol Surv. 2001 Aug;56(8):483–91.
17. Kroon B, Johnson N, Chapman M, Yazdani A, Hart R. Fibroids in infertility—consensus statement from ACCEPT (Australasian CREI Consensus Expert Panel on Trial evidence). Aust N Z J Obstet Gynaecol. 2011 Aug;51(4):289–95.
18. Agarwal A, Aponte-Mellado A, Premkumar BJ, Shaman A, Gupta S. The effects of oxidative stress on female reproduction: a review. Reprod Biol Endocrinol. 2012 Jun 29;10:49.
19. Gleicher N, Barad D. Unexplained infertility: does it really exist? Hum Reprod. 2006;21:1951–5.
20. Siristatidis C, Bhattacharya S. Unexplained infertility: does it really exist? Does it matter? Hum Reprod. 2007 Aug;22(8):2084–7.
21. Boivin J, Bunting L, Collins JA, Nygren KG. International estimates of infertility prevalence and treatment-seeking: potential need and demand for infertility medical care. Hum Reprod. 2007 Jun;22(6):1506–12.
22. Mascarenhas MN, Flaxman SR, Boerma T, Vanderpoel S, Stevens GA. National, regional, and global trends in infertility prevalence since 1990: a systematic analysis of 277 healthsurveys. PLoS Med. 2012;9(12):e1001356.
23. Schmidt L, Munster K, Helm P. Infertility and the seeking of infertility treatment in a representative population. Br J Obstet Gynaecol. 1995;102:978–84.
24. Buckett W, Bentick B. The epidemiology of infertility in a rural population. Acta Obstet Gynecol Scand. 1997;76:233–7.
25. Stephen EH, Chandra A. Updated projections of infertility in the United States: 1995–2025. Fertil Steril. 1998 Jul;70(1):30–4.
26. Stephen EH, Chandra A. Use of infertility services in the United States: 1995. Fam Plann Perspect. 2000 May-Jun;32(3):132–7.
27. Moreau C, Bouyer J, Ducot B, Spira A, Slama R. When do involuntarily infertile couples choose to seek medical help? Fertil Steril. 2010 Feb;93(3):737–44. doi:10.1016/j.fertnstert.2008.10.011.
28. Cates W, Farley TM, Rowe PJ. Worldwide patterns of infertility: is Africa different? Lancet. 1985;2:596–8.
29. Smith S, Pfiefer, SM, Collins J, Diagnosis and management of female infertility. JAMA. 2003;290(13):1767–70.
30. Aboulghar MA, Mansour RT, Serour GI, Al-Inany HG. Diagnosis and management of unexplained infertility: an update. Arch Gynecol Obstet. 2003 Feb;267(4):177–88.
31. Isaksson R, Tiitinen A. Present concept of unexplained infertility. Gynecol Endocrinol. 2004 May;18(5):278–90.
32. Polyzos NP, Tzioras S, Mauri D, Tsappi M, Cortinovis I, Tsali L, Casazza G. Treatment of unexplained infertility with aromatase inhibitors or clomiphene citrate: a systematic review and meta-analysis. Obstet Gynecol Surv. 2008b;63(7):472–479.
33. Guzick DS, Sullivan MW, Adamson GD, Cedars MI, Falk RJ, Peterson EP, Steinkampf MP. Efficacy of treatment for unexplained infertility. Fertil Steril. 1998;70(2):207–13.
34. Maheshwari A, Hamilton M, Bhattacharya S. Effect of female age on the diagnostic categories of infertility. Hum Reprod. 2008 Mar;23(3):538–42.
35. Kovacs G, Editor. The subfertility handbook: a clinician's guide, 2nd ed. Cambridge: Cambridge University Press; 2010.

Part II
Pathophysiology: Male

Sperm Biology from Production to Ejaculation

5

Damayanthi Durairajanayagam, Anil K. Rengan, Rakesh K. Sharma and Ashok Agarwal

Introduction to the Male Reproductive System

The male reproductive system is a complex and intricate system that produces spermatozoa or sex cells to carry the genetic material of the male. The components of the male reproductive system include the hypothalamic–pituitary–gonadal (HPG) axis, and both the external and internal sexual organs. The male reproductive system forms during the early stages of embryonic development, becomes fertile during puberty and maintains the masculinity of the adult male. The external genitalia include the scrotum, testes, and penis whereas the internal genitalia include the epididymis, seminal ducts, spermatic cords, seminal vesicles, ejaculatory ducts, bulbourethral or Cowper's glands, and the prostate gland. The testes produce the male gametes (spermatozoa). The excurrent duct system matures, stores, and transports the gametes to the penis for expulsion, and the accessory glands produce and modify the contents of the semen.

The Scrotum and the Regulation of Testicular Temperature

The testes are the only organs in the human body located externally. Each testis is individually housed in a sac-like structure called the scrotum. The temperature of the underlying testes is reflected by the temperature of the scrotum. The process of spermatogenesis is optimal at temperatures 2–4 °C lower than that of core body temperature [1]. In order to maintain a hypothermic testis, the scrotum has several integral properties that facilitate the dissipation of heat. These include thin scrotal skin, minimal subcutaneous fat, sparse distribution of hair, and a large number of sweat glands. In addition, the scrotal skin hangs loose and wrinkled with a large, total surface area that adjusts according to the ambient temperature.

The cremaster and dartos muscles in the testis also help to regulate testicular temperature. The cremaster muscle is a thin layer of skeletal muscle that surrounds each testis and spermatic cord. When this muscle contracts, the testes rise closer to the abdomen, keeping them warm when ambient temperature is low. The dartos muscle is a thin layer of smooth muscle fiber beneath the scrotal skin. When contracted, the dartos muscle causes the exposed scrotal skin surface area to decrease and heat to be conserved. Conversely, when both these muscles are in a relaxed state, the testis hangs further from the abdomen, enveloped by the scrotal skin. This aids in keeping the temperature of the testes lower than that of the core body. Furthermore, rising external temperatures activate the cutaneous receptors on the scrotal skin to initiate sweat secretion and active heat loss through the evaporation of sweat [2].

The Testes

The human testes are a pair of ovoid (ellipsoid) structures measuring approximately 4.5–5 cm in length by 2.5–4 cm in width and about 15–25 mL in volume (Fig. 5.1). The tunica albuginea, the outer capsule of the testes, is composed of a thick and flexible (though not stretchable) fibrous layer of connective tissue [3]. The parenchyma of the testis is divided by the septa (connective tissue) into 250–300 conical lobules. Each of these lobules consists of masses of highly convoluted seminiferous tubules. Both ends of the seminiferous tubules connect at the hilus to form the rete testis [4]. The seminiferous tubules secrete fluid that flows into the rete testis to be collected and delivered to the excurrent ductal system of the epididymis [5].

Each testis is composed of two distinct compartments: (1) the tubular compartment that contains the seminiferous tubules and (2) the intertubular compartment that lies

D. Durairajanayagam (✉) · A. K. Rengan · R. K. Sharma · A. Agarwal
Center for Reproductive Medicine, Cleveland Clinic, Cleveland, OH, USA
e-mail: agarwaa@ccf.org

A. K. Rengan
7 Setter Place, Kendall Park, NJ 08824, USA

G. L. Schattman et al. (eds.), *Unexplained Infertility*, DOI 10.1007/978-1-4939-2140-9_5,

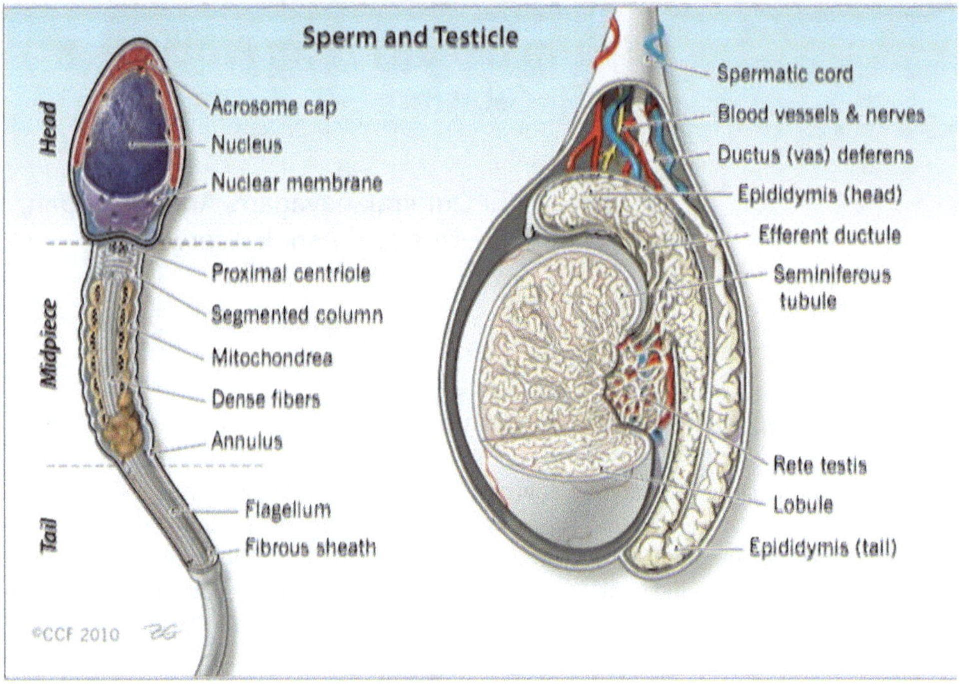

Fig. 5.1 The human spermatozoa, testis, and epididymis. To the *left* is a mature human spermatozoon showing the components that make up the *head*, midpiece and *tail* sections. To the *right* is a view of the human testis and the seminiferous tubules, as well as the epididymis, showing the corpus (*head*) and caudal (*tail*) sections. (Reprinted with permission, Cleveland Clinic Center for Medical Art & Photography © 2010–2013. All rights reserved.)

between the seminiferous tubules and contains the interstitial tissue. Each of these compartments is anatomically separate but remains closely linked together. Within the seminiferous tubules are the spermatogonial germ and Sertoli cells. The Sertoli cells provide a hormonally active environment for the evolution of primitive germ cells into mature male gametes or spermatozoa.

The bulk (90 %) of the testicular volume is made up of the seminiferous tubules and the germ cells that lie within the invaginations of the Sertoli cells, which make up the germinal epithelium. The seminiferous tubules also consist of peritubular tissue or lamina propria [6]. The peritubular tissue contains myofibroblasts that cause peristaltic contractions of the seminiferous tubules. This movement helps to transport the developing, immotile germ cells to the rete testis [7]. The intertubular spaces within the lobules contain clusters of Leydig or interstitial cells that make up the endocrine portion of the testis. The interstitial tissue consists primarily of blood and lymph vessels, nerve and collagenous fibers, macrophages, and a variety of connective tissue cells. The spermatogenic process is dependent on intra- and extra-testicular hormonal regulatory processes, the functions of the intertubular microvasculature, Leydig cells, and other cellular components in the interstitium (intertubular space) [8].

The testis is responsible for synthesizing (steroidogenesis) and secreting androgens (i.e., testosterone), which is directly interrelated to its second function, producing spermatozoa (spermatogenesis). These functions are under hormonal control via the pituitary gonadotropins—luteinizing hormone (LH), and follicle-stimulating hormone (FSH).

Hormonal Control of Spermatogenesis (Extrinsic Influences)

The hormonal regulation of spermatogenesis is under the control of the hypothalamus–pituitary–gonadal (HPG) axis. This axis begins as the higher center sends signals to the hypothalamus, which acts as the integrating center. The hypothalamus releases gonadotropin releasing hormone (GnRH) in discrete pulses that peak every 1.5 h. GnRH acts on the anterior pituitary to stimulate gonadotropin production (LH and FSH). A continuous production of GnRH will cause gonadotrophin desensitization, which will diminish LH and FSH release. LH is released in a similar pulsatile pattern to that of GnRH while FSH release is influenced by inhibin. LH and FSH act on the testes to produce testosterone and inhibin, respectively. LH acts on the Leydig cells in the testes to stimulate testosterone production through the conversion of cholesterol. When testosterone levels accumulate, it exerts a negative feedback effect at the pituitary (short loop) to suppress the release of LH and at the hypothalamus (long loop), which ultimately suppresses GnRH production and thereby regulates testosterone levels. FSH acts on the Sertoli cells to stimulate inhibin and androgen-binding protein (ABP) secretion. Accumulating inhibin levels exert a negative feedback effect at the pituitary to suppress FSH release, thereby regulating inhibin levels.

FSH is required at the onset of puberty to initiate spermatogenesis as its action on Sertoli cells is necessary for germ cell maturation. Testosterone is essential for maintaining the spermatogenic process. Its actions are facilitated by the Sertoli cells. Spermatocytes have ABP receptors but not androgen receptors whereas the Sertoli cells have androgen receptors. The binding of ABP to testosterone may assist testosterone movement toward the lumen of the seminiferous tubule onwards to the epididymis. FSH also induces the conversion of testosterone to 5α-dihydrotestosterone (5α-DHT) and 17β-estradiol. 5α-DHT is more active than testosterone and along with 17β-estradiol, is involved in the development and function of the penis, scrotum, accessory sex glands, secondary sex characteristics, libido and potency.

Leydig Cells

Leydig cells are embedded in groups that surround the connective tissue between seminiferous tubules in the testicle. These endocrine cells are the principal source of testosterone, the production of which is stimulated by LH (Table 5.1). In adults, testosterone in circulation is kept within the physiological range of 300–1200 ng/dL while intratesticular levels of testosterone are far higher. In the testes, testosterone levels are highest at the basement membrane of the seminiferous tubules.

Testosterone

Testosterone, the major male androgen in circulation and in the Leydig cells, is responsible for primary and secondary sex characteristics. It is synthesized from cholesterol in the Leydig cells. Primary sex characteristics are structures responsible for promoting the development, preservation, and delivery of sperm cells while secondary sex characteristics are structures and behavioral features that externally differentiate men from women.

Sertoli Cells

Sertoli cells, also known as sustentacular or nurse cells, are highly specialized cells that regulate the development of spermatogonia into spermatozoa (Table 5.1). They originate from the tubular basement membrane and extend up toward the lumen of the seminiferous tubules. The basement membrane acts as a barrier that prevents large molecules in the interstitial fluid from entering the tubule but allows the entry of testosterone. Sertoli cells provide sustenance for developing spermatogonia and are involved in germ cell phagocytosis. The formation of lipid droplets in Sertoli cells is associated with this phagocytosis [9]. The number of lipid droplets found in Sertoli cells increases as the testes advance in age [10]. They also produce and secrete anti-Müllerian hormone (AMH), inhibin, activin, growth factors, enzymes, and ABP. AMH is involved in embryonic development and contributes to the regression of Müllerian ducts. Inhibin, another hormone, helps to regulate FSH secretion from the anterior pituitary. When FSH binds to high-affinity FSH receptors on the Sertoli cells, ABP is secreted (by Sertoli cells) into the lumen of the seminiferous tubule, where it binds to testosterone (secreted by Leydig cells). This causes testosterone to become less lipophilic and more concentrated within the luminal fluid.

Neighboring Sertoli cells have membrane specializations at the basolateral side that forms a band, sealing the cells together and forming a tight junction. The blood–testis barrier prevents molecules in the blood from moving past the tight junctions toward the lumen of the seminiferous tubules. This ensures that the germ cells in the later stages of development remain inaccessible to any harmful molecules in circulation.

The Blood–Testis Barrier

In the mammalian testes, the blood–testis barrier is composed of specialized junctions that are tightly bound between adjacent Sertoli cells in the epithelium of the seminiferous tubule. This barrier is also known as the Sertoli cell seminiferous epithelium barrier. The strong intercellular junctional complexes that link two adjacent Sertoli cells in the tubule form an additional barrier between the tubular lumen and the interstitial fluid outside the tubule. This divides the seminiferous tubule space into two parts: the basal (basement membrane) compartment that is in contact with blood and lymph vessels and the adluminal (lumen) compartment that is isolated from these fluids. The blood and lymph vessels and

Table 5.1 Functions of the Leydig and Sertoli cells

Functions of the Leydig cells	Functions of the Sertoli cells
Initiation and maintenance of spermatogenesis	Maintains the integrity of seminiferous tubules epithelium
Activation of the hypothalamus–pituitary–gonadal axis	Secretion of hormones—inhibin and androgen-binding protein (ABP)
Production of testosterone—manifestation of male secondary sex characteristics	Secretes tubular fluid into the tubular lumen for transport of sperm within the duct
Differentiation of male genital organs	Delivery of nutrients to germ cells
Masculinization of the brain and sexual behavior	Steroidogenesis and steroid metabolism
–	Aids in process of phagocytosis and elimination of cytoplasm
–	Regulates the spermatogenic cycle
–	Acts as a hormonal target for LH, FSH, and testosterone

nerves are located in the interstitium between the tubules and do not penetrate the seminiferous tubules [11]. The Sertoli cells are surrounded by closely aligned myoid or peritubular cells. These arrangements collectively form the blood–testis barrier, which provides an immunologically privileged site for spermatogenesis to thrive.

The fluid found in the tubular compartment of the testes differs from that in found in the interstitium as the former contains low concentrations of glucose and high concentrations of potassium ions and steroid hormones. The tight junctions of the blood–testis barrier break and reform around the migrating cells to ensure that the barrier remains intact.

Intrinsic Regulation

The process of spermatogenesis is also regulated independently from within the testis. The Leydig cells secrete (1) testosterone, (2) neuroendocrine substances that serve as neurotransmitters, and (3) growth factors for neighboring Leydig cells, blood vessels, lamina propria of the seminiferous tubules, and Sertoli cells [12–14]. Leydig cells also contribute toward the nutrition of the Sertoli cells and help to regulate blood flow in the intertubular microvasculature [3]. The cells of the peritubular tissue influence myofibroblast contractility and regulate spermatozoa transportation via peristaltic movements of the seminiferous tubules. The Sertoli cells deliver different growth factors, and various germ cells participate in the development and regulation of other germ cells.

Spermatogenesis

Spermatogenesis is an extremely intricate process of cell differentiation, starting with germ cell (spermatogonia) development and culminating in the production of highly specialized spermatozoa. This process produces the genetic material required for species replication. Spermatogenesis occurs in the lumen of the seminiferous tubules. It was classically believed that human spermatogenesis takes about 64 days in the testis (from spermatogonium to spermatid) with an additional 10–14 days in the epididymis for maturation of spermatozoa. Thus, the entire process took about 70 ± 4 days to complete [15]. However, a more recent report suggests that the entire process from production to ejaculation of spermatozoa is completed within a shorter period: an average of 64 ± 8 days (with a range of 42–76 days) [16]. Spermatogenesis begins at puberty and occurs continually throughout the entire male adult life span in contrast to oogenesis, which is finite in women. The baseline number of precursor cells in the testes is regulated by FSH. Early in embryonic development, the gonocytes, which precede the formation of spermatogonial germ cells, undergo active mitotic replication [17].

Spermatogenesis involves a series of cellular events that begin in the basal compartment and end in the apical compartment. The basal and the luminal compartments are kept separate by tight junctions. In the seminiferous tubules, the developing cells are arranged in a highly ordered sequence from the basement membrane toward the lumen (Fig. 5.2). Spermatogonia are positioned directly on the basement membrane. Primary spermatocytes, secondary spermatocytes, and spermatids lie closest to the lumen. Spermatogonia and primary spermatocytes are found in the basal compartment whereas secondary spermatocytes and spermatids are found in the adluminal compartment.

During spermatogenesis, two events occur in the basal compartment outside the blood–testis barrier: (1) the renewal and proliferation of spermatogonia via mitosis and differentiation and (2) the cell cycle progression from type B spermatogonia to preleptotene spermatocytes. The following three events occur in the adluminal or apical compartment behind the blood–testis barrier: (1) the cell cycle progression from zygotene to pachytene and then to diplotene spermatocytes, followed by meiosis I and meiosis II; (2) spermiogenesis, during which the round spermatids develop into elongated spermatids and eventually spermatozoa; and finally (3) spermiation, which involves spermatozoa maturation and subsequent release into the lumen (Table 5.2).

The following is an overview of the spermatogenic events. First, the primary spermatocytes undergo two meiotic divisions. The first division gives rise to two haploid secondary spermatocytes, which is followed by the second division, which gives rise to four haploid spermatids (1n, 23 chromosomes). Two of these spermatids carry the X maternal chromosome while the other two spermatids carry the Y paternal chromosome. Each spermatid will subsequently undergo spermiogenesis, a metamorphosis into spermatozoa. The spermatozoa are then released into the lumen of the seminiferous tubule (Fig. 5.3).

Spermatogoniogenesis

Spermatogonia are a population of long-living primordial germ cells that undergo mitosis to provide a renewing stem cell population and meiosis for spermatozoa production. Germ cells are named according to their morphological appearance and can be categorized into two classes: Type A and Type B. In humans, Type A cells, the most rudimentary of cells, can be further classified as "pale Type A (A_p)" and "dark Type A (A_d)" spermatogonia. A_p spermatogonia can divide mitotically into more A_p cells or Type B spermatogonia. Type A spermatogonia comprise the stem cell pool whereas Type B spermatogonia continue to develop into spermatids.

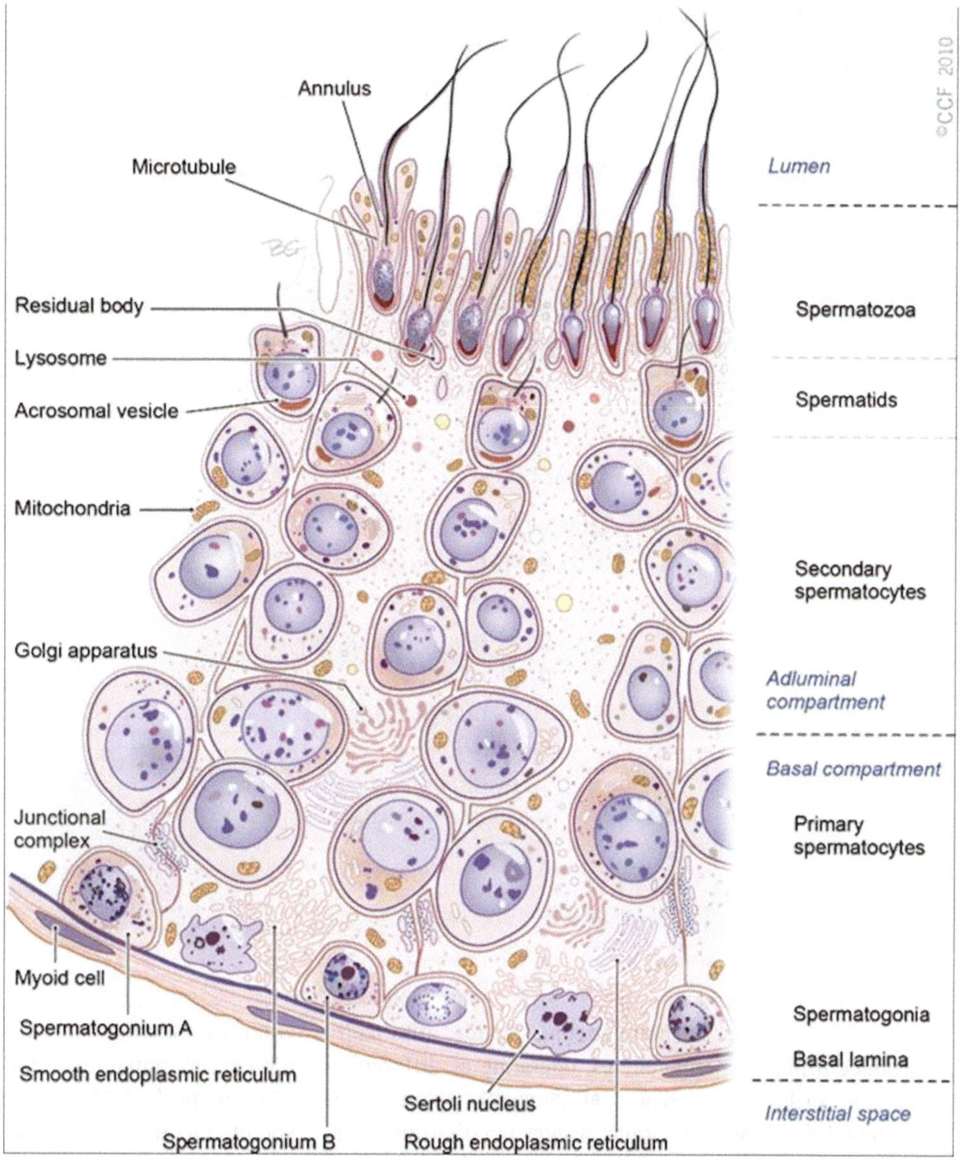

Fig. 5.2 Seminiferous tubule. A cross section of the germinal epithelium in the seminiferous tubule. The germinal epithelium is divided by the Sertoli cell into two compartments, i.e., the basal and adluminal compartments. Fully formed spermatozoa are released into the lumen. (Reprinted with permission, Cleveland Clinic Center for Medical Art & Photography © 2010–2013. All rights reserved.)

Table 5.2 Terminology in spermatogenesis

Process	Description
Spermatogoniogenesis	Process of producing spermatogonia through multiple mitoses to amass a large population of stem cells, most of which undergo meiosis to produce spermatozoa
Spermatogenesis	Process of differentiation of a spermatogonium into a spermatid Purpose: to produce (via mitosis and meiosis) the necessary genetic material for species replication
Spermatocytogenesis	Process of producing spermatocytes that occurs in the basal compartment of the seminiferous tubules
Spermiogenesis	A complex metamorphosis that transforms round spermatids (from the final division of meiosis) into a complex structure spermatozoon
Spermiation	Process whereby a mature spermatid frees itself from the Sertoli cell and enters the tubular lumen

A_p spermatogonia remain attached to the basal membrane and continue to replenish its numbers, allowing the spermatogenic process to persist despite the aging process. Spermatogonia continuously increase in number via successive, but usually incomplete, mitosis. On the other hand, A_d cells seldom divide, potentially serving as a dormant reserve or nonproliferative stem cells that give rise to A_p spermatogonia [15].

Type B spermatogonia have more chromatin within the inner nuclear envelope than to the intermediate or type A

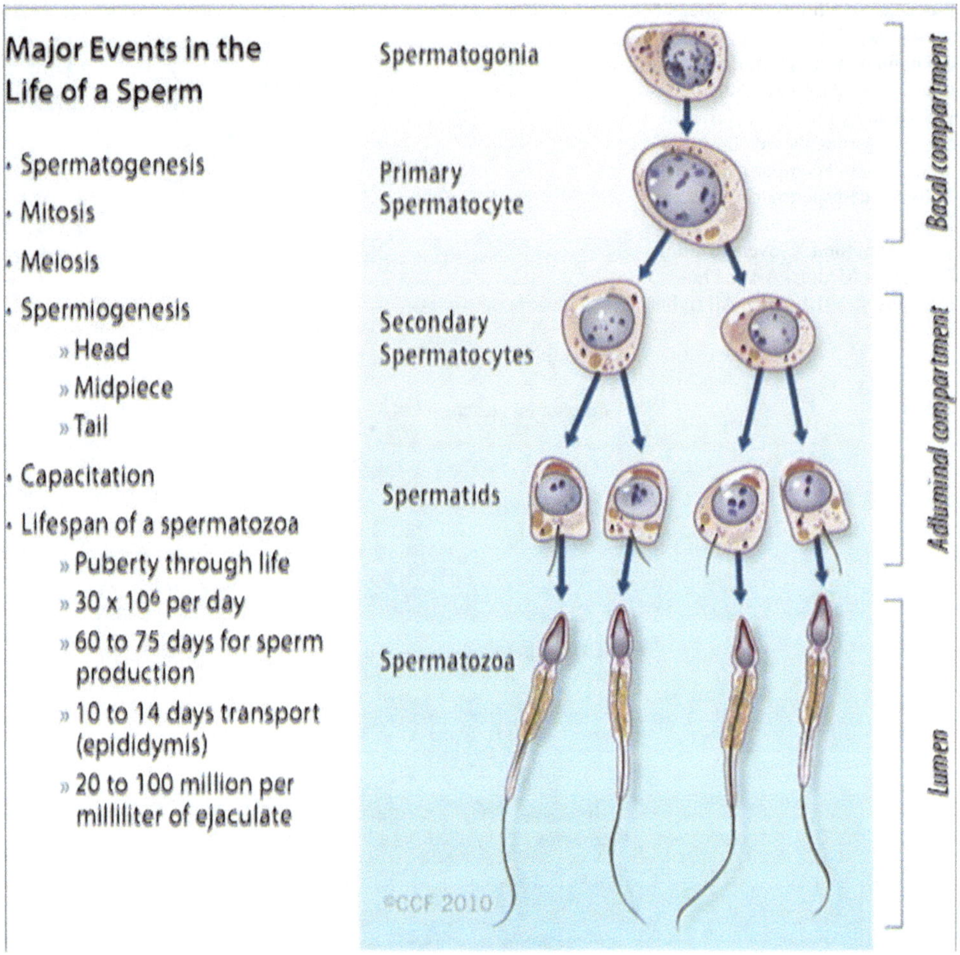

Fig. 5.3 Spermatogenesis. Major events in the life of a sperm involving spermatogenesis, spermiogenesis, and spermiation. (Reprinted with permission, Cleveland Clinic Center for Medical Art & Photography © 2010–2013. All rights reserved.)

spermatogonia. Type B spermatogonia divide mitotically to produce primary spermatocytes, operating as differential precursors to the preleptotene spermatocytes. Spermatogonia remain joined by intercellular bridges but dissolve in the advanced phases of spermatid development. The synchrony of germ cell maturation is thus maintained [18], which is likely to aid in its biochemical interactions.

Spermatocytogenesis

Spermatocytogenesis involves the formation of spermatocytes and takes place in the basal compartment of the seminiferous tubule. The process begins with the primary spermatocytes undergoing meiosis I to form secondary spermatocytes. The prophase of the first meiotic division is very long and thus, the primary spermatocyte has the longest lifespan. Secondary spermatocytes then undergo the meiosis II to produce spermatids. Secondary spermatocytes have a comparably shorter lifespan of 1.1–1.7 days.

Spermatogenesis, from spermatogonium division to spermatozoa release into the tubule, takes about 64 days to complete. Sperm released into the lumen of the seminiferous tubules are immature and incapable of moving on their own. They are pushed through the lumen both by other developing sperm cells moving toward the lumen and by the bulk flow of fluid secreted by Sertoli cells. Sperm cells entering the epididymis complete maturation after 10–14 days of transit, aided by protein secretions from epididymal cells.

Disruption of Spermatogenesis

Type A spermatogonia are necessary for spermatogenesis, and in cases of reduced spermatogenesis, it is likely that A_d spermatogonia are absent [8]. When Type A or Type B spermatogonia are absent and the germinal epithelium is made up only of Sertoli cells, then spermatogenesis will not occur. This "Sertoli Cell Only Syndrome" may be congenital (absence of spermatogonia from birth) or acquired (spermatogonia destroyed by exposure to radiation, etc.). Spermatogenic arrest at the spermatogonial stage occurs when A_p spermatogonia fail to develop into Type B spermatogonia [19].

Mitosis (Cytodifferentiation of Spermatids)

Mitosis involves nuclear division and separation of duplicated chromosomes to form two daughter cells with genetic content exactly identical to its parent cell (diploid, $n=46$). Mitosis is vital for proliferation and maintenance of spermatogonial cells. Meiosis involves an intricate series of events that encompass the duplication of chromosomes, nuclear envelope breakdown, and equal division of chromosomes and cytoplasm that leads to the formation of two daughter cells. Specific regulatory proteins interact on DNA loop domains during cellular replication [20, 21]. The germ cells involved in the mitotic phase are the Type A spermatogonia, which first form the Type B spermatogonia and later the primary spermatocytes. Through a series of mitotic divisions, developing germ cells, which are interconnected by intracellular bridges, produce primary spermatocytes—the largest germ cell of the germinal epithelium. The baseline number of spermatogonia is established after puberty. Mitosis then supplies the precursor cells and initiates the differentiation and maturation processes.

Meiosis

Meiosis is a complex process during which chromosomal exchange of genetic material occurs to form four daughter cells with half the number of chromosomes (haploid, $n=23$) compared to their parent cells. The purpose of meiosis is to ensure genetic diversity. The germ cells involved in the meiotic phase are the primary spermatocytes, secondary spermatocytes, and spermatids. Meiosis occurs twice in succession as meiosis I and meiosis II; each meiotic process consists of prophase, metaphase, anaphase, and telophase. Prophase itself is made up of four stages: leptotene, zygotene, pachytene, and diplotene. Leptotene takes place in the basal compartment while the remaining three take place in the adluminal compartment. Meiosis I is the reducing division in which the number of chromosomes are halved (i.e., the replicated chromosomes in one cell is split between two diploid cells). Meiosis II is the division in which there is no DNA replication and the sister chromatids are split, resulting in four halpoid cells.

The meiotic process is regulated by its own specific mechanisms [22]. In the seminiferous tubules, meiosis begins with the detachment of Type B spermatogonia from the basement membrane to form preleptotene primary spermatocytes. In theory, each primary spermatocyte yields four spermatids, but the actual yield is lower as some of these germ cells are lost in the process. After meiosis I, each daughter cell (secondary spermatocyte) contains one half of the homologous chromosome pair. The secondary spermatocytes then quickly undergo meiosis II, during which time the chromatids separate at the centromere, yielding early round spermatids with haploid chromosomes "22X" or "22Y." During the entire meiotic phase, homologous chromosomes pair up, cross over, and exchange genetical material to form an entirely new genome. Defects during meiosis include apoptotic spermatocytes and spermatogenic arrest of primary spermatocytes. These germ cells bordering the seminiferous tubules cease to develop further and disintegrate [8].

Spermiogenesis

In spermiogenesis, haploid spermatids undergo complete differentiation or morphogenesis to form highly specialized spermatozoa with fully compacted chromatin. These morphological changes begin after meioses I and II. In humans, there are eight different stages (S_{a-1}, S_{a-2}, S_{b-1}, S_{b-2}, S_{c-1},S_{c-2}, S_{d-1},and S_{d-2}) involved in the maturation of spermatids to spermatozoa. Each stage is identifiable by the maturing cell's morphological characteristics. In the postmeiotic phase, there is progressive condensation of the nuclear chromatin (to about 1/10 the volume of an immature spermatid) with the inactivation of the genome. In addition, the Golgi apparatus forms the acrosome cap, and the flagellum structures begin to develop [8]. Histones—alkaline proteins that condense the DNA—are converted into transitional proteins, and protamines are converted into well-developed disulfide bonds. Defects during spermiogenesis include acrosomal and flagellar defects, absence of the acrosome or the midpeice of the flagellum, and impaired nuclear condensation in malformed spermatids [8].

Nuclear Development

The nucleus and its contents undergo several changes during spermatogenesis. During the first eight steps of spermiogenesis [23], the nucleus elongates and flattens, giving the head its characteristic oval shape. This nuclear compaction is believed to facilitate oocyte penetration and help to optimize spermatozoa swimming capacity [24]. This nuclear compaction includes chromatin remodeling. During the last postmeiotic phase of spermiogenesis, histone molecules, around which DNA is organized, are converted to translational proteins that are then converted to protamines [25]. Protamines contain large amounts of cysteine, which aids in disulfide bond formation as the sperm cells mature in the epididymis [26–28]. Protamines in the chromatin of the spermatozoa are replaced by histones from the oocyte within 2–4 h of fertilization.

Spermiation

During spermiation, the mature sperm cell releases itself from the Sertoli cell and moves into the lumen of the seminiferous tubule [28]. Spermatids originating from the same spermatogonia remain attached to each other by bridges, facilitating the transfer of cytoplasmic products. Spermiation may also involve the movement of spermatids as they progress toward the lumen of the seminiferous tubules [28]. Mature spermatids close their intracellular bridges and disconnect from the germinal epithelium, becoming free cells (spermatozoa). At this stage, portions of the sperm cell cytoplasm, known as the cytoplasmic droplet, are eliminated. However, the cytoplasmic droplet may remain in immature spermatozoa during the process of spermiation, becoming "excess residual cytoplasm" [29].

The Cycle or Wave of Seminiferous Epithelium

Spermatogenesis involves the division of primitive spermatogonial cells into germ cell types through the process of meiosis. At any given time, groups of cells in different developmental phases are present within the germinal epithelium of the seminiferous tubule. Germ cells are localized in spatial units known as stages, designated by Roman numerals. Each stage is distinguished by (1) acrosome development, (2) meiotic phase, (3) nucleus shape, and (4) spermatozoa release into the lumen of the seminiferous tubule [30] (Fig. 5.4). The same typical aspects of germ cell epithelium appear every 16 days [8]. The time it takes for Type A spermatogonial to divide is shorter than that required for the entire process of spermatogenesis. The development of Type A spermatogonia into mature spermatids followed by the delivery of mature spermatozoa through the epididymal duct system takes anywhere between 42 and 76 days [16].

Rete Testis and Epididymis

Spermatozoa in the lumen of the seminiferous tubules leave the testis through the rete testis and several vasa (ductuli) efferentia. The ductuli combine to form a single, highly convoluted duct at the head of the epididymis. The epididymis, located along the dorsolateral edge of each testis, allows for post-testicular maturation and storage of spermatozoa during their passage from the testis to the vas deferens. It is divided into three unique segments: the caput epididymis (head) for spermatozoa concentration, corpus epididymis (body) for spermatozoa maturation, and cauda epididymis (tail) for spermatozoa storage. As they pass through the epididymis, spermatozoa attain their full maturity, fertilizing ability, and motility, although they typically do not move under their own control until after ejaculation. The epididymal epithelium is sensitive to androgen stimulation and possesses both absorptive and secretory abilities. As they journey through the epididymis, spermatozoa undergo changes in membrane protein composition, phospholipid and fatty acid content, net surface charge, immunoreactivity, and adenylate cyclase activity. At the caput, a significant amount of the fluid that carries spermatozoa from the seminiferous tubules is reabsorbed, greatly increasing spermatozoa concentration. Spermatozoa remain motionless in the male genital tract and are transported by the flow of fluid in the testes, and thereafter by contraction of the organs.

Spermatozoa mature outside the testes, leaving those within the testes with poor motility and fertilization ability. The cauda epididymis stores mature spermatozoa, permitting repetitive, rich ejaculations. Sperm cell storage capacity diminishes distally. At the cauda epididymis, spermatozoa lose fertilizing potential first, motility second, and vitality last. These cells, along with nearly half of all spermatozoa released from the testes, will disintegrate and undergo reabsorption by the epididymal epithelium. This includes older gametes that must be eliminated from the male reproductive tract regularly to ensure high quality of the ejaculate.

Vas Deferens

The vas deferens is a muscular tube adjacent to the prostate that extends from the epididymis, passing through the inguinal canal into the peritoneal cavity and opening into the urethra. Near the prostate end, the vas deferens enlarges and forms a gland called the ampulla. This portion, along with excretory canals of the seminal vesicles, forms the ejaculatory ducts and joins the urethra. The ampulla is where the majority of sperm cells are stored for ejaculation. Few spermatozoa find their way from the caudal epididymis into the seminal vesicle where they will then degenerate. These cells are generally found in the terminal portion of the ejaculate.

Accessory Sex Glands

The seminal vesicles, prostate gland, and Cowper's (bulbourethral) gland are collectively known as the accessory sex glands. These glands secrete fluids that act as the medium for sperm transport and sustenance (Table 5.3). These secretions make up the seminal plasma of the ejaculate. The seminal vesicles join the ampullary portion of the vas deferens and produce fructose and coagulating proteins. The prostate gland is located at the junction of the vas deferens and the urethra. Fluid produced by the prostate contains zinc, citric acid, and acid phosphatase, which give semen its typical odor. In addition, the prostate secretes enzymes that liquefy

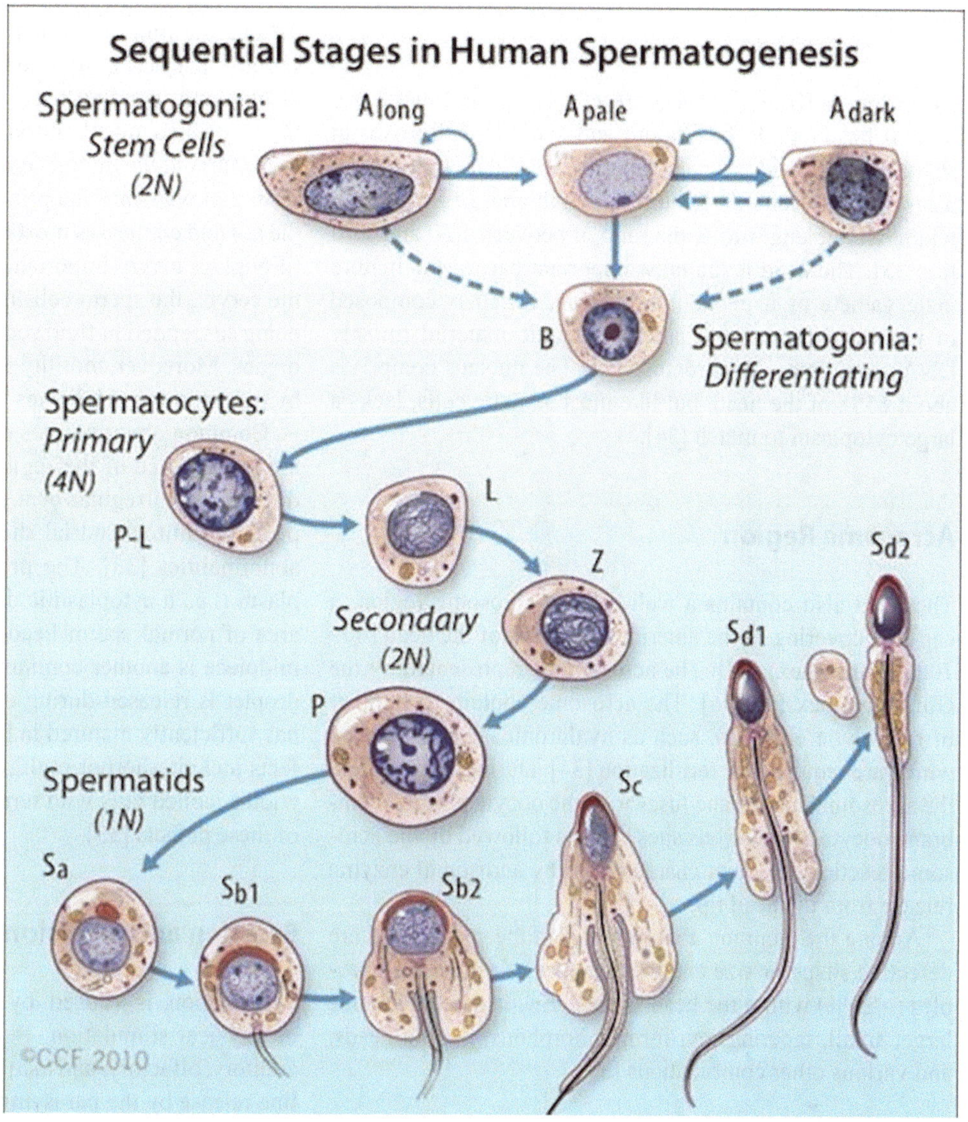

Fig. 5.4 Stages in spermatogenesis. The sequential stages of differentiation during spermatogenesis: from a diploid germ cell into a fully functional spermatozoon. (Reprinted with permission, Cleveland Clinic Center for Medical Art & Photography © 2010–2013. All rights reserved.)

Table 5.3 Composition of semen

Component	Function	Source
Sperm	Carries the paternal genetic material	Seminiferous tubules
Mucus	Acts as a lubricant	Bulbourethral glands
Water	Provides a liquid medium	All accessory glands
Buffers	Neutralizes the acidic environment of the vagina	Prostate, bulbourethral glands
Nutrients		
L-carnitine	Nourishes the spermatozoa	Epididymis
Fructose Vitamin C		Seminal vesicles
Citric acid		Prostate
Enzymes	Forms coagulum in vagina, then liquefies	Seminal vesicles and prostate
Prostaglandins	Smooth muscle contraction; aids sperm transport within both the male and female reproductive tract	Seminal vesicles

the seminal coagulum. The Cowper's gland is situated distal to the prostate gland and empties into the bulbous urethra. Fluid from the Cowper's gland lubricates the urethra prior to ejaculation.

Structure of Spermatozoon

A morphologically normal sperm cell is about 45–50 μm in length and consists of a head and tail.

Head

According to Kruger's strict criteria [31], a morphologically normal head should be smooth and symmetrically oval in shape with a broad base and tapering apex. The sperm head measures between 4.0–5.5 μm in length and 2.5–3.5 μm in width, with a length-to-width ratio of between 1.50 and 1.70 [32, 33]. The head is the most important part of the mature male gamete as it contains a nucleus, which is composed of packed chromosomal paternal genetic material (mostly DNA) containing 23 chromosomes. The nucleus comprises about 65 % of the head, but like most somatic cells, lacks a large cytoplasm to match [34].

Acrosome Region

The head also contains a well-defined acrosome region, a cap-like covering of the anterior two thirds of the head (40–70 % of the apex) [33]. The acrosome is represented by the Golgi complex [35, 36]. The acrosome contains a number of hydrolytic enzymes, such as hyaluronidase and acrosin, which are required for fertilization [34]. During fertilization, the acrosomal membrane fuses with the oocyte plasma membrane oocyte at numerous sites. This is followed by the acrosome reaction, an event characterized by acrosomal enzyme release from the head tip.

Among the common abnormalities of the sperm head are defective shape or size and the presence of numerous vacuoles (>20 %) within the head surface. Shape defects include large, small, tapering, pyriform, amorphous, double heads, and various other combinations [33].

Neck

The neck is formed by the fragile junction between the head and tail portion.

Tail

The tail measures 40–50 μm in length (nearly ten times the length of the head) and provides motility for the cell. The sperm cell's entire motility apparatus is contained in the tail, propelling the sperm body via waves generated in the neck region that pass along distally in a whiplash manner.

The tail can be divided into the midpiece (anterior portion), principal piece, and endpiece (posterior portion). Ideally, the midpiece supports the head at exactly the center position. It should be slender as well (maximum width of 1 μm), yet thicker than the rest of the tail and between 7.0 and 8.0 μm in length. The tail diameter should be between 0.4 and 0.5 μm, measuring about 50 μm in length. The tail should have a well-defined endpiece, without any coiling or abnormal bending (over 90°). The midpiece consists of tightly packed mitochondria surrounded by a sheath. The mitochondria in the midpiece supply energy in the form of ATP for tail movement. The principal piece is the longest part of the tail and comprises most of the propellant machinery. Motility plays a very important role in sperm transport through the cervix; the sperm cells need to maintain motility despite being suspended in fluid secreted by the female reproductive organs. Moreover, motility is required to avoid phagocytosis by polymorphonucleocytes found in female body fluid.

Common abnormalities of the neck and midpiece region are the absence of the regions themselves, thickened neck, distended or irregular/bent midpiece, abnormally thin midpiece (no mitochondrial sheath), or a combination of these abnormalities [33]. The presence of excess residual cytoplasm (i.e., a cytoplasmic droplet greater than one third the area of normal sperm head) at the posterior portion of the midpiece is another common abnormality. The cytoplasmic droplet is released during ejaculation as long as the sperm has sufficiently matured in the epididymis. Common tail defects include short or multiple hairpin broken tails, irregular widths, coiled tails with terminal droplets, or a combination of these defects [33].

Erection and Emission

An erection is caused by sexually related psychic and/or physical stimulation. Before an erection occurs, visual, auditory, olfactory, and tactile stimulation triggers acetylcholine release by the parasympathetic nervous system. Acetylcholine causes vasodilation of the pudendal arteries, which leads to increased blood flow to the corpus cavernosum and corpus spongiosum of the penis. As the venous outflow is compressed, the penis becomes engorged with blood and grows more turgid, leading to an erection. Penile erection is required for penetration into the vagina for sperm deposition. Erectile dysfunction is the repeated inability to achieve or maintain an erection rigid enough for sexual intercourse.

Semen, the mixture of sperm and fluids, is expelled via a neuromuscular reflex in two sequential phases: emission and ejaculation. At the start of emission, a series of coordinated sequential contractions begins in the testis efferent ducts, the cauda epididymis and the convoluted portion of the vas deferens. The contractions advance in an assimilated manner, propelling the sperm from the cauda epididymis forward into the prostatic urethra. Here, the prostatic fluid, the sperm-rich fraction from the ampulla, and the fluid from the seminal vesicle are deposited into the prostatic urethra. This action propels sperm from the efferent ducts, through the ejaculatory ducts, and into the urethra. The filling of the urethra with sperm initiates sensory signals that travel to the sacrospinal region of cord. The internal urethral sphincter is closed by sympathetic discharge to prevent retrograde ejaculation into the urinary bladder. During the emission phase, when spermatozoa pass into the urethra, sympathetic stimulations release adrenaline and initiate contraction of the smooth muscles surrounding the ampulla, deferens ducts, and the cauda epididymis.

Ejaculation

Ejaculation is initiated after emission, and the process expels semen from the penile urethra. It includes external sphincter relaxation and rhythmic prostate contractions. The bulbospongiosus muscle propels the semen in an antigrade manner out of the external urethral meatus. Sperm that is not ejaculated will gradually die and undergoes cytolysis. Ejaculation involves both the sympathetic and parasympathetic nervous systems. Parasympathetic fibers initiate the contraction of the bulbospongiosus muscle, which leads to forcible expulsion of the semen from the urethra. Ascending impulses contribute simultaneously toward the sensation of orgasm.

The ejaculate, or semen, is freshly produced at the time of ejaculation. Ejaculation normally occurs in a definite sequence. First, a small amount of Cowper's gland fluid is extruded followed by prostatic fluid and the sperm-rich fraction from the ampulla, and finally secretions from the seminal vesicle (Table 5.3). These secretions form the seminal coagulum, a gel-like substance that normally liquefies in about 20 min. Sperm cells are trapped within the gel matrix of the coagulum and remain immotile until activation upon liquefaction.

Once the ejaculate is expelled, detumescence of the penis begins under sympathetic control. Noradrenaline is secreted, causing dilation of the penile vasculature and penile flaccidity.

Capacitation and Acrosome Reaction

The spermatozoa undergoes several chemical changes during capacitation, which occurs in the cervix, uterine cavity, and the fallopian tubes during the estrogenic phase. Capacitation allows the acrosome reaction to occur as the sperm and oocyte come into contact with one another. As with epididymal maturation, capacitation is also required before fertilization can occur. Capacitation takes place after ejaculation into the female reproductive tract. During capacitation, spermatozoa undergo a sequence of biochemical changes that ultimately enable them to fertilize an ovum. The sperm plasmalemma is reorganized to support the subsequent acrosome reaction; seminal plasma factors are removed and modifications are made to the sperm membrane, sterols, lipids, glycoproteins, outer acrosomal membrane, and surface charge. The concentration of intracellular free Ca^{2+} increases as well [37]. In particular, it is the removal of cholesterol from the surface membrane that allows for the acrosome reaction to occur [38].

The acrosome reaction is a form of exocytosis that gives spermatozoa the ability to advance through the zona pellucida and prepares them for fusion with the ovum membrane. This process helps to dispel the contents of the acrosome, including surface antigens and enzymes, for successful fertilization. D-mannose binding lectins on the sperm surface, for example, have been shown to help bind spermatozoa to the zona pellucida [39, 40]. The acrosomal enzymes digest the outer acrosomal membrane and the plasma membrane to which it is attached. At this point, the head is covered only by the inner acrosomal membrane. The posterior region of the head is enclosed by a single membrane known as the postnuclear cap. The acrosome and postnuclear cap overlap to form the equatorial segment, which does not take part in the acrosome reaction. The spermatozoon progresses forward and rapidly penetrate the three layers of the oocyte, moving through the cumulus oophorus, corona radiate, and zona pellucida, respectively. Once inside the perivitelline space, the cortical reaction is induced, triggering the completion of meiosis II in the oocyte. Next, the spermatozoon attaches to the vitelline membrane at the postnuclear cap area and fuses with the oocyte membrane. Consequently, its tail breaks off at the midpiece, detaching from the head, and is followed by axoneme and head decondensation to free the male chromatids. Epididymal maturation, capacitation, and the acrosome reaction induce cellular and chromatin modifications in germ cells for their transformation into fully functional spermatozoa (Fig. 5.5).

Spermatogenic Efficiency

In humans, it takes a spermatogonium approximately 64 days to differentiate into four mature spermatids and into mature spermatozoa [41]. The daily production rate of spermatozoa is 3–4 million per gram of testicular tissue [42], which is meager in comparison to that of laboratory animals. More than 75 % of the developed sperm cells perish due to apoptosis or degeneration, and more than 12.5 % of the remaining cells are abnormal. In the end, the spermatogenetic potential for reproduction amounts to approximately 12 % [13]. Daily sperm production gradually decreases with advancing age. This reduction could be attributed to the loss of Sertoli cells, increase in germ cell degeneration during prophase of meiosis, loss of primary spermatocytes, and the loss of Leydig cells, non-Leydig interstitial cells, and myoid cells [30].

Initial information regarding the success of spermatogenesis is obtained by evaluating ejaculate under light

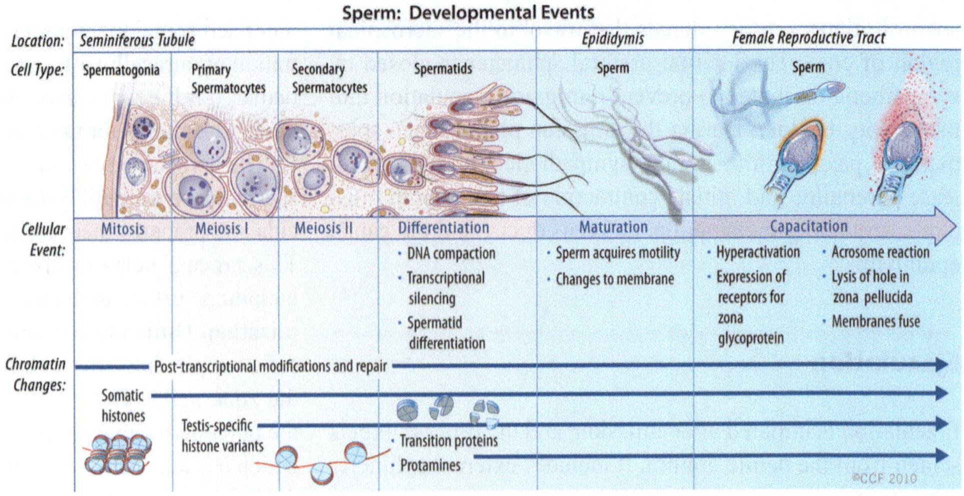

Fig. 5.5 Sperm developmental events. Changes that occur during the development of a germ cell into a spermatozoon leading to its release and subsequent maturation and storage in the epididymis, prior to its journey into the female reproductive tract. (Reprinted with permission, Cleveland Clinic Center for Medical Art & Photography © 2010–2013. All rights reserved.)

microscopy to assess the number, shape, and motility patterns of spermatozoa and to assess other cellular components present in the ejaculate [10].

Immune Status

Despite their biological necessity, spermatozoa are not recognized by the immune system. While immune function is established shortly after birth, surface markers found in late pachytene spermatocytes, spermatids, and spermatozoa develop during puberty. The spermatozoa are protected, however, by the blood–testis barrier, a microenvironment in the seminiferous epithelium that renders them free from immunological attack [43]. Despite the barrier, an immune monitoring system still exists in both the testes and epididymis that defends against autoimmune disease [44].

Disturbances to Spermatogenesis

Several factors can potentially disturb gamete proliferation or differentiation and the intra- or extratesticular mechanisms that regulate spermatogenesis. These include exposure to physical agents such as heat or chemical substances, poor nutrition, obesity, nicotine use, alcohol consumption, ingestion of therapeutic and recreational drugs, bacterial infections, hormonal imbalances, varicocele, cryptorchidism, testicular cancer and radiation [45, 46]. Environmental toxicants such as pesticides, phthlates, polychlorinated biphenyls (PCBs) and endocrine disrupting chemicals (EDCs) can also negatively impact the spermatogenic process [45, 47, 48].

Semen Parameters and Reference Range

A routine semen analysis is the "gold standard" for the initial investigation of male fertility. The following factors are assessed in the seminal ejaculate: physical characteristics (e.g., color, volume, pH, odor, viscosity, and liquefaction time), sperm concentration, motility, progression, viability, and morphology and leukocyte count. Semen parameters such as sperm concentration, motility, and morphology can act as markers of male fertility and may reflect testicular causes of infertility. However, semen analysis must be performed on two or three separate occasions (owing to its large individual biological variability) before any conclusion can be made [49]. The World Health Organization (WHO) normal cutoff values for semen characteristics are shown in Table 5.4.

Conclusion

Spermatogenesis is a highly organized, complex sequence of differentiation events, both mitotic and meiotic, that yields genetically distinct male gametes for fertilization with the female ovum. In a broader scope, it helps to propagate a species and contributes to genetic diversity. In human males, spermatogenesis begins at puberty and persists throughout life. Sperm production is a continuous process that occurs in the seminiferous tubules within the blood–testis barrier of the testis—an immune privileged site. Spermatogenesis involves the transformation of spermatogonial germ cells into spermatids via proliferation and cellular remodeling. The process is regulated by various intrinsic and extrinsic factors. Spermiogenesis converts the spermatids to motile spermatozoa, which are highly specialized haploid cells. Spermatozoa are released along the seminiferous tubules into the epididymis where post-testicular maturation and storage take place.

Table 5.4 Reference values for semen characteristics according to the WHO, 4th (1999) and 5th (2010) edition

Parameter	WHO 1999 (4th edition) [33]	WHO 2010 (5th edition)[33] (Lower reference limits obtained from lower 5th centile values)
Volume (mL)	≥2	1.5
Sperm concentration (10^6 per mL)	≥20	15
Total sperm count (10^6)	≥40	39
Total motility (% motile)	≥50	40
Progressive motility[a](%)	≥25 % (grade a)	32 (grade a+b)
Vitality (% alive)	≥75	58
Morphology (% normal forms)	14	4
Peroxidase-positive leukocytes (10^6 per mL)	<1.0	<1.0

[a] Grade a=rapid progressive motility (>25 µm/s), grade b, slow/sluggish progressive motility (5–25 µm/s); normal, 50 % motility (grade a+b) or 25 % progressive motility (grade a) within 60 min of ejaculation

Before fertilization can occur, spermatozoa must undergo further biochemical changes via capacitation and the acrosome reaction, both of which occur after ejaculation. The entire sperm production process can be inhibited by numerous factors, such as poor nutrition, hormonal imbalances, and therapeutic drug side effects.

References

1. Agger P. Scrotal and testicular temperature: its relation to sperm count before and after operation for varicocele. Fertil Steril. 1971;22(5):286–97.
2. Candas V, Becmeur F, Bothorel B, Hoeft A. Qualitative assessment of thermal and evaporative adjustments of human scrotal skin in response to heat stress. Int J Androl. 1993;16(2):137–42.
3. Middendorff R, Muller D, Mewe M, Mukhopadhyay AK, Holstein AF, Davidoff MS. The tunica albuginea of the human testis is characterized by complex contraction and relaxation activities regulated by cyclic GMP. J Clin Endocrinol Metab. 2002;87(7):3486–99.
4. Roosen-Runge EC, Holstein AF. The human rete testis. Cell Tissue Res. 1978;189(3):409–33.
5. Holstein AF, Schafer E. A further type of transient cytoplasmic organelle in human spermatids. Cell Tissue Res. 1978;192(2):359–61.
6. Davidoff MS, Breucker H, Holstein AF, Seidl K. Cellular architecture of the lamina propria of human seminiferous tubules. Cell Tissue Res. 1990;262(2):253–61.
7. Holstein AF, Maekawa M, Nagano T, Davidoff MS. Myofibroblasts in the lamina propria of human semi-niferous tubules are dynamic structures of heterogeneous phenotype. Arch Histol Cytol. 1996;59(2):109–25.
8. Holstein AF, Schulze W, Davidoff M. Understanding spermatogenesis is a prerequisite for treatment. Reprod Biol Endocrinol. 2003;1:107.
9. Wang H, Xiong W, Chen Y, Ma Q, Ma J, Ge Y, et al. Evaluation on the phagocytosis of apoptotic spermatogenic cells by Sertoli cells in vitro through detecting lipid droplet formation by Oil Red O staining. Reproduction. 2006;132(3):485–92.
10. Holstein AF. Spermatogenese beim Menschen: Grundlagenforschung und Klinik. Ann Anat. 1999;181:427–36.
11. Cheng CY, Mruk DD. A local autocrine axis in the testes that regulates spermatogenesis. Nat Rev Endocrinol. 2010;6(7):380–95.
12. DeKretser DM, Kerr JB. The cytology of the testis. In: Knobill E, Neil JD, Editors. The physiology of reproduction. New York: Raven; 1994. p. 1177–290.
13. Sharpe RM. Regulation of spermatogenesis. In: Knobill E, Neil JD, Editors. The physiology of reproduction. New York: Raven; 1994. p. 1363–434.
14. Jegou B. The Sertoli cell. Baillieres Clin Endocrinol Metab. 1992;6(2):273–311.
15. Clermont Y. Kinetics of spermatogenesis in mammals: seminiferous epithelium cycle and spermatogonial renewal. Physiol Rev. 1972;52(1):198–236.
16. Missell LM, Holochwost D, Boban D, Santi N, Shefi S, Hellerstein MK, Turek PJ. A stable isotop-mass spectrometric method for measuring human spermatogenesis kinetics in vivo. J Urol. 2006;175:242–6.
17. Culty M. Gonocytes, the forgotten cells of the germ cell lineage. Birth Defects Res C Embryo Today. 2009;87(1):1–26
18. Dym M, Fawcett DW. Further observations on the numbers of spermatogonia, spermatocytes, and spermatids connected by intercellular bridges in the mammalian testis. Biol Reprod. 1971;4(2):195–215.
19. Holstein AF, Roosen-Runge EC, Schirren C. Illustrated pathology of human spermatogenesis. Berlin: Grosse; 1988.
20. Izaurralde E, Kas E, Laemmli UK. Highly preferential nucleation of histone H1 assembly on scaffold-associated regions. J Mol Biol. 1989;210(3):573–85.
21. Adachi Y, Kas E, Laemmli UK. Preferential, cooperative binding of DNA topoisomerase II to scaffold-associated regions. EMBO J. 1989;8(13):3997–4006.
22. Giroux CN. Meiosis: components and process in nuclear differentiation. Dev Genet. 1992;13(6):387–91.
23. Auger J, Schoevaert D, Negulesco I, Dadoune JP. The nuclear status of human sperm cells by TEM image cytometry: nuclear shape and chromatin texture in semen samples from fertile and infertile men. J Androl. 1993;14(6):456–63.
24. Miller D, Brinkworth M, Iles D. Paternal DNA packaging in spermatozoa: more than the sum of its parts? DNA, histones, protamines and epigenetics. Reproduction. 2010;139(2):287–301.
25. Braun RE. Packaging paternal chromosomes with protamine. Nat Genet. 2001;28(1):10–2.
26. Balhorn R. The protamine family of sperm nuclear proteins. Genome Biol. 2007;8(9):227.
27. Bedford JM, Calvin H, Cooper GW. The maturation of spermatozoa in the human epididymis. J Reprod Fertil Suppl. 1973;18:199–213.
28. Russell LD, Griswold MD. The Sertoli cells. Clearwater: Cache Press; 1993.
29. Breucker H, Schafer E, Holstein AF. Morphogenesis and fate of the residual body in human spermiogenesis. Cell Tissue Res. 1985;240(2):303–9.
30. Sharma R, Agarwal A. Spermatogenesis: An Overview. In: Zini A, Agarwal A, Editors. Sperm chromatin: biological and clinical applications in male. New York: Springer; 2011. p. 19–44.

31. WHO. WHO laboratory manual for the examination of human semen and sperm-cervical mucus interaction. 5. ed. Cambridge: Cambridge University Press; 2010.
32. Katz DF, Overstreet JW, Samuels SJ, Niswander PW, Bloom TD, Lewis EL. Morphometric analysis of spermatozoa in the assessment of human male fertility. J Androl. 1986;7(4):203–10.
33. WHO. WHO laboratory manual for the examination of human semen and sperm-cervical mucus interaction. 4. ed. Cambridge: Cambridge University Press; 1999.
34. Hafez ES. The human semen and fertility regulation in the male. International Conference in Andrology. J Reprod Med. 1976;16(2):91–6.
35. Menkveld R, Stander FS, Kotze TJ, Kruger TF, van Zyl JA. The evaluation of morphological characteristics of human spermatozoa according to stricter criteria. Hum Reprod. 1990;5(5):586–92.
36. Kruger TF, Menkveld R, Stander FS, Lombard CJ, Van der Merwe JP, van Zyl JA, et al. Sperm morphologic features as a prognostic factor in in vitro fertilization. Fertil Steril. 1986;46(6):1118–23.
37. Langlais J, Roberts KD. A molecular membrane model of sperm capacitation and the acrosome reaction of mammalian spermatozoa. Gamete Res. 1985;12(2):183–224.
38. Osheroff JE, Visconti PE, Valenzuela JP, Travis AJ, Alvarez J, Kopf GS. Regulation of human sperm capacitation by a cholesterol efflux-stimulated signal transduction pathway leading to protein kinase A-mediated up-regulation of protein tyrosine phosphorylation. Mol Hum Reprod. 1999;5(11):1017–26.
39. Song X, Li F, Cao G, Zhang J, Han Y. Distribution of alpha-D-mannose residues on zona pellucida and their role(s) in fertilization in pigs. Sci China C Life Sci. 2007;50(2):170–7.
40. Benoff S, Hurley I, Cooper GW, Mandel FS, Hershlag A, Scholl GM, et al. Fertilization potential in vitro is correlated with head-specific mannose-ligand receptor expression, acrosome status and membrane cholesterol content. Hum Reprod. 1993;8(12):2155–66.
41. Heller CH, Clermont Y. Kinetics of the germinal epithelium in man. Recent Prog Horm Res. 1964;20:545–75.
42. Schulze W, Rehder U. Organization and morphogenesis of the human seminiferous epithelium. Cell Tissue Res. 1984;237(3):395–407.
43. Filippini A, Riccioli A, Padula F, Lauretti P, D'Alessio A, De Cesaris P, et al. Control and impairment of immune privilege in the testis and in semen. Hum Reprod Update. 2001;7(5):444–9.
44. Mahi-Brown CA, Yule TD, Tung KS. Evidence for active immunological regulation in prevention of testicular autoimmune disease independent of the blood-testis barrier. Am J Reprod Immunol Microbiol. 1988;16(4):165–70.
45. Sharpe RM. Environmental/lifestyle effects on spermatogenesis. Philos Trans R Soc Lond B Biol Sci. 2010;365(1546):1697–712.
46. Magelssen H, Brydoy M, Fossa SD. The effects of cancer and cancer treatments on male reproductive function. Nat Clin Pract Urol. 2006;3(6):312–22.
47. Yeung BH, Wan HT, Law AY, Wong CK. Endocrine disrupting chemicals: multiple effects on testicular signaling and spermatogenesis. Spermatogenesis. 2011;1(3):231–9.
48. Mathur PP, D'Cruz SC. The effect of environmental contaminants on testicular function. Asian J Androl. 2011;13(4):585–91.
49. Esteves SC, Zini A, Aziz N, Alvarez JG, Sabanegh ES, Jr., Agarwal A. Critical appraisal of World Health Organization's new reference values for human semen characteristics and effect on diagnosis and treatment of subfertile men. Urology. 2012;79(1):16–22.

Idiopathic Infertility: Survival and Function of Sperm in the Female Reproductive Tract

6

Michelle van der Linde and Stefan S. du Plessis

Introduction

Spermatozoa are highly specialized cells with very unique characteristics and an equally unique purpose. Being the smallest cell in the human body, they have arguably the single biggest responsibility—successfully fertilizing the oocyte. To accomplish this, the sperm must be able to remain viable outside of the male reproductive tract for a certain amount of time, while producing sufficient energy to sustain their metabolic processes, final maturational steps, and motility.

Spermatogenesis occurs in the male reproductive tract over a ± 74 day [1] period through both mitotic and meiotic cell division, followed by dynamic maturation processes [2]. Spermatozoa are deposited in the female reproductive tract during sexual intercourse, after which they have to function independently and with limited resources to ultimately accomplish successful fertilization. As human spermatozoa face tremendous obstacles during their lifespan, spermatogenesis is geared toward producing cells that are specifically designed to cope with and overcome these challenges. Some of the complications that a sperm may encounter in the female reproductive tract include a hostile environment in terms of acidity and female immune cells, factors that thwart progressive movement such as gravity and high viscosity of female secretions, as well as physical barriers that may prevent their advancement entirely. Simultaneously, these challenges faced by the spermatozoa most probably act as a natural selection process, allowing only the most physiologically superior spermatozoa to reach the site of fertilization.

This chapter will discuss the many challenges that human spermatozoa face in the female reproductive tract as they make their way toward the oocyte, as well as the functions they have to fulfill and the various means by which they are adapted to survive these hostile circumstances.

M. van der Linde (✉) · S. S. du Plessis
Division of Medical Physiology, Department of Biomedical Sciences, Stellenbosch University, Parow, Western Cape, South Africa
e-mail: 15076202@sun.ac.za

Spermatogenesis and Seminal Plasma

In order to grasp the ability of the spermatozoa to survive the various challenges faced in the female reproductive tract, it is important to understand the origin, composition, and purpose of spermatozoa and seminal plasma (see Table 6.1).

Following spermatogenesis in the testes, the sperm are stored and they undergo further maturation in the epididymis, where the principle cells secrete glycerophosphocholine, inhibiting both motility and premature capacitation [3]. In this metabolically-suppressed state, spermatozoa can survive in the male reproductive tract for many weeks.

A normal, mature spermatozoon consists of a head, midpiece, and flagellum. The head, containing a haploid set of DNA material, is covered with a cap-like structure known as the acrosome. The midpiece houses the mitochondria, which provide ATP via oxidative phosphorylation, and the flagellum is used to propel the spermatozoa and contains glycolytic enzymes for ATP production by glycolysis.

During ejaculation, as the spermatozoa pass through the ejaculatory ducts, the accessory sex glands contribute various secretions that ultimately constitute the bulk of the seminal plasma. The seminal plasma consists of several components intended to sustain and promote survival of the spermatozoa. Key features of semen include its high buffering capacity, maintaining its pH to almost neutral in acidic environments, as well as a substantially high osmolarity in comparison to blood plasma (hypertonic) [4], a feature which is influenced greatly by the concentrations of sugars, ionic salts, and other organic compounds [5] and which has been noted to increase significantly with age [6]. Seminal plasma contains more than 50 different chemical compounds, each of which assists sperm survival and function in the female reproductive tract.

Ejaculation comprises of two phases: during the first phase, the emission stage, the spermatozoa are transported from the epididymis to the urethra via smooth muscle contraction; while during the second phase, the true ejaculatory phase, seminal plasma is moved through the urethra and, along with the sperm, expelled from the body as semen [7].

G. L. Schattman et al. (eds.), *Unexplained Infertility*, DOI 10.1007/978-1-4939-2140-9_6,

Table 6.1 Constituents of seminal plasma and their functions

Gland	Secretion	Function
Principle cells [3] (epididymus)	Glycerophosphocholine	Inhibits motility and premature capacitation
Seminal vesicles [3]	Viscous fluid rich in fructose and glucose, several proteins, including fibrinogen and prostaglandins	Substrates for anaerobic metabolism; fibrinogen initiates postejaculatory coagulation; prostaglandins contribute to make the female environment more hospitable
Prostate [3]	Alkaline secretion containing calcium, albumin, proteolytic enzymes, acid phosphatase, fibrinogenase, profibrinolysine, zinc, citric acid, and lipids	Neutralisation; fibrinogenase for postejaculatory coagulation; profibrinolysine for liquefaction; zinc stabilizes the DNA; citrate contributes to the pH buffering capacity
Bulbourethral glands [3]	Clear fluid	Lubrication for easy expulsion of the semen; neutralization; aids the mobility of spermatozoa by creating less viscous channels
Epididymis [7]	Lymphocytes and macrophages	Reactive oxygen species [55] (ROS) which has beneficial functions at physiological levels
Prostate and seminal vesicles	Granulocytes [7]	

The seminal vesicles are the first to add their secretion to the seminal plasma, producing a viscous fluid rich in nutrients such as fructose (274 mg/100 ml) [8] and glucose, at an average concentration of (102 mg/100 ml) [4], as well as several proteins, including fibrinogen and prostaglandins [3]. The sugars serve as substrates for anaerobic metabolism (fructolysis and glycolysis), which the spermatozoa will utilize as soon as they gain motility. Fibrinogen initiates postejaculatory coagulation of the seminal plasma, while the prostaglandins help to make the female environment more hospitable to the spermatozoa in terms of pH-buffering [3].

The prostate gland contributes an alkaline secretion containing calcium, albumin, proteolytic enzymes, acid phosphatase, fibrinogenase, profibrinolysine, zinc, citric acid, and lipids [3]. Since spermatozoa are extremely susceptible to an acidic environment, the most important function of the prostatic secretion is neutralisation of (i) the vas deference, which is acidic due to metabolic waste such as increased CO_2 and lactic acid produced by the spermatozoa, and (ii) the vagina, which is acidic due to the natural bacteria it contains. The fibrinogenase assists in postejaculatory coagulation, and the profibrinolysine leads to liquefaction [3]. Zinc helps to stabilize the DNA-containing chromatin [9]; citrate contributes to the pH buffering capacity and is also believed to be the major regulator of ionized calcium levels in the seminal plasma [10, 11]. The calcium concentration is a key factor in sperm motility, metabolism, acrosome reaction, and fertilization [12].

Additional cells that may be found in seminal plasma are lymphocytes and macrophages, which originate mainly from the epididymis, as well as granulocytes that are derived from both the prostate and seminal vesicles [13]. Activated granulocytes release reactive oxygen species (ROS), which have beneficial functions at physiological levels, but can become detrimental when elevated, in which case it disrupts the spermatozoa's membranes and compromises DNA integrity [13].

Finally, the bulbourethral glands secrete a clear fluid into the lumen of the urethra, providing lubrication for easy expulsion of the semen [3], as well as buffers to assist in neutralization of the acidic vaginal pH [14]. This mucus furthermore aids the mobility of spermatozoa in both the vagina and cervix as it creates channels that are less viscous through which the spermatozoa can swim.

The World Health Organization describes normal human semen as having a volume of at least 1.5 ml, pH of around 7.2, sperm concentration greater than 15×10^6 spermatozoa/ml, and total motility of at least 40 % with forward progression of 32 % within 60 min of ejaculation [15].

Function of Spermatozoa in the Female Reproductive Tract

Introduction

Despite being motile once inside the female reproductive tract, spermatozoa are not yet capable of fertilizing an oocyte at this stage. Spermatozoa require a species-dependant amount of time to travel from the site of deposition, in the vagina, to the site of fertilization, in the fallopian tubes [16], while simultaneously acquiring fertilizing ability by undergoing a series of complex changes along the way, collectively referred to as capacitation [16].

Capacitation

The process of capacitation has been defined as a "functional maturation of the spermatozoon" [17]. Capacitation involves considerable alterations to the surface of the plasma membrane, with various molecules being removed, rearranged, or revealed. These changes are facilitated by the removal of cholesterol and glycoproteins, resulting in a more fluid plasma membrane with an increased permeability to Ca^{2+}[16]. The subsequent upsurge in Ca^{2+} leads to increased intracellular cAMP levels and, consequently, increased motility [3].

The uterus aids in the steps of capacitation by secreting sterol binding albumin, lipoproteins, and glycosidases such as heparin [18]. Sterol binding albumin promotes cholesterol efflux from the sperm plasma membrane [19], while heparin [20] and lipoproteins [21] have been shown to accelerate the initiation of both capacitation and the acrosome reaction in vitro. Extracellular Ca^{2+} plays an important role as a signalling molecule during capacitation and the acrosome reaction, and is a prerequisite for both processes [16]. The acrosomal area also undergoes changes during capacitation in preparation for a possible acrosome reaction closer to fertilization.

As a result of the increased intracellular Ca^{2+} levels mentioned before, and by the time the fallopian tubes are reached, the spermatozoa become hyperactivated, indicating the successful completion of the capacitation process.

Hyperactivation

Hyperactivation is a motility pattern usually occurring in vivo in the fallopian tubes [22], and is characterized by increased amplitude and asymmetrical flagellar beating [23] together with increased amplitude of lateral head displacement (ALH) [24]. Hyperactivation is triggered by a rise in intracellular flagellar Ca^{2+} and requires an increase in both pH and ATP production [23]. Since, hyperactivation is normally only displayed at the site of fertilization, it may therefore be modulated by chemotactic signals to direct and turn spermatozoa toward the oocyte [23], while the increased sideways displacement of the head increases the spermatozoon's chances of encountering the egg [22]. Furthermore, hyperactivation enhances the ability of the spermatozoa to traverse the viscous fluids in the fallopian tubes, affording increased flexibility and facilitating the penetration of the spermatozoon through the cumulus complex and zona pellucida [22].

Acrosome Reaction

The oocyte is surrounded by various external structures; the outermost is the cumulus oophorus, a gel-like hyaluronic acid that the spermatozoa encounters initially and needs to penetrate first. Inside of the cumulus is the zona pellucida, to which sperm must bind. This acts as the final mechanical barrier for spermatozoa before fertilization. In order for the spermatozoa to fuse with the oolemma, it must bind to the zona pellucida, reorientate, and finally, penetrate the oocyte [25]. The zona pellucida consists predominantly of glycoproteins, among which ZP1, ZP2, ZP3, and ZP4 [26] are highly species-specific and complimentary to glycoproteins on the surface of the head of the spermatozoa. The zona glycoproteins ZP1, ZP3, and ZP4 are primarily responsible for the tight binding of capacitated, acrosome-intact spermatozoa and initiating a cascade of cellular interactions that culminate in fertilization. In vivo, the acrosome reaction is initiated when the spermatozoon comes into contact with or in very close proximity to the oocyte's cumulus layer. The purpose of the acrosome reaction is the release of the enzymes (hyaluronidase and acrosin [27]) contained inside the acrosomal cap, which is responsible for digestion of the zona pellucida and oolemma in order to allow the spermatozoon to penetrate the oocyte. The enzymes that are released digest the cumulus cells surrounding the oocyte, exposing the oocyte to the acrosin attached to the inner membrane of the sperm. Acrosin digests the zona pellucida and membrane of the oocyte. Progesterone, secreted by the cumulus cells, is an important cofactor for the initiation of this process [27], as is the increase in calcium permeability due to successful capacitation [28].

Upon completion of the acrosome reaction, the inner membrane of the spermatozoa subsequently fuses with the oolemma and the contents of the sperm head enter the oocyte during a process termed penetration [29].

Fertilization

Upon penetration, the oocyte becomes activated. It completes its secondary meiotic division and the two haploid nuclei—paternal and maternal—fuse to form a diploid zygote. In order to prevent polyspermy and minimize the possibility of producing a triploid zygote, several changes to the oocytes' membranes render them impenetrable shortly after the first sperm enters the egg through a process called the zona reaction [29].

Metabolism

Being independent living cells, spermatozoa must sustain themselves and support their functions and motility for an extended period of time under varying conditions [30], and as they are not directly attached to the female body or linked to the bloodstream, they must survive on very limited resources. Spermatozoa are maintained at a low energy consumption state during epididymal storage, conserving energy and favoring long-term cell survival [3]. Despite being very small cells, spermatozoa require a substantial amount of energy in the form of ATP in order to support cellular processes and functions such as protein phosphorylation and motility [30]. The preferred metabolic pathway for ATP production varies greatly between species.

In humans, immature spermatids seem to favor the substrates lactate and pyruvate, indicating that oxidative phosphorylation is the main energy source during early spermatogenesis. However, as spermatozoa undergo maturation in the epididymis, they expand their energy production ability to furthermore utilize glycolysis as an alternative source [30].

While the acrosome reaction utilizes lactate and pyruvate for ATP production by oxidative phosphorylation, gamete fusion requires glucose to produce NADPH by the pentose pathway. Normal sperm motility appears to be sustained by relatively low ATP levels, but increased ATP levels are required for tyrosine phosphorylation linked to hyperactivation. Thus, each individual process and event requires a different substrate and metabolic pathway [30], although it is important to note that utilization of these two metabolic pathways is not mutually exclusive.

Glycolysis appears to be indispensable to the spermatozoa of all species and has been shown to compensate for a lack of oxidative phosphorylation, thereby leading to the recovery of most sperm functions. Spermatogenic glycolytic enzymes may be more flexible in the use of substrates, and able to adapt to unexpected conditions in the female reproductive tract [30].

Ultimately, it appears that the metabolic pathway utilized in vivo is greatly influenced by the conditions of the female reproductive tract [31], which, in turn, may be influenced by a variety of factors, not the least of which is the menstrual cycle.

Motility/Swimming Patterns

After sperm have been in the epididymis for 18–24 h, they develop the capability of motility, even though several inhibitory proteins in the epididymal fluid still prevent final motility until after ejaculation. Smooth muscle contractions of the female reproductive tract, ciliary beats, fluid currents, and flagellar activity of sperm are primary mechanisms of sperm movement and transport [32]. Sperm can live for many weeks in the suppressed state in the male reproductive tracts, but the life expectancy of ejaculated sperm in the female genital tract is only about 5 days [3].

Normal motile, fertile spermatozoa are capable of flagellated movement at velocities of up to104 mm/min. The motility of sperm is significantly enhanced in a neutral and slightly alkaline medium, as it exists in the ejaculated seminal plasma, but it is greatly suppressed in even a slightly acidic medium. The activity of spermatozoa accelerates markedly with increased temperature, but so does the rate of metabolism, leading to a reduction in the lifespan of the spermatozoa.

Activated motility as seen in freshly ejaculated spermatozoa refers to the low amplitude symmetric waves propagating along the length of the flagellum and resulting in linear propulsion of the sperm cell [33]. Hyperactivated motility, as seen at the site of fertilization occurs when the flagellar movement becomes asymmetrical with higher amplitude, resulting in highly curved trajectories [34].

Survival of Spermatozoa in the Female Reproductive Tract

Introduction

The passage of sperm through the female reproductive tract is regulated to maximize the chance of fertilization and ensure that morphologically and functionally normal spermatozoa will be the ones to succeed. A single spermatozoon is about 60 μm long, and needs to swim a distance of approximately 20 cm to reach the oocyte. Millions of spermatozoa are produced by the male as a first attempt to increase the chance of successful fertilization, as many spermatozoa die along the way. Spermatozoa must survive the journey independently and without the benefit of reparative mechanisms available as is the case with somatic cells [35], while being subjected to various physical and chemical stressors (refer to Fig. 6.1). In humans, it has been observed that sperm are still viable and fertile in the female up to 5 days after intercourse.

The remainder of this chapter will be dedicated to the obstacles spermatozoa face in the female reproductive tract, and, more importantly, the mechanisms that exist to aid in the survival of the spermatozoa in this hostile environment.

Vagina

During intercourse, semen deposition is usually confined to the anterior vaginal region, near the cervical os. Spermatozoa deposited in the vagina face two major complications: gravity and a sudden acidic environment. Upon ejaculation, the semen immediately coagulates in the vagina and liquefies after 30–60 min. This initial clotting of the semen inside the vagina not only prevents sperm loss and leaking due to gravity, but it furthermore provides the spermatozoa with a pH buffered and substrate rich milieu in the interim. During the sequential liquefaction process mucus molecules present in the seminal plasma arrange themselves to form channels that help guide the motile spermatozoa out of the plasma coagulum and toward the opening of the cervix. This process serves as the first selection step toward a viable sperm fraction, as immature/immotile sperm will not be able to migrate efficiently from the seminal plasma [35].

Being exposed to the external environment, the vagina is susceptible to infections, and is therefore well equipped with antimicrobial defenses, which, in addition to the acidic pH,

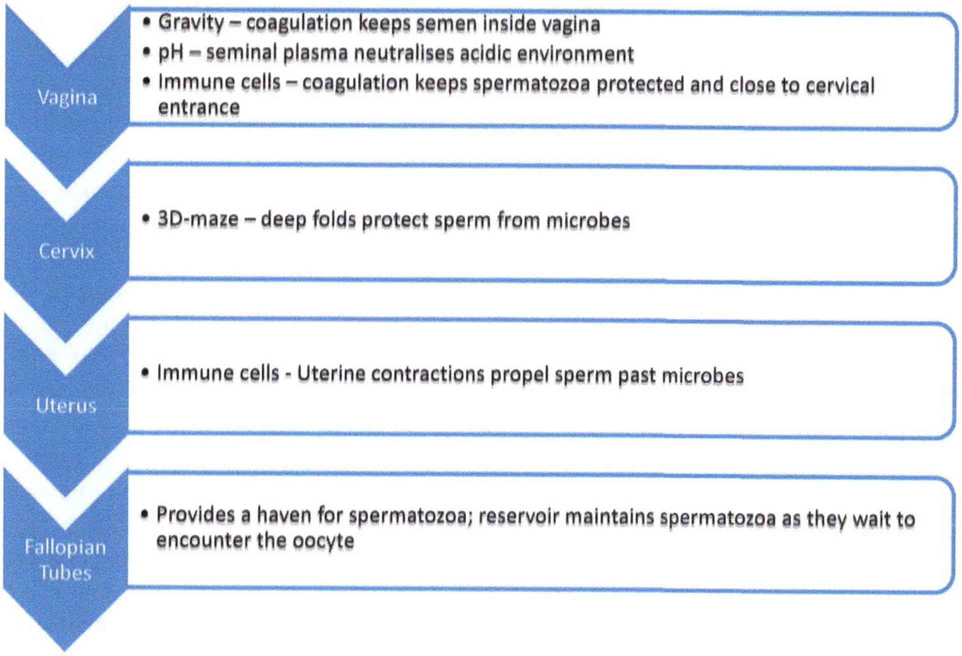

Fig. 6.1 Anatomical pathway, challenges and surviving mechanisms of spermatozoa in the female reproductive tract

includes high incidence of immune cells [35]. However, due to the prostaglandins' immune-suppressing effects and pH buffering of the seminal plasma, spermatozoa can survive in the vagina for 24–48 h before they are removed by the female immune cells [3].

Cervix

The entrance to the cervix is practically impermeable throughout most of the menstrual cycle due to the compact microarchitecture of the cervical mucus, effectively acting as a plug. Under the influence of the sex steroidal hormones around the time of ovulation, the mucus becomes thin and hydrated, often exceeding 96 % water, while estrogen causes the cervical canal to widen, allowing sperm-penetration [35]. In addition to being a three-dimensional maze, the cervix is also filled with cervical mucus, which is thick and very viscous. Once in the cervix, the cervical mucus presents a great obstacle to abnormal or immature spermatozoa that are not sufficiently motile or present poor hydrodynamic profiles, while normal, vigorously motile spermatozoa have less trouble traversing through the mucus [35].

It has been observed that, during the follicular phases of the menstrual cycle, the composition of the mucus deep in the channels is different and less dense than that in the central area of the cervical canal. Female immune cells are also more concentrated in the central portions of the canal. This indicates that the cervix may support the movement of normal motile spermatozoa in the deeper regions of the canal, while restraining passage of microbes and spermatozoa with abnormal morphology or motility. In addition to this protection, the cervix may furthermore aid in guiding the spermatozoa toward the uterus through the microarchitecture of the cervical mucus. Mucins are the primary glycoproteins comprising the cervical mucus, and are long, flexible molecules that arrange themselves to become aligned, allowing spermatozoa to orient themselves along these molecules. Human spermatozoa have been observed to swim in a more linear path in cervical mucus when compared to suspension in seminal plasma or culture medium [35]. Sperm recovered from cervical mucus 24 h after intercourse are greatly outnumbered by leukocytes, indicating that the cervix is not a suitable storage site for spermatozoa [36].

The prostaglandins, secreted by the seminal vesicles, have a three-fold function [3]: firstly, to react with the cervical mucus to make it more hospitable to the sperm; secondly, they are involved in suppressing the female's immune response against the seminal proteins and spermatozoa; and thirdly, they stimulate reversed peristalsis in the uterus and fallopian tubes to promote the movement of spermatozoa to the ovum.

Uterus

The human uterine cavity is only a few centimeters in length, and could be traversed in a few minutes by mature spermatozoa with normal motility abilities. In the uterus, spermatozoa are propelled mainly by the rhythmic contractions of the uterus. These contractions may be inspired by stimulatory secretions from the seminal plasma, as well as by hormonal changes in the female. The menstrual cycle may affect the transport of spermatozoa through the uterus, as ultrasonography of the uterus has revealed cranially directed waves of uterine smooth muscle contractions that increase in intensity during the late follicular phase [36], when spermatozoa can be rapidly transported from the cervix into the uterus and even into the tubal isthmus. This rapid transport of the spermatozoa through the uterus can improve survival of spermatozoa by propelling them past the immunological defense system of the female, instead of allowing the spermatozoa to accumulate, along with leucocytes and macrophages, in the restricted space of the uterine cavity [35]. The contractile activity of uterine muscle may further serve to draw watery midcycle cervical mucus into the uterus along with the spermatozoa, providing the spermatozoa with an aqueous medium to swim [35].

Another difficult point is the transition from the uterus to the fallopian tubes. This opening is fairly narrow and opens only periodically, allowing merely limited numbers of spermatozoa to pass through, half of which will enter the oviduct where an oocyte has not been released. It has been observed that several surface proteins are required for spermatozoa to pass through the uterotubal junction, and that spermatozoa lacking these proteins are not only unable to cross the junction, but are also incapable of fertilizing the oocyte [35]. Therefore, normal morphology and motility do not seem to be sufficient for sperm to pass through the junction, and a stringent selection process based on extended criteria is made to ensure that the spermatozoa that ultimately manage to make it through display virtually no abnormalities [37].

Fallopian Tubes

Yanagimachi and Chang (1963) were the first to describe a reservoir of sperm in the tubal isthmus of hamsters [38]. Since then, formation of sperm reservoirs has been observed in many species. Unlike the uterus, cervix, and vagina, the fallopian tubes do not respond to the presence of the spermatozoa with an influx of leukocytes, and therefore the fallopian tubes provide some refuge for the spermatozoa that finally reach them. In animals, the storage reservoir maintains the viability and fertilizing capacity of spermatozoa until ovulation. The tubal reservoir is created when spermatozoa bind to the epithelial lining of the first segments of the tube, stabilizing the sperm membranes and simultaneously serving to delay capacitation and prevent polyspermic fertilization by only allowing a few spermatozoa to reach the oocyte in the ampulla at a time.

In vitro studies have shown that incubation of human spermatozoa with human epithelial cells prolong the viability of spermatozoa, but no in vivo models have been able to prove the existence of these reservoirs in humans. However, this does not necessarily mean that the reservoirs do not exist, as it might indicate that, in humans, the binding of the spermatozoa to the epithelium does not have to be as quick or as tight as is the case in other species. Even though a visibly distinct sperm reservoir has not been observed in the fallopian tubes of humans, a functional reservoir could be present that leads to detention of the spermatozoa in the tubal isthmus, slowing their progress toward the ampulla. Mucus in the lumen of the tube may also contribute to slowing the progress, together with the mucosal folds that increase in both height and complexity toward the ovary, delaying the advancement of the spermatozoa into and through the ampulla. The slowing of the advancement of spermatozoa could serve the function of a reservoir that is prolonging the availability of viable sperm in the fallopian tube and avoiding polyspermic fertilization. Nevertheless, since pregnancies can result from intercourse as early as 5 days prior to ovulation, human spermatozoa must be stored somewhere in the female tract. It has been observed that spermatozoa can survive and remain fertile in the fallopian tubes for up to 85 h [39]. Spermatozoa that reach the fallopian tubes have been reported to have a higher amount of morphologically normal cells than is seen lower in the female reproductive tract [40], supporting the theory that the natural barriers sperm encounter in the female serve to select for the most viable spermatozoa capable of successfully fertilizing the oocyte.

However, when in vitro fertilization (IVF) techniques are performed, much of these barriers are bypassed and spermatozoa are often selected based on normal morphology, vitality and/or superior motility, even though none of these are reflective of the inherent DNA integrity of the spermatozoa. In addition, many of the currently employed sperm preparation techniques for IVF can induce even further damage to the spermatozoa through increased oxidative stress levels and concurrent DNA damage [41]. The injection of superficially normal spermatozoa with damaged chromatin during intracytoplasmic sperm injection (ICSI) can be related to the high spontaneous abortion rates that are associated with ICSI. In vitro studies have found that, in addition to surviving longer, spermatozoa that adhere to the fallopian epithelium are of higher quality in terms of motility, morphology, and DNA integrity than those who do not [42]. This implies that fallopian tube epithelium can be utilized in vitro as a method to isolate both physiologically and biochemically high-quality spermatozoa for clinical fertilization procedures. Furthermore, as spermatozoa from neat, uncentrifuged preparations have been seen to bind to fallopian epithelial cell cultures (Ellington, unpublished observations), the need for centrifugation is negated, and the DNA integrity of the spermatozoa is preserved.

Female Response to Spermatozoa

Introduction

The female body is constantly changing as it prepares for potential conception. In the event of successful fertilization, the body must adapt in order to support the subsequent pregnancy, and in the absence of fertilization, the body must return to its former state and start preparing for the release of a new oocyte. This cycle is termed the menstrual cycle, and it necessitates physical, hormonal, and thermogenic alterations in the female body (see Table 6.2). Physical changes include the development and shedding of the endometrium, which is associated with hormonal changes such as a surge in the oestrogen and pituitary gonadotropins LH and FSH around ovulation and a progesterone surge in the mid-luteal phase [43]. These hormonal fluctuations bring about changes in the pH, and there is an elevation in the basal body temperature for the duration of the luteal phase. These changes significantly impact the survival of the spermatozoa in the female reproductive tract, seemingly promoting the survival and even transport of the spermatozoa closer to ovulation, and preventing their advancement when the oocyte is not ready to be released.

Since spermatozoa are allogenic to the female, they may encounter immune cells that are meant to fight off infectious diseases in many regions of the female body [35]. Spermatozoa are phagositosed by lymphocytes and macrophages, which greatly diminish their numbers in the vagina, cervix, and uterus, where their presence often results in an influx of the immunological cells to these regions.

Therefore, it is important to note that the normal functioning of the female body, such as the menstrual cycle and immune system, also has an effect on the survival of the spermatozoa.

Inflammation and Antibodies

Spermatozoa remaining in the vagina are destroyed mostly by the acidic pH, although some are also phagositosed by leukocytes [35]. Spermatozoa that stay behind in the cervix or uterus are cleared mainly by leukocytes, the infiltration of which is often induced by coitus. In animals, these leukocytes have been shown to be primarily neutrophils [44].

In rare cases spermatozoa may be presented to the defense system of the female and a defense reaction is set in motion as the immune system of the female forms antibodies against her partner's spermatozoa [37]. Although the precise etiology of sperm immunity in women is unknown, there are a few proposed mechanisms. The most probable of these is the theory that if a woman expresses antibodies to her male partner's spermatozoa, it is very likely that he already has sperm autoantibodies in his semen [45], and that it was exchanged during intercourse where they were both exposed to the same microbes. Another theory is that, since the uterine cervix is a highly efficient mucosal immune site, many IgA-positive plasma cells are located in the epithelial layers. Secretory IgA antibodies can immobilize spermatozoa [46] through cross-linkage to the cervical mucus, essentially preventing their progress to the upper regions of the female reproductive tract [47]. Therefore, high levels of these antibodies can effectively prevent fertilization. Witkins et al. (1988) reported that in about 30 % of their cases, women seemed to react to their partner's sperm antigens, rather than to sperm-specific antigens [48] while Blum et al. (1989) observed significant similarities between Chlamydia antibodies and sperm antibodies in young women [49]. It is also possible that, in addition to antibodies for sperm membrane antigens, antibodies can also be formed for some internal sperm components [50]. Finally, another study suggested that antibody-coated spermatozoa may stimulate interferon-gamma (IFN-γ) synthesis by female lymphocytes, which ultimately leads to T-cell recruitment and subsequent initiation of sperm antibody production by B-lymphocytes [51].

Table 6.2 The menstruation cycle [43, 56]

Cycle phase	Days	Events	Hormones	Temperature	pH	Affect	Other
Early follicular	1–4	Menstrual phase; shedding of endometrium	Decline in oestrogen and progesterone	Stable	Increase (alkaline)		Abdominal pain Breast tenderness
Late follicular	5–13	Follicle maturation, endometrium regrows	LH and FSH gradually increases	Stable	Decrease (acidic)	Increased sexual interest	
Ovulation	14	Follicle released	LH and FSH peaks	Stable	Decrease (acidic)		Increased appetite
Luteal	15–28	Uterine milk secretion	Increase in estrogen and progesterone	Increased	Decrease (acidic)	Fluctuating mood; irritability tension anxiety depression	Abdominal pain Breast tenderness Headaches Fatigue Increased appetite

Menstrual Cycle

One of the major factors that influence the survival of spermatozoa is the composition of the cervical fluid, the amount and composition of which varies with the menstrual cycle under hormonal influence [52]. Spermatozoa often remain surrounded by cervical mucus for most of their journey toward the oocyte, as cervical mucus also enters the uterus and sometimes the isthmus due to the uterine muscle contractions. The composition of the cervical fluid shortly before ovulation supports spermatozoa by providing an alkaline environment and metabolic substrates such as carbohydrates, and also by creating mucin channels that guide the spermatozoa in the right direction [53]. Spermatozoa can survive in the presence of this favorable cervical fluid for 3–5 days. During and after ovulation the cervical mucus becomes dehydrated, viscous and practically impenetrable, and passage of spermatozoa through the female reproductive tract becomes near impossible.

Chemotaxis and Thermotaxis in Fallopian Tubes

There is an evidence for the existence of two complementary guidance mechanisms at work within the fallopian tube. These mechanisms are geared toward guiding capacitated spermatozoa toward the oocyte. The longer range thermotaxis is based on the relative temperature difference between the cooler tubal isthmus region and the warmer tubal ampulla region, where the spermatozoa swim toward the slightly higher temperature. Once they are in the tubal ampulla and in closer proximity to the oocyte, a second, shorter-range chemotactic mechanism may serve to guide spermatozoa closer to the oocyte. Spermatozoa are equipped with a mechanism for turning toward the oocyte in response to chemotactic factors, as they can alternate between symmetrical flagellar beating and asymmetrical (hyperactivated) flagellar beating. Odorant receptors unique to mammalian spermatozoa have been localized to a spot on the base of the flagellum of human spermatozoa [35]. Spermatozoa that were placed in a gradient of the pleasant-smelling odorant *bourgeonal* in vitro were reported to reorient themselves into the gradient while a simultaneous calcium- and cAMP-mediated signalling cascade was triggered [54]. Identifying the chemotactic odorant present in the oviduct could be useful during IVF treatments.

Conclusion

In conclusion, to enable fertilization to take place, both the male and the female have adopted mechanisms for protecting spermatozoa on their journey toward the oocyte. This means that, in addition to the inherent female processes that affect sperm function, there are many other obstacles that the spermatozoa encounter in the female reproductive tract, all of which may exist for one reason: to naturally select for physiologically superior spermatozoa to reach the site of fertilization, thereby increasing the chance of successful conception.

References

1. Johnson L. Spermatogenesis and aging in the human. J Androl. 1986;7(6):331–51.
2. Cobb M. Heredity before genetics: a history. Nat Rev Genet. 2006;7(12). doi:10.1038/nrg1948.
3. Hall JE. Reproductive and hormonal functions of the male (and function of the pineal gland). In: Textbook of medical physiology. 12th ed. Philadelphia: Saunders Elsevier; 2011. p. 973–986.
4. Owen DH, Katz DF. A review of the physical and chemical properties of human semen and the formulation of a semen simulant. J Androl. 2005;26(4). doi:10.2164/jandrol.04104.
5. Mandal A, Bhattacharyya AK. Differences in osmolality, pH, buffering capacity, superoxide dismutase and maintenance of sperm motility in human ejaculates according to the degree of coagulation. Int J Androl.1987b;11:45–51.
6. Velazquez A, Pedron N, Delgado NM, Rosado A. Osmolality and conductance of normal and abnormal human seminal plasma. Int J Fertil. 1977;22:92–7.
7. Encyclopædia Britannica. Ejaculation. http://www.britannica.com/EBchecked/topic/181568/ejaculation. Accessed 13 Dec 2012.
8. Carpino A, Siciliano L. Unaltered protein pattern/genital tract secretion marker levels in seminal plasma of highly viscous human ejaculates. Arch Androl. 1998;41:31–5.
9. Canale D, Bartelloni M, Negroni A, Meschini P, Izzo PL, Bianchi B, Menchini-Fabris GF. Zinc in human semen. Int J Androl. 1986;9(6). doi:10.1111/j.1365-2605.1986.tb00909.x.
10. Fong JC, Lin CH, Wei YH, Ho LT, Hong CY. Calcium buffering capacity of human seminal plasma: the role of EGTA in stimulating sperm motility. Chin J Physiol. 1986;29:7–12.
11. Magnus O, Abyholm T, Kofstad J, Purvis K. Ionized calcium in human male and female reproductive fluids: relationships to sperm motility. Hum Reprod. 1990;5:94–98.
12. Sorensen MB, Bergdahl IA, Hjollund NHI, Bonde JPE, Stoltenberg M, Ernst E. Zinc, magnesium and calcium in human seminal fluid: relations to other semen parameters and fertility. Mol Hum Reprod. 1999;5:331–7.
13. Wolff H. The biologic significance of white blood cells in semen. Fertil Steril. 1995;63(6). (PubMed PMID:7750580).
14. Sirigu P, Turno F, Usai E, Perra MT. Histochemical study of the human bulbourethral (Cowper's) glands. Andrologia. 1993;25(5). doi:10.1111/j.1439-0272.1993.tb02728.x.
15. World Health Organization. WHO laboratory manual for the examination and processing of human semen, 6th ed. Geneva: World Health Organization; 2010.
16. Fraser LR. Sperm capacitation and the acrosome reaction. Hum. Reprod. 1998;13(suppl 1): 9–19. doi:10.1093/humrep/13.suppl_1.9 (1998).
17. McPartlin LA. Taking a molecular approach to a clinical problem: sperm capacitation as the missing link for successful in vitro fertilization in the horse [Doctoral dissertation]. Cornell University; 2010.
18. Early, R. Male reproductive system. In: Online Learning Package. University of the West of England. http://www.google.co.za/url20early&source=web&cd=1&cad=rja&ved=0CDAQFjAA&url=htt

p%3A%2F%2Fhsc.uwe.ac.uk%2Fnet%2Fstudent%2FData%2FSites%2F1%2FGalleryImages%2Fwelcome%2Fmale%2520repro.docx&ei=F07hUIuPJ8iShgeNn4HABw&usg=AFQjCNGujRRqwIsW6_RCiuFAYNQgruEW7A&bvm=bv.1355534169,d.ZG4. Accessed 13 Dec 2012.

19. Langlais J, Kan FWK, Granger L, Raymond L, Bleau G, Roberts KD. Identification of sterol acceptors that stimulate cholesterol efflux from human spermatozoa during in vitro capacitation. Gamete Res. 2005;20(2). doi:10.1002/mrd.1120200209.
20. Varner DD, Bowen JA, Johnson, L. Effect of heparin on capacitation/acrosome reaction of equine sperm. Syst Biol Reprod Med [Internet]. 1993;31(3):199–207. http://informahealthcare.com/doi/abs/10.3109/01485019308988400. Accessed 13 Dec 2012.
21. Lane ME, Therien I, Moreau R, Manjunath P. Heparin and high-density lipoprotein mediate bovine sperm capacitation by different mechanisms. Biol Reprod. 1999;60(1). doi:10.1095/biolreprod60.1.169.
22. Stauss CR, Votta TJ, Suarez SS. Sperm motility hyperactivation facilitates penetration of the hamster zona pellucida. Biol Reprod. 1995;53(6). doi:10.1095/biolreprod53.6.1280.
23. Suarez SS. Control of hyperactivation in sperm. Hum Reprod Update. 2008;14(6). doi:10.1093/humupd/dmn029.
24. Mazzilli F, Rossi T, Delfino M, Dondero F, Makler A. A new objective method for scoring human sperm hyperactivation based on head axis angle deviation. Int J Androl. 2001;24(4). doi:10.1046/j.1365-2605.2001.00271.x.
25. Baltz JM, Katz DF, Cone RA. Mechanics of sperm-egg interaction at the zona pellucida. Biophys J. 1988;54(4). doi:10.1016/S0006-3495(88)83000-5.
26. Conner SJ, Lefievre L, Hughes DC, Barratt CLR. Cracking the egg: increased complexity in the zona pellucida. Hum. Reprod. 2005;20(5). doi:10.1093/humrep/deh835.
27. Patrat C, Serres C, Jouannet P. The acrosome reaction in human spermatozoa. Biol Cell. 2000;92(3-4). doi:10.1016/S0248-4900(00)01072-8.
28. Brucker C, Lipford GB. The human sperm acrosome reaction: physiology and regulatory mechanisms. an update. Hum Reprod [Internet]. 1994;1(1):51–62. http://humupd.oxfordjournals.org/content/1/1/51.short. Accessed 13 Dec 2012.
29. Kim NH, Funahashi H, Abeydeera LR, Moon SJ, Prather RS, Day BN. Effects of oviductal fluid on sperm penetration and cortical granule exocytosis during fertilization of pig oocytes in vitro. J Rreprod Fertil. 1996;107(1). doi:10.1530/jrf.0.1070079.
30. Miki K, Roldan ERS, Gomendio M. Energy metabolism and sperm function. In: Spermatology. Proceedings of the 10th International Symposium on Spermatology; 2006;17–22; El Escorial, Madrid, Spain. Nottingham University Press; 2007. p. 309–25.
31. Storey BT. Mammalian sperm metabolism: oxygen and sugar, friend and foe. Int J Dev Biol. 2008;52(5):427.
32. Hawk HW. Sperm survival and transport in the female reproductive tract. J Dairy Sci. 1983;66(12). doi:10.3168/jds.S0022-0302(83)82138-9.
33. Curtis P, Lindsay P, Jackson AE, Shaw RW. Adverse effects on sperm movement characteristics in women with minimal and mild endometriosis. Int J Obstet Gynaecol. 1993;100(2). doi:10.1111/j.1471-0528.1993.tb15215.x165-169.
34. Ishijima S, Baba SA, Mohri H, Suarez SS. Quantitative analysis of flagellar movement in hyperactivated and acrosome-reacted golden hamster spermatozoa. Mol Reprod Dev. 2002;61(3). doi:10.1002/mrd.10017.
35. Suarez SS, Pacey AA. Sperm transport in the female reproductive tract. Hum Reprod Update. 2006;12(1). doi:10.1093/humupd/dmi047.
36. Thompson LA, Barratt CLR, Bolton AE, Cooke ID. The leukocytic reaction of the human uterine cervix. Am J Reprod Immunol. 1992;28(2). (PubMed PMID: 1285856).
37. UZ Leuven Fertility Clinic. Fertility in men. www.uzleuven.be/node/17230. Accessed 13 Dec 2012.
38. Yanagimachi R, Chang MC. Fertilization of hamster eggs in vitro. Nature. 1963;200:281–2. doi:10.1038/200281b0.
39. Ahlgren M. Sperm transport to and survival in the human fallopian tube. Gynecol Invest [Internet]. 1975;6(3–4):206–214. http://content.karger.com/ProdukteDB/produkte.asp?Doi=301517. Accessed 13 Dec 2013.
40. Mortimer, D, Leslie, EE, Kelly, RW, Templeton, AA. Morphological selection of human spermatozoa in vivo and in vitro. J Reprod Fertil. 1982;64(2):391–9.
41. Twigg, J, Irvine, DS, Houston, P, Fulton, N, Michael, L, Aitken, RJ. Iatrogenic DNA damage induced in human spermatozoa during sperm preparation: protective significance of seminal plasma. Mol Hum Reprod. 1998;4(5), 439–45.
42. Ellington, JE, Evenson, DP, Wright Jr, RW, Jones, AE, Schneider, CS, Hiss, GA, et al. Higher-quality human sperm in a sample selectively attach to oviduct (fallopian tube) epithelial cells in vitro. Fertil Steril. 1999;71(5):924–9.
43. Sanders, D, Warner, P, Bäckström, T, Bancroft, J. Mood, sexuality, hormones and the menstrual cycle. I. changes in mood and physical state: description of subjects and method. Psychosom Med. 1983;45(6), 487–501.
44. Austin CR. Fate of spermatozoa in the uterus of the mouse and rat. J Endocrinol 1957;14,335–42.
45. Witkin SS, Chaudhry A. Relationship between circulating antisperm antibodies in women and autoantibodies on the ejaculated sperm of their partners. Am J Obstet Gynecol. 1989;161:900–3.
46. Ingerslev HJ, Moller NP, Jager S, Kremer J. Immunoglobulin class of sperm antibodies in cervical mucus from infertile women. Am J Reprod Immunol. 1982;2:296–300.
47. Kremer J, Jager S. The significance of antisperm antibodies for spermcervical mucus interaction. Hum Reprod. 1992;7:781–4.
48. Witkin SS, Vogel-Roccuzzo R, David SS, Berkeley A, Goldstein M, Graf M. Heterogeneity of antigenic determinants on human spermatozoa: relevance to antisperm antibody testing in infertile couples. Am J Obstet Gynecol. 1988;159:1228–31.
49. Blum, M, Pery, J, Blum, I. Antisperm antibodies in young oral contraceptive users. Adv Contracept. 1989;5(1):41–6.
50. Witkin SS. Production of interferon gamma by lymphocytes exposed to antibody-coated spermatozoa: a mechanism for sperm antibody production in females. Fertil Steril. 1988;50:498–502.
51. Witkin SS. Production of interferon gamma by lymphocytes exposed to antibody-coated spermatozoa: a mechanism for sperm antibody production in females. Fertil Steril. 1988;50:498–502.
52. Fordney-Settlage D. A review of cervical mucus and sperm interactions in humans. Int J Fertil. 1981;26(3). (PubMed PMID: 6118336).
53. Hafez ES. In vivo and in vitro sperm penetration in cervical mucus. Acta Eur Fertil. 1979 10(2). (Pubmed PMID: 397707).
54. Spehr, M, Gisselmann, G, Poplawski, A, Riffell, JA, Wetzel, CH, Zimmer, RK, et al. Identification of a testicular odorant receptor mediating human sperm chemotaxis. Science. 2003;299(5615):2054–58.
55. Shekarriz M, Thomas AJ, Agarwal A. Incidence and level of seminal reactive oxygen species in normal men. Urology. 1995;45(1). doi:10.1016/S0090-4295(95)97088-6.
56. Laessle, RG, Tuschi, RJ, Schweiger, U, Pirke, KM. Mood changes and physical complaints during the normal menstrual cycle in healthy young women. Psychoneuroendocrinology 1990;15(2):131–8.

7 Potential Male Etiologies of Unexplained Infertility

Brent M. Hardin and Edward D. Kim

Introduction

Male factor infertility contributes to one-half of all infertile couples. Of these, approximately 40% have an unknown cause. This subgroup can be divided into two categories based on the results of two properly obtained semen analyses (SA): idiopathic male infertility (IMI) and unexplained male infertility (UMI). Both groups exhibit normal physical exam findings and endocrine evaluations, but they are different in the fact that men with IMI have abnormal semen analyses while men with UMI have normal semen parameters.

The semen analysis is an important laboratory test and a cornerstone for the assessment of male fertility, but normal semen parameters do not guarantee fecundity. Basic semen analysis testing does not assess the functional capabilities of sperm. Understanding this concept is critical in the management of the subfertile male population.

An understanding of recent changes in the 2010 World Health Organization (WHO) reference values for semen analyses is of importance. The WHO examined seminal parameters of roughly 2000 men from eight nations who had conceived children in 12 months or less after stopping contraceptive measures. As compared to the reference values from the 4th ed., the 2010 update lowered the reference values for sperm concentration and total seminal volume by 25%, which in effect increases the number of infertile men that now have normal semen parameters [1]. Many of these men, who were previously identified as idiopathic male infertility, now fall into the category of UMI that is defined as an infertile man with normal semen analyses, a normal physical exam, a normal endocrine profile, and no identifiable female cause. It is estimated that 6–27% of infertile men fall into the category of UMI [2].

E. D. Kim (✉) · B. M. Hardin
Division of Urology, Department of Surgery, University of Tennessee Graduate School of Medicine, 1928 Alcoa Highway, Suite 222, Knoxville, TN 37920, USA
e-mail: ekim@utmck.edu

Initial Investigation

A critical step in the initial management of a male patient with unexplained infertility is determining if he truly qualifies to be diagnosed as such. Therefore, the clinician must eliminate readily identifiable causes of infertility at presentation. The basic male infertility evaluation starts with a history and physical examination. Conditions, such as varicocele, obvious reproductive tract anomalies, and sexual behavior, are also discovered on this initial visit. Two properly collected semen analyses with 2–3 days of abstinence should be obtained and an initial hormonal evaluation should include a serum follicle stimulating hormone (FSH) and testosterone level.

The following must be confirmed for a patient to be classified as UMI:

1. Absence of a female factor
2. Proper coital technique and timing
3. Normal semen analyses

These three facets are usually examined before the couple meets with the andrologist. In short, the female should be questioned and examined to confirm a normal ovulatory cycle and patency of her fallopian tubes. The topics involving the female evaluation will be discussed in much greater detail in other chapters of this book.

Proper technique and timing of sexual intercourse is centered around ensuring that viable sperm are present in the female reproductive tract during the 12–24 h time frame when the ovum is present in the fallopian tube and capable of being fertilized. To allow for this to occur, experts recommend having intercourse every 2 days around the time of ovulation [3]. Avoidance of artificial lubrication will also increase the likelihood of proper sperm delivery. Penile anatomic abnormalities, such as hypospadias and erectile dysfunction, can also affect the delivery of the ejaculate to the cervix.

G. L. Schattman et al. (eds.), *Unexplained Infertility,* DOI 10.1007/978-1-4939-2140-9_7,

Table 7.1 Potential causes of UMI

Potential etiologies of unexplained male infertility
Poor sexual function and/or technique
Immunologic: antisperm antibodies
Errors in spermatogenesis
Genetic causes: mutations, chromosomal nondisjunction, damage to DNA integrity
Oxidative stress
Defects in sperm fertilization potential: poor ZP binding/penetration, defects in capacitation

Potential Causes

Immunologic Causes

The topic of antisperm antibodies (ASA) and immunologic infertility remain controversial among some experts in andrology, but it is certainly worth mentioning in the discussion of UMI (Table 7.1). An in-depth discussion on this subject will occur in a later chapter, but an overview of antisperm antibodies and their potential deleterious effects will be covered here. Antisperm antibodies have historically been implicated in 4% of male infertility patients and up to 40% of males with unexplained infertility [4, 5]. Our understanding of immunologic infertility stems from the knowledge that the testis, and therefore, the developing spermatozoa are within the privileged blood–testis barrier. Any insult that disrupts this barrier has the potential to damage sperm by exposing antigens on the spermatozoa, which the body then attacks.

One can divide the broader topic of immunologic infertility into the two categories of basic immunology: humoral and cellular. Humoral immunity accounts for ASA, which are present in 10% of infertile men versus only 2% of fertile men [6]. These antibodies can usually be found in three locations: serum, seminal plasma, and bound to sperm. The sperm-bound antibodies are the most clinically relevant [7]. In addition, sperm antibodies can be found in cervical fluid in 7–17% of infertile women [8, 9].

While commonly associated with low sperm motility, antisperm antibodies can be present in men with normal semen parameters. The diagnosis of immunologic infertility should be suspected in all cases of UMI, in addition to the following scenarios [10]:

1. Sperm agglutination or clumping in the absence of infection
2. Low sperm motility in a patient with a history of testis trauma or surgery
3. Confirmation of increased number of leukocytes on SA
4. Sperm "shaking" on sperm–cervical mucus testing
5. Poor penetration of mucus on a postcoital test

Our knowledge of cellular immunity and male infertility is based on studies of testes with a history of testicular torsion and testes that had undergone orchidopexy for failure to descend into the scrotum. Multiple studies have examined the testis before and after testicular torsion for the presence of ASA, and have concluded that despite a preexisting defect in spermatogenesis in some of the torsed testes, the torsion event itself does not increase the incidence of antisperm antibodies [11–13].

However, in the circumstance of orchidopexy, evidence exists of an increased risk of ASA that is even higher with increasing age toward puberty at the time of orchidopexy [14]. Other potential disease states that have been linked to ASA include vasectomy, vasectomy reversal, epididymal and ejaculatory obstruction, orchitis, prostatitis, malignancies of the lower urinary tract, varicoceles, testis biopsy, and sexual trauma [10].

Errors in Spermatogenesis

The biologic pathway and physiologic function of sperm will be explored in subsequent chapters, but a brief mention regarding the basics of sperm function is worth noting. The first major step in sperm development is when Type B spermatogonia undergo mitosis to give rise to diploid primary spermatocytes. The primary spermatocyte crosses over the blood–testis barrier of the Sertoli cell tight junctions to begin the differentiation process of spermatogenesis within the immune-privileged adluminal compartment. Meiosis then occurs to give rise to haploid secondary spermatocytes, which undergo a second meiotic division with the entire process resulting in four haploid spermatids [15].

Genetic Causes

There are three basic genetic causes of UMI, and will be discussed separately as: alterations in chromosomal complement, gene mutations and polymorphisms, and DNA integrity defects.

Genetic recombination is a necessary step in spermatogenesis as it provides genetic variation and prepares for chromosomal separation later on in meiosis. An error in this process has been reported in 10% of patients with nonobstructive azoospermia, and in one-half of men with specific diagnosis of maturation arrest [16]. Errors of recombination are commonly known as nondisjunction events, which result in either a missing or an extra chromosome. An abnormal number of chromosomes is simply referred to as aneuploidy. Increased paternal age, ingestion of alcohol, and previous treatment with chemotherapy have been implicated in cases of aneuploidy; although, the exact cause has yet not been discovered [17]. Further, testing for this condition is expensive and therapeutic options are limited.

The role of specific gene mutations on UMI has been extrapolated from multiple animal studies on mice. These studies have identified 300 null mutations and 50 additional deletions that produce murine infertility [17]. In human studies, DNA microarray analysis has demonstrated underexpression of specific genes in normospermic infertile males compared to fertile controls [18]. Further studies are needed in this area before any definitive conclusion can be made.

Damage to the integrity of DNA may also affect sperm function. It has been observed that increased DNA damage leads to inferior outcomes with IVF and ICSI [19], and it is estimated that 8% of infertile men have DNA damage despite a normal semen analysis [20]. Potential contributors to DNA damage can be classified as either extrinsic or intrinsic factors. Examples of extrinsic causes, include heat, tobacco exposure, alcohol exposure, radiation, and other gonadotoxins. Intrinsic factors identified, include protamine deficiency, specific genetic mutations, reactive oxygen species, and aging [17]. One can examine for DNA damage by testing for chromatin compaction (assesses DNA susceptibility to gonadotoxins) or by testing for DNA fragmentation [21]. However, routine use of these assays is controversial and not yet endorsed by society guidelines.

Oxidative Stress

Oxidative stress is known as the effect induced on cells by reactive oxygen species (ROS), and is a known contributor to male infertility in up to 80% cases [22, 23]. There are many documented causes of oxidative stress, most of which contribute to damaging the DNA integrity as discussed previously. Smoking tobacco has been shown to significantly increase ROS, both, by increasing leukocyte concentration and ROS generation in semen and also by decreasing the level of seminal superoxide dismutase, an antioxidant enzyme that combats ROS [24]. Varicoceles have also been shown to cause increased ROS levels, and surgical repair by varicocelectomy leads to a decline in ROS in the testes as well as in the seminal fluid in addition to an improvement in overall sperm quality [25].

ROS have the potential to cause infertility without affecting commonly measured semen parameters. Thus, many men with infertility secondary to ROS fall into the category of UMI as they have normal semen analyses. Finally, the presence of increased ROS is an independent marker of male factor infertility [26].

If oxidative stress is suspected as a cause of UMI, one can test for it either by directly detecting ROS via chemiluminescence or flow cytometry, or indirectly via colorimetry [17]. A later chapter is dedicated to the topic of ROS and will discuss these methods in further detail.

Sperm Fertilization Defects

Sperm function may be affected by each of the previous listed causes of UMI. Antisperm antibodies can affect the fertilizing capability of the mature spermatid by diminishing sperm motility and decreasing the ability of the spermatid to pass through the cervical mucus and the remainder of the female reproductive tract to interact with the oocyte. This is highlighted by the following processes associated with ASA [10]:

1. Agglutination of sperm, rendering them immobile and incapable of penetrating cervical mucus
2. Immobilization of sperm by female-derived ASA encountered in cervical mucus
3. Opsonization of the sperm-antibody complex within the female reproductive tract
4. Prevention of binding of sperm to the zona pellucida (ZP)
5. Prevention of penetration of the oocyte

Thus, sperm function is hindered by the activity of antisperm antibodies in multiple fashions.

Sperms may also have isolated defects in either capacitation or ZP binding and penetration. Each of these topics will be discussed in brief detail accordingly.

Capacitation is actually the summation of two separate events in sperm function: hyperactivation and acrosomal reaction [27]. Hyperactivation describes the process by which a sperm acquires a less-progressive and more haphazard motility, while the acrosomal reaction is the process whereby the sperm plasma membrane fuses with the acrosomal membrane at the time of ZP binding [17]. Errors in either mechanism prevent sperm from reaching and binding to the ZP.

Defects in ZP binding have been documented in 13% of subfertile men with normal semen analyses [28]. It has been demonstrated that there are four distinct ZP glycoproteins expressed on the human ZP to make up its outer shell and to provide the attachment points by which capacitated sperm bind to the ZP to undergo the acrosomal reaction [29]. Specific genes for each glycoprotein provide for the expression of the respective glycoprotein. Genetic mutations could play an additional role in UMI via defective production of the ZP glycoproteins. Finally, acrosome-reacted sperm must undergo proper fusion with the plasma membrane of the ZP.

Conclusions

With the recent modification to the WHO classification of male infertility based on semen analyses [1], larger number of men will present to andrologists with UMI. Treatment strategies are modified according to findings on subsequent evaluation. Assisted reproductive techniques remain an option for most couples with UMI. Further studies are needed to provide better insight in regards to cost-benefit analyses and success of various interventions.

References

1. World Health Organization. WHO laboratory manual for the examination and processing of human semen. 5th ed. Geneva: WHO press; 2010.
2. Moghissi K, Wallach E. Unexplained infertility. Fertil Steril. 1983;39(1):5–21.
3. Wilcox A, Weinberg C, Baird D. Timing of sexual intercourse in relation to ovulation: effect on the probability of conception, survival of the pregnancy, and sex of the baby. N Engl J Med. 1995;333:1517–21.
4. Dohle G, Diemer T, Giwercman A, et al. Guidelines of male infertility. European Association of Urology. 2010. http://www.uroweb.org/gls/pdf/Male%20Infertility%202010.pdf. Accessed 19 Nov 2012.
5 Moghissi K, Sacco A, Borin K. Immunologic infertility. I. Cervical mucus antibodies and postcoital test. Am J Obstet Gynecol. 1980;136(7):941–50.
6. Gusick D, Overstreet J, Factor-Litvak P, et al. Sperm morphology, motility, and concentration in fertile and infertile men. N Engl J Med 2001;345(19):1388–93.
7. Turek P. Male infertility. In: Tanagho E, editor. Smith's general urology. 17th ed. New York: McGraw-Hill; 2008. pp 684–716.
8. Jones W. The use of antibodies developed by infertile women to identify relevant antigens. Karolinska Symposia on Research Methods in Reproductive Endocrinology Immunological Approach to Fertility Control. 1974; Stockholm, Karolinska Instititute.
9. Beer A, Neaves W. Antigenic status of semen from the viewpoints of the female and male. Fertil Steril. 1978; 29(1):3–22.
10. Walsh T, Turek P. Immunologic Infertility. In: Lipshultz L, Howards S, Niederberger C, editors. Infertility in the male. 4th ed. Cambridge: Cambridge University Press; 2009. p 277–94.
11. Anderson M, Dunn J, Lipshultz L, et al. Semen quality and endocrine parameters after acute testicular torsion. J Urol. 1992; 147(6):1545–50.
12. Fraser I, Slater N, Tate C, et al. Testicular torsion does not cause autoimmunization in man. Br J Surg. 1985; 72:237–8.
13. Arap M, Vincentini F, Cocuzza M, et al. Late hormonal levels, semen parameters, and presence of antisperm antibodies in patients treated for testicular torsion. J Androl. 2007;28(4):528–32.
14. Sinisi A, Pasquali D, Papparella A, et al. Antisperm antibodies in cryptorchidism before and after surgery. J Urol. 1998;160(5):1834–7.
15. Alukal J, Lamb D, Neiderberger C, et al. Spermatogenesis in the adult. In: Lipshultz L, Howards S, Iederberger C, editors. Infertility in the male. 4th ed. Cambridge: Cambridge University Press; 2009. p 74–89.
16. Gonsalves J, Sun F, Schlegel P, Turek P, et al. Defective recombination in infertile men. Hum Mol Genet. 2004;13(22):2875–83.
17. Hamada A, Esteves S, Agarwal A. The role of contemporary andrology in unraveling the mystery of unexplained male infertility. Open Reprod Sci J. 2011;4:27–41.
18. Garrido N, Martinez-Conjero J, Jauregui J, et al. Microarray analysis in sperm from fertile and infertile men without basic sperm analysis abnormalities reveals a significantly different transcriptome. Fertil Steril. 2009;91(4):1307–10.
19. Saley R, Agarwal A, Nada E, et al. Negative effects of increased sperm DNA damage in relation to seminal oxidative stress in men with idiopathic and male factor infertility. Fertil Steril. 2003;79:1591–1605.
20. Practice Committee of the American Society for Reproductive Medicine. The clinical utility of sperm DNA Integrity testing. Fertil Steril. 2006;86(1):35–7.
21. Yeung C. Sperm quality and function tests. In: Nieschlag E, Behre HM, Nieschlag S, editors. Andrology, male reproductive health and dysfunction. Heidelberg: Springer-Verlag; 2010. pp 139–54.
22. Kefer J, Agarwal A, Sabanegh E. Role of antioxidants in the treatment of male infertility. Int J Urol. 2009;16(5):449–57.
23. Auger J, Eustache F, Andersen A, et al. Sperm morphological defects related to environment, lifestyle and medical history of 1001 male partners of pregnant women from four European cities. Hum Reprod. 2001;16(12):2710–7.
24. Vine M. Smoking and male reproduction: a review. Int J Androl. 1996;19:323–7.
25. Zini A, Blumenfield A, Libman J, et al. Beneficial effect of microsurgical varicocelectomy on human sperm DNA integrity. Hum Reprod. 2005;20;1018–21.
26. Agarwal A, Sharma R, Nallela K, et al. Reactive oxygen species as an independent marker of male factor infertility. Fertil Steril. 2006;86(4):878–85.
27. Esteves S, Sharma R, Thomas A, et al. Effect of *in vitro* incubation on spontaneous acrosomal reaction in fresh cryopreserved human spermatozoa. Int J Fertil Womens Med. 1998;43(5):235–42.
28. Liu D, Liu M, Garrett C, et al. Comparison of the frequency of defective sperm-zona pellucida (ZP) binding and the ZP-induced acrosome reaction between subfertile men with normal and abnormal semen. Hum Reprod. 2007;22(7):1878–84.
29. Lefievre L, Conner S, Salpekar A, et al. Four zona pellucida glycoproteins are expressed in the human. Hum Reprod. 2004;19(7):1580–6.

Genetic Basis of Unexplained Male Infertility

8

Ricardo Miyaoka and Sandro C. Esteves

Introduction

Infertility is determined by the inability of a couple to achieve pregnancy after 1 year of noncontraception and regular intercourse [1]. In this scenario, it is expected that 84 % of healthy young couples attain pregnancy within 1 year [2]. Nevertheless, 13–15 % of couples remain childless after this period, which represents approximately 140 million people in a global perspective [3]. As such, several societies' guidelines recommend that investigation start at this point or even earlier in the presence of risk factors including advanced maternal (> 35 years) or paternal (> 45 years) age, history of urogenital surgery, cancer, cryptorchidism, varicocele, orchitis, genital infection, etc., [4].

Concerning males in reproductive age, it is estimated that 8 % seek medical counseling for infertility-related problems [5]. However, in spite of the proper diagnostic workup, and as our knowledge of all events involved in normal conception is still limited, we fail to determine the cause of infertility in nearly half of these cases. Also, it remains difficult to find a threshold from which fertile or infertile ejaculates can be identified based on the results of conventional semen analysis [6]. Likewise, it is impossible to make a final diagnosis of infertility solely based on conventional approaches [7, 8].

Despite the evolving advances in assisted reproductive technology (ART) as a therapeutic option to overcome infertility, the use of genetically compromised spermatozoa in ART has been associated with a wide range of adverse outcomes including abnormal embryo development, which may either fail to implant or result in an increased risk of miscarriage and defects in the offspring [9]. In fact, embryogenesis and development of a full-term pregnancy depend on the integrity of the genetic information of both male and female gametes.

Infertile men with unexplained infertility (UI) present with normal semen analysis parameters according to the World Health Organization (WHO) criteria [10] and no obvious fertility problems detected on initial workup [11]. Abnormalities are likely to be present but are not detected by conventional approaches. Genetic defects may be partly or entirely involved in the true cause of infertility in such men. In this chapter, we first present basic genetic concepts and discuss the genetic background of male infertility. Then, we specifically discuss the genetic disorders associated with unexplained male infertility. Finally, we outline the testing performed to diagnose genetic conditions associated with male UI and propose a workup plan for genetic evaluation of men with UI.

Genetic Concepts: A Brief Overview

Somatic cells harbor the human genome comprised of 23 pairs of nuclear chromosomes. These, in turn, result from the combination of 22 pairs of autosomes and 1 pair of sex chromosomes. These nonreproductive cells are the very basic units of all human tissues. Germ cells (oocytes and spermatozoa), on the other hand, contain solely 23 chromosomes (not pairs) and are haploid. The human genome also includes mitochondrial chromosomes originated from the cytoplasm of the fertilized ovum, thus inherited from the mother's side [12]. Mitochondrial chromosomes are only 16 Kb long (less than 0.03 % the length of the smallest nuclear chromosome) and encode 13 key structural genes as well as several structural ribonucleic acid genes (RNA) [13].

Nuclear chromosomes are composed of chromatin, a complex of unbroken long double-stranded helical DNA carrying genes and proteins. Chromatin basic subunits are called nucleosomes, which are composed by DNA wrapped around proteins (histones). The DNA single strand is formed

R. Miyaoka (✉) · S. C. Esteves
ANDROFERT, Andrology and Human Reproduction Clinic, Referral Center for Male Reproduction, Avenida Dr. Heitor Penteado, 1464, Campinas, SP 13075-460, Brazil
e-mail: rmiyaoka@medreprodutiva.com.br

S. C. Esteves
e-mail: s.esteves@androfert.com.br

G. L. Schattman et al. (eds.), *Unexplained Infertility,* DOI 10.1007/978-1-4939-2140-9_8,

from units called nucleotides, a composition of nitrogenous bases (adenine, guanine, cytosine, and thymine or A, G, C, and T, respectively), deoxyribose and phosphate. Nucleotides polymerize in long polynucleotide chains through 5′-3′ phosphodiester bonds between adjacent deoxyribose units. Hydrogen bridges interconnect base pairs through specific nitrogen bases to form the DNA double helix. It is estimated that the human genome contains 6 to 7 billion base pairs in its diploid form. There are five main types of histones designated H1, H2A, H2B, H3, and H4. They play a major role in chromatin fiber storage. Two copies of each of these histones form an octamer around which DNA wraps itself. Approximately 140 DNA base pairs are associated with a histone center [12]. After a short "spacing" DNA segment of 20–60 base pairs another DNA complex center is formed (Fig. 8.1).

Genes can be defined as stretches of DNA sequence that encode different functions including protein synthesis after mRNA transcription and functional RNA synthesis. There are about 40 million genes in the human genome [12]. Very few genes exist as continuous coding sequences (called "exons"); the vast majority is interrupted by noncoding regions called "introns." Introns are initially transcripted to RNA in the nucleus; however, mature mRNA is not found in the cell cytoplasm and therefore introns are not represented in the protein end product. Although some genes lack introns, the majority contains at least one or several of them [13]. Interestingly, introns rather than exons constitute the greater part of the gene length. Introns are removed from synthesized RNA by splicing. This process also joins exons to form mRNA that codes-specific protein synthesis.

The term "locus" defines the exact position a gene occupies on a chromosome while the term "allele" stands for a variant form of a specific gene. A gene is represented by two alleles. When both alleles are identical the individual is termed homozygous for that gene. However, when they are different the individual is termed heterozygous for such gene.

Genotype is the genetic code that determines physical and functional traits of an individual. The genotype is not sensitive to environmental factors. In contrast, phenotype refers to the peculiar characteristics and traits of an individual such as external appearance, biochemical or molecular properties, and behavior. In other words, phenotype is the sole expression of the genotype, and this correlation may be altered by environmental factors.

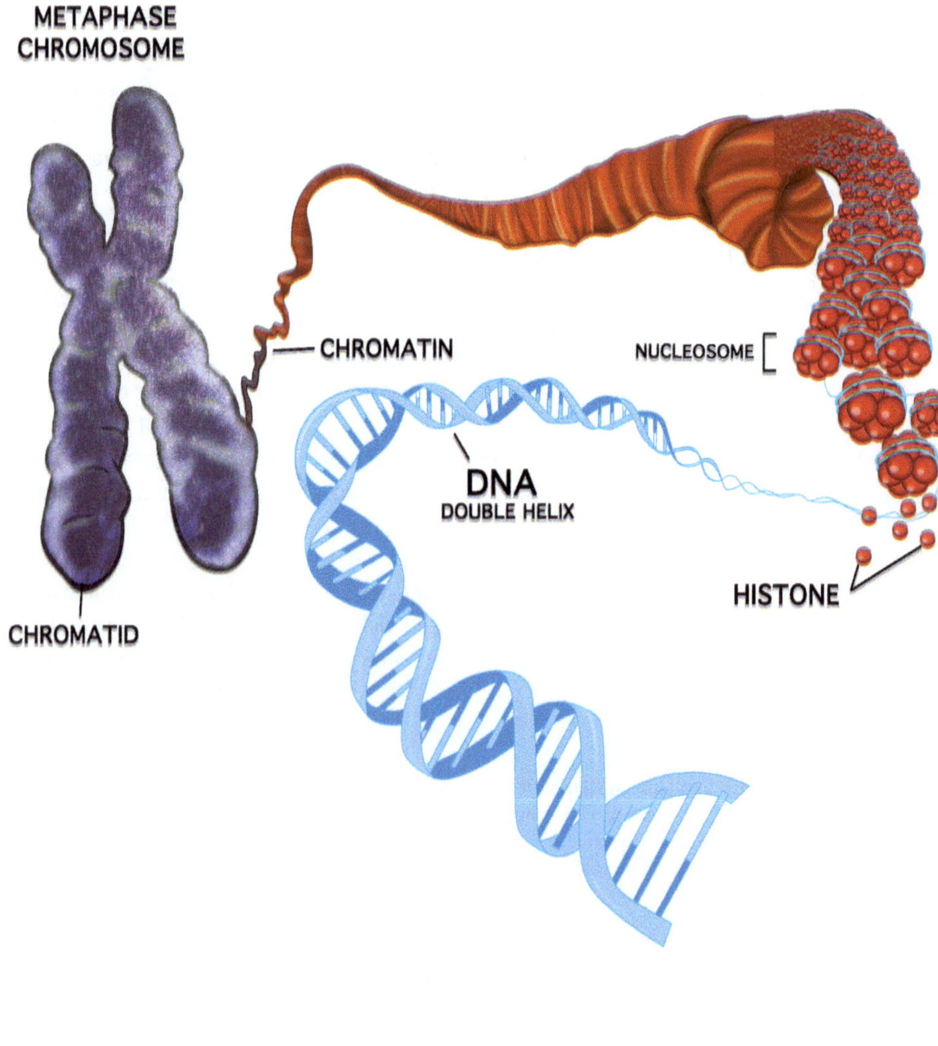

Fig. 8.1 Structure of nuclear metaphase chromosome. The chromatin is a complex of unbroken long double-stranded helical DNA carrying genes and proteins. The nucleosome is the basic chromatin subunit composed of DNA wrapped around histones. (Reprinted from [12], p. 114. With permission from Jaypee Brothers Med. Publishers Ltd.)

There are basically four DNA nucleotide sequence variations [12]. The first is the single-nucleotide polymorphism (SNP), which is a single-nucleotide alteration along the DNA sequence that occurs at a rate of 1 in every 1250 bases throughout the 3 billion base pairs of the human genome. Up to 20 million SNP exist, although not evenly distributed. As an example, SNP may alter the DNA nucleotide sequence from AAGGTAA to ATGGTAA, which is a variation found in at least 1 % of the human population, and that may occur in both coding (exons) and noncoding regions (introns). Most SNPs have no pathological significance; however, very few code for new amino acids or have a role as stop codon, that is, signal a termination in translation. The second variation of DNA nucleotide sequence is a mutation. Mutations are considered as a type of SNP by Hamada et al. [12]. However, unlike SNPs, mutations affect less than 1 % of the general population and most of them correlate with harmful events. The term "mutation" refers to a novel genetic change which was not previously known in a family and, sometimes, may allude to an abnormal allele. Alterations in DNA sequence may contribute to diseases or adverse effects on the host or offspring. Mutations may occur in germ cells during gametogenesis (sperm or oocyte formation) and are usually transmitted to the offspring or render the host infertile. Transmitted mutations may determine different degrees of disease severity ranging from minor physiologic modifications to death. Somatic mutations usually alter the genetic load after conception and play a key role in the pathogenesis of human diseases, notably cancer. In other cases, mutations solely represent phenotype variations. The third variation of DNA nucleotide sequence is short tandem repeats (STR), or in other words, sequences of two to four base pairs such as CG and CAG that repeat in tandems and may occur in exons, introns, and 5′ genomic sequences. Expansion of such repeats may be associated with neurodegenerative disorders and fragile X syndrome [12]. Finally, the last one is the copy number variation (CNV), a relatively common type of structural genetic sequence change that affects 8–12 % of human genome [14]. The CNV requires a long DNA segment of over 1000 bases to be inserted or deleted. The CNV may affect one gene or a complete set of genes and usually results in an increased frequency of its expression or in the amount of the coded protein. Although harmless in the vast majority of cases, CNV has been associated with cancer and increased susceptibility to systemic lupus erythematous [12].

Genetic diseases can be didactically classified in four major categories: chromosomal disorders, single-gene mutation-related disorders, multifactorial disorders, and mitochondrial genetic disorders [12]. Chromosomal disorders are chromosomal numeric abnormalities (aneuploidy) or structural changes. Single-gene disorders occur in a Mendelian fashion or can be sex linked. Multifactorial disorders involve alterations in the expression of multiple genes and are likely influenced by environmental factors affecting the resulting phenotype. Mitochondrial genetic disorders are maternal related and contribute to certain debilitating states.

Role of Genetics in Male Fertility

Sperm production is controlled by genetic factors and involves three distinct phases: (i) mitotic proliferation of spermatogonial cells into primary spermatocytes; (ii) meiotic division of spermatocytes generating haploid secondary spermatocytes after the first meiotic division, and haploid spermatids after second meiotic division; and (iii) spermiogenesis of the haploid spermatids. Hence, a single-diploid spermatocyte will eventually generate four haploid spermatids (Fig. 8.2). Spermatogonial series are kept in a latent state inside the fetal testis until puberty when they increase in number by repeated mitotic divisions. The full process of spermatogenesis starts in adolescence (between 13 and 16 years). It has been estimated that 2000 genes are essential for spermatogenesis and spermiogenesis, from which only 30 genes are present in the Y chromosome [15, 16].

Genetic diversity takes place during the prophase of the first meiotic division. Sister chromatids of paired homologous chromosomes form areas of synaptonemal contact during the pachytene stage. These contacts enable chromatids to exchange segments of genetic material between homologous chromosomes resulting in the formation of new chromosomes. Next, separation of the homologous chromosomal pairs is followed by the second round of meiotic division which results in spermatid formation. During the last phase of spermatogenesis, round spermatids undergo cytologic transformations in a process called "spermiogenesis" to form elongated spermatozoa. Nuclear chromatin condensation, acrosomal cap formation and midpiece and flagellar structure development are the three essential steps of spermiogenesis [12].

Chromatin modification and condensation during spermiogenesis are essential for sperm function. The coiling of human sperm DNA material is mediated by specific proteins which control condensation and decompression in a time-dependent manner. During the condensation process, 90–95 % of histones are replaced by protamines [17]. Protamination of sperm chromatin not only facilitates the nuclear compaction necessary for adequate sperm motility but also helps to protect the genome from oxidizing and harmful molecules within both the male and female reproductive tracts [17]. It also diminishes DNA transcriptional activity. Transition proteins 1 and 2 (TP1 and TP2) are proteins of intermediate basicity that bind to the DNA and facilitate removal of histones. Finally, transitional proteins are completely replaced by protamines [18].

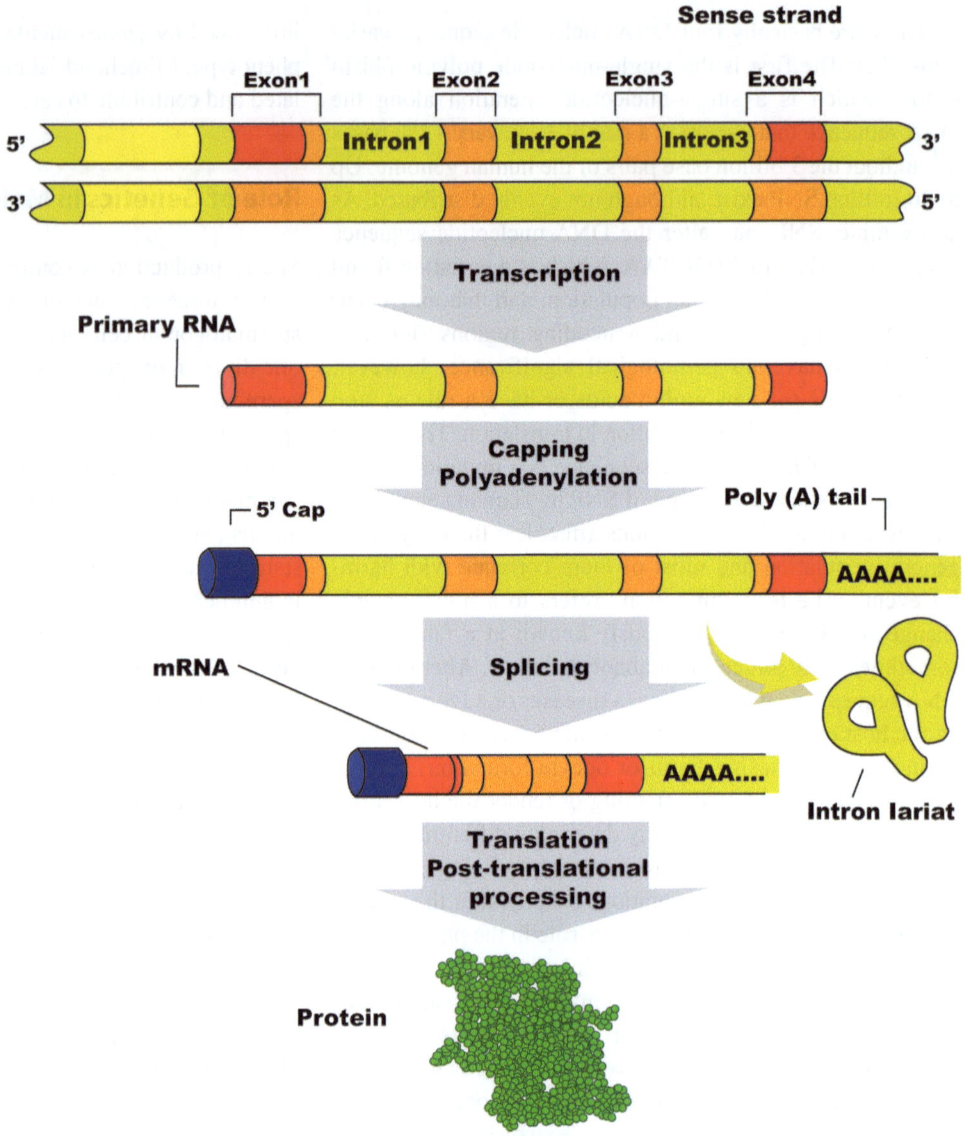

Fig. 8.2 Gene organization, splicing process, and post-translational protein synthesis. (Reprinted from [12], p. 115. With permission from Jaypee Brothers Med. Publishers Ltd.)

Two types of protamines (P1 and P2) are expressed in humas in an equally balanced amount [19]. Improper processing of protamine transcripts and altered P1/P2 ratio are associated with subfertility [20, 21]. Chromatin compaction is the result of disulfide bonds among protamines, which provide the formation of toroid chromatin structures with high resistance to mechanical disruption [22]. Protamines contain large bands of positively charged arginine residues which neutralize the negative phosphodiester backbone of the DNA. Such configuration minimizes DNA repulsion allowing it to double back and fold up onto itself, thus creating the highly compact toroid [23]. Toroids are the most compressed form of sperm DNA. They are stacked side-by-side in a way to provide maximum surface area allocation (Fig. 8.3). Tight condensation makes the DNA resistant to endonuclease digestion [24]. Matrix attachment regions (MARs) are located between each protamine toroid, anchoring them in place (toroid linkers). MARs are very sensitive to nuclease activity as they contain histones. In addition to providing the link between DNA and the nuclear matrix, MARs also serve as a checkpoint for sperm DNA integrity. Protamination not only protects sperm chromatin from damage during transport but also plays an epigenetic role in silencing protamine-bounded genomic regions until time comes for transcription [25]. Once the spermatozoon fuses with the oocyte, protamines are completely replaced by histones from the oocyte within the first 4 h.

The second most prevalent form of sperm DNA structure is histone-bound DNA, accounting for about 4 % of the DNA in mature sperm. Histones are primarily found in association with gene promoter sites. Genes vital for spermiogenesis and early fertilization events are preferentially associated with histones [26, 27]. Human histones are more precisely associated with miRNA clusters, HOX gene clusters, and the promoters of stand-alone developmental transcription and signaling factors [26]. Since sperm DNA histones are not

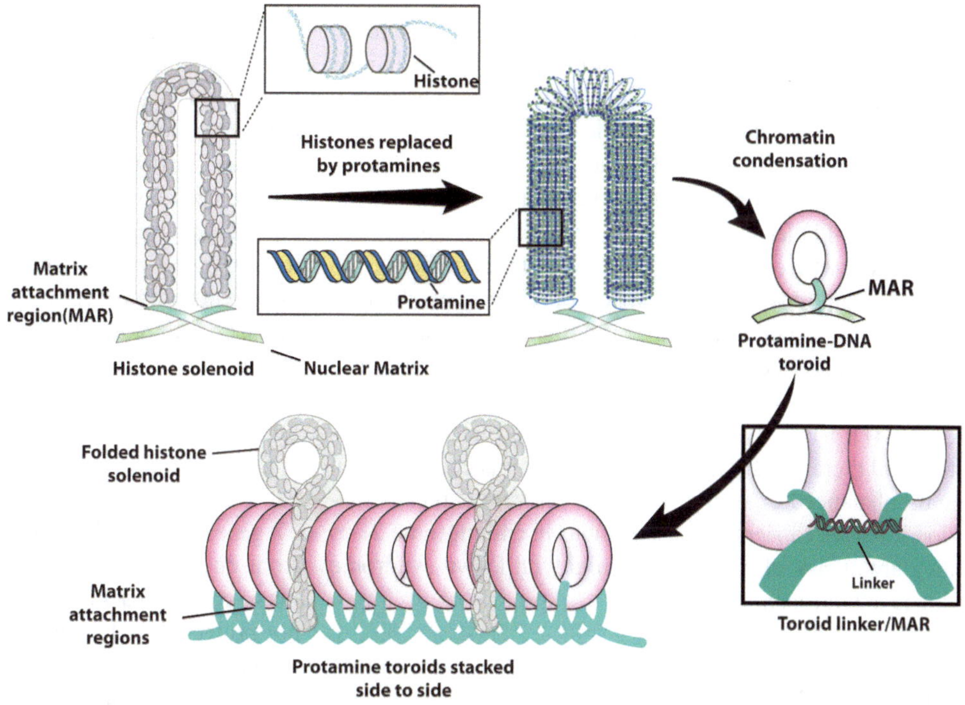

Fig. 8.3 Sperm DNA structure. (Adapted from [12], p. 119. With permission from Jaypee Brothers Med. Publishers Ltd.)

replaced by those of the oocyte after fertilization, it is likely that inflicted damage to histone-bound sperm DNA will be transmitted to the embryo without detection and possible modification.

Genetic abnormalities including chromosomal aberrations and monogenic diseases have been estimated to respond for 10–15% of human infertility cases [28]. Infertile men with genetic alterations usually present with impaired spermatogenesis, genital structural abnormalities, reduced testicular size, hypogonadism and sperm dysfunction, although no detectable abnormalities can also be seen. One important genetic aspect associated with infertility and normal phenotype is sperm chromatin damage [29–33]. A wide range of clinical scenarios may arise from sperm DNA damage including infertility, miscarriage, and increased risk of defects in the offspring [34–37]. Infertile males usually have high rates of sperm DNA damage which are mainly associated with oxidative stress (OS). A chapter in this book is dedicated to OS in unexplained male infertility.

Genetic Disorders Associated with UI

Genetic abnormalities with possible roles in unexplained male infertility can be grouped into five main categories: (i) chromosomal defects in the somatic cells, (ii) gene mutations and polymorphisms in the somatic cells, (iii) sperm DNA damage, (iv) sperm chromosomal abnormalities, and (v) epigenetic disorders. The first two categories affect individuals with abnormal genotypes in somatic cells while sperm DNA damage and epigenetic disorders affect individuals with normal genotypes in somatic cells. Sperm chromosomal abnormalities can be originated from both individuals with abnormal and normal genotypes.

Chromosomal Defects

Chromosomal defects are the most common genetic abnormalities in infertile males, accounting for 2.1–15.5% of cases [38]. Klinefelter syndrome, chromosome translocations, inversions, and deletions fall in this category, and the vast majority of affected individuals display severely compromised semen quality. Translocation carriers, however, may present with different sperm production phenotypes, varying from normal spermatogenesis to inability to produce spermatogonia [39]. Chromosomal translocations occur when nonhomologous chromosomes exchange segments. Translocations involve both sex chromosomes and autosomes, which can be either balanced or unbalanced; most often they are either associated with severe sperm abnormalities or lethal for fetuses. Robertsonian translocation (RT) represents a translocation category in which two acrocentric chromosomes fuse at the region next to the centromere causing loss of their short arms. The resulting balanced karyotype has only 45 chromosomes including the chromosome with the translocation, which is actually constituted by long arms of two chromosomes. As the short arms of the five acrocentric chromosomes (chromosomes 13, 14, 15, 21, and 22) harbor multiple copies of ribosomal RNA, the loss of their short arms is not harmful. RTs are the most frequent structural chromosome abnormalities in humans, affecting the fertility status of one in 1000 men [28]. Although their prevalence in subfertile males is estimated to be only 0.8 %, it is nine times higher than in the general population [40]. In heterozygous carriers, RT chromosomes and their acrocentric homologues may undergo either alternate segregation or adjacent segregation at meiosis. Alternate segregation results in the formation of balanced gametes carrying either RT or normal karyotype, whereas adjacent segregation leads to the formation of aneuploidy gametes. Carriers of RTs may exhibit normal phenotype but otherwise be infertile due to more or less severe oligozoospermia [38]. In addition, RT may predispose to abnormal embryo development that account for few cases of UI [41]. There is also a risk of unbalanced gamete production and therefore an increased risk of spontaneous abortion and unbalanced offspring. The most relevant clinical situation involves carriers of translocations in chromosome 21 as they are at risk of producing a child with Down syndrome due to a 21q trisomy inheritance.

Gene Mutations

Like chromosomal defects, gene mutations are usually related to severely abnormal sperm production phenotypes. Microdeletions in the Y chromosome azoospermia factor (AZF) region, mutations in the cystic fibrosis gene, and mutations and polymorphisms of the androgen receptor gene are classic examples of genetic abnormalities in this disease category. In the context of UI, however, abnormalities of interest include mutations of cation channel of sperm (CatSper) and sperm mitochondrial genes.

CatSper Gene In humans, sperm hyperactivation is not as well defined as it is for other species, and only a small part of the sperm population undergoes hyperactivation at each time. The proportion of sperm exhibiting hyperactivated motility is positively correlated with the extent of zona binding, acrosome reaction, zona-free oocyte penetration, and fertilization capacity in vitro. Studies have demonstrated that voltage-gated calcium channels (Cation CatSpe; CatSper 1–4) and proton pumps located in the principal piece of the sperm flagellum regulates hyperactivation [42, 43]. Intracellular calcium entry is induced by intracellular alkalinization secondary to H^+ extrusion through voltage-gated proton pumps [43]. Variations in intracellular pH and calcium also regulate the sperm ability to fertilize the egg [42]. CatSper ion channel is a recently discovered protein complex composed of six subunits. Among these, four are α subunits (CatSper 1-4) with calcium-selective pore while two are transmembrane proteins with large extracellular domains and unknown function (CatSper beta and CatSper gamma) [44]. In a study involving infertile men with normal semen parameters, Avenarius et al. noted that patients with mutated CatSper1 gene had an abnormally low proportion of sperm exhibiting hyperactivation [45]. In addition, a study in mice has shown that mutations in each CatSper (1–4) ion channel protein led to infertility despite normal seminal parameters and testicular development [46]. CatSper 1, 2, 3, and 4 have been mapped to chromosomes 11q12.1, 15q13-q15, 5q31.2, and 1p35.3, respectively. Further studies are needed to clarify the genetic and molecular nature of fertilization in patients with defective hyperactivation and UI. Also, the impact of minor mutations in human CatSper (1–4) genes in men with UI is yet to be determined.

Sperm Mitochondrial DNA (mtDNA) Mutations Spermatozoa mitochondria are located around the midpiece in a helical arrangement containing 1–2 mtDNA. mtDNA encodes 37 genes that regulate oxidative phosphorylation. It differs from nuclear DNA in respect to replication, repair mechanism, genome packing, and position. In addition, mtDNA is not protected by histones and is physically associated with the inner mitochondrial membrane, where highly mutagenic oxygen radicals are generated in the respiratory chain [47, 48]. The leakage of these free radicals makes mitochondria a major source of reactive oxygen species (ROS). These features may explain why mtDNA is more prone to mutations than nuclear DNA [38, 49]. Besides, excess production of ROS may induce the opening of the membrane permeability transition pore and release of free radicals, cytochrome C, and other factors that may ultimately lead to sperm apoptosis.

Most studies focusing on sperm mtDNA mutations and infertility have shown that sperm phenotypes display motility abnormalities related to dysfunctional axonemes [50]. However, Jensen et al. studied the mtDNA polymerase gamma gene (POLG) in patients with UI and found that CAG repeat lengths ranged from 8 to 13 triplets. Homozygotes with ten repeats in both alleles (10/10) were the most common, and constituted 75 % of all subjects. These authors found that 14.3 % of men with UI were homozygous not10/not10 compared with only 2.3 % in the unselected control group ($P=0.001$) and 0.9 % in the fertile group ($P=0.0001$). The odds ratio of having not10/not10 and being normozoospermic and infertile was 18.1 (95 % CI 3.3–184) [51]. Despite the undefined role of determining mtDNA mutations as a marker of male infertility, prognosis for pregnancy is good in cases treated with ART since mtDNA is not transmitted to the offspring [38].

Sperm DNA Damage

Sperm chromatin integrity is crucial to normal reproductive outcomes and its disturbance has been associated with infertility, decreased embryo quality and implantation in ART, and increased miscarriage [30, 31, 34–36]. A normally packaged chromatin in the nucleus of mature spermatozoa is important not only for DNA accommodation but also DNA protection. DNA-strand breaks are often seen as a result of oxidative stress during sperm DNA packaging; however, such breaks are corrected by a complex mechanism involving phosphorylation and polymerization. It has been hypothesized that OS may disrupt spermiogenesis and result in the production of sperm with poorly remodeled chromatin [52]. These defective gametes are released from the testes carrying a tendency to undergo apoptotic events that include the activation of free radical generation by mitochondria. As a consequence, lipid peroxidation and oxidative DNA fragmentation are induced, ultimately resulting in cell damage. Although the likely result is infertility, these defective cells may still fertilize oocytes.

In general, oocytes have repair mechanisms that can alleviate the mutational load to be carried by the embryo. However, the effectiveness of such repair mechanisms is negatively affected by female age [53]. When sperm DNA fragmentation repair fails, de novo genetic mutation will be transmitted to the embryo. Such mutations may lead to different scenarios including embryo development arrest, increased risk of miscarriage, and increased risk of infertility, childhood cancer and imprinting diseases in the offspring [54].

DNA damage may result from both intrinsic and extrinsic disturbances usually associated with OS. Intrinsic causes include, for example, protamine deficiency and DNA packaging defects [55]. A small, nonclinically significant percentage of spermatozoa from fertile men possess detectable levels of DNA damage. However, sperm DNA damage is increased in infertile men [31, 56]. It has been shown that approximately 5–15 % of the latter have complete protamine deficiency thus rendering DNA vulnerable to attacks such as those inflicted by ROS [17, 20]. External factors include genital inflammation, heat, radiation, chemotherapy, and cigarette smoking [57]. Cigarette smoking generates high levels of OS, directly increasing seminal leukocyte concentrations and seminal ROS generation, which are known to induce OS. Smoking also reduces the concentration of antioxidants in the seminal plasma thus decreasing its oxidant scavenging capacity [58–60].

Rybar et al. studying sperm DNA fragmentation index (DFI), found that the proportion of sperm with fragmented DNA was significantly higher in normozoospermic men from couples with UI compared with young men with no infertility history (DFI 17.4 % ± 10.8 % versus 12.2 % ± 7.3 %; $P<0.01$) [7]. Earlier studies have also suggested that sperm chromatin damage in male partners from couples with UI was higher than fertile males (1.9 % ± 1.1 % versus 0.3 % ± 0.4 %, $P<0.05$), but its association with semen quality as conventionally assessed had been ambiguous [61–63]. Abnormally elevated levels of sperm DNA damage have been observed in approximately 5 % of infertile men with normal semen analysis in comparison with 25 % of counterparts with abnormal semen analysis. At present, it seems sound to assume that the poor-quality sperm chromatin is indicative of male subfertility regardless of number, motility, and morphology of spermatozoa [31, 32, 56, 64]. In fact, in a prospective study involving 165 couples (presumably fertile) seeking fertility counseling in the USA, sperm chromatin structural assay (SCSA), which is one of the methods for sperm DNA integrity assessment, has proved to be the best predictor for successful pregnancy in first pregnancy planners as well as in couples undergoing intrauterine insemination (IUI) [30]. Currently, sperm DNA fragmentation assessments are considered useful tools in the investigation, counseling, and treatment of infertile couples [65].

Sperm Chromosomal Abnormalities

It has been estimated that there is a threefold increase in sperm aneuploidy frequencies in infertile men compared with fertile men [66]. Sperm aneuploidies have been associated with severe sperm defects, infertility, miscarriage, in vitro fertilization (IVF) failure and increased risk of chromosome abnormalities in newborns. Albeit counterintuitive, there is little or no evidence to support the argument that an aneuploidic spermatozoon is at disadvantage in fertilizing an oocyte compared with normal haploid sperm [67]. There is, however, an obvious correlation between the increased frequency of aneuploidy observed in sperm (around 3 % in infertile men) and paternally derived de novo chromosome abnormalities in embryos, fetuses, and newborns conceived using intracytoplasmic sperm injection (ICSI)). This increase in de novo abnormalities after ICSI is estimated to affect 2–3 % of conceptions [68, 69], which represents an approximate threefold increase compared with natural conceptions.

Studies from the past decade using the fluorescent in situ hybridization (FISH) technique showed that the rate of sperm aneuploidies was inversely correlated to sperm quality. Moreover, sperm disomy (two pairs of a single chromosome), diploidy (two pairs of all chromosomes), and polyploidy positively correlated to sperm morphological abnormalities including macrocephalic, multinucleated, and multiflagellate sperm [70–73]. This knowledge highlights the importance of implementing techniques to detect sperm aneuploidy at the time of sperm selection for ICSI.

Epigenetic Disorders

Epigenetics is defined as "the study of mitotically and/or meiotically heritable changes in gene function that cannot be explained by changes in DNA sequence" [74]. Epigenetic components have a profound impact on developmental processes and affect diverse areas of biology and medicine, including cancer biology, environmental effects, and aging [75]. Concerning male fertility, epigenetics describes all types of molecular information that are transmitted from the spermatozoon to the embryo. Epigenetic regulatory mechanisms required for proper embryogenesis include: (i) functional role of centrosome, (ii) DNA methylation, (iii) histone modifications, (iv) chromatin remodeling, and (v) role of RNA transcripts and telomere length.

DNA segments that are tightly compacted are called heterochromatin and are transcriptionally inactive. In contrast, regions that are bound loosely to histones are called euchromatin and are transcriptionally active. Compactness of DNA in a determined region is regulated by epigenetics. While the genetic code is considered to be static in every cell for an organism's entire life, the epigenetic code is rather dynamic and tissue specific [76]. It is a dynamic imprint to fine tune the phenotype according to environmental and other factors [12].

The sperm centrosome is critical for fertilization, chromosome segregation, and cell division [77]. Abnormal centrosome morphology and sperm aster formation have been associated with decreased fertilization and increased miscarriage rates [78]. Immature sperm, as the ones harvested from the testicles, may not have fully functional centrosomes, and their use for assisted conception may result in the formation of mosaic and aneuploid embryos due to abnormal chromosome segregation [79, 80]. Altered centrosomes have also been associated with embryo cleavage arrest [78].

Methylation is the best example of the sperm epigenetic contribution to the embryo. Human embryos cannot develop without proper paternal DNA methylation, it determines which genes from both parental genomes will be expressed [81]. Methylation occurs at the 5-carbon position of cytosines found in cytosine–phosphate–guanine dinucleotides (CpGs). CpGs are found in high concentrations near the gene promoter and are termed "CpGs islands." Decreased methylation of the paternal IGF2/H19 imprinting control region 1 (ICR1) and GTL2 have been found in spermatozoa of men with disturbed spermatogenesis [82]. In a recent study by Poplinsky et al., the degree of methylation of the IGF2/H19 ICR1 and mesoderm-specific transcript (MEST) locus was determined in swim-up purified spermatozoa from 148 infertile men and 33 normozoospermic controls [83]. All control individuals had high- and low-methylation degree of IGF2/H19 ICR1 and MEST, respectively. However, MEST hypermethylation imprinting defect was strongly associated with infertility [83]. DNA imprinting regions are reset at every reproductive cycle thus allowing renewing of parental imprints in parental germ cells [84]. Imprinting activation is a result of differential marking of DNA regions with histone modifications, methylation, or a combination of both, to allow only one allele to remain active [85]. It has been hypothesized that some ART procedures might be compromised because of using sperm not fully matured and therefore, without a fully established epigenetic code. Besides, immature sperm have been associated with other fertilization defects related to centrosome abnormalities [86], sperm nuclear protein abnormalities, and inability to activate the oocyte [87]. If the sperm are too immature or abnormal, chances are higher for the offspring to inherit an imprinting disorder [78].

Histones also play an important role in the transmission of paternal epigenetic information. Histone covalent modifications are associated with several nuclear functions including transcriptional control, chromatin packaging, and DNA methylation. The transcriptional control of gene expression is regulated by the addition of acetyl, methyl, ubiquitin, and phosphate groups to histones [88]. During chromatin packaging, 85 % of histones are replaced by protamines [89]. In an intermediate phase of the replacement process, TPs are inserted into the chromatin structure. It is known that disruption of TPs (TP1 and TP2) encoding genes can produce infertile phenotypes, as well as unbalanced P1/P2 ratios and early transcription of mRNA of P1 [90–92]. Histones are more easily extracted from DNA than protamines, and histone-bound DNA is more susceptible to DNA-damaging agents than protamine counterparts [93]. If abnormally modified, histones are candidates for impeding normal embryogenesis [94].

Finally, telomeres have also been targeted as potential candidates to explain some infertile phenotypes. Telomere function includes protection of the genetic information encoded on the chromosome, localization of chromosomes in the nucleus, and support for DNA replication [81]. Abnormal telomere shortening has been associated with male factor infertility [95]. Studies in mice have suggested that there is a protective mechanism that degrades spermatocytes with reduced telomere length to prevent their maturation [96]. However, this process may eventually fail, as shown by Liu et al., who found that spermatocytes with shortened telomeres had reached reached the meiosis I, thus indicating that they had passed the checkpoint without being degraded [97]. Despite these insights, the role of telomere length on male infertility remains to be further investigated [81].

In conclusion, current epigenetic knowledge on reproductive sperm biology indicates that inheritance is much more complex than the transmission of information provided by the paternal DNA. It means that a series of epigenetic signals coming from the paternal chromatin is needed for the proper execution of the DNA-encoded genetic program [93].

Genetic Testing for Males with UI

There are basically five groups of tests that can be used to detect genetic and epigenetic diseases in men with UI: (i) cytogenetic tests to detect chromosomal alterations; (ii) specific gene sequencing for mutational and polymorphism analysis; (iii) chromatin integrity assays for measurement of sperm DNA damage; (iv) FISH to detect sperm aneuploidies; and (v) next-generation sequencing technologies to detect epigenetic changes (Table 8.1).

Cytogenetic analysis is carried out by karyotyping, which evaluates the number and appearance of chromosomes in the nucleus of a eukaryotic cell. There are several cytogenetic techniques to visualize different aspects of chromosomes. The classic karyotype is mostly used, in which a dye, often Giemsa (G-banding), is used for stain bands on the chromosomes that are then examined under light microscopy. In brief, it involves the collection of heparinized peripheral blood samples and the isolation of a plasma lymphocyte suspension. Lymphocytes are cultured to promote mitosis stimulation, and then division is arrested at the metaphase [12, 38]. Each chromosome has a characteristic-banding pattern that helps its identification. Structural chromosome abnormalities such as translocations can be easily detected by cytogenetic techniques.

For specific-gene sequencing and mutational analyses, the "dye terminator sequence" method is usually performed. It also involves the collection of peripheral blood. Its principle is the premature termination of four separate sequencing reactions that contain all standard deoxynucleotides (dATP, dGTP, dCTP, and dTTP) and the DNA polymerase. Only one of the four dideoxynucleotides (ddATP, ddGTP, ddCTP, or ddTTP), which are chain-terminating nucleotides that lack the 3′-OH group required for the formation of a phosphodiester bond between two nucleotides, is added to each reaction. Thus, DNA strand extension is terminated, resulting in DNA fragments of varying lengths. Next, these labeled DNA fragments are separated by gel electrophoresis on a denaturing polyacrylamide-urea gel and read in a specific manner from the shortest to the longest [12].

Measurement of DNA damage is carried out by sperm chromatin assays and expressed by DFI. Assays to evaluate sperm chromatin/DNA integrity can be didactically divided in three groups: (i) sperm chromatin probes using nuclear dyes (e.g., microscopic acridine orange test, sperm chromatin structure assy [SCSA], aniline blue test, chromomycin-A3 and toluidine blue); (ii) tests for direct assessment of sperm DNA fragmentation (e.g., terminal deoxynucleotidyl trasnferase mediated dUTP nick end labeling assay [TUNEL] and single-cell gel electrophoresis assay [COMET]); and (iii) sperm nuclear matrix assays (e.g., sperm chromatin dispersion [SCD] test) [98]. These tests differ in their ability to detect chromatin compaction and single- or double-strand DNA breaks. Common limitations of these tests are that they provide limited information on the nature of the DNA lesions detected and do not allow the identification of the causative etiology of DNA damage. In general, aliquots of liquefied ejaculates are used for testing. More detailed information on each method is provided in Chap. 11.

FISH combines the classic karyotype method with molecular techniques using fluorescent DNA probes to bind selectively to a specific single-stranded chromosomal region after denaturation. The fluorochromes are then visualized by fluorescent microscopy. FISH can be used to detect chromosomal aneuploidy and structural abnormalities both in eukaryotic cells and sperm [12, 38]. Unlike karyotype that requires metaphase cells, FISH can be applied to interphase nuclei.

The availability of next-generation sequencing technologies has recently allowed the survey of genome-wide epigenetic variation at high resolution. Bisulfite sequencing (Bi-seq), reduced-representation Bi-seq (RRBS), methylated DNA immunoprecipitation sequencing (MeDIP-seq), methylated DNA capture by affinity purification sequencing (MeCAP-seq), methylated DNA binding domain sequencing (MBD-seq), and ethylation-sensitive restriction enzyme sequencing (MRE-seq) are the methods for detecting DNA methylation problems. Chromatin immunoprecipitation followed by sequencing (ChIP-seq) is the standard approach used to detect histone-tail modifications while long noncoding RNAs can be detected using RNA-sequencing studies [99].

Table 8.1 Genetic tests for males with unexplained infertility (UI)

Test	Principle	Specimen tested
Cytogenetic test (Karyotype)	Assess number and appearance of eukaryotic cells	Peripheral blood
Gene sequencing for mutational and polymorphism analysis	Determine gene sequencing and mutation occurrence using dye terminator sequence	Peripheral blood
Chromatin integrity assays	Measure sperm DNA damage	Sperm
Fluorescence in situ hybridization (FISH)	Detect chromosomal aneuploidy and structural abnormalities both in eukaryotic cells and spermatozoa	Peripheral blood; sperm
Microarray technology	Analyze mRNA transcripts pool expressed by sperm	Sperm
Next-generation sequencing technologies	Detect DNA methylation problems	Peripheral blood

Workup Plan for Genetic Diagnosis in the Male with Unexplained Infertility

Genetic testing not only allows clarifying an obscure infertility diagnosis but also helps to prevent the occurrence of miscarriage and iatrogenic transmission of genetic defects to the offspring via assisted reproductive techniques. The latter can be achieved by means of either genetic counseling prior to ART or preimplantational genetic diagnosis (PGD). Yet, the widespread use of genetic testing in cases of UI has been limited by the massive use of ART to overcome infertility. Other limitations include tests' costs, availability, clinical relevance, and endorsement by societies' guidelines, to cite a few. The most important strengths of genetic testing in this scenario lies on its ability to identify men with genetically defective sperm who have decreased reproductive potential thus aiding couples make informed reproductive decisions.

Our opinion is that a cost-effective genetic evaluation should be an integral part of the workup of couples with UI. At Androfert, we routinely include karyotyping and sperm DNA damage assessment during the infertility workup of such men. We found SCD to be a simple, cost-effective, fast, reliable, and accurate test that has been shown to provide results highly correlated to those obtained by SCSA [100, 101]. Assessment of sperm DNA chromatin provides a relatively independent measure of sperm quality that yields diagnostic and prognostic information complementary to, but distinct and more significant than, standard sperm parameters [100].

The usefulness of sperm chromatin evaluation in the context of unexplained male infertility is manifold, as listed below:

1 It aids in selecting the best treatment strategy and prevents the use of suboptimal ART techniques in cases of elevated levels of sperm DNA fragmentation. In fact, current evidence indicates that a cut-off value of 30 % for SCSA has been recommended as a maximum limit to anticipate an acceptable chance of natural conception [30, 31] and IUI [33] success. Sperm samples containing more than 12 % spermatozoa with fragmented DNA by TUNEL assay, on the other hand, resulted in no pregnancies following IUI [102]. Moreover, significant lower number of pregnancies has been achieved by conventional IVF compared with ICSI in cases of elevated DNA fragmentation (26 % versus 42 %, respectively; $P<0.05$) [33].
2. It can be used as a counseling toll for couples already enrolled in ART programs whose male partners have elevated levels of DNA fragmentation. As mentioned earlier, sperm DNA defects that are not repaired by the oocyte can be promutagenic and potentially increase the chance of diseases in the offspring [9]. To date, there is evidence suggesting that babies conceived after ART have higher risk of low birth weight, developmental delay, increased incidence of congenital malformations, sex chromosomal abnormalities, and structural chromosomal abnormalities [103]. In addition, a sixfold increase in the incidence of imprinting defects has been reported for babies conceived by IVF/ICSI, which may be partially explained by the use of epigenetically immature spermatozoa [104]. Moreover, a recent meta-analysis of 16 cohort studies involving 2969 couples indicated that there was a significant risk of miscarriage in couples undergoing IVF/ICSI with high-sperm DNA damage compared with normal DNA damage levels (risk ratio = 2.16; 95 % confidence interval: 1.54–3.03; $P<0.001$) [105]. Even though the chance of pregnancy is higher in ICSI compared with IVF in cases of elevated DNA fragmentation, the incidence of DNA damage is lower in testicular sperm compared with ejaculated ones [106]. Therefore, ICSI using testicular spermatozoa may be considered to infertile men with elevated sperm DNA fragmentation.
3. Given the importance of OS-induced DNA damage, men with high-DNA fragmentation should be counseled towards strategies that may alleviate damage, including lifestyle modifications (weight loss, quitting smoking, and antioxidant-rich food diet) and varicocele repair, if clinically detectable [60, 107–109].

Sperm aneuploidy assessment is left for selected cases of UI with repeated IVF failures or recurrent pregnancy loss. Sperm aneuploidy screening is not technically demanding or prohibitively expensive in terms of materials; however, it is costly regarding training and operator time to score the large number of cells required, between 5000 and 20,000. One other point of sperm aneuploidy assessment concerns its prognostic value, that is, how to determine the impact of sperm aneuploidy in terms of risk to fetuses and newborns since it is not possible to test the individual sperm to be used in the ICSI treatment. To date, very few studies have provided direct correlations between sperm aneuploidy and ICSI outcomes, thus making it difficult to establish any threshold to predict the success of ICSI [67]. Although somatic and sperm chromosomal abnormalities, as well as mutations, cannot be treated, knowledge of such defects, together with genetic counseling, allows couples to evaluate their options and make informed decision that may include using PGD, using donor sperm or remaining childless.

Conclusions and Future Perspectives

Male fertility, including spermatogenesis and sperm function, is regulated by thousands of genes. There is an ongoing research effort to identify specific gene loci regulating early and late stages of spermiogenesis. It has been possible to create models of male infertility in studies involving mice, with up to 300 null mutations and 50 conditional targeted deletions. As men with UI can harbor genetic abnormalities that may compromise their reproductive potential, efforts should be made to identify such conditions. Currently, few diagnostic tools are available for routine use and their usefulness is not yet completely clear. Chromosomal abnormalities in somatic cells can be detected by karyotyping. Sperm aneuploidy assessment in couples with UI experiencing either repeated IVF failures or recurrent pregnancy loss can be performed by FISH, while mutations and polymorphisms are identified by specific gene sequencing and mutational analyses methods. However, diagnostic tests are not available for each gene, thus making the accurate genetic diagnosis a challenge. Yet, existing data justify the clinical use of testing to measure sperm DNA fragmentation, despite the claims that current evidence is insufficient to provide clinical ground for its routine use in infertility evaluation. Assessment of sperm DNA chromatin provides a relatively independent measure of sperm quality that yields diagnostic and prognostic information complementary to, but distinct and more significant than, standard sperm parameters. While treating cytogenetic abnormalities and genetic aberrations is still out of reach, sperm oxidative DNA damage to a large extent can be either prevented or decreased by lifestyle changes and specific treatments.

Major advances in biomolecular techniques have led to the development of new analytical tools such as DNA sequencing and DNA microarrays that will likely become part of the male infertility investigation [110]. Microarray technology can yield information about thousands of mRNAs' expression in a single experiment, enabling the analysis and comparison of complete sperm expression profiles. The integration of these novel techniques with proteomics may unravel the mysteries of sperm function in UI [111]. An example of what the future holds is the recent work of Bonache and colleagues, who described a genetic sperm expression profile able to reflect the fertilizing potential of spermatozoa with better predictive value than classical semen parameters. Analyzing the semen samples of 68 normozoospermic donors used for therapeutic IUI, the authors developed a model to classify the fertility status based on the expression signature of four genes (EIF5A, RPLI3, RPL23A, and RPS27A) with a sensitivity and specificity of 82 and 90 %, respectively, to discriminate donors resulting in low pregnancy rates [112].

Other approaches to molecular evaluation of spermatozoa are under investigation, including array comparative genomic hybridization (aCGH), whole-genome sequencing, and noncoding RNA arrays [113]. Concerning sperm epigenetics, there is still a lot to be learned but this field bears the promise of reversing the effect due to its dynamic nature. As such, deeper understanding of the epigenetic processes could shed light on therapies based on epigenome modifications. This has an advantage over genetic studies, since cure may be offered to the individuals bearing epigenetic changes in contrast to those harboring genetic modifications.

Acknowledgment The authors are grateful to Fabiola C. Bento for her help in language revision.

References

1. World Health Organization. WHO manual for standardised investigation and diagnosis of the infertile couple. Cambridge: Cambridge University Press; 2000.
2. Kamel RM. Management of the infertile couple: an evidence-based protocol. Reprod Biol Endocrinol. 2010;8:21–8.
3. Right Diagnosis.com [homepage on the internet]. Statistics by country for infertility. Health Grades Inc. [updated: 23rd August 2011; cited 24th December 2011]. Available from: http://www.rightdiagnosis.com/i/infertility/stats-country.htm. Accessed 5 June 2012.
4. Esteves SC, Miyaoka R. Male infertility—when and how to start the evaluation. In: Rizk B, Aziz N, Agarwal A, Sabanegh E, editors. Male infertility practice. New Delhi: Jaypee Brothers Pvt Ltd; 2013, pp. 33-45.
5. Vital and health statistics, series 23, no. 26, CDC. http://www.cdc.gov [cited 24th December 2011]. Accessed 5 June 2012.
6. Esteves SC, Zini A, Aziz N, Alvarez JG, Sabanegh ES Jr, Agarwal A. Critical appraisal of World Health Organization's new reference values for human semen characteristics and effect on diagnosis and treatment of subfertile men. Urology. 2012;79:16–22.
7. Rybar R, Markova P, Veznik Z, et al. Sperm chromatin integrity in young men with no experiences of infertility and men from idiopathic infertility couples. Andrologia. 2009;41:141–9.
8. Guzick DS, Overstreet JW, Factor-Litvak P, et al. National cooperative reproductive medicine network. Sperm morphology, motility, and concentration in fertile and infertile men. N Engl J Med. 2001;345:1388–93.
9. Aitken RJ, Koopman P, Lewis SE. Seeds of concern. Nature. 2004;432:48–52.
10. World Health Organization. WHO laboratory manual for the examination and processing of human semen, 5th ed. Geneva: WHO Press; 2010. p. 287.
11. Sigman M, Lipshultz L, Howard S. Office evaluation of the subfertile male. In: Lipshultz LI, Howards SS, Niederberger CS, editors. Infertility in the male. 4th ed. Cambridge: Cambridge University Press; 2009. pp. 153–76.
12. Hamada A, Esteves SC, Agarwal A. Genetics and male infertility. In: Dubey AK, editor. Infertility diagnosis, management and IVF, 1st ed. New Delhi, Jaypee-Highlights Medical Publishers Inc; 2012. pp. 113–57.
13. Thompson MW, McInnes RR, WillardHF. Estrutura e função dos cromossomos e genes. In: Thompson MW, editors. Thompson e Thompson: Genética Médica, Quinta edição. Rio de Janeiro, editora Guanabara Koogan S.A; 1993. pp. 22–38.
14. Bailey JA, Gu Z, Clark RA, et al. Recent segmental duplications in the human genome. Science. 2002;297:1003–7.
15. Hargreave TB. Genetic basis of male infertility. Br Med Bull. 2000;56:650–71.
16. Matzuk MM, Lamb DJ. Genetic dissection of mammalian fertility pathways. Nat Cell Biol. 2002; 4 Suppl:s41–9.
17. Oliva R. Protamines and male infertility. Hum Reprod Update. 2006;12:417–35.
18. Meistrich ML, Mohapatra B, Shirley CR, Zhao M. Roles of transition nuclear proteins in spermiogenesis. Chromosoma. 2003;111:483–8.

19. Corzett M, Mazrimas J, Balhorn R. Protamine 1: protamine 2 stoichiometry in the sperm of eutherian mammals. Mol Reprod Dev. 2002;61:519–27.
20. Carrell DT, Liu L. Altered protamine 2 expression is uncommon in donors of known fertility, but common among men with poor fertilizing capacity, and may reflect other abnormalities of spermiogenesis. J Androl. 2001;22:604–10.
21. Torregrosa N, Domingues-Fandos D, Camejo MI, et al. Protamine 2 precursors, protamine 1/protamine 2 ratio, DNA integrity and other sperm parameters in infertile patients. Hum Reprod. 2006;21:2084–9.
22. Cree LH, Blahorn R, Brewer LR. Single molecule studies of DNA-protamine interactions. Protein Pept Lett. 2011;18:802–10.
23. Ward WS. Function of sperm chromatin structural elements in fertilization and development. Mol Hum Reprod. 2010;16:30–6.
24. Dominguez K, Arca CDR, Ward WS. The relationship between chromatin structure and DNA damage in mammalian spermatozoa. In: Zini A, Agarwal A, Editors. Sperm chromatin: biological and clinical applications in male infertility and assisted reproduction. New York: Springer; 2011. pp. 61–8.
25. Carrell DT, Emery BR, Hammoud S. The aetiology of sperm protamine abnormalities and their potential impact on the sperm epigenome. Int J Androl. 2008;31:537–45.
26. Hammoud SS, Nix DA, Zhang H, et al. Distinctive chromatin in human sperm packages genes for embryo development. Nature. 2009;460:473–8.
27. Arpanahi A, Brinkworth M, Iles D, et al. Endonuclease-sensitive regions of human spermatozoa chromatin are highly enriched in promoter and CTCF binding sequences. Genome Res. 2009;19:1338–49.
28. Ferlin A, Raicu F, Gatta V, Zuccarello D, Palka G, Foresta C. Male infertility: role of genetic background. Reprod Biomed Online. 2007;14:734–45.
29. Sun JG, Jurisicova A, Casper RF. Deletion of deoxyribonucleic acid fragmentation in human sperm: correlation with fertilization in vitro. Biol Reprod. 1997;56:602–7.
30. Evenson DP, Jost LK, Marshall D, et al. Utility of sperm chromatin structure assay as a diagnostic and prognostic tool in the human fertility clinic. Hum Reprod. 1999;14:1039–49.
31. Spano M, Bonde JP, Hjollund HI, Kolstad HA, Cordelli E, Leter G. Sperm chromatin damage impairs human fertility. Fertil Steril. 2000;73:43–50.
32. Agarwal A, Said TM. Role of sperm chromatin abnormalities and DNA damage in male infertility. Hum Reprod Update. 2003;9:331–45.
33. Bungum M, Humaidan P, Axmon A, et al. Sperm DNA integrity assessment in prediction of assisted reproduction technology outcome. Hum Reprod. 2007;22:174–9.
34. Virant-Klun I, Tomazevic T, Meden-Vrtovec H. Sperm single stranded DNA, detected by acridine orange staining, reduces fertilization and quality of ICSI derived embryos. J Assist Reprod Genet. 2002;19:319–28.
35. Gaspari L, Chang SS, Santella RM, et al. Polycyclic aromatic hydrocarbon-DNA adducts in human sperm as a marker of DNA damage and infertility. Mutat Res. 2003;535:155–60.
36. Frydman N, Prisant N, Hesters L, et al. Adequate ovarian follicular status does not prevent the decrease in pregnancy rates associated with high sperm DNA fragmentation. Fertil Steril. 2008;89:92–7.
37. Aitken RJ, de Iullis GN, McLachlan RI. Biological and clinical significance of DNA damage in the male germ line. Int J Androl. 2009;32:46–56.
38. Dada R, Thilagavathi J, Venkatesh S, et al. Genetic testing in male infertility. Open Reprod Sci J. 2011;3:42–56.
39. Georgiou I, Syrrou M, Pardalidis N, et al. Genetic and epigenetic risks of intracytoplasmic sperm injection method. Asian J Androl. 2006;8:643–73.
40. De Braekeeler M, Dao TN. Cytogenetic studies in male infertility: a review. Hum Reprod. 1991;6:245–50.
41. Conn CM, Cozzi J, Harper JC, Winston RM, Delhanty JD. Preimplantation genetic diagnosis for couples at high risk of Down syndrome pregnancy owing to parental translocation or mosaicism. J Med Genet. 1999;36:45–50.
42. Lishko PV, KirichokY. The role of Hv1 and CatSper channels in sperm activation. J Physiol. 2010;588:4667–72.
43. Carlson AE, Burnett LA, Del Camino D, et al. Pharmacological targeting of native CatSper channels reveals a required role in maintenance of sperm hyperactivation. PLoS ONE. 2009;4:e6844.
44. Wang H, Liu J, Cho KH, et al. A novel, single, transmembrane protein CATSPERG is associated with CATSPER1 channel protein. Biol Reprod. 2009;81:539–44.
45. Avenarius MR, Hildebrand MS, Zhang Y, et al. Human male infertility caused by mutations in the CATSPER1 channel protein. Am J Hum Genet. 2009;84:505–10.
46. Qi H, Moran MM, Navarro B, et al. All four CatSper ion channel proteins are required for male fertility and sperm cell hyperactivated motility. Proc Natl Acad Sci U S A. 2007;104:1219–23.
47. Venkatesh S, Deecaraman M, Kumar R, et al. Role of reactive oxygen species in the pathogenesis of mitochondrial DNA (mtDNA) mutations in male infertility. Indian J Med Res. 2009;129:127–37.
48. Richter C, Suter M, Walter PB. Mitochondrial free radical damage and DNA repair. Biofactors. 1998;7:207–8.
49. Wallace DC, Brown MD, Lott MT. Mitochondrial genetics. London: Churchill Livingstone; 1997.
50. Shamsi MB, Kumar R, Bhatt A, et al. Mitochondrial DNA mutations in etiopathogenesis of male infertility. Indian J Urol. 2008;24:150–4.
51. Jensen M, Leffers H, Petersen JH, et al. Frequent polymorphism of the mitochondrial DNA polymerase gamma gene (*POLG*) in patients with normal spermiograms and unexplained infertility. Hum Reprod. 2004;19:65–70.
52. Aitken RJ, Koppers AJ. Apoptosis and DNA damage in human spermatozoa. Asian J Androl. 2011;13:36–42.
53. Tease C, Fisher G. The influence of maternal age on radiation-induced chromosome aberrations in mouse oocytes. Mutat Res. 1991;262:57–62.
54. Aitken RJ, De Iullis GN. Value of DNA integrity assays for fertility evaluation. Soc Reprod Fertil. 2007;65(Suppl):81–92.
55. Bianchi PG, Manicardi GC, Bizzaro D, Bianchi U, Sakkas D. Effect of deoxyribonucleic acid protamination on fluorochrome staining and in situ nick-translation of murine and human mature spermatozoa. Biol Reprod. 1993;49:1083–8.
56. Zini A, Bielecki R, Phang D, Zenzes MT. Correlations between two markers of sperm DNA integrity, DNA denaturation and DNA fragmentation, in fertile and infertile men. Fertil Steril. 2001;75:674–7.
57. Potts RJ, Newbury CJ, Smith G, Notarianni LJ, Jefferies TM. Sperm chromatin damage associated with male smoking. Mutat Res. 1999;423:103–11.
58. Rajpurkar A, Jiang Y, Dhabuwala CB, Dunbar JC, Li H. Cigarette smoking induces apoptosis in rat testis. J Environ Pathol Toxicol Oncol. 2002;21:243–8.
59. Sepaniak S, Forges T, Gerard H, Foliguet B, Bene MC, Monnier-Barbarino P. The influence of cigarette smoking on human sperm quality and DNA fragmentation. Toxicology. 2006;223:54–60.
60. Esteves SC, Agarwal A. Novel concepts in male infertility. Int Braz J Urol. 2011;37:5–15.
61. Host E, Lindenberg S, Kahn JA, Christensen F. DNA strand breaks in human spermatozoa: a possible factor to be considered in couples suffering from unexplained infertility. Obstet Gynecol Scand. 1999;78:622–5.
62. Zini A, Fischer MA, Sharir S, Shayegan B, Phang D, Jarvi K. Prevalence of abnormal sperm DNA denaturation in fertile and infertile men. Urology. 2002;60:1069–72.

63. Saleh RA, Agarwal A, Nada EA, et al. Negative effects of increased sperm DNA damage in relation to seminal oxidative stress in men with idiopathic and male factor infertility. Fertil Steril. 2003;79:1597–605.
64. Kodama H, Yamaguchi R, Fukuda J, et al. Increased oxidative deoxyribonucleic acid damage in the spermatozoa of infertile male patients. Fertil Steril. 1997;68:519–24.
65. Bungum M, Bungum L, Giwercman A. Sperm chromatin structure assay (SCSA): a tool in diagnosis and treatment of infertility. Asian J Androl. 2011;13:69–75.
66. Moosani N, Pattinson H, Carter M, et al. Chromosomal analysis of sperm from men with idiopathic infertility using sperm karyotyping and fluorescence in situ hybridization. Fertil Steril. 1995;64:111–8.
67. Tempest HG, Martin RH. Cytogenetic risks in chromosomally normal infertile men. Curr Opin Obstet Gynecol. 2009;21:223–7.
68. Bonduelle M, Van Assche E, Jris H, et al. Prenatal testing in ICSI pregnancies: incidence of chromosomal anomalies in 1586 karyotypes and relation to sperm parameters. Hum Reprod. 2002;17:2600–14.
69. Devroey P, Van Steirteghem A. A review of ten years experience of ICSI. Hum Reprod Update. 2004;10:19–28.
70. Tempest HG, Griffin DK. The relationship between male infertility and increased levels of sperm disomy. Cytogenet Genome Res. 2004;107:83–94.
71. Benzacken B, Gavelle FM, Martin-Pont B, et al. Familial sperm polyploidy induced by genetic spermatogenesis failure: case report. Hum Reprod. 2001;16:2646–51.
72. Devillard F, Metzler-Guillemain C, Pelletier R, et al. Polyploidy in large head sperm: FISH study of three cases. Hum Reprod. 2002;17:1292–8.
73. Lewis-Jones I, Aziz N, Sheshadri S, et al. Sperm chromosomal abnormalities are linked to sperm morphological deformities. Fertil Steril. 2003;79:212–5.
74. Riggs AD, Martinssen RA, Russo VEA. Introduction. In: Russo VEA, Martienssen A, Riggs AD (eds) Epigenetic mechanism of gene regulation. Cold Spring Harbor: Cold Spring Harbor Press; 1996. pp. 1–4.
75. Herceg Z, Vaissiere T. Epigenetic mechanisms and cancer: an interface between the environment and the genome. Epigenetics. 2011;6:804–19.
76. Li ZX, Ma X, Wang ZH, et al. A differentially methylated region of the DAZ1 gene in spermatic and somatic cells. Asian J Androl. 2006;8:61–7.
77. Sathanathan AH, Ratnasooryia WD, de Silva PK, et al. Characterization of human gamete centrosomes for assisted reproduction. Ital J Anat Embryol. 2001;106:61–73.
78. Rawe VY, Terada Y, Nakamura S, et al. A pathology of the sperm centriole responsible for defective sperm aster formation, syngamy and cleavage. Hum Reprod. 2002;17:2344–9.
79. Palermo G, Munne S, Cohen J. The human zygote inherits its mitotic potential from the male gamete. Hum Reprod. 1994;9:1220–5.
80. Obasaju M, Kadam A, Sultan K, et al. Sperm quality may adversely affect the chromosome constitution of embryos that result from intracystoplasmic sperm injection. Fertil Steril. 1999;72:1113–5.
81. Emery BR, Carrell DT. The effect of epigenetic sperm abnormalities on early embryogenesis. Asian J Androl. 2006;8:131–42.
82. Kobayashi H, Sato A, Otsu E, et al. Aberrant DNA methylation of imprinted loci in sperm from oligospermic patients. Hum Mol Genet. 2007;16:2542–51.
83. Poplinsky A, Tüttelmann K, Kanber D, Horsthemke B, Gromoll J. Idiopathic male infertility is strongly associated with aberrant methylation of MEST and IGF2/H19 ICR1. Int J Androl. 2010;33:642–9.
84. Hajkova P, Erhardt S, Lane N, et al. Epigenetic reprogramming in mouse primordial germ cells. Mech Dev. 2002;117:15–23.
85. Reik W, Dean W, Walter J. Epigenetic reprogramming in mammalian development. Science. 2001;293:1089–93.
86. Sofikitis N, Miyagawa I, Yamamoto Y, et al. Micro-and macro-consequences of ooplasmic injections of early haploid male gametes. Hum Reprod Update. 1998;4:197–212.
87. Kimura Y, Yanagimachi R. Mouse oocytes injected with testicular spermatozoa or round spermatids can develop into normal offspring. Development. 1995;121:2397–405.
88. Martin C, Zhang Y. Mechanisms of epigenetic inheritance. Curr Opin Cell Biol. 2007;19:266–72.
89. Carrell DT, Emery BR, Hammoud S. Altered protamine expression and diminished spermatogenesis: what is the link? Hum Reprod Update. 2007;13:313–27.
90. Yu YE, Zhang Y, Unni E, et al. Abnormal spermatogenesis and reduced fertility in transition nuclear protein-1-deficient mice. Proc Natl Acad Sci U S A. 2000;97:4683–8.
91. Lee K, Haugen HS, Clegg CH, et al. Premature translation of protamine 1 mRNA causes precocious nuclear condensation and arrests spermatid differentiation in mice. Proc Natl Acad Sci U S A. 1995;92:12451–5.
92. Cho C, Jung-Ha H, Willis WD, et al. Protamine 2 deficiency leads to sperm DNA damage and embryo death in mice. Biol Reprod. 2003;69:211–7.
93. Yamauchi Y, Shaman JA, Ward WS. Non-genetic contributions of the sperm nucleus to embryo development. Asian J Androl. 2011;13:31–5.
94. Nanassy L, Carrell DT. Paternal effects on early embryogenesis. J Exp Clin Assist Reprod. 2008;5:2.
95. Zalenskaya IA, Zalensky AO. Telomeres in mammalian male germline cells. Int Rev Cytol. 2002;218:37–67.
96. Hemann MT, Rudolph KL, Strong MA, et al. Telomere dysfunction triggers developmentally regulated germ cell apoptosis. Mol Biol Cell. 2001;12:2023–30.
97. Liu L, Blasco M, Trimarchi J, et al. An essential role for functional telomeres in mouse germ cells during fertilization and early development. Dev Biol. 2002;249:74–84.
98. Erenpreiss J, Spano M, Erenpreiss J, Bungum M, Giwercman A. Sperm chromatin structure and male fertility: biological and clinical aspects. Asian J Androl. 2006;8:11–29.
99. Bell JT, Spector TD. A twin approach to unraveling epigenetics. Trends Genet. 2011;27:116–25.
100. Fernandes JL, Muriel L, Goyanes V, et al. Simple determination of human sperm DNA fragmentation with an improved sperm chromatin dispersion test. Fertil Steril. 2005;84:833–42.
101. Absalan F, Ghannadi A, Kazerooni M, et al. Value of sperm chromatin dispersion test in couples with unexplained recurrent abortion. J Assist Reprod Genet. 2012;29:11–4.
102. Duran EH, Morshedi M, Taylor S, Oehninger S. Sperm DNA quality predicts intrauterine insemination outcome: a prospective cohort study. Hum Reprod. 2002;17:3122–8.
103. Hansen RS, Laird CD. A new regulatory pathway for fragile syndrome? Nat Med. 2002;8:1204–5.
104. Edwards RG. Genetics, epigenetics and gene silencing in differentiating mammalian embryos. Reprod Biomed Online. 2006;13:732–53.
105. Robinson L, Gallos ID, Rajkhowa M, et al. The effect of sperm DNA fragmentation on miscarriage rates: a systematic review and meta-analysis. Hum Reprod. 2012;27: 2908–17.
106. Grecco E, Scarselli F, Iacobelli M, et al. Efficient treatment of infertility due to sperm DNA damage by ICSI with testicular spermatozoa. Hum Reprod. 2005;20:226–30.
107. Dada R, Shamsi MB, Venkatesh S. Attenuation of oxidative stress & DNA damage in varicocelectomy: implications in infertility management. Indian J Med Res. 2010;132:728–30.
108. Esteves SC, Oliveira FV, Bertolla RP. Clinical outcome of intracystoplasmic sperm injection in infertile men with treated and untreated clinical varicocele. J Urol. 2010;184:1442–6.

109. Esteves SC, Hamada A, Kondray V, et al. What every gynecologist should know about male infertility: an update. Arch Gynecol Obstet. 2012;286:217–29.
110. Ostermeier GC, Dix DJ, Miller D, et al. Spermatozoal RNA profiles of normal fertile men. Lancet. 2002;360:772–7.
111. Garrido N, Martínez-Conejero JA, Jauregui J, et al. Microarray analysis in sperm from fertile and infertile men without basic sperm analysis abnormalities reveals a significantly different transcriptome. Fertil Steril. 2009;91:1307–10.
112. Bonache S, Mata A, Ramos MD, Bassas L, Larriba S. Sperm gene expression profile is related to pregnancy rate after insemination and is predictive of low fecundity in normozoospermic men. Hum Reprod. 2012;27:1556–67.
113. Garrido N, Garcia-Herrero S, Meseguer M. Assessment of sperm using mRNA microarray technology. Fertil Steril. 2013;99:1008–22.

Role of the Immune System in Unexplained Male Infertility

9

Rajesh K. Naz and Walter K. H. Krause

Immune System and Spermatogenesis

The testis is an immunologically privileged organ. During puberty, when spermatogenesis starts, several "nonself" antigens develop on the later stages of germ cell formation (secondary pachytene stage onwards) that were not present when the immune system was developing a recognition of the "self" antigens in the fetal life. These "nonself" antigens/sperm are sequestered from the immune attack by the development of the blood–testis barrier, which is primarily formed by tight Sertoli cell junctions. Besides the blood–testis barrier, there are additional mechanisms that contribute toward the uniquely protected environment of the testis [1]. When the blood–testis barrier is compromised by factors such as infection and/or inflammation, "nonself" antigens present on sperm could induce an autoimmune response. The mechanism involved in this may be equated to the "danger model" [2]. This model proposes that stressed and necrotic cells release "danger" signals such as heat shock proteins (HSP) that could trigger an autoimmune response. Indeed, HSP60 and HSP70 have been identified as autoantigens in the testis. Dendritic cells (DCs) are usually involved in the antigen presentation for activation of naive B and T cells. It is hypothesized that immature DCs, that are normally involved in maintaining immune privilege, mature under inflammatory pathological conditions and overcome the immune privilege/tolerance by the local activation and expansion of autoreactive T cells [1]. In the experimental autoimmune orchitis (EAO) of rats, the number of DCs in the testicular interstitium was found to increase during the course of EAO [3]. Several T cell subsets (CD4+ and CD8+ αβ T cells and γδ T cells) and natural killer (NK) cells exist in normal testicular interstitium. These cells are involved in the regulation of immune response and immune modulation in the testis [3]. Testicular mast cells (MCs) are found adjacent to the seminiferous tubules in the testis. Activated MCs also coincide with elevated numbers of several types of immune cells in the testis of infertile men and may, therefore, also be involved in the pathogenesis of testicular inflammatory process [4].

Sertoli cells are one of the most interesting cell types, playing a role both in reproduction and immunological reaction in the testis. They act as nutritive cells for the developing spermatogenetic cell lineage and are responsible for the formation of blood–testis barrier. There is also increasing evidence of their role in immunoregulatory function in the testis [5]. Sertoli cells produce a number of immunoregulatory mediators including TGF-β, which is thought to play a major role in immunosuppression. The communication between germ and Sertoli cells appears to involve the same mechanism(s) that overlap with the inflammatory processes in infectious diseases. This link may partly explain how the immunologic spermatogenic disruption may be caused by inflammation and infection.

Finally, the apoptosis of spermatogenic cells, which is an integral part of normal spermatogenesis, is enhanced during the breach of the immune privilege of the testis such as in EAO. Proinflammatory cytokines (TNF-α and IL-6) and

R. K. Naz (✉)
Department of Obstetrics and Gynecology, West Virginia University School of Medicine, HSC North, Room 2085, 1 Medical Center Drive, Morgantown, WV 26506, USA
e-mail: rnaz@hsc.wvu.edu

W. K. H. Krause
Deptartment of Dermatology and Allergology, University Hospital, Philipp University, Deutschhausstr. 9, 35033 Marburg, Germany
e-mail: krause@med.uni-marburg.de

G. L. Schattman et al. (eds.), *Unexplained Infertility*, DOI 10.1007/978-1-4939-2140-9_9,

Fas ligand, produced by interstitial mononuclear cells during EAO development, may contribute to the increased germ cell apoptosis [3]. Although EAO is not commonly observed in humans, some of the mechanisms observed in the experimental condition may be the basis of spermatogenic failure observed in male infertile patients.

Antisperm Antibodies (ASAs)

The phenomenon most commonly observed in immune infertility is the antibodies directed against fertility-related antigens of sperm proteome. ASAs are found in 9–12.8% of infertile couples. The presence of ASAs indicates a relative decrease of fertility. However, ASAs are also present in approximately 1–2.5% of fertile men and in 4% of fertile women [6, 7]. The presence of ASAs in the fertile population suggests that not all ASAs cause infertility [8–10]. These antibodies may be called "sperm-reactive" immunoglobulins since they do not contribute to the phenomenon of immune infertility. ASAs are usually sperm-specific; thus, the presence of ASAs does not exert in most cases any harmful effect on patients, except for infertility.

The formation of fertility-related ASAs requires an immune reaction directed against sperm antigens, which are involved in the sperm motility, function, and fertilization process. The antigens which are present on the sperm surface, externalized on the surface after sperm acrosome exocytosis, and/or involved in oocyte binding and penetration are most relevant in immunoinfertility. The fertility-related sperm antigens are proteins/glycoproteins that develop during later stages of spermatogenesis and/or those which are absorbed on the surface during the transit in the genital tract. These antigens are not present during fetal development when the immune tolerance was developing by clonal selection and propogation. They develop later in life during puberty, thus, are recognized as "nonself" and able to induce an immune response.

ASAs can be directed to the peptide moiety or carbohydrate epitopes of the sperm proteins/glycoproteins. The antigenic component of sperm immobilizing antibodies that are primarily detected in the serum of infertile women is in the carbohydrate moieties of CD52, a GPI anchor glycoprotein, expressed in lymphocytes and various components of the male genital tract, including sperm and seminal plasma [11].

The site of formation in the genital tract of the spontaneously occurring ASAs in infertile men is unclear. However, some indications can be drawn from the findings on the risk factors involved in ASAs induction (Table 9.1). ASAs can be present circulating in the serum and/or locally in the genital tract secretions such as seminal plasma, cervical mucus, vaginal secretion, and fallopian fluid. The immunoglobulin G (IgG) antibodies in semen and other genital tract secretions are mainly transudate of the serum IgG. The immunoglobulin A (IgA) antibodies, however, can originate locally and/or transudate from serum [12].

Risk Factors of ASAs Formation

The obstruction/leakage/infection/inflammation of the testis, and especially the epididymis and vas deferens, frequently induces high titers of ASAs [13–17]. Between 50 and 100% of men that undergo vasectomies subsequently develop ASAs in serum and semen [17]. Following vasectomy, sperm granuloma frequently develops in epididymal distension results due to increased intraluminal pressure. The sperm granuloma is a dynamic structure where active phagocytosis occurs by macrophages. It is plausible that the immune process inducing ASAs production initiates here, since T cells have also been observed.

ASAs can penetrate from circulation into the male genital tract via rete testis, epididymis, vas deferens, and accessory glands. They can attach to sperm at any of these regions after transudation. In spermatozoa retrieved directly from the distal end of the vas deferens in patients undergoing vasectomy reversal (vasovasostomy), ASAs, both IgG and IgA, were present in 78.6 and 32.1% of the patients, respectively [18].

The infection and/or inflammation of the male genital tract can cause ASAs formation; however, the data are inconsistent. Jarow et al. [19] described a positive association between prostatitis and ASAs using the gel agglutination assay in serum. In a series of 365 patients with documented inflammation/infection of the male genital tract,

Table 9.1 Risk factors involved in the development of antisperm antibodies (ASAs) in men. (Based on data from ref. [98])

Condition	Induction of ASAs	Site of induction
Chronic obstruction of genital tract/vasectomy	Proven	Epididymis/vas deferens
Varicocele	Doubtful	Testis
Cryptorchidism	Doubtful	Testis
Testis trauma, testis surgery	No risk factor	–
Testicular torsion	No risk factor	–
Testis tumor	Doubtful	Testis
Intrarectal sperm contact	Doubtful	Rectal mucosa

suffering from—in accordance to the American Urological Association definition—chronic bacterial prostatitis, inflammatory chronic prostatitis/chronic pelvic pain syndrome, noninflammatory chronic pelvic pain syndrome, chronic urethritis, and chronic epididymitis, no association between ASAs formation/titers and the intensity of these diseases was demonstrable [20].

Immunological cross-reactivity between antigens of the sperm membrane and *Chlamydia trachomatis* may occur and explain some cases of an association between infections and ASAs formation [20]. Epitopes of chlamydial HSP60 protein cross-react with those of human HSP60. However, clinical data fail to detect an association between chlamydial infections and the presence of ASAs in seminal plasma [21].

It is unclear whether varicocele, testicular trauma, surgery, or testicular torsion can induce ASAs formation. Also, the association between cryptorchidism and ASAs remains controversial [17].

Although suggested by epidemiologic studies, the direct proof of ASAs as a cause of infertility is difficult to obtain, since prospective studies comparing pregnancies in patients with and without ASAs are limited [22–24]. In the retrospective studies, the degree of sperm autoimmunization showed a significant inverse correlation with the incidence of spontaneous pregnancies. In the first report by Rumke et al. [25] using a 10-year follow-up of 254 infertile men with serum sperm-agglutinating activity, the ASAs titers were found to be inversely correlated with the occurrence of spontaneous pregnancies. If only normozoospermic men were included, no pregnancy was observed with very high ASAs titers. In a cohort of 108 infertile couples, the pregnancy rates were significantly higher when males had low antibody titers than in those with high titers [6]. In another set of 157 infertile couples, the cumulative spontaneous pregnancy rates over 6 years were higher (~50%) when the IBT results were < 0.50%; lower (~30%) when test results were 50–90%; and very low (~15%) when the test showed > 90% ASAs binding in IBT [26]. A significant inverse correlation between the degree of sperm autoimmunization and pregnancy rates after vasovasostomy was observed in a follow-up study of 216 men [27]. However, this observation was not confirmed by others [28].

Tests for ASAs

Mixed Antiglobulin Reaction (MAR) Test

The MAR test detects antibodies bound to spermatozoa. The technique is simple: a semen sample is mixed with a suspension of particles, which are conjugated to immunoglobulins, which is a second antibody against human immunoglobulins present on sperm. If ASAs are present on spermatozoa, the particles get attached to the spermatozoa, which can be easily seen under the microscope. As a test result, the percentage of motile sperm bearing the particles is counted. A MAR test is considered positive when > 10% of sperm are attached to a particle and is of clinical significance when > 80% binding is present.

The MAR test is easy to perform, reproduce, and the results are apparent within a few minutes. Different IgG classes can be detected using this test. The test has some limitations; it is difficult to perform when the sperm are fewer in number and immotile, such as in oligozoospermia and asthenozoospermia, and it requires fresh semen samples [29]. Commercially available SpermMar kits are based on an antiserum against human IgG to induce mixed agglutination between antibody-coated and latex beads conjugated with antihuman immunoglobulin [30].

The MAR test can also be used to detect ASAs present in biological fluids such as serum and seminal plasma. In the first step, donor sperm are mixed with the fluid and then the sperm undergo the MAR test as described above (indirect MAR test). The reproducibility of the indirect MAR test using different donor sperm is poor [31].

Quality control of the MAR test comprises inter- and intra-assay variations. It was shown that the intra-assay variation is minimum if different tests are performed using the same spermatozoa. However, an interassay comparison of tests using spermatozoa from different donors' reveals poor congruence [31].

Immunobead Binding Test (IBT)

The IBT is similar to the MAR test and is easy to perform. The IBT allows determination of the antibody class attached to spermatozoa, the subcellular localization of the antibodies attached, and the percentage of antibody-coated sperm. When performing the test, sperm concentration is usually adjusted to $10–25 \times 10^6$ motile sperm/ml to optimize the microscopic evaluation. Like the MAR test, the IBT can also be performed indirectly using biological fluids. It was shown that the indirect IBT has a low intra-assay and a high interassay variation [32].

Both the MAR test and IBT are recommended by the World Health Organization (WHO) manual [33]. The MAR test does not require washing spermatozoa of the seminal plasma, which makes it easier and faster than IBT. It requires less semen volume and could be applied to samples with a lower sperm concentration compared to IBT [34]. Comparison of IBT and MAR tests has shown a high degree of agreement [30, 35]. The sensitivity and specificity are comparable between these two tests [36].

The existing consensus indicates that a semen sample having > 50% of spermatozoa showing binding in MAR test or IBT is suggestive of ASAs-mediated immunoinfertility [33]. There is no correlation between the test positivity and the sperm concentration, motility, and morphology and leukocyte concentration in the semen. However, ASAs levels are usually higher in men with abnormal sperm parameters than in those with normozoospermia. The MAR test results were found positive in 48 of 484 men (10%) with normal sperm counts, 18 of 78 of men (23%) with low sperm motility, and 19 of 128 of men (15%) with low counts. The presence of antibodies in about 10% of men may provide additional information besides the semen parameters in some cases of unexplained infertility [37].

Enzyme-Linked Immunosorbent Assay (ELISA)

The visualization of antigen–antibody binding by chromogens amplified by an enzyme is an elegant method to demonstrate the presence of specific antibodies and also allows the determination of an antibody titer. In ELISA, either the antigen or the antibody is fixed to a solid phase. It requires information on the specificity of antibodies and antigens. This prerequisite is not completely fulfilled in the determination of ASAs using ELISA, since all antigens against which the ASAs are directed to have not been defined. The tests that are marketed measure the binding of antibodies to sperm extracts containing several antigens. Thus, they are of limited application for the diagnosis of ASAs-associated infertility since only the antigens relevant to fertility are important in immunoinfertility. This is also true for radioimmunoassay (RIA), which requires the use of radioactive materials [36].

Flow Cytometry

Flow cytometry is used to detect, isolate, and quantitate the percentage of sperm bound with antibodies [38]. However, flow cytometry requires expensive laboratory instruments and reveals limited results without providing specificity of ASAs for fertility-related antigens.

Treatment of Immune Infertility

Immunosuppressive Therapy with Glucocorticosteroids

Although an interesting concept, the use of glucocorticosteroids to lower the antibody titer could have potential adverse effects, associated with generalized immunosuppression. To minimize the side effects, it is usually restricted to the first 7–10 days of the female cycle, irrespective of whether the steroids are given to a male or female partner of an infertile couple. Steroid therapy to suppress ASAs was first recommended by Hendry et al. [39]. They reported an increased conception rate in the steroid-treated group compared to the placebo group. Later on, several studies were published in which corticosteroids did not show an effect on ASAs titers, sperm parameters, or conception rate [9, 38–46] (Table 9.2).

Table 9.2 Randomized trials measuring the effect of corticosteroids on antisperm antibodies (ASAs). (Based on data from ref. [98])

Patient number	Treatment	Effect on ASAs	Effect on fertility	Adverse effect(s)	Reference
10	T: Prednisolone, 1 mg/kg/d, 9 d C: Placebo	None	No difference in CR	No data	De Almeida et al. [40]
43	T: Methylprednisolone, 96 mg/d, 9 d C: Placebo	None	No difference in CR	No data	Haas and Manganiello [41]
43	T: Prednisolone, 20 mg/d cyclic C: Placebo	No data	9 conceptions 1 conception	~60% mild reaction	Hendry et al. [39]
20	T: Prednisolone, 40 mg cyclic+TI C: Placebo	Significant reduction	0 conceptions 0 conceptions	~40% mild reaction	Bals-Pratsch et al. [42]
30	T: corticosteroids+IUI C: corticosteroids+TI	Significant reduction	11 pregnancies 2 pregnancies	No data	Robinson et al. [43]
46	T: Prednisolone, 20 mg/d+IUI C: Prednisolone, 20 mg/d+TI	–	9 pregnancies 1 pregnancy	No data	Lahteenmaki et al. [44]
ND	T: Prednisolone, 20 mg/d C: Placebo	Significant reduction	No data	No data	Räsänen et al. [38]
36	T: Corticosteroids+IUI C: IUI only	No data	16.1% CR 21.2% CR	No data	Grigoriou et al. [45]
53	T: Prednisolone, 20 mg/d, 2 weeks prior to IVF C: no treatment	None	29% CR 32% CR	No data	Lahteenmaki et al. [46]
77	T: Prednisolon, 5 mg/d C: no treatment	No data	20% CR 5% CR	None	Omu et al. [9]

ND not defined, *T* treatment group, *C* control group, *CR* conception rate, *IUI* intrauterine insemination, *TI* timed intercourse

For this reason, the therapy is no longer used for treatment of immune infertility.

In-Vitro Techniques

The following in-vitro techniques have been tried to inhibit binding or remove the antibodies bound to the sperm surface.

Prevention of ASAs Binding to Sperm

The assumption that ASAs bind to sperm during and/or just after ejaculation and that the antibodies are mostly present in the secretions of prostate and seminal vesicles prompted trials with split ejaculations. However, this technique has been proven ineffective in decreasing ASAs binding to sperm [47]. It was examined if the collection of semen into insemination medium containing a high concentration of fetal cord/maternal serum would decrease the antibody binding to sperm. Two studies [48, 49] observed that semen collection into serum-supplemented medium resulted in increased fertilization rates in in vitro fertilization (IVF) procedure, and one of these studies also showed an increase in pregnancy rates [50]. Experimental studies [50] showed that the antibodies preferentially transude into the epididymis (especially corpus or caudal regions) and vas deferens, and not into testes to bind to sperm cells [50]. These findings indicate that in men, ASAs bind to sperm before ejaculation via transudation through epididymis, vas deferens, and probably rete testis.

Immunomagnetic Separation Technique

This technique has been tried to separate the antibodies bound on the sperm surface [51]. The sperm with antibodies are tagged with anti-immunoglobulin antibodies coupled to magnetic microspheres, and then the magnetic field is applied. However, limited success in isolating a sufficient number of ASAs-free sperm having good motility makes this procedure theoretically interesting, but clinically unacceptable.

Removing ASAs Bound on Sperm Surface

There are mixed reports on simple sperm washing on ASAs elution from various laboratories. Adeghe found that washing decreased IgG bound on the sperm surface [52]. Other groups did not find the similar positive effects [53], even after subjecting the sperm to multiple washings [54]. Antibodies were also not reduced by passing sperm through a percoll gradient [55].

The protease treatment can be used to degrade antibodies on the sperm surface [56]. IgA1 protease treatment was effective in reducing IgA on sperm [57]. In another study, incubation of sperm with chymotrypsin before intrauterine insemination (IUI) resulted in a 25% cycle fecundity versus 3% in controls [58]. IUI with protein digestive enzyme treatment was more effective than IUI without enzymatic therapy. However, IVF with ICSI provided three times the pregnancy rate for males with sperm coated in ASAs than IUI with chymotrypsin-treated sperm [59].

The clinical efficacy of proteolytic enzymes has to be examined since it may affect proteins present on the sperm surface, especially the oocyte binding receptors.

The use of immunobeads has been suggested as a treatment to remove the sperm-bound antibodies. It has been reported that simple incubation of ASAs-positive sperm from immunoinfertile men with immunobeads results in a time-dependent decrease in antibody concentration on sperm surface [51] and even enhanced pregnancies [60]. The explanation that the antibodies are removed from the sperm surface after incubation with immunobeads is not widely accepted. It is generally believed that the immunobeads just select ASAs-positive sperm, leaving ASAs-free sperm. This procedure does not remove the antibodies from the sperm surface.

Immunoelution of Bound ASAs Using Defined Sperm Antigens

Fertilization antigen-1 (FA-1) antigen is a well-defined sperm-specific surface molecule that is evolutionarily conserved on sperm of various mammalian species, including men [50]. Antibodies to an FA-1 antigen inhibit human sperm–zona interaction, and also block human sperm capacitation/acrosome reaction by inhibiting tyrosine phosphorylation [61]. The cDNA encoding for mouse FA-1 and human FA-1 have been cloned and sequenced [62]. Vaccination of female mice with recombinant FA-1 antigen causes a long-term reversible contraception by raising sperm-specific immune response [63].

FA-1 antigen is involved in human immunoinfertility in both men and women. The antibodies are found in sera as circulating antibodies and also locally in genital tract secretions, such as seminal plasma of men, and cervical mucus and vaginal secretions of women [64]. The lymphocytes from immunoinfertile, but not fertile, men and women are sensitized against FA-1 antigen and proliferate on incubation with the antigen in vitro [65].

The presence of these antibodies inhibits fertilization in IVF procedure. The involvement of FA-1 antigen in human involuntary immunoinfertility has been confirmed in several laboratories by leading investigators working in the field of ASAs. Based upon these findings, a clinical trial was conducted at the University of Michigan Medical School to determine whether immunoadsorption with FA-1 antigen would remove autoantibodies from sperm surface of immunoinfertile men [66]. Adsorption with FA-1 antigen increased immunobead-free swimming sperm on an average of 50 and 76% for IgA ASAs and IgG ASAs, respectively. The acrosome reaction rates increased significantly and showed improvement in 78% of the sperm samples after FA-1 adsorption. The IUI of FA-1 treated antibody-free sperm resulted in normal pregnancies and healthy babies, indicating that the antigen treatment does not have a deleterious effect on implantation or embryonic and fetal development. This study needs to be extended to a larger number of ASAs-positive infertile men and constitutes an exciting therapeutic modality using well-defined sperm antigens.

Assisted Reproductive Techniques (ART)

Various ART have been used for the treatment of immunoinfertility.

Intrauterine Insemination Procedure

IUI has been found to enhance the pregnancy rates in some cases of ASAs-positive infertile men. The results are summarized in Table 9.3 [58, 67–69]. The results do not indicate a definite advantage of the procedure. It is not clear how IUI can improve fertility outcome when ASAs are present in men. Washing the sperm in the incubation medium should not elute the antibodies bound to the sperm surface proteins. It appears likely that the procedure is of benefit because the subfertility has another etiology rather than the presence of ASAs.

In Vitro Fertilization Procedure

The IVF procedure has been used for the treatment of immunoinfertility. A number of studies have been published comparing the outcome of IVF in men with or without ASAs. They are summarized in Table 9.4 [51, 70–84]. Several studies have shown decreased fertilization rates in immunoinfertile patients in IVF procedure. Some studies also found a correlation of the effect of antibodies on the fertilization rates with the antibody class/subclass and the sperm-binding sites of ASAs. The quality of embryos obtained after IVF using sperm from ASAs-positive men is generally poor compared to those obtained after fertilization with sperm from ASAs-negative men.

Intracytoplasmic Sperm Injection (ICSI) Procedure

The ICSI procedure has been used to treat immunoinfertility in men. Several studies have been conducted to compare the fertilization rates after ICSI in men with or without ASAs. The Table 9.5 [85–92] summarizes the studies reported in the literature. Most of these studies did not find a difference in

Table 9.3 Studies comparing the pregnancy rates after intrauterine insemination (IUI) with sperm from men with or without antisperm antibodies (ASAs)

Number of patients/cycles	Pregnancy rate with ASAs	Pregnancy rate without ASAs	Reference (#)
59 couples	56%	83%	Check and Bollendorf [67]
110 cycles	0%	25.6%	Francavilla et al. [68]
159 couples	33%	21%	Agarwal [58]
804 cycles	8.6%	1.7% with timed intercourse	Mahmoud et al. [69]

Table 9.4 Studies comparing the outcome in in vitro fertilization (IVF) using sperm from men with or without antisperm antibodies (ASAs)

Number of couples/cycles	Fertilization/pregnancy rate with ASAs	Fertilization/pregnancy rate without ASAs (%)	Reference (#)
17 couples	27%	72	Clarke et al. [70]
40 couples	34%	74	Mandelbaum et al. [71]
20 couples	14%	60	de Almeida et al. [72]
36 couples	50.5%	72.7	Rajah et al. [73]
67 cycles	41.9%	73.1	Acosta et al. [74]
63 couples	25%	68	Ford et al. [51]
72 couples	Significantly reduced ($p > 0.001$)	–	Junk et al. [75]
137 couples	Significantly reduced	–	Chang et al. [76]
67 couples	18%	0	Witkin et al. [77]
343	59%	52	Pagidas et al. [78]
160 couples	75%	69.3	Sukcharoen and Keith [79]
181 oocytes	44.2%	84.4	Vazquez-Levin et al. [80]
52 couples	28.6%	28.9	Vujisić et al. [81]
Not described	No significant difference	–	Janssen et al. [82]
24 cycles	No significant difference	–	Zouari et al. [83]
80 cycles	No significant difference	–	Yeh et al. [84]

Table 9.5 Studies comparing the outcome in intracytoplasmic sperm injection (ICSI) using sperm from men with or without antisperm antibodies (ASAs)

Number of couples/cycles	Fertilization/pregnancy rate with ASAs (%)	Fertilization/pregnancy rate without ASAs (%)	Reference (#)
48 couples	79	68	Zini et al. [91]
55 cycles	75.0	69.2	Nagy et al. [85]
179 couples	62	58	Clarke et al. [86]
60 cycles	60.3	60.7	Jun et al. [87]
279 cycles	36	39	Mercan et al. [88]
351 cycles	82.4	80.0	Javed and Naz. [92]
87 couples	56	55	Check et al. [89]
Not described	42	52	Zini et al. [90]

the fertilization rates after ICSI using sperm from men with or without ASAs. It may be concluded from the studies that ICSI is the most effective therapy for male immunoinfertility. The conclusion is also drawn by Zini et al. [91].

One study is worth discussing here; it included 29 ASAs-positive infertile couples, where 22 of them were tested before IVF procedure and had a poor fertilization rate (6%) [93]. These couples were then subjected to ICSI procedure. After ICSI, the fertilization (79%) and cleavage (89%) rates in the ASAs-positive group were similar to those (68 and 93%, respectively) in the ASAs-negative group. Surprisingly, 46% of the pregnancies in the ASAs-positive group ended in spontaneous pregnancy loss, compared with none in the ASAs-negative group. This indicates that ICSI can bypass the ASAs involved in fertilization, but can still affect postfertilization events.

Some ASAs can have deleterious postfertilization effects on developing preimplantation embryos [94–96]. ASAs can affect early embryonic development if: (1) an oocyte is fertilized with a sperm cell which carries these specific antibodies into the ooplasm, and/or (2) these antibodies are cross reactive with the antigens present on the developing embryos. Some of these antigens and antibodies have been characterized, and the cDNA encoding for a few of these antigens has also been cloned and sequenced [92]. Using the ICSI procedure in immunoinfertile men, one can achieve higher fertilization rates than using the IVF procedure. However, the fertilized zygotes show higher degeneration and mortality and decreased embryonic development [97].

Conclusion

In conclusion, the immune system plays an important role in male infertility. The testis is an immune-privileged site. Sperm cell has several "nonself" antigens that develop during later stages of spermatogenesis. These "nonself" antigens are sequestered from the immune attack by the blood–testis barrier. The most frequent phenomenon of immune pathology in infertility is the development of antibodies directed to these "nonself" antigens that are relevant to sperm motility, function, fertilization, and fertility. There are several etiological factors and sites in the male genital tract that can induce antibodies to sperm. The ASAs can be detected by various methods, including the MAR test, IBT, and ELISA [98]. The presence of ASAs has been shown to reduce fertilization rates in the IVF procedure used for the treatment of male infertility. For the treatment of immunoinfertility, the suppression of antibody production using steroids (glucocorticoids) has not yielded successful results. Several in-vitro methods have been used to remove antibodies bound to sperm for treatment. The ICSI technique has been successfully used to bypass sperm antibodies that are relevant to fertilization. However, the embryos may degenerate even after successful fertilization. The available data indicates that immunological factors, including ASAs, play an important role in pathogenesis of unexplained male infertility. As additional fertility-related sperm antigens and mechanisms become delineated, a larger subgroup of "unexplained infertility" is becoming a part of "immunoinfertility."

References

1. Fijak M, Bhushan S, Meinhardt A. Immunoprivileged sites: the testis. Methods Mol Biol. 2011;677:459–70.
2. Matzinger, P. Tolerance, danger, and the extended family. Annu Rev Immunol. 1994;12:991–1045.
3. Jacobo P, Guazzone VA, Theas MS, Lustig L. Testicular autoimmunity. Autoimmun Rev. 2011 Feb;10(4):201–4. (Epub 2010 Oct 14).
4. Haidl G, Duan YG, Chen SJ, Kohn FM, Schuppe HC, Allam JP. The role of mast cells in male infertility. Expert Rev Clin Immunol. 2011 Sep;7(5):627–34.
5. Bhushan S, Schuppe HC, Fijak M, Meinhardt A. Testicular infection: microorganisms, clinical implications and host-pathogen interaction. J Reprod Immunol. 2009 Dec;83(1–2):164–7.
6. Ayvaliotis B, Bronson RA, Rosenfeld D, et al. Conception rates in couples where autoimmunity to sperm is detected. Fertil Steril. 1985;43(5):739–42.

7. Collins JA, Burrows EA, Yeo J, et al. Frequency and predictive value of antisperm antibodies among infertile couples. Hum Reprod. 1993;8(4):592–8.
8. Heidenreich A, Bonfig R, Wilbert DM, et al. Risk factors for antisperm antibodies in infertile men. Am J Reprod Immunol. 1994;31(2–3):69–76.
9. Omu AE, al-Qattan F, Abdul Hamada B. Effect of low dose continuous corticosteroid therapy in men with antisperm antibodies on spermatozoal quality and conception rate. Eur J Obstet Gynecol Reprod Biol. 1996;69(2):129–34.
10. Sinisi AA, Di Finizio B, Pasquali D, et al. Prevalence of antisperm antibodies by SpermMARtest in subjects undergoing a routine sperm analysis for infertility. Int J Androl. 1993;16(5):311–4.
11. Hasegawa A, Koyama K. Sperm-immobilizing antibody and its target antigen (CD52). In: Krause WKH, Naz RK, Editors. Immune infertility. Berlin: Springer Verlag; 2009. pp. 131–42.
12. Yin X, Ouyang S, Xu W, et al. YWK-II protein as a novel G(o)-coupled receptor for Müllerian inhibiting substance in cell survival. J Cell Sci. 2007;120(Pt 9):1521–8.
13. Gubin DA, Dmochowski R, Kutteh WH. Multivariant analysis of men from infertile couples with and without antisperm antibodies. Am J Reprod Immunol. 1998;39(2):157–60.
14. Jarow JP, Sanzone JJ. Risk factors for male partners antisperm antibodies. J Urol. 1992;148(6):1805–7.
15. Lee R, Goldstein M, Ullery B, et al. Value of serum antisperm antibodies in diagnosing obstructive azoospermia. J Urol. 2009;181(1):264–9.
16. Marconi M, Nowotny A, Pantke P, et al. Antisperm antibodies detected by mixed agglutination reaction and immunobead test are not associated with inflammation and infection of the seminal tract. Andrologia. 2008;40(4):227–34.
17. Marconi M, Weidner W. Site and risk factors of antisperm antibodies production in the male population. In: Krause WKH, Naz RK, Editors. Immune infertility. Berlin: Springer Verlag; 2009. pp. 97–110.
18. Wen RQ, Li SQ, Wang CX, et al. Analysis of spermatozoa from the proximal vas deferens of vasectomized men. Int J Androl. 1994;17(4):181–5.
19. Jarow JP, Kirkland JA, Assimos DG. Association of antisperm antibodies with chronic non bacterial prostatitis. Urology. 1990;36(2):154–6.
20. Marconi M, Pilatz A, Wagenlehner F, et al. Are really antisperm antibodies associated with proven chronic inflammatory and infectious diseases of the male reproductive tract? Eur Urol. 2009;56(4):708–15.
21. Eggert-Kruse W, Rohr G, Demirakca T, et al. Chlamydial serology in 1303 asymptomatic subfertile couples. Hum Reprod. 1997;12(7):1464–75.
22. Witkin SS, David SS. Effect of sperm antibodies on pregnancy outcome in a subfertile population. Am J Obstet Gynecol. 1988;158(1):59–62.
23. Eggert-Kruse W, Christmann WM, Gerhard I. Circulating antisperm antibodies and fertility prognosis: a prospective study. Hum Reprod. 1989;4(5):513–20.
24. Francavilla F, Baronetti A. Male autoimmune infertility.In: Krause WKH, Naz RK, Editors. Immune infertility. Berlin: Springer Verlag; 2009. pp. 145–54.
25. Rumke PH, Van Amstel N, Messer EN, et al. Prognosis of fertility of men with sperm agglutinins in the serum. Fertil Steril. 1974;25(5):393–8.
26. Abshagen K, Behre HM, Cooper TG, et al. Influence of sperm surface antibodies on spontaneous pregnancy rates. Fertil Steril. 1998;70(2):355–6.
27. Meinertz H, Linnet L, Fogh-Andersen P, et al. Antisperm antibodies and fertility after vasovasostomy: a followup study of 216 men. Fertil Steril. 1990;54(2):315–21.
28. Matson PL, Junk SM, Masters JR, et al. The incidence and influence upon fertility of antisperm antibodies in seminal fluid following vasectomy reversal. Int J Androl. 1989;12(2):98–103.
29. Jager S, Kremer J, van Slochteren-Draaisma T. A simple method of screening for antisperm antibodies in the human male. Detection of spermatozoal surface IgG with the direct mixed antiglobulin reaction carried out on untreated fresh human semen. Int J Fertil. 1978;23(1):12–21.
30. Kay DJ, Boettcher B. Comparison of the SpermMar test with currently accepted procedures for detecting human sperm antibodies. Reprod Fertil Dev. 1992;4(2):175–81.
31. Bohring C, Krause W. The intra- and inter-assay variation of the indirect mixed agglutination reaction test: is a quality control suitable? Hum Reprod. 1999;14(7):1802–5.
32. Franco JG Jr., Schimberni M, Rojas FJ, et al. Reproducibility of the indirect immunobead assay for detecting sperm antibodies in serum. J Reprod Med. 1989;34(4):259–63.
33. World Health Organization. WHO laboratory manual for the examination of human semen and sperm–cervical mucus interaction. Cambridge: Cambridge University Press; 2004.
34. Ackerman S, McGuire G, Fulgham DL, et al. An evaluation of a commercially available assay for the detection of antisperm antibodies. Fertil Steril. 1988;49(4):732–4.
35. Mahmoud A, Comhaire F. Antisperm antibodies: use of the mixed agglutination reaction (MAR) test using latex beads. Hum Reprod. 2000;15(2):231–3.
36. Haas GG Jr., D'Cruz OJ, DeBault LE. Comparison of the indirect immunobead, radiolabeled, and immunofluorescence assays for immunoglobulin G serum antibodies to human sperm. Fertil Steril. 1991;55(2):377–88.
37. Fichorova RN, Boulanov ID. Anti-seminal plasma antibodies associated with infertility: I. Serum antibodies against normozoospermic seminal plasma in patients with unexplained infertility. Am J Reprod Immunol. 1996;36(4):198–203.
38. Räsänen M, Lahteenmaki A, Saarikoski S, et al. Comparison of flow cytometric measurement of seminal antisperm antibodies with the mixed antiglobulin reaction and the serum tray agglutination test. Fertil Steril. 1994;61(1):143–50.
39. Hendry WF, Hughes L, Scammell G, et al. Comparison of prednisolone and placebo in subfertile men with antibodies to spermatozoa. Lancet. 1990;335(8681):85–8.
40. De Almeida M, Feneux D, Rigaud C, et al. Steroid therapy for male infertility associated with antisperm antibodies. Results of a small randomized clinical trial. Int J Androl. 1985;8(2):111–7.
41. Haas GG Jr., Manganiello P. A double-blind, placebocontrolled study of the use of methylprednisolone in infertile men with sperm-associated immunoglobulins. Fertil Steril. 1987;47(2):295–301.
42. Bals-Pratsch M, Doren M, Karbowski B, et al. Cyclic corticosteroid immunosuppression is unsuccessful in the treatment of sperm antibody-related male infertility: a controlled study. Hum Reprod. 1992;7(1):99–104.
43. Robinson JN, Forman RG, Nicholson SC, et al. A comparison of intrauterine insemination in superovulated cycles to intercourse in couples where the male is receiving steroids for the treatment of autoimmune infertility. Fertil Steril. 1995;63(6):1260–6.
44. Lahteenmaki A, Rasasnen M, Hovatta O. Low-dose prednisolone does not improve the outcome of in-vitro fertilization in male immunological infertility. Hum Reprod. 1995;10(12):3124–9.
45. Grigoriou O, Vitoratos N, Papdias C, et al. Intrauterine insemination as a treatment of infertility in women with antisperm antibodies. Int J Gynecol Obstet. 1991;35(2):151–6.
46. Lahteenmaki A, Veilahti J, Hovatta O. Intra-uterine insemination versus cyclic, low-dose prednisolone in couples with male antisperm antibodies. Hum Reprod. 1995;10:142–7.
47. Lenzi A, Gandini L, Claroni F, et al. Immunological usefulness of semen manipulation for artificial insemination homologous (AIH)

in subjects with antisperm antibodies bound to sperm surface. Andrologia. 1988;20(4):314–21.
48. Bronson R, Cooper G, Rosenfeld D. Sperm antibodies: their role in infertility. Fertil Steril. 1984;42(2):171–83.
49. de Almeida M, Herry M, Testart J, et al. In-vitro fertilization results from thirteen women with anti-sperm antibodies. Hum Reprod. 1987;2(7):599–602.
50. Naz RK. Modalities for treatment of antisperm antibody mediated infertility: novel perspectives. Am J Reprod Immunol. 2004;51(5):390–7.
51. Ford WC, Williams KM, McLaughlin EA, Harrison S, Ray B, Hull MG. The indirect immunobead test for seminal antisperm antibodies and fertilization rates at in-vitro fertilization. Hum Reprod. 1996 Jul;11(7):1418–22.
52. Adeghe AL. Effect of washing on sperm surface autoantibodies. Br J Urol. 1987;60(4):360–3.
53. Windt ML, Menkveld R, Kruger TF, et al. Effect of sperm washing and swim-up on antibodies bound to sperm membrane: use of immunobead/sperm cervical mucus contact tests. Arch Androl. 1989;22(1):55–9.
54. Haas GG, D'Cruz OJ, Denum BM. Effect of repeated washing on sperm-bound immunoglobulin G. J Androl. 1988;9(3):190–6.
55. Almagor M, Margalioth EJ, Yaffe H. Density differences between spermatozoa with antisperm autoantibodies and spermatozoa covered with antisperm antibodies from serum. Hum Reprod. 1992;7(7):959–61.
56. Bronson RA, Cooper GW, Rosenfeld DL, Gilbert JV, Plaut AG. The effect of an IgA1 protease on immunoglobulins bound to the sperm surface and sperm cervical mucus penetrating ability. Fertil Steril. 1987 Jun;47(6):985–91.
57. Kutteh WH, Kilian M, Ermel LD, Byrd EW, Mestecky J. Antisperm antibodies (ASAs) in infertile males: subclass distribution of IgA antibodies and the effect of an IgA1 protease on sperm-bound antibodies. Am J Reprod Immunol. 1994 Mar–Apr;31(2–3):77–83.
58. Agarwal A. Treatment of immunological infertility by sperm washing and intrauterine insemination. Arch Androl. 1992;29(3): 207–13.
59. Check HJ. Antisperm antibodies and human reproduction. Clin Exp Obstet Gynecol. 2010;37(3):169–74.
60. Foresta C, Varotto A, Caretto A. Immunomagnetic method to select human sperm without sperm surface-bound autoantibodies in male autoimmune infertility. Arch Androl. 1990;24(2):221–5.
61. Naz RK, Bhargava KK. Antibodies to sperm surface fertilization antigen (FA-1): their specificities and site of interaction with sperm in male genital tract. Mol Reprod Dev. 1990;26(2):175–83.
62. Zhu X, Naz RK. Fertilization antigen-1: cDNA cloning, testis-specific expression, and immunocontraceptive effects. Proc Natl Acad Sci, USA. 1997;94:4704–9.
63. Naz RK, Zhu RK. Recombinant fertilization-1 causes a contraceptive effect in actively immunized mice. Biol Reprod. 1998;59:1095–1100.
64. Naz RK, Menge AC. Antisperm antibodies: origin, regulation, and sperm reactivity in human infertility. Fertil Steril. 1994;61(6):1001–13.
65. Naz RK, Chaudhry A, Witkin SS. Lymphocyte proliferative response to fertilization antigen in patients with antisperm antibodies. Am J Obstet Gynecol. 1990;163(2):610–3.
66. Menge AC, Christman GM, Ohl DA, et al. Fertilization antigen-1 removes antisperm autoantibodies from spermatozoa of infertile men and results in increased rates of acrosome reaction. Fertil Steril. 1999;71(2):256–60.
67. Check JH, Bollendorf A. Effect of antisperm antibodies on post-coital results and effect of intrauterine insemination on pregnancy outcome. Arch Androl. 1992;28(1):25–31.
68. Francavilla F, Romano R, Santucci R, Marrone V, Corrao G. Failure of intrauterine insemination in male immunological infertility in cases in which all spermatozoa are antibody-coated. Fertil Steril. 1992 Sep;58(3):587–92.
69. Mahmoud AM, Tuyttens CL, Comhaire FH. Clinical and biological aspects of male immune infertility: a case-controlled study of 86 cases. Andrologia. 1996 Jul–Aug;28(4):191–6.
70. Clarke GN, Lopata A, McBain JC, Baker HW, Johnston WI. Effect of sperm antibodies in males on human in vitro fertilization (IVF). Am J Reprod Immunol Microbiol. 1985 Jun;8(2):62–6.
71. Mandelbaum SL, Diamond MP, DeCherney AH. Relationship of antisperm antibodies to oocyte fertilization in in vitro fertilization-embryo transfer. Fertil Steril. 1987 Apr;47(4):644–51.
72. de Almeida M, Gazagne I, Jeulin C, Herry M, Belaisch-Allart J, Frydman R, Jouannet P, Testart J. In-vitro processing of sperm with autoantibodies and in-vitro fertilization results. Hum Reprod. 1989 Jan;4(1):49–53.
73. Rajah SV, Parslow JM, Howell RJ, Hendry WF. The effects on in-vitro fertilization of autoantibodies to spermatozoa in subfertile men. Hum Reprod. 1993 Jul;8(7):1079–82.
74. Acosta AA, van der Merwe JP, Doncel G, Kruger TF, Sayilgan A, Franken DR, Kolm P. Fertilization efficiency of morphologically abnormal spermatozoa in assisted reproduction is further impaired by antisperm antibodies on the male partner's sperm. Fertil Steril. 1994 Oct;62(4):826–33.
75. Junk SM, Matson PL, Yovich JM, Bootsma B, Yovich JL. The fertilization of human oocytes by spermatozoa from men with antispermatozoal antibodies in semen. J In Vitro Fert Embryo Transf. 1986 Dec;3(6):350–2.
76. Chang TH, Jih MH, Wu TC. Relationship of sperm antibodies in women and men to human in vitro fertilization, cleavage, and pregnancy rate. Am J Reprod Immunol. 1993 Sep–Oct;30(2–3):108–12.
77. Witkin SS, Viti D, David SS, Stangel J, Rosenwaks Z. Relation between antisperm antibodies and the rate of fertilization of human oocytes in vitro. J Assist Reprod Genet. 1992 Feb;9(1): 9–13.
78. Pagidas K, Hemmings R, Falcone T, Miron P. The effect of antisperm autoantibodies in male or female partners undergoing in vitro fertilization-embryo transfer. Fertil Steril. 1994 Aug;62(2):363–9.
79. Sukcharoen N, Keith J. The effect of the antisperm auto-antibody-bound sperm on in vitro fertilization outcome. Andrologia. 1995 Sep–Oct;27(5):281–9.
80. Vazquez-Levin MH, Notrica JA, Polak de Fried E. Male immunologic infertility: sperm performance on in vitro fertilization. Fertil Steril. 1997 Oct;68(4):675–81.
81. Vujisić S, Lepej SZ, Jerković L, Emedi I, Sokolić B. Antisperm antibodies in semen, sera and follicular fluids of infertile patients: relation to reproductive outcome after in vitro fertilization. Am J Reprod Immunol. 2005 Jul;54(1):13–20.
82. Janssen HJ, Bastiaans BA, Goverde HJ, Hollanders HM, Wetzels AA, Schellekens LA. Antisperm antibodies and in vitro fertilization. J Assist Reprod Genet. 1992 Aug;9(4):345–9.
83. Zouari R, De Almeida M, Rodrigues D, Jouannet P. Localization of antibodies on spermatozoa and sperm movement characteristics are good predictors of in vitro fertilization success in cases of male autoimmune infertility. Fertil Steril. 1993 Mar;59(3):606–12.
84. Yeh WR, Acosta AA, Seltman HJ, Doncel G. Impact of immunoglobulin isotype and sperm surface location of antisperm antibodies on fertilization in vitro in the human. Fertil Steril. 1995 Jun;63(6):1287–92.
85. Nagy ZP, Verheyen G, Liu J, Joris H, Janssenswillen C, Wisanto A, Devroey P, Van Steirteghem AC. Results of 55 intracytoplasmic sperm injection cycles in the treatment of male-immunological infertility. Hum Reprod. 1995 Jul;10(7):1775–80.
86. Clarke GN, Bourne H, Baker HW. Intracytoplasmic sperm injection for treating infertility associated with sperm autoimmunity. Fertil Steril. 1997 Jul;68(1):112–7.

87. Jun JH, Lim CK, Park YS, Lee YS, Seo JT, Son IP, Lee HJ, Kang IS. Efficacy of intracytoplasmic sperm injection (ICSI) treatment in the immunological infertile patients. Am J Reprod Immunol. 1997 Apr;37(4):310–4.
88. Mercan R, Oehninger S, Muasher SJ, Toner JP, Mayer J Jr., Lanzendorf SE. Impact of fertilization history and semen parameters on ICSI outcome. J Assist Reprod Genet. 1998 Jan;15(1):39–45.
89. Check ML, Check JH, Katsoff D, Summers-Chase D. ICSI as an effective therapy for male factor with antisperm antibodies. Arch Androl. 2000 Nov–Dec;45(3):125–30.
90. Zini A, Lefebvre J, Kornitzer G, Bissonnette F, Kadoch IJ, Dean N, Phillips S. Anti-sperm antibody levels are not related to fertilization or pregnancy rates after IVF or IVF/ICSI. J Reprod Immunol. 2011 Jan;88(1):80–4.
91. Zini A, Fahmy N, Belzile E, Ciampi A, Al-Hathal N, Kotb A. Antisperm antibodies are not associated with pregnancy rates after IVF and ICSI: systematic review and meta-analysis. Hum Reprod. 2011 Jun;26(6):1288–95. (Epub 2011 Mar 23).
92. Javed AA, Naz RK. Human cleavage signal-1 protein: cDNA cloning, transcription and immunological analysis. Gene. 1992; 112(2):205–11.
93. Lahteenmaki A, Reima I, Hovatta O. Treatment of severe male immunological infertility by intracytoplasmic sperm injection. Hum Reprod. 1995;10(11):2824–8.
94. Ahmad K, Naz RK. Antibodies to sperm surface antigens and the c-myc proto-oncogene product inhibit early embryonic development in mice. Biol Reprod. 1991;45(6):841–50.
95. Ahmad K, Naz RK. Effects of human antisperm antibodies on development of preimplantation embryos. Arch Androl. 1992;29(1):9–20.
96. Naz RK. Effects of antisperm antibodies on early cleavage of fertilized ova. Biol Reprod. 1992;46(1):130–9.
97. Esteves SC, Schneider DT, Verza S Jr. Influence of antisperm antibodies in the semen on intracytoplasmic sperm injection outcome. Int Braz J Urol. 2007 Nov–Dec;33(6):795–802.
98. Krause W, Naz RK. Immunology of male infertility. In: Dubey A, Editor. Infertility: diagnosis, management and IVF. New Dehli: Jaypee Brothers Medical Publishers; 2012. pp. 79–89.

Oxidative Stress in Unexplained Male Infertility

10

Sejal B. Doshi, Rakesh K. Sharma and Ashok Agarwal

Introduction

Despite advances in modern reproductive technologies, infertility remains a common problem for couples worldwide. It is defined as the inability to conceive after one of year of unprotected sexual intercourse [1, 2]. In as many as 50% of infertile couples, a male factor has been implicated as the sole or partial cause [3, 4]. Although there are specific male-related etiologies that can be addressed to correct the issue, in many cases, the cause of infertility cannot be identified, leading to a diagnosis of unexplained infertility (UMI). In fact, the diagnosis of unexplained infertility accounts for 10–30% of infertility cases [5]. This chapter aims to shed light on the concept of UMI, particularly focusing on the diagnosis, treatment, and implicating factors involved in the pathogenesis of this condition, including oxidative stress.

Unexplained vs. Idiopathic Male Infertility

Unexplained male infertility is the inability to reproduce despite having a normal sexual history, physical exam, and semen analysis on two or more occasions as well as no harmful toxin exposure. Its reported prevalence ranges from 6–27% [2, 6]. Unexplained infertility is often loosely interchanged with its counterpart, idiopathic infertility. Idiopathic infertility is defined as having an abnormal semen analysis in the absence of any identifiable cause [7]—this second category accounts for 40–50% of male infertility cases [3]. For unknown reasons, the semen analysis of those with this type of infertility shows decreased sperm motility and sperm number and/or an increased number of spermatozoa with abnormal morphology [3].

Due to the similarities in their definitions, studies often categorize unexplained and idiopathic infertility as one and the same [8]. However, further research on this topic has shown that there are significant distinctions between the two types of infertility (Table 10.1). Newer tests involving cytogenetic analysis and molecular genetics highlight these differences, which lie primarily in their specific etiologies [3]. Specifically, UMI has been associated with the following contributory factors: sperm dysfunction, auto-antibodies directed against sperm antigens, certain coital factors interfering with successful fertilization, and oxidative stress [9]. On the other hand, idiopathic infertility is suggested to be caused by age, environmental pollutants, mitochondrial alterations, and infective agents such as *Chlamydia trachomatis*, herpes virus, and adenovirus [10, 11]. Additionally, post-testicular organs such as the epididymis have been shown to cause DNA methylation of cytosine–guanine nucleotides. This can lead to transcription repression and eventual idiopathic infertility [10, 12]. Interestingly, recent reports state that sperm DNA damage and oxidative stress in the seminal plasma do not exist in certain males with idiopathic infertility due to differential expression of gene polymorphisms, such as the GSTM1 genotype. Specifically, males with this gene alteration have been associated with increased levels of oxidative-induced DNA damage [13, 14].

Although a singular cause of unexplained infertility cannot be identified in many cases, it is of great importance that a systematic infertility workup be performed (Table 10.1). This prevents the oversight of an underlying etiology of UMI [2]. Amidst the modern reproductive technologies of today, this chapter aims to shed light on the concept of UMI, particularly focusing on the diagnosis, treatment, and implicating factors involved in the pathogenesis of this condition.

A. Agarwal (✉) · S. B. Doshi · R. K. Sharma
Center for Reproductive Medicine, Cleveland Clinic, 10681 Carnegie Avenue, Desk X11, Cleveland, OH 44195, USA
e-mail: sharmar@ccf.org

G. L. Schattman et al. (eds.), *Unexplained Infertility*, DOI 10.1007/978-1-4939-2140-9_10,

Table 10.1 Unexplained male infertility versus idiopathic male infertility

Parameter	Unexplained male infertility	Idiopathic male infertility
Semen analysis [1, 2, 6]	Normal	Abnormal
History, physical exam, and endocrine assessment [2, 3, 14]	Normal	Normal
Female factor infertility [2, 6]	Ruled out (no tubal patency, no cervical hostility, or good endometrial receptivity)	Ruled out (no tubal patency, no cervical hostility, or good endometrial receptivity)
Percentage of total cases of male infertility [1, 3, 5]	10–30 %	40–50 %
Contributory causes [9–12]	1. Sperm dysfunction 2. Auto-antibodies directed against sperm antigens 3. Coital factors interfering with successful fertilization 4. Oxidative stress	1. Age 2. Environmental pollutants 3. Mitochondrial alterations 4. Infective agents (i.e., *Chlamydia trachomatis*, herpes virus, and adenovirus)
History of harmful toxin exposure [6, 7]	None	None
Infertility Status [3–5]	Unknown	Known
Categorized under [1, 2]	Male infertility of unknown origin	Male infertility of unknown origin

Assessment of Males with Unexplained Infertility

When a couple seeks assistance for infertility issues, a thorough clinical evaluation of both partners should be performed to rule out identifiable causes and focus the investigation [15, 16]. The initial infertility workup includes a detailed history with an emphasis on the couple's previous fertility record. This may include a history of recurrent miscarriages and ectopic pregnancies, the period of time in which the patient has been infertile, successful previous pregnancies, and any complications that may have occurred before, during, or after delivery [2, 17]. Furthermore, a thorough coital history from both partners is necessary to reveal any difficulties in regard to intercourse, such as improper sexual technique or inappropriate timing of intercourse [18]. In addition to male infertility evaluation, the female partner should undergo a separate workup, in order to assess the patency of both fallopian tubes, consistency of the cervical mucus, and receptivity of the endometrium to blastocyst implantation [2, 6].

Once a thorough sexual and fertility history has been completed, a comprehensive physical exam should be performed, which can help to exclude anatomical causes of infertility [2]. The physician should carefully examine the male patient for any physical aberrations within the structures of the male reproductive system. The penis, in addition to the epididymis, testis, and spermatic cord, should be palpated in order to rule out conditions such as epididymitis, orchitis, and varicocele [19–21]. In particular, all of these conditions promote the aggregation of free radicals or reactive oxygen species (ROS), eventually leading to sperm dysfunction and infertility [19].

Routine Semen Analysis

After the completion of an extensive medical history and physical examination, a routine semen analysis should be the first laboratory test conducted in the infertility workup. This is a cost-effective, non-invasive test that has been integral in the evaluation of male factor infertility for decades [22]. The efficacy of this test lies in the parameters for which it tests, which include pH, volume, color, total count, motility, concentration, and morphology.

Sperm count and motility are the first and most important predictors of fertility potential [23]. Normal values for all semen parameters have been highly associated with improved fertility outcomes and therefore are used for the assessment of infertility [24]. Although semen analysis is the first diagnostic step routinely employed in the evaluation of UMI, it does not identify the exact cause behind the infertility [23, 25].

Therefore, in addition to a comprehensive history, clinical examination, and initial lab assessment, sperm function tests should be performed [26, 27]. Moreover, etiologies related to endocrine or genetic abnormalities should also be explored in the infertile individual [28]. Overall, it is clear that a routine semen analysis cannot be used alone to diagnose infertility. Additional tests are required for the investigation and evaluation of the subfertile male [4].

Upon obtaining a normal semen analysis concurrent with an unremarkable history and physical examination, the physician can make the diagnosis of UMI. At this point, the physician should then explore potential contributing factors implicated in the pathogenesis of the UMI [2, 4]. This includes immunologic factors, genetic integrity defects, fertilization defects, and oxidative stress. The former three are explained in greater detail in subsequent chapters whereas oxidative-induced UMI is the prominent focus of this chapter.

Immunologic Factors

The immune system of the human body naturally protects its cells from the harmful effects of an autoimmune reaction and various pathogens [29]. One such defense mechanism is the blood-testis-barrier, which protects sperm cells undergoing the process of spermatogenesis from an autoimmune attack [30]. However, if this barrier is broken, sperm antigens will come into contact with the immune system and lead to the formation of antisperm antibodies and eventually autoimmune infertility [31].

In regard to the role of autoimmunity in infertility, studies have shown that antisperm antibodies penetrate the blood-testis-barrier, bind to spermatozoa, and reduce their fertilization capacity. These antibodies may also inhibit the acrosome reaction, activate the complement cascade system to lyse sperm cells, and interfere with the sperm's ability to recognize particular binding sites on the zona pellucida [32]. Furthermore, they enter the cervical mucus and inhibit the ability of spermatozoa to penetrate it. Overall, the improper cellular or humoral immune response against sperm antigens causes dysfunction of spermatozoa and is a possible contributing factor to the unexplained infertility seen in males.

Defects in Genetic Integrity

Compromises in genetic integrity have been significantly correlated with UMI. Such compromises in DNA can take the form of insertion or deletion of bases, cross-linkage of strands, chromosomal anomalies, as well as single or double-stranded breaks [33]. Current research suggests that there is a causal relationship between defective spermatozoa DNA and male infertility [34]. This was demonstrated in a study that performed microarray analyses on spermatozoa mRNA, which illustrated differential expression of many genes between normozoospermic infertile men and fertile men. This indicates that males with unexplained infertility have distinct genome expression profiles specific only to UMI [35–37].

Overall, it is evident that large amounts of DNA damage in spermatozoa can interfere with a man's ability to achieve a natural, viable pregnancy. Further research needs to be conducted on the effects of DNA damage on pregnancy outcomes as well as the threshold of damage that allows for normal functioning of spermatozoa [33].

Fertilization Defects

Fertilization of the oocyte is a complex and arduous process carried out by spermatozoa. It is a multi-step event beginning with (1) capacitation, (2) hyperactivation, (3) sperm-zona pellucida binding, (4) acrosome reaction, (5) penetration of the zona pellucida, (6) sperm-oocyte fusion, (7) cortical and zona reaction, and finally (8) post-fertilization events. Each component of this process must be carried out in a precise manner because interference with any of these steps can potentially lead to infertility [38]. Specifically, those with UMI have been shown to have reduced levels of protein phosphorylation, which is necessary for the process of capacitation [39]. Moreover, normozoospermic infertile men have demonstrated decreased hyperactivation of spermatozoa as well as defects in the proteins necessary for the zona pellucida induced-acrosome reaction [40–42]. Overall, a variety of anomalies can take place during the process of fertilization and contribute to unexplained infertility in males.

Oxidative Stress

Oxidative stress is defined as an imbalance between reactive oxygen species (ROS) and antioxidant defense mechanisms in the body [43]. ROS comprise a class of radical and non-radical oxygen derivatives [44]. Not only do ROS include oxygen radicals such as the hydroxyl radical, superoxide radical, and hydrogen peroxide but also a subclass of nitrogen-containing compounds collectively known as reactive nitrogen species (RNS). Examples of RNS include peroxynitrite anion, nitroxyl ion, nitrosyl-containing compounds, and nitric oxide [44, 45]. The most common ROS that is produced by spermatozoa is the superoxide anion radical; this is turn forms hydrogen peroxide (strong oxidizer) on its own or by the action of superoxide dismutase (SOD).

Physiologic Role of Free Radical Species Studies have shown that physiological levels of ROS are required for many baseline bodily functions [44]. Moreover, appropriate concentrations of ROS allow for proper signal transduction, mediation of cytotoxic events, and facilitation of inflammation via prevention of platelet aggregation and neutrophil adherence to endothelial cells [44]. These free radical species also serve as signaling molecules or second messengers, as well as aid in the production of hormones, regulation of tight junctions, and mediation of apoptosis. In regard to the male reproductive system, low ROS levels are necessary for capacitation, hyperactivation, acrosome reaction, zona pellucida binding and fertilization capacity of spermatozoa and promote normal semen parameters, such as sperm motility, morphology, and viability [19, 28, 46].

Detrimental Role of Reactive Oxygen Species Although ROS are necessary for normal physiological functions, excess levels overwhelm the body's natural antioxidant capacity. Due to the unpaired electron in their outer orbit, ROS are highly reactive and interact with a variety of lipids, proteins, and nucleic acids in the body. Such reactions are extremely harmful for reproductive potential and possibly contribute to testicular dysfunction, decreased gonadotropin secretion, and abnormal semen parameters [47]. While ROS affect a variety of reproductive functions, their reactive nature leads to the generation of more free radicals. This, in turn, perpetuates a chain of reactions creating tissue damage in the form of oxidative stress [45].

In the male reproductive system, ROS are mainly produced by immature spermatozoa, macrophages, and polymorphonuclear leukocytes. Specifically, the latter two represent the majority of seminal leukocytes that generate ROS [48]. Conditions such as varicocele and leukocytospermia stimulate these leukocytes, among other inflammatory cells, to produce large amounts of ROS. Moreover, lifestyle habits such as smoking are strongly correlated with increased ROS production [49]. Additionally, these free radical species have been associated with cardiovascular disease due to the oxidation of low density lipoprotein (LDL) within the vascular endothelium. Oxidative stress also contributes to reperfusion injury following ischemia well as tissue injury after radiation therapy. Furthermore, infections such as *Helicobacter pylori* and neurodegenerative diseases such as Alzheimer's and Huntington's disease have been also been linked to the accumulation of oxidative stress [48].

Role of Oxidative Stress in Unexplained Infertility In addition to contributing to a variety of conditions, there is growing evidence that oxidative stress is involved in many aspects of UMI (Fig. 10.1). Studies have shown that when compared to fertile men, normozoospermic infertile males have elevated ROS levels measured by the malonaldehyde levels and protein carbonyl groups. [1, 50]. This is also evident by lower reactive oxygen species-total antioxidant capacity (ROS-TAC) scores in patients with UMI, which indicates elevated levels of seminal oxidative stress [51, 52]. Moreover, studies report high ROS dysfunction in UMI patients. This dysfunction can be in the form of reduced fertilization capacity, impairment of sperm metabolism, and lipid peroxidation of polyunsaturated fatty acids within the sperm plasma membrane [53]. Detrimental effects of high ROS on semen parameters such as motility, viability, morphology have been demonstrated by numerous studies [54, 55]. Not only does oxidative stress have negative consequences on sperm parameters but also on the DNA of sperm cells [50]. Studies have shown that patients with UMI have a significantly higher DNA fragmentation index (>30 %) induced by toxic levels of ROS when compared to those who are fertile [56]. Specifically, a fragmentation index>30 % is associated with lower chances of achieving pregnancy by natural conception or by insemination [57]. This finding of increased ROS levels may indicate that seminal oxidative stress may be involved in the pathogenesis of sperm DNA damage in these patients [56]. It has also been suggested that specific

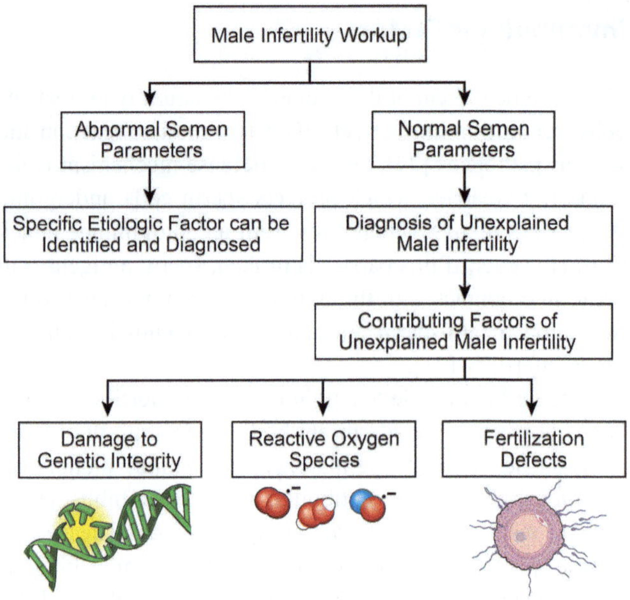

Fig. 10.1 Schematics of unexplained male infertility resulting in production of reactive oxygen species, genetic defects as well as fertilization defects

genetic polymorphisms can promote the accumulation of oxidative stress within the seminal plasma, such as the glutathione S-transferase Mu-1 (GSTM1) gene polymorphism. Studies have reported that men with idiopathic and unexplained infertility who have the GSTM1 null genotype had significantly higher levels of seminal oxidative stress than those who possessed the GSTM1 gene. Therefore, in patients suffering from infertility, the GSTM1 polymorphism might be integral to determining the susceptibility of spermatozoa to oxidative damage [58]. Additionally, studies report that UMI patients with excess levels of ROS have numerous mutations on genetic analysis of sperm mitochondrial DNA. Examples of such alterations include nucleotide changes in the ATPase and nicotinamide adenine dinucleotide dehydrogenase genes. These DNA mutations may be the underlying etiology of a male's unexplained infertility [59]. Furthermore, reactive oxygen species-induced DNA damage may accelerate the process of germ cell apoptosis, leading to the decline in sperm counts associated with male infertility [60]. Overall, it is clear that the oxidative stress may play a role in UMI via the mechanism of spermatozoa DNA damage.

Measurement of Oxidative Stress

A number of methods have been utilized in the laboratory setting to measure ROS [45]. Direct methods include cytochrome c reduction, electron spin resonance, and nitroblue tetrazolium technique (NBT, and xyenol orange-based assay). Indirect methods of measurement include the Endtz test, redox potential (GSH/GSSG), measurement of lipid peroxidation levels, chemokines and measurement of DNA damage, and measurement of reactive nitrogen species by Greiss reaction and fluorescence spectroscopy [61].

Assessment of ROS by Chemiluminescence The chemiluminescence assay is one of the most commonly used techniques to measure seminal ROS levels in clinical andrology laboratories. The two commonly used probes are luminol (5-amino-2,3-dihydro-1,4-phthalazinedione and 3-aminophthalic hydrazide) and lucigenin (*N, N'*-dimethyl-9,9'-biacridinium dinitrate). Both H_2O_2 and $O_2^{\bullet-}$ are involved in luminol-dependent chemiluminescence because both catalase and SOD can disrupt the luminol signal very efficiently. A luminescent signal is produced with luminol through a one-electron oxidative event mediated by hydrogen peroxide (H_2O_2) and either endogenous peroxidase or by addition of horse radish peroxidase. Superoxide anion ($O_2^{\bullet-}$)is an essential intermediate for the luminol-dependent chemiluminescence. Also, the redox cycling activity associated with this probe allows the significant amplification of the signal and allows easy measurement of H_2O_2. There are a variety of luminometers available and these may be single tube or multiple tube luminometers [61].

Luminol measures both intracellular and extracellular ROS such as hydrogen peroxide, and superoxide anion, on the other hand, lucigenin measures only extracellular ROS, and in particular superoxide anion.

For the actual assay, luminol (5 millimolar) is used to measure ROS in a clinical andrology lab setting. Chemiluminescence is measured using an instrument called luminometer (Fig. 10.2). Luminol is sensitive to light and the assay is performed in indirect light or in the dark. The samples are run in duplicate or in triplicate with appropriate negative and positive controls. Test samples are comprised of 400 μL of completely liquefied seminal ejaculate +10 μL luminol; positive control: 400 μL of phosphate buffered saline (PBS) and 50 μL hydrogen peroxide (30%)+10 μL luminol; and negative control: 400 μL PBS and 10 μL luminol. (Fig. 10.3) The measurement is for 15 min. The results are expressed as relative light units (RLU)/s/10^6 sperm. ROS levels >20(RLU)/s/10^6 sperm are considered as positive.

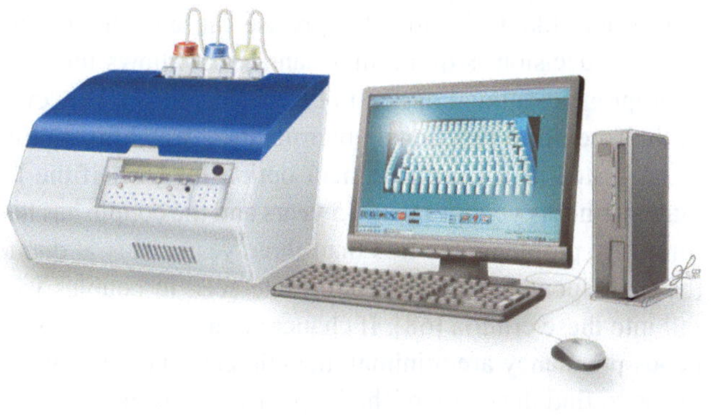

Fig. 10.2 A multitube Autolumat 953 plus luminometer used in the measurement of ROS by chemiluminescence assay. Multiple tubes can be loaded simultaneously for measuring ROS. (Reprinted with permission, Cleveland Clinic Center for Medical Art & Photography © 2011–2013. All rights reserved)

Flow Cytometry Flow cytometry is a laboratory method used for analyzing the expression of cell surface markers and intracellular molecules. Oxidation of 2, 7 dichlorofluorescein diacetate (DCFH-DA) by ROS, which is generated within the cell, makes them highly fluorescent and can be used to measure formation of intracellular levels of hydrogen peroxide. Hydroethidine (HE) is another fluorescent probe that can be used for the measurement of intracellular levels of superoxide [61, 62].

Griess Test and Spectrophotometry The Griess test is one of the most sensitive methods for detecting ROS in the form of nitrite or nitrous acid. Specifically, the presence of these NO-containing compounds can be assessed by reacting them with sulfanilic acid. The resulting product is a diazonium compound, which combines with alpha-naphthylamine to produce pink azo dye that is highly absorbent. In particular, the formation of this dye can be used to measure amounts of any substance that will yield nitrite in known proportions. The amount of nitrogenous compounds absorbed by the azo dye is measured colorimetrically [63, 64].

Measurement of Other Parameters of Oxidative Stress

Total antioxidant capacity In addition to measuring levels of ROS, total antioxidant capacity and DNA damage can also be evaluated to study the impact of oxidative stress on UMI. Total antioxidant capacity can be measured in the seminal plasma samples using an antioxidant assay kit (Cayman Chemical Company, Ann Arbor, Michigan). Its principle is based on the ability of aqueous and lipid-based antioxidants in seminal plasma to inhibit oxidation of the ABTS (2,2'-Azino-di-[3-ethylbenzthiazoline sulphonate]) to $ABTS^{\bullet+}$. Under the reaction conditions used, the antioxidants in the seminal plasma suppress absorbance at 750 nm to a degree that is proportional to their concentration. The capacity of the antioxidants in the sample to prevent ABTSoxidation can be compared with that of Trolox, a water-soluble tocopherol analog, and the results are reported as micromolar trolox equivalents [65].

Measurement of DNA damage DNA damage can be measured by the terminal deoxynucleotidyl transferase-mediated fluorescein-dUTP nick end labeling (TUNEL) assay. In

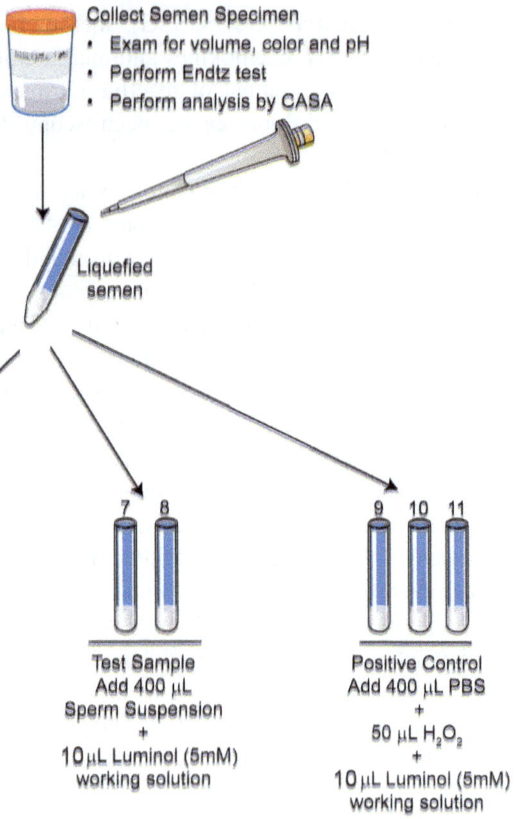

Fig. 10.3 Schematics of sample preparation for the ROS measurement. A total of 11 tubes are labeled from S1–S12: blank, negative control, patient sample, and positive control. Luminol is added only to all tubes except blank. Hydrogen peroxide is added only to the positive control

this assay, sperm DNA fragmentation is evaluated using a TUNEL assay with an Apo-Direct^{TM} kit (Pharmingen, San Diego, CA) as described earlier [66, 67]. An aliquot of well liquefied seminal ejaculate is used to assess DNA damage using the TUNEL assay. Briefly, 1–2 million spermatozoa are washed in (PBS) and resuspended in 3.7 % paraformaldehyde; the sperm concentration is adjusted to $1–2 \times 10^6$ sperm/mL. Spermatozoa are washed to remove the paraformaldehyde and then resuspended in 70 % ice-cold ethanol. Positive and negative kit controls provided by the manufacturer are run in addition to the lab internal control specimen (specimens from donors and patients with known DNA damage) with each run. Following a second wash with "Wash buffer" to remove ethanol, the sperm pellets are resuspended in 50 μL of freshly prepared staining solution for 60 min at 37 °C [66, 67]. The staining solution contains terminal deoxytransferase (TdT) enzyme, TdT reaction buffer, fluorescein isothiocynate tagged deoxyuridine triphosphate nucleotides (FITC-dUTP) and distilled water. After washing in "Rinse buffer" they are re-suspended in 0.5 mL of propidium iodide/RNase solution, and incubated for 30 min in the dark at room temperature followed by flow cytometric analysis. The samples are next analyzed within an hour after PI/RNase staining.

All fluorescence signals of labeled spermatozoa are analyzed by the flow cytometer FACScan (Becton Dickinson, San Jose, CA). About 10,000 spermatozoa are examined for each assay at a flow rate of < 100 cells/s. The excitation wavelength is set at 488 nm supplied by an argon laser at 15 mW. Green fluorescence (480–530 nm) is measured in the FL-1 channel and red fluorescence (580–630 nm) in the FL-2 channel. The percentage of positive cells (TUNEL-positive) is calculated on a 1023-channel scale using the flow cytometer software FlowJo Mac version 8.2.4 (FlowJo, LLC, Ashland, OR) [66, 67] (Fig. 10.4). Samples with > 19 % DNA damage are considered as positive or abnormal.

Therapeutic Options for UMI

Upon receiving a diagnosis of UMI, a couple must decide if they would like to identify the precise cause of the infertility. This decision is quite important, for it allows the most appropriate treatment option to be considered [7]. However, in the face of no functional abnormalities, watchful waiting is suggested as a valid treatment option for UMI if the female partner is younger than 35 years and the couple has had infertility problems for less than three years. This is due to the high spontaneous conception rate seen in couples who fall into these criteria [68]. If chances of achieving a spontaneous pregnancy are minimal, the clinician should continue trying to find the cause of the infertility via testing.

The tests for determining infertility are quite specific and manifold. Thus, in order to save the patient time and money, it is essential to narrow down the underlying cause of UMI so that unnecessary tests are not performed [69]. Subsequent

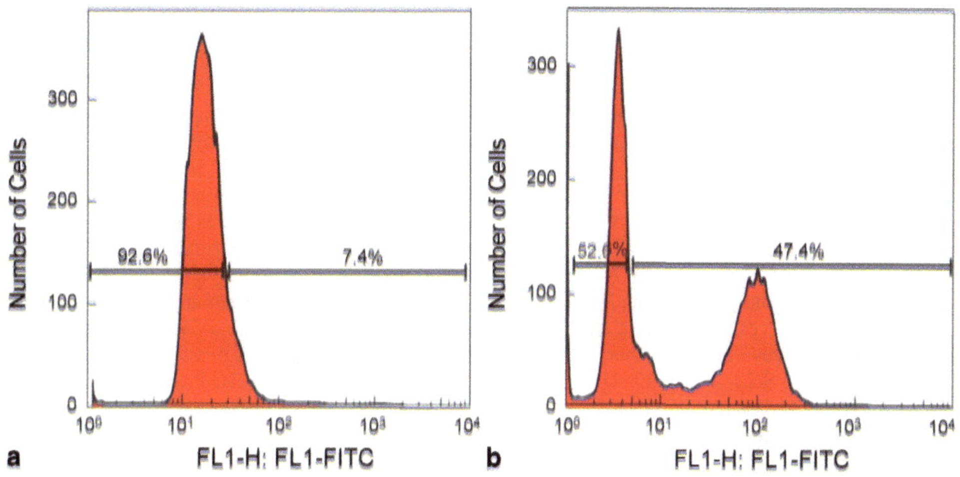

Fig. 10.4 A typical curve showing sample with **a**: Negative DNA damage and **b**: positive DNA damage

chapters will go into further details regarding the battery of tests available for detecting the functionality of spermatozoa, defects in genetic integrity, as well as the fertilization potential of sperm [70, 71].

Once the contributing cause has been determined, a variety of treatment options can be used. Specifically, when considering infertile males with antisperm antibodies, DNA damage, fertilization defects, or oxidative stress, studies have shown that intracytoplasmic sperm injection (ICSI) is the most successful treatment of choice [1]. In this assisted reproductive technique (ART), a spermatozoon is directly injected into an oocyte's cytoplasm. This allows for direct fertilization of the oocyte and bypasses any barriers that spermatozoa may encounter during the natural fertilization process [72]. Nevertheless, this technique does not come without its risks. If a defective sperm happens to be selected for ICSI, the resulting pregnancy has a risk of giving rise to mutations after fertilization. This is because damage to the spermatozoa, often in the form of compromised genetic integrity, cannot be fixed during the early stages of embryonic development as ICSI directly injects the spermatozoon into the egg. As a result, there are no natural protections available to the spermatozoa on its journey to the oocyte [73]. Although ICSI is a promising treatment for UMI due to a myriad of causes, further research is still needed on the complications of this technique in regard to embryo development and pregnancy outcomes [72].

When considering oxidative stress as the sole cause of man's unexplained infertility, a multitude of treatment options exist. One such treatment includes dietary antioxidant supplementation. Specifically, antioxidants neutralize ROS and prevent subsequent tissue damage as a result of oxidative stress [74]. Helpful antioxidants include carnitine, selenium, zinc, lycopene, vitamin E, and vitamin C. Adding these antioxidants to the diet of males with unexplained infertility has shown to substantially improve sperm DNA damage, pregnancy rates, semen parameters, and live birth outcomes [75]. However, more research needs to be done to determine the dose and duration of antioxidant therapy that will eliminate oxidative stress without causing any harmful side effects.

Other helpful methods for ROS-induced UMI include a variety of lifestyle modifications: consuming more fruits and vegetables, exercising, and avoiding tobacco products [2, 75].

Conclusion

Upon reviewing the literature, it can be concluded that normal sperm parameters do not guarantee full fertilization capacity of spermatozoa. Only after performing a thorough history and physical exam of both partners in the face of a normal semen analysis should UMI be considered. Specifically, doing this can help rule out female infertility factors, coital and genetic problems, as well as any physical aberrations. It is also important to fully comprehend the process of fertilization and the various components required for maximum fertilization potential of sperm. Upon confirming a diagnosis of UMI, a variety of factors should be explored as suggestive causes of infertility. These include autoimmune antibodies, DNA damage, fertilization defects, and oxidative stress. Modern andrology has developed innovative treatment options specific to the case of UMI. Overall, further molecular and genetic studies are needed to better understand the physiology of spermatozoa and the overall fertilization process. Finally, long-term clinical trials need to be performed in order to assess the effects of various reproductive techniques on pregnancy rates and embryo outcomes.

References

1. Aktan G, Doğru-Abbasoğlu S, Küçükgergin C, Kadıoğlu A, Ozdemirler-Erata G, Koçak-Toker N. Mystery of idiopathic male infertility: is oxidative stress an actual risk? Fertil Steril. 2013; 99:1211–5.
2. Hamada A, Esteves SC, Nizza M, Agarwal A. Unexplained male infertility: diagnosis and management. Int Braz J Urol. 2012;38:576–94.
3. Hamada A, Esteves SC, Agarwal A. Unexplained male infertility: potential causes and management. Hum Androl. 2011;1:2–16.
4. Hamada A, Esteves SC, Agarwal A. The role of contemporary andrology in unraveling the mystery of unexplained male infertility. Open Repro Sci J. 2011;4:27–41.
5. Templeton AA, Penney GC: The incidence, characteristics and prognosis of patients whose infertility is unexplained. Fertil Steril. 1982;37:175–82.
6. Sigman M, Lipshultz L, Howard S. Office evaluation of the subfertile male. In: Lipshultz LI, Howards SS, Niederberge CS, editors. Infertility in the male. 4th ed. Cambridge: Cambridge University Press; 2009. p. 153–176.
7. Hamada A, Esteves SC, Agarwal A. Unexplained infertility-looking beyond routine semen analysis. Eur Urol Rev. 2012;7:90–6.
8. Dohle GR, Colpi GM, Hargreave TB, Papp GK, Jungwirth A, Weidner W. EAU guidelines on male infertility. Eur Urol. 2005;48: 703–11.
9. Moghissi KS, Wallach EE: Unexplained infertility. Fertil Steril. 1983;39:5–21.
10. Cavallini G. Male idiopathic oligoasthenoteratozoospermia. Asian J Androl. 2006;8:143–157.
11. Silber SJ. Evaluation and treatment of male infertility. Clin Obstet Gynecol. 2000;43:854–88.
12. Ariel M, Cedar H, McCarrey J. Developmental changes in methylation of spermatogenesis-specific genes include reprogramming in the epididymis. Nat Gen. 1994;7:59–63.
13. Hughes CM, Lewis SE, McKelvery-Martin VJ, Thompson W. A comparison of baseline and induced DNA damage in human spermatozoa from fertile and infertile men, using a modified comet assay. Mol Hum Reprod. 1996;2:613–619.
14. Verit FF, Verit A, Kocyigit A, Ciftci H, Celik H, Koksal M. No increase in sperm DNA damage and seminal oxidative stress in patients with idiopathic infertility. Arch Gynecol Obstet. 2006;274:339–44.
15. Jarrow JP. Diagnostic approach to the infertile male patient. Endrocrinol Metab Clinc North Am. 2007;36:297–311.
16. Kamischke A, Cordes T, Nieschlag E. The diagnostic of male infertility—an important part of reproductive medicine. Ther Umsch. 2009;66:789–95.
17. Lewis SE: Is Sperm evaluation useful in predicting human fertility? Reproduction. 2007;134:31–40.
18. Kamel RM. Management of the infertile couple: an evidence-based protocol. Reprod Biol Endocrinol. 2010;8:21. doi:10.1186/1477-7827-8-21.
19. Agarwal A, Prabakaran S, Allamaneni SS. Relationship between oxidative stress, varicocele and infertility: a meta analysis. Reprod Biomed Online. 2006;12:630–3. Published online 2010 March 6. doi:10.1186/1477-7827-8-21
20. Jørgensen N, Rajpert-De Meyts E, Main KM, Skakkebaek NE. Testicular dysgenesis syndrome comprises some but not all cases of hypospadias and impaired spermatogenesis. Int J Androl. 2010;33:298–303.
21. Devine CJ Jr, Horton CE. Chordee without hypospadias. J Urol. 1973;110:264–71.
22. Jurema MB, Vieira AD, Bankowski B, Petrella C, Zhao Y, Wallach E, et al. Effect of ejaculatory abstinence period on the pregnancy rate after intrauterine insemination. Fertil Steril. 2005;84:678–81.
23. Khalil AA, Hussein HM, Sarhan EM. Oxidative stress induces idiopathic infertility in Egyptian males. Afr J Biotechnol. 2011;11: 1516–22.
24. Polanksy FF, Lamb EJ. Do the results of semen analysis predict future fertility? A survival analysis study. Fertil Steril. 1998;49:1059–65.
25. Safi J, Sharma RK, Agarwal A. Intrauterine insemination. In: Seli E, editors. Infertility. Oxford: Blackwell; 2011. 114–26.
26. Esteves SC, Zini A, Aziz N, Alvarez JG, Sabanegh ES Jr, Agarwal A. Critical appraisal of Word Health's Organization's new reference values for human semen characteristics and effect on diagnosis and treatment of subfertile men. Urology. 2012;79:16–22.
27. World Health Organization. WHO Laboratory Manual for the examination and processing of human semen. 5th ed. Geneva: WHO Press; 2010.
28. Agarwal, A, Sharma, RK, Nallella, KP, Thomas, AJ. Jr., Alvarez, JG, Sikka, SC. Reactive oxygen species as an independent marker of male factor infertility. Fertil Steril. 2006;86:878–85.
29. Haas GG JR, Cines DB, Schreiber AD. Immunologic infertility: identification of patients with antisperm antibody. N Eng J Med. 1980;303:722–7.
30. Pelletier RM. The blood-testis barrier: the junctional permeability, the proteins and the lipids. Prog Histochem Cytochem. 2011;46: 49–127.
31. Mazumdar S, Levine AS. Antisperm antibodies: etiology, pathogenesis, diagnosis, and treatment. Fertil Steril. 1998;70:799–810.
32. Chiu WW, Chamley LW. Clinical Associations and mechanisms of action of antisperm antibodies. Fertil Steril. 2004;82:529–35.
33. Bungum M, Humaidan P, Axmon A, Spano M, Bungum L, Erenpreiss J, et al. Sperm DNA integrity assessment in prediction of assisted reproduction technology out come. Hum Reprod. 2007;22:174–9.
34. Evenson DP, Larson KL, Jost LK. Sperm chromatin structure assay: its clinical use for detecting sperm DNA fragmentation in male infertility and comparison with other techniques. J Androl. 2002;23:25–43.
35. Garrido N, Martinex-Conejero JA, Jauregui J, Horcajadas JA, Simon C, Remohi J, Mesequer M. Microarray analysis in sperm from fertile and infertile men without basic sperm analysis abnormalities reveals a significantly different transcriptome. Fertil Steril. 2009;91:1307–10.
36. Jensen M, Leffers H, Petersen JH, Nyboe Andersen A, Jørgensen N, Carlsen E, et al. Frequent polymorphism of mitochondrial DNA polymerase gamma gene (POLG) in patients with normal spermiograms and unexplained subfertility. Hum Reprod. 2004;19:65–70.
37. Fraser L. Structural damage to nuclea DNA in mammalian spermatozoa: its evaluation techniques and relationship with male infertility. Pol J Vet Sci. 2004;7:311–21.
38. Mackenna A. Contribution of the male factor to unexplained infertility: a review. Int J Androl.1995;18:58–61.
39. Visconti PE, Galantino-Homer H, Moore GD, Bailey JL, Ning, Fornes M, et al. The molecular basis of capacitation. J Androl. 1998;19:242–6.
40. Suarez SS: Control of hyperactivation in sperm. Hum Reprod Update. 2008;14:647–57.
41. Liu DY, Clark GN, Martic M, Garrett C, Baker HW. Frequency of disordered zona pellucida (ZP)-induced acrosome reaction in infertile men with normal semen analysis and normal spermatozoa-ZP binding. Hum Reprod. 2001;16:1185–90.
42. Liu de Y Liu ML Garrett C Baker HW. Comparison of the frequency of defective sperm zona pellucida (ZP) binding and the ZP-induced acrosome reaction between subfertile men with normal and abnormal semen. Hum Reprod. 2007;22:1878–84.
43. Agarwal A, Prabakaran SA. Mechanism, measurement, and prevention of oxidative stress in male reproductive physiology. Indian J Exp Biol. 2005;43:963–974.

44. Doshi SB, Khullar K, Sharma RK, Agarwal A. Role of reactive nitrogen species in male infertility. Reprod Biol Endocrinol. 2012;10:109.
45. Sikka SC. Relative impact of oxidative stress on male reproductive function. Curr Med Chem. 2001;8:851–62.
46. Kothari S, Thompson A, Agarwal A, du Plessis SS. Free radicals: their beneficial and detrimental effects on sperm function. Indian J Exp Biol. 2010;48:425–35.
47. Griveau JF, Le Lannou D. Reactive oxygen species and human spermatozoa: physiology and pathology. Int J Androl. 1997;20: 61–9.
48. Thomas J, Fishel SB, Hall JA, Green S, Newton TA, Thornton SJ. Increased polymorphonuclear granulocytes in seminal plasma in relation to sperm morphology. Hum Reprod. 1997;12:2418–21.
49. Esteves SC. Effect of cigarette smoking on levels of seminal oxidative stress in infertile men: a prospective study. Int Braz J Urol. 2002;38:484–5.
50. Venkatesh S, Shamsi MB, Deka D, Saxena V, Kumar R, Dada R. Clinical implications of oxidative stress and sperm DNA damage in normozoospermic infertile men. Indian J Med Res. 2011;134: 369–8.
51. Benedetti S, Tagliamonte MC, Catalani S, Primiterra M, Canestrari F, De Stefani S, et al. Differences in blood and semen oxidative status in fertile and infertile men, and their relationship with sperm quality. Reprod Biomed Online. 2012;25:300–6.
52. Pasqualotto FF, Sharma RK, Kobayashi H, Nelson DR, Thomas AJ Jr, Agarwal A. Oxidative stress in normospermic men undergoing infertility evaluation. J Androl. 2001;22:316–22.
53. Kreeger KY, Rubbo H, Radi R, Trujillo M, Telleri R, Kalyanaraman B, Barnes S, Kirk M, Freeman BA. Nitric oxide regulation of superoxide and peroxynitrite-dependent lipid peroxidation. J Biol Chem. 1994;269:26066–75.
54. Agarwal A, Saleh RA, Bedaiwy MA. Role of reactive oxygen species in the pathophysiology of human reproduction. Fertil Steril. 2003;79:829–843.
55. Mahfouz RZ, du Plessis SS, Aziz N, Sharma R, Sabanegh E, Agarwal A. Sperm viability, apoptosis, and intracellular reactive oxygen species levels in human spermatozoa before and after induction of oxidative stress. Fertil Steril. 2010;93:814–21.
56. Saleh RA, Agarwal A, Nada EA, El-Tonsy MH, Sharma RK, Meyer A, Nelson DR, Thomas AJ. Negative effects of increased sperm DNA damage in relation to seminal oxidative stress in men with idiopathic and male factor infertility. Fertil Steril. 2003;79:1597–605.
57. Oleszczuk K, Augustinsson L, Bayat N, Giwercman A, Bungum M. Prevalence of high DNA fragmentation index in male partners of unexplained infertile couples. Andrology. 2013;1:357–60.
58. Aydemir B, Onaran I, Kiziler AR, Alici B, Akyolcu MC. Increased oxidative damage of sperm and seminal plasma in men with idiopathic infertility is higher in patients with glutathione S-transferase Mu-1 null genotype. Asian J Androl. 2007;9:108–15.
59. Kumar R, Venkatesh S, Kumar M, Tanwar M, Shasmsi MB, Kumar R, et al. Oxidative stress and sperm mitochondrial DNA mutation in idiopathic oligoasthenozoospermic men. Indian J Biochem Biophys. 2009; 46:172–7.
60. Agarwal A, Saleh RA, Bedaiwy MA. Role of reactive oxygen species in the pathophysiology of human reproduction. Fertil Steril. 2003;79:829–43.
61. Benjamin D, Sharma RK, Moazzam A, Agarwal A: Methods for the detection of ROS in human sperm samples. In: Agarwal Ashok, Aitken Robert J, Alvarez Juan G, editors. Studies on men's health and fertility. New York: Springer; 2012, Chap. 13, pp 257–273.
62. Mahfouz R, Sharma R, Lackner J, et al. Evaluation of chemiluminescence and flow cytometry as tools in assessing production of hydrogen peroxide and superoxide anion in human spermatozoa. Fertil Steril. 2009;92:819–827.
63. Beckman JS, Conger K. Direct measurement of nitric oxide in solution with an ozone based chemiluminescent detector. Methods. 1995;7:35–39.
64. Giustarini D, Rossi R, Milzani A, Dalle-Donne I. Nitrite and nitrate measurement by griess reagent in human plasma: evaluation of interferences and standardization. Methods Enzymol. 2008;440:361–380.
65. Mahfouz R, Sharma R, Sharma D, Sabanegh E, Agarwal A. Diagnostic value of the total antioxidant capacity (TAC) assay in human seminal plasma. Fertil Steril. 2009;91:805–811.
66. Sharma RK, Sabanegh E, Mahfouz R, Gupta S, Thiyagarajan A, Agarwal A. TUNEL as a test for sperm DNA damage in the evaluation of male infertility. Urology. 2010;76:1380–1386.
67. Sharma RK, Agarwal A. Laboratory evaluation of sperm chromatin: TUNEL assay. In: Zini Armand, Agarwal Ashok, editors. Sperm chromatin: biological and clinical applications in male infertility and assisted reproduction. New York: Springer; 2011, Chap. 14, pp 201–15.
68. Brandes M, Hamilton CJ, van der Steen JO, de Bruin JP, Bots RS, Nelen WL, et al. Unexplained infertility: overall ongoing pregnancy rate and mode of conception, Hum Reprod. 2011;26:360–8.
69. Beltsos AN, Fisher S, Uhler ML, Clegg ED, Zinaman M. The relationship of the postcoital test and semen characteristics to pregnancy rates in 200 presumed fertile couples. Int J Fertil Menopausal Stud. 1996;41:405–11.
70. Eimers JM, te Velde ER, Gerritse R, van Kooy RJ, Kremer J, Habbema JD. The validity of the postcoital test for estimating the probability of conceiving. Am J Obstet Gynecol. 1994;171:65–70.
71. Margalioth EJ, Feinmesser M, Navot D, Mordel N, Bronson RA. The long-term predictive value of the zona-free hamster ova sperm penetration assay. Fertil Steril. 1989;52:490–4.
72. Sadeghi MR, Lakpour N, Heidari-Vala H, Hodjat M, Amirjannati N, Hossaini Jadda H, et al. Relationship between sperm chromatin status and ICSI outcome in men with obstructive azoospermia and unexplained infertile normozoospermia. Rom J Morphol Embryol. 2011;52:645–51.
73. Feng C Wang LQ, Dong MY, Huang HF. Assisted reproductive technology may increase clinical mutation detection in male offspring. Fertil Steril. 2008;90:92–6.
74. Choudhary R, Chawala VK, Soni ND, Kumar J, Vyas RK: Oxidative stress and role of antioxidants in male infertility. Pak J Physiol. 2010;6:54–59.
75. Showell MG, Brown J, Yazdani A, Stankiewicz MT, Hart RJ. Antioxidants for male subfertility. Cochrane Database Syst Rev. 2011;19:CD007411.

Role and Significance of Sperm Function in Men with Unexplained Infertility

11

Sandro C. Esteves, Sidney Verza Jr., Rakesh K. Sharma, Jaime Gosálvez and Ashok Agarwal

Introduction

Semen analysis has traditionally been one of the first steps in the evaluation of the infertile male [1]. Conventional semen analysis assesses the physical characteristics of semen, specimen volume, sperm concentration, sperm motility and progression, sperm morphology, and the number of leukocytes. It provides information on the functional status of the seminiferous tubules, epididymis, and accessory sex glands, and its results are often taken as a surrogate measure of his ability to father a pregnancy. Although helpful, conventional semen analysis cannot alone be used to predict the male fertility potential. It is significantly modulated by internal and external factors, such as abstinence period, overall health status, and environmental exposure to toxicants, to cite a few, thus leading to difficulties in the interpretation and management of infertile men with normal and abnormal results. Therefore, the male infertility evaluation must go far beyond a simple semen analysis, as it has to be complemented with a proper physical examination, a comprehensive history taking, and relevant endocrine, genetic, and other investigations, including laboratory sperm functional tests [2]. The importance of semen analysis in the management of men with unexplained infertility (UI) is covered in greater detail in Chap. 3.

When all semen parameters are normal and after ruling out female infertility, there is a role for using specific laboratory tests which may identify the potential causes of male infertility in couples otherwise classified as having UI. In this scenario, possible factors in males that might explain difficulties to conceive include the presence of elevated antisperm antibodies (ASA) levels, increased sperm DNA damage, elevated levels of reactive oxygen species (ROS) in the seminal plasma and/or sperm, and sperm dysfunctions that impair the fertilization process as a whole, including the sperm ability to penetrate the cervical mucus, capacitation, acrosome reaction (AR), and sperm penetration into the oocyte and fusion with the oolemma.

In an attempt to quantitatively and/or qualitatively measure these aforesaid factors, some tests are available, as listed in Table 11.1.

For many years, tests that assessed ASA, AR, capacitation, sperm–zona, and ovum–membrane binding, and penetration were used not only to investigate males with UI but also to predict the fertilizing potential of sperm. Unfortunately, clinicians do not have effective clinical treatment to offer their patients when defects in the aforementioned steps are found. Still, with the advent of intracytoplasmic sperm injection (ICSI), these issues are no longer a concern as these critical steps are bypassed by ICSI. As such, many of the tests have been abandoned or are rarely used. In contrast, modern Andrology testing involving genetics, proteomics, and metabolomics holds much more promise since there is an opportunity for treatment in the face of abnormal results. Examples of tests in these categories, which have already been made available in the clinical setting, include sperm DNA chromatin tests (genetics) and quantification of oxidative stress markers (metabolomics). Sperm DNA integrity tests are of particular interest provided they are low cost and easy-to-implement. Moreover, results correlate with spontaneous, conventional in vitro fertilization (IVF), and ICSI

S. C. Esteves (✉) · S. Verza Jr.
ANDROFERT, Referral Center for Male Reproduction, Andrology and Human Reproduction Clinic, Avenida Dr. Heitor Penteado 1464, Campinas, Sao Paulo 13075-460, Brazil
e-mail: s.esteves@androfert.com.br

S. Verza Jr.
e-mail: sidney.labfiv@androfert.com.br

R. K. Sharma · A. Agarwal
Center for Reproductive Medicine, Cleveland Clinic
10681 Carnegie Avenue, Desk X-11, Cleveland, OH 44195, USA
e-mail: sharmar@ccf.org

A. Agarwal
e-mail:agarwaa@ccf.org

J. Gosálvez
Biology Department, Genetics Unit, Universidad Autónoma de Madrid, C/Dawin 2, 28049 Madrid, Spain
e-mail: jaime.gosalvez@uam.es

G. L. Schattman et al. (eds.), *Unexplained Infertility*, DOI 10.1007/978-1-4939-2140-9_11,

Table 11.1 Laboratory tests to assess sperm function

Target of investigation	Available tests
Antisperm antibodies	Mixed agglutination reaction (MAR) test
	Direct immunobeads binding test (direct IBT)
Fertilization defects	Hemizona assay
	Sperm–zona binding ratio test
	Hyperactivation (HA) motility
	Acrosome reaction assays
	Sperm penetration assay (SPA)
Oxidative stress	Thiobarbituric acid reactive substances (TBARS) assay
	Chemiluminescence assays
	Superoxide anion by nitroblue tetrazolium (NBT) reduction test
Sperm DNA integrity	Terminal deoxy nucleotidyl transferase mediated dUTP nick end labeling (TUNEL) assay
	Comet assay
	Sperm chromatin structure assay (SCSA)
	Sperm chromatin dispersion (SCD) test

outcomes, thus hindering sperm chromatin testing a valid sperm biomarker.

In this chapter, we describe the tests clinically available to investigate males with UI, including the traditional and novel ones, and discuss their utility in practical terms. We also present our experience in using some of these tests in our laboratories.

Antisperm Antibodies

ASA, the hallmark of autoimmune male infertility, are implicated in sperm dysfunction by their direct effect on various sperm antigens. ASA may induce sperm apoptosis and untimely AR [3]. ASA may also hinder fertilization by interfering with sperm penetration into the cervical mucus, zona pellucida (ZP) binding, and sperm–oocyte fusion. Furthermore, ASA may alter chaperone function, protein folding, and disulphide bonds [4]. These alterations ultimately decrease the chances of achieving a natural conception [5]. As a matter of fact, Ayvaliotis et al. reported a significantly lower spontaneous conception rates (15.3 %) in couples where autoimmunity to sperm was detected compared with those without clinically relevant levels of ASA (66.7 %, $p<0.05$) [5].

Sperm agglutination and/or immobilization is usually observed in association with ASA, and may limit sperm progression through the female genital tract [6]. The findings of sperm agglutination, "shaking motility," or both, during conventional semen analysis are highly suggestive of elevated ASA titers [7]. The term "agglutination" describes spermatozoa that are stuck to each other by antibodies. Sperm agglutination usually occurs in specific manners such as head-to-head, midpiece-to-midpiece, tail-to-tail, or tail-tip-to-tail-tip [8]. On the other hand, "shaking motility" is a pattern of sperm movement characterized by a very strong tail movement associated with a nonprogressive motility that results in immobilization [8].

Although immunoglobulin subclasses IgA, IgG, and IgM can be found in human ejaculates, IgA seems to be the most important one from a biological standpoint [9, 10]. IgA bound to the sperm surface significantly impair sperm progression through the cervical mucus [10]. Nevertheless, immunoglobulins can adhere to various sperm sites regardless of their subclasses [5].

It is out of our scope to provide a comprehensive review on immunologic male infertility since it is discussed in Chap. 9. Our focus is otherwise to present the tests to determine ASA, as well as their advantages and limitations.

Laboratory Tests to Detect Antisperm Antibodies

Concerning the testing for ASA in UMI, the specimen of interest is the semen. ASA can also be assessed in the seminal plasma when low sperm counts and/or motility limits the applicability of the assay. However, such conditions are associated with abnormal semen analysis results, and therefore do not meet the criteria of UMI. The immunobeads binding test (IBT) and the mixed agglutination reaction (MAR) test are the most commonly used among andrology laboratories performing ASA determination (Table 11.2) [11].

Mixed Agglutination Reaction Test

The MAR test is an inexpensive, quick, and sensitive screening test in which sheep erythrocytes or latex particles coated with human IgG or IgA are used to detect and localize antibody-bound sperm [12, 13]. The formation of mixed agglutinates between the particles/red blood cells and motile spermatozoa indicates the presence of IgG or IgA antibodies on the spermatozoa.

Table 11.2 Methods for assessing antisperm in men with unexplained male infertility

Assay	Principle	Advantage	Disadvantage	Specimen	How results are expressed	Normal limits	Clinical significance in unexplained male infertility
Direct immunobeads test (IBT)	Polyacrylamide beads coated with antihuman immunoglobulin antibodies against α-, γ-, and μ-chains that bound to antibodies present in spermatozoa	Identify the proportion of antibody-bound sperm, the antibody class, and the location of the antibodies on the sperm surface	More time consuming than the MAR test; ASA-positive spermatozoa and ASA-negative spermatozoa should be included as controls in each test	Ejaculated sperm	Percentage of motile spermatozoa with beads bonded to their membrane	≤50 % of motile sperm bounded to the beads	Significantly lower (15.3 %) conception rates in couples with sperm autoimmunity compared to couples without clinically relevant levels of ASA (66.7 %, $p<0.05$) [5]
Mixed agglutination reaction (MAR) test	A "bridging" antibody (anti-IgG or anti-IgA) is used to bring the antibody-coated beads into contact with unwashed spermatozoa in semen bearing surface IgG or IgA	Inexpensive, quick and sensitive screening test; agglutination between beads serves as a positive control for antibody–antigen recognition	Provides less information than the direct immunobead test				

Immunobeads Binding Test

IBT is more time consuming than the MAR test, but it identifies the proportion of antibody-bound sperm in a given sample, the antibody class, and the location of antibodies on the sperm surface. IBT is our preferred approach to determine the levels of ASA in the semen, seminal plasma, and cervical mucus. IBT involves the use of poliacrilamide microspheres coated with human anti-immunoglobulin combined IgA, IgG, and IgM classes. These treated beads adhere to light or heavy antibody chains [14]. The test is termed "direct" when it investigates the presence of ASA on the surface of motile spermatozoa in ejaculates (direct IBT), and is termed "indirect" when used to test for ASA in the seminal plasma or cervical mucus (indirect IBT). First, a screening test is performed to determine the percentage of spermatozoa with surface antisperm-bound, regardless of immunoglobulin subclasses. In case of positive results, ASA subclasses can be assessed and quantified. The method involves the incubation of an aliquot of liquefied semen containing 8–10 million motile sperm with a suspension of immunobeads diluted with protein-supplemented phosphate buffer saline (PBS). The mixture is then washed by centrifugation and resuspended in PBS supplemented with 5 % bovine serum albumin (BSA). An aliquot of 8 μL of sperm suspension and immunobeads is placed on a glass microscope slide, and checked for the presence of ASA. Slides are analyzed under phase-contrast microscope at 400× magnification to determine the presence of beads bounded to the sperm surface (Fig. 11.1). Only motile spermatozoa are evaluated and at least 200 cells are analyzed. Results are based on the percentage of spermatozoa with beads bounded to their membrane [6, 15]. The cutoff value for normality is ≤50 % of motile sperm bounded to the beads according to the World Health Organization (WHO) guidelines for assessing the human sperm [16].

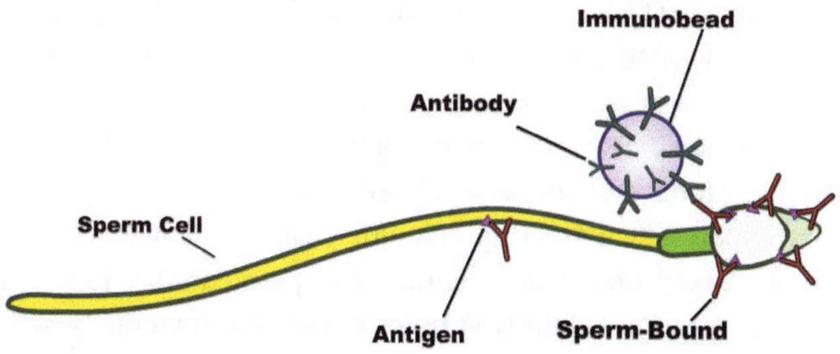

Fig. 11.1 Illustration depicting the immunobeads binding test (IBT). Human anti-immunoglobulin-coated beads are mixed with motile spermatozoa. Anti-immunoglobulins (antibodies) combine with the immunoglobulins (sperm-bound) present on the sperm surface. The presence of beads bounding to the sperm surface is examined under phase-contrast microscopy

Fertilization Defects

The sperm fertilizing potential is related to its ability of undergoing capacitation, ZP binding, and AR, which ultimately leads to sperm penetration into the oocyte and fusion with the oolema.

In vivo, ejaculated spermatozoa from all Eutherian mammals are unable to fertilize until they have undergone capacitation, which allows the AR to take place, when they approach or contact the oocyte [17]. Capacitation has been recognized as a time-dependent phenomenon, with the absolute time course being species-specific [18]. Capacitation prepares the sperm to undergo AR with the accompanying release of lytic enzymes and exposure of membrane receptors, which are required for sperm penetration through the ZP and for fusion with the oolema [18]. Sperm transport through the female genital tract can occur quite rapidly (times as short as 15 to 30 min have been reported in humans), whereas the capacitation process can take from 3 to 24 h [18]. It is speculated, therefore, that capacitation is not completed until after spermatozoa have entered the cumulus oophorus. This delay is physiologically beneficial because spermatozoa do not respond to AR-inducing signals until they have approached the ZP, thus preventing premature AR that ultimately leads to sperm inability to timely penetrate the egg vestments [18, 19]. Sperm capacitation is a postejaculatory modification of the sperm surface, which involves the mobilization and/or removal of certain surface components of the sperm plasma membrane, such as glycoproteins, decapacitation factor, acrosome-stabilizing factor, and acrosin inhibitor. Sperm capacitation involves major biochemical and biophysical changes in the membrane complex and energy metabolism. The presence of high concentrations of cholesterol in the seminal plasma, which maintains high cholesterol concentration in the sperm membranes, seems to be the most important factor for inhibition of capacitation [20]. Capacitation is associated with increased membrane fluidity caused by removal of cholesterol from sperm plasma membrane via sterol acceptors from the female tract secretions [21, 22]. A marked change in sperm motility, named hyperactivation (HA), is the first step in this complex process. Hyperactivated spermatozoa exhibit an extremely vigorous but nonprogressive motility pattern, as a result of a Ca^{2+} influx, which causes increased flagellar curvature [23] and extreme lateral movement of the sperm head [8]. Proteasome participates in activating calcium channels that also leads to increased membrane fluidity and permeability [24–27]. These events are followed by or occur simultaneously with (i) a decrease in net surface charge, (ii) the absence of intramembrane protein and sterols area, and (iii) increased concentrations of anionic phospholipids [27, 28]. Hyperactivated motility is essential for sperm penetration into the intact oocyte-cumulus complexes in vitro and in vivo [29, 30]. Various components of the female reproductive tract act as physiological stimuli for HA, such as progesterone, ions, and secretions in the oviduct luminal fluid [31]. The extent of which sperm is hyperactivated is positively correlated with the sperm's ability of zona binding, AR, zona-free oocyte penetration, and thus fertilizing capacity in vitro [31].

The spermatozoon binds to the ZP with its intact plasma membrane after capacitation and penetration into the cumulus oophorous. Sperm binding occurs via specific receptors to ZP glycoproteins located over the anterior sperm head [32]. Glycosylation of ZP glycoproteins is important in sperm-ZP interaction. It is believed that human ZP glycoprotein-3 (ZP3) has a central role in initiating the AR [33]. However, human ZP1 and ZP4 are also implicated in the process [21, 22, 34–37]. ZP3-induced AR involves the activation of T-type voltage operated calcium channels (VOCCs), whereas ZP1- and ZP4-induced ARs involve both T- and L-type VOCCs. Chiu et al. [38] reported that glycodelin-A, a glycoprotein present in the female reproductive tract, sensitizes spermatozoa to undergo ZP-induced AR. The process involves the activation of the adenylyl cyclase/PKA pathway along with up-regulation of ZP-induced calcium influx and suppression of extracellular signal-regulated kinase activation. It is, therefore, suggested that glycodelin-A may be important in vivo to ensure full responsiveness of human spermatozoa to the ZP. Defective ZP-bound sperms are present in approximately 15 % of subfertile men with normal semen analysis, and it may explain the low success of IVF and intrauterine insemination (IUI) when these methods are applied in certain cases of UI [39, 40]. The presence of defective sperm–ZP binding in infertile men with normal semen parameters may be due to either a defective signal transduction pathways upstream of protein kinases A and C, or downstream disorders, structural defects, or absence of sperm receptors for ZP binding [12]. Such defects are not identified unless specialized sperm function tests are used [41].

The AR is a stimulus-induced process that involves fusion of the sperm plasma membrane with the outer acrosomal membrane. This process leads to the release of exocytotic proteolytic enzymes in response to sperm–ZP binding [42, 43]. The mammalian sperm head is composed of two main structures, the acrosome and the nucleus. The acrosome is a membrane-bound organelle derived from the Golgi complex located in the anterior portion of the sperm head. In humans, the acrosome occupies 40–70 % of the sperm head and its contents include proteases such as proacrosin, hyaluronidase, and phospholipase A2. Spermatozoa bind to the ZP with intact acrosomes. Then, multiple fusions between the outer acrosomal membrane and the plasma membrane result in the release of hydrolytic enzymes (mostly acrosin) and exposure of new membrane domains, both of which essential for fertilization. The released hydrolytic enzymes digest the ZP, allowing the spermatozoa to penetrate the oocyte [32].

The AR seems to be physiologically induced by natural stimulants such as follicular fluid (FF), progestin, progesterone, and hydroxy progesterone, all of which bind to sperm receptors [28]. FF and cumulus cells have protein-bound progesterone, and this hormone is considered among the most important AR-inducing agents [43, 44]. However, other sperm-deriving factors may also play a role in this process. For instance, a link between estradiol locally produced by ejaculated spermatozoa, sperm capacitation, and AR have been demonstrated [45]. These stimulatory signals are intracellularly transduced via second messengers ultimately leading to exocytosis [46]. A number of second-messenger pathways have been identified in human spermatozoa, including those that result in the activation of cyclic adenosine monophosphate (cAMP), cyclic guanosine monophosphate (cGMP), and phospholipid dependent protein kinases [27, 47–49]. These kinases are called, respectively, protein kinases A, G, and C. It is possible that these pathways interact to assure an optimal response at the correct place and time during the fertilization process.

The AR is a time-dependent phenomenon that cannot take place prematurely or too late [47]. As such, acrosome integrity is crucial for normal fertilization both in vivo and in vitro. In fact, a high proportion of sperm with intact acrosomes is seen in ejaculates of normal men. In such individuals, ~5–20 % sperm cells exhibit spontaneous AR devoid of clinical significance [48]. In contrast, abnormal conditions affecting the sperm may lead to decreased fertilization ability. One example is acrosomeless round-headed spermatozoa (globozoospermic spermatozoa) that are unable to fertilize. Increased percentages of morphologically abnormal acrosomes have also been related to fertilization failure in assisted conception using conventional IVF [49]. In addition, premature AR and sperm inability to release the acrosomal contents in response to proper stimuli (AR insufficiency) have been associated with unexplained male infertility [50]. Although the cause of premature AR is unknown, the premature (stimulus independent) initiation of acrosomal exocytosis seems to be related to a perturbation of the plasma membrane stability. In this context, the AR may not involve a premature activation of the receptor-mediated process, but rather reflect an inherent fragility of the sperm membrane, leading to a receptor-independent acrosomal loss [51].

ASA may also adversely affect the ability of sperm to undergo capacitation and AR [15]. Chang et al. [52] reported a reduction in fertilization either by the action of IgG directly bound to sperm or IgM present in the female serum. Moreover, the combination of IgG and IgA has synergistic negative effects on fertilization [53–56]. Gonadotoxic substances can also influence AR. High concentrations of dietary phytochemicals, such as genistein isoflavone and β-lapachone, were shown to suppress the AR in a dose- and time-dependent manner in the rat model [57]. Inhibition of AR by genistein seems to involve the protein kinase C pathway while β-lapachone has a direct cytotoxic effect on the sperm cell membrane. It is suggested that genistein and β-lapachone may impact male fertility via AR suppression in high doses and AR induction in low doses [57]. Calcium channel blockers may also interfere with the AR exocytic event. Sperm incubation with different blockers, such as trifluoperazine (calmodulininhibitor), verapamil (Ca^{2+} channel inhibitor), and nifedipine (voltage-dependent Ca^{2+} channel inhibitor) significantly reduces the ability of hamster sperm to undergo AR [58]. The frequency of acrosome-reacted spermatozoa is also increased by the recreational use of marijuana [59]. Falzone et al. [60], studying the effect of pulsed 900-MHz GSM mobile phone radiation on the AR of human sperm, observed that despite not adversely affecting the AR rate, radiofrequency electromagnetic fields (RF-EMF) exposure significantly impaired sperm morphometry and the ability of sperm binding to the hemizona. Finally, Mukhopadhyay et al. evaluated the in vitro effect of benzo[a]pyrene, a substance present in cigarettes, on sperm HA and acrosome status of normozoospermic semen specimens. They observed a significant increase in sperm HA as well as in the premature AR rates in the presence of benzo[a]pyrene [61]. In conclusion, exogenous factors may affect the sperm's ability to undergo timely AR, thus hindering such gametes infertile.

Laboratory Tests to Measure Fertilization Defects

Several tests can be used to measure sperm fertilization defects at different levels, as summarized in Table 11.3.

Assessment of Sperm Binding Using Human ZP Assays

The hemizona assay and the sperm–zona binding ratio test are used to evaluate sperm binding to the human ZP [12]. The hemizona assay uses human oocytes from which a single ZP is isolated and split in half. One half is incubated with fertile donor sperm (positive control) and the other half is incubated with patient sperm (Fig. 11.2). In the sperm–zona binding ratio test, a complete zona is incubated with equal numbers of motile spermatozoa from control and test populations, each labeled with a different fluorescent dye [67]. Irrespective of the method, the number of spermatozoa bounded to the zona is counted and results are expressed as a ratio of the number of test sperm to that of control, with less than 30 % considered abnormal [18]. These tests are clinically useful in cases of UI and low or failed fertilization after conventional IVF [12, 62, 68].

Table 11.3 Functional in vitro tests for measuring sperm fertilization defects at different levels

Level of assessment	Assay	Principle	Specimen	How results are expressed	Normal limits	Clinical relevance
Sperm binding to the human zona	Hemizona assay (HZA)	In HZA, a single ZP is split in half; one half is incubated with donor sperm (positive control) and the other half is incubated with patient sperm	Ejaculated sperm	Ratio of patient and control spermatozoa bound to the zona	≥30%	Men with defective ZP-binding showed a reduced chance of achieving successful fertilization when undergoing IVF [62]
	Sperm–zona binding ratio test (SZBT)	In SZBT, a complete zona is incubated with equal numbers of motile spermatozoa from control and test populations, each labeled with a different fluorescent dye	Ejaculated sperm	Identical to HZA assay	≥30 %	Two of eighteen men with unexplained infertility showed lack of sperm binding to the zona despite having sperm morphology and hyperactivation status similar to fertile individuals [41]
Capacitation	Hyperactivated motility	Assessment of sperm motility using computerized motion analysis in conjunction with kinematics module	Washed sperm incubated under capacitating conditions	Percentage of motile sperm exhibiting hyperactivation motility	≥20%	Significant decrease in the percentage of hyperactivated sperm in infertile men compared to fertile controls after overnight incubation with capacitating conditions [63] Follicular fluid (FF)-induced hyperactivation significantly lower in patients with unexplained infertility in comparison with normal fertile men [41]
Acrosome	ZP-induced AR (ZPIAR)	Assessment of the human sperm acrosome using lectins, monoclonal antibodies, or staining techniques to distinguish the proportions of cells with intact and reacted acrosomes after exposure to zona pellucida	Washed sperm incubated under capacitating conditions	A score is calculated by subtracting the baseline frequency of AR from the values obtained following incubation with zona pellucida	≥15%	Patients with unexplained infertility in whom sperm-ZP binding is normal may have a defective ZP-induced AR (ZPIAR), which will result in reduced sperm–ZP penetration and fertilization failure [64]

Table 11.3 (continued)

Level of assessment	Assay	Principle	Specimen	How results are expressed	Normal limits	Clinical relevance
	Acrosome reaction to ionophore challenge (ARIC)	Assessment of the human sperm acrosome using lectins, monoclonal antibodies, or staining techniques to distinguish the proportions of cells with intact and reacted acrosomes after exposure of stimulants	Washed sperm incubated under capacitating conditions	A score is calculated by subtracting the baseline frequency of AR from the values obtained following stimulant challenge	Baseline frequency of AR above 15 % indicates spontaneous and premature AR	Defective ZPIAR was found in 25 % of normozoospermic subfertile men [65]
Fusogenic ability of the acrosome-reacted sperm with the oolema	Sperm penetration assay (SPA)	Sperm incubation with capacitation media and acrosome reaction stimulants, and assessment of the number of sperm that penetrate zona-free hamster oocytes	Washed sperm incubated under conditions that stimulates capacitation and acrosome reaction	Percentage of eggs penetrated by at least one spermatozoon and the number of spermatozoa per penetrated egg	>10 % of eggs penetrated	34.1 % of patients with unexplained infertility showed less than 10 % oocyte penetration compared to none in a control group of fertile men [66]

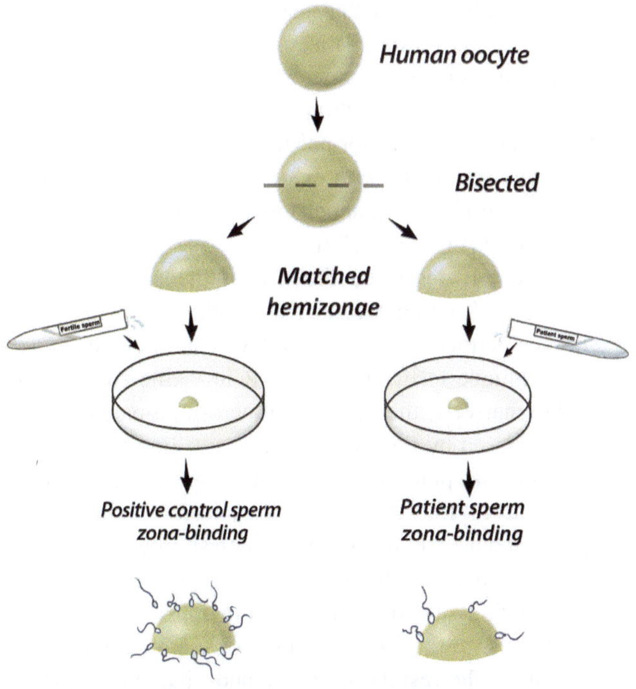

Fig. 11.2 Illustration depicting the hemizona assay. A single zona is bisected and each half is incubated with control and patient sperm suspensions. The number of spermatozoa from each population is counted and the number of test sperm is expressed as a ratio of that of the control

Assessment of Sperm Capacitation by Hyperaticvation Motility

Assessment of HA motility in vitro involves the use of computerized motion analysis in conjunction with a kinematics module to distinguish different subpopulations of motile spermatozoa. Populations of motile sperm are first incubated under capacitating conditions. This step can be carried out by the swim-up method. Briefly, liquefied semen is diluted with an equal volume of culture media (e.g., modified Biggers–Whitten Whittingham [BWW]. After centrifugation at 300*g* for 10 min, the supernatant is removed and the pellet resuspended in 2–3 mL of BWW. A second centrifugation is followed by resuspension to a final volume of approximately 600 μL of BWW supplemented with 0.3 % bovine serum albumin (BSA) factor V. This resuspension, which contains a large number of spermatozoa, is divided in aliquots of 200 μL that are underlayered beneath 800 μL of protein-supplemented BWW. The tubes are loosely capped and placed in a 37 °C incubator under 5 % carbon dioxide in the air, at a 45° angle for 1 h. Motile sperm migrates from the sperm suspension to the upper portion of the culture medium. After this period, the supernatant containing the subpopulation of active motile sperm is removed [69]. Then, these spermatozoa are incubated under capacitating conditions in a BWW

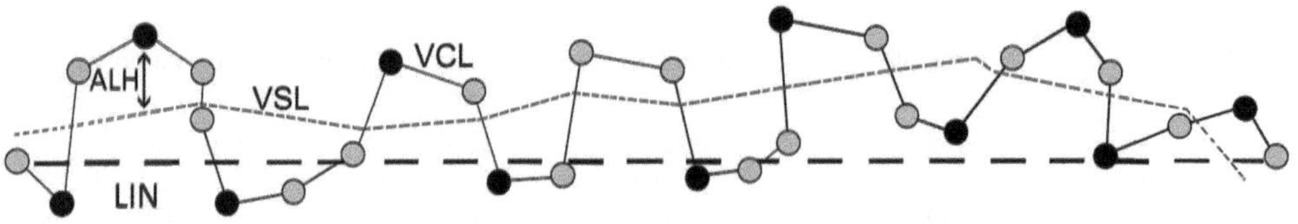

Fig. 11.3 The illustration depicts sperm motion characteristics as assessed by computer-assisted analyzers. VCL = curvilinear velocity, ALH = amplitude of lateral head displacement, and LIN = linearity (see text for definitions)

medium supplemented with 3 % BSA, under 5 % carbon dioxide in the air, for a minimum of 3 h [51]. To assess the HA status of such sperm, aliquots are analyzed on a computer-assisted semen analyzer (CASA) to assess their motion characteristics. This system reconstructs sperm trajectories in successive video frames, and movement parameters are derived. Then, the analyzer segregates the subpopulation of spermatozoa that meets operator-defined kinematics criteria. Hyperactivated spermatozoa can be distinguished from nonhyperactivated ones by their greater curvilinear velocity (VCL; μm/s) and amplitude of the lateral head displacement (ALH; μm), and lower linearity (LIN; %). Curvilinear velocity is the total distance between two points in a given sperm trajectory during the acquisition period, divided by the lime elapsed. The amplitude of lateral head displacement measures sperm head oscillation whereas linearity (calculated as straight line velocity [VSL] /VCL×100 with 100 % representing an absolute straight track; VSL being the straight-line distance between two points divided by the acquisition time) measures linear progression [70] (Fig. 11.3). The definition of HA, as proposed by Burkman, is commonly used and includes all the following criteria: VCL≥100 μm/s, LIN≤65 %, and ALH≥7.5 μm) [71]. In a previous report using this algorithm and the Hamilton–Thorn sperm analyzer, we noted that the proportion of sperm exhibiting HA under capacitating conditions was 21.4 % in normal men [72].

The clinical significance of determining sperm HA is reflected by its correlation with IVF outcomes and natural pregnancy rates [73]. A significant decrease in the percentage of hyperactivated sperm was observed in infertile men compared with sperm from fertile donors [63]. Moreover, computerized assessment of follicular fluid (FF)-induced HA was shown to be significantly lower in patients with UI in comparison with normal fertile men [74]. In fact, the absence of HA after the addition of FF was observed in 39 % of patients with UI. It is, therefore, possible that spermatozoa from such patients have reduced ability to penetrate through the oocyte vestments a result of this abnormal HA response to FF. Despite the aforementioned evidence supporting the role of HA in UI, some authors argue that the determination of HA using "snapshot" of sperm trajectories, as routinely performed by computer-aided sperm analysis instruments, is limited in their ability to truly assess the multiphasic nature of HA [75].

Assessment of Sperm Acrosome Using Lectins

Assessment of the sperm's ability to undergo AR has been used as a test of sperm function for more than two decades [76]. Several techniques have been described to visualize the sperm acrosome including those using stains (fluorescent lectins), monoclonal antibodies, and electron microscopy [76]. Fluorescent lectins are often used; such stains bind to either the outer membrane or the acrosomal contents thus discriminating sperm populations with intact or reacted acrosomes [32, 48, 76–81].

Fluorescein isothiocyanate-conjugated peanut agglutinin (FITC-PNA) and fluorescein isothiocyanate-conjugated Pisum sativum (FITC-PSA) are the most used probes to assess the sperm acrosome. FITC-PNA binds specifically to the outer acrosomal membrane (beta-fraction of D-galactose) while FITC-PSA binds to the alpha-methyl mannose and labels the acrosome contents [79]. Because acrosomal loss can result from sperm death, AR testing is usually performed in conjunction with a test to monitor sperm viability. This strategy allows the distinction of reacted acrosomes in nonviable and viable spermatozoa; the latter represents the population of sperm with "true" AR. In a report using ejaculated specimens from normal men, Esteves et al. showed that the percentage of sperm exhibiting AR would have been overestimated if a simultaneous assessment of viability had not been used (Fig. 11.4) [79].

Cross et al. described the use of the supravital stain Hoechst-33258, a fluorescent DNA-binding dye with limited membrane permeability, combined with an immune-fluorescence technique to evaluate the AR in viable spermatozoa [78]. Alternatively, the viability of acrosome-reacted sperm can be assessed by the hypo-osmotic swelling test (HOST) [82]. HOST has potential advantages over protocols involving the use of fluorochrome-dye exclusion techniques. It precludes the use of an additional fluorescence filter cube to simultaneously assess the acrosome and to monitor viability thus reducing assay costs. We have previously demonstrated the usefulness of the HOST to monitor sperm viability [83]. In our study, the results of HOST and vital staining (Hoescht-33258 and eosin-nigrosin) were highly correlated in fresh sperm (r = 0.95) but not in frozen-thawed ones (r = 0.22) [83]. In a subsequent study, we confirmed that HOST can be used in conjunction with lectins to simultaneously assess viability and acrosome status of fresh sperm (Fig. 11.5) [79].

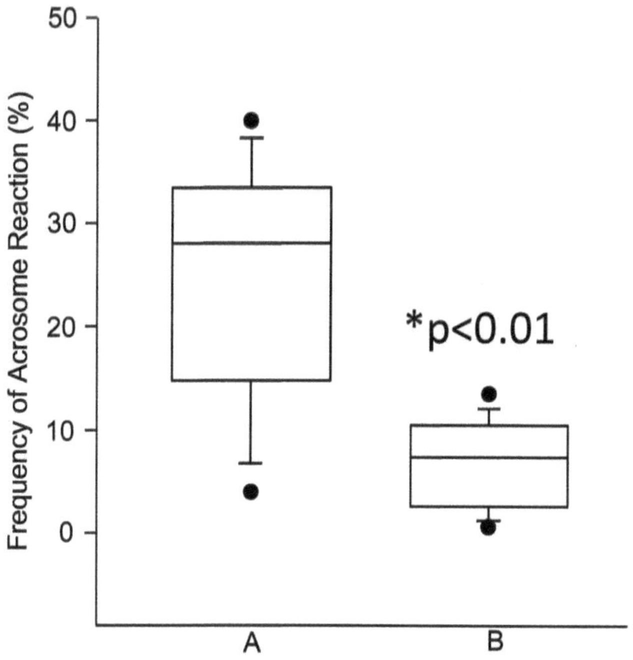

Fig. 11.4 Frequency of acrosome reaction (AR) in semen specimens of fertile donors. AR was determined by FITC-PNA, and sperm viability by Hoechst-33258 staining. **a** Total AR (normal reacted cells plus postmortem degeneration of the acrosomes). **b** AR in live human spermatozoa ($^*p<0.01$). Box covers the middle 50 % of the data values, between the lower and upper quartile. The central line is the median and the whiskers extend out to 80 % of the data. Bars represent values between the 5th and 95th percentile. (Reprinted from Esteves SC, Sharma RK, Thomas AJ Jr, Agarwal A. Evaluation of acrosomal status and sperm viability in fresh and cryopreserved specimens by the use of fluorescent peanut agglutinin lectin in conjunction with hypo-osmotic swelling test. Int Braz J Urol 2007; 33:364–74. With permission from International Brazilian Journal of Urology)

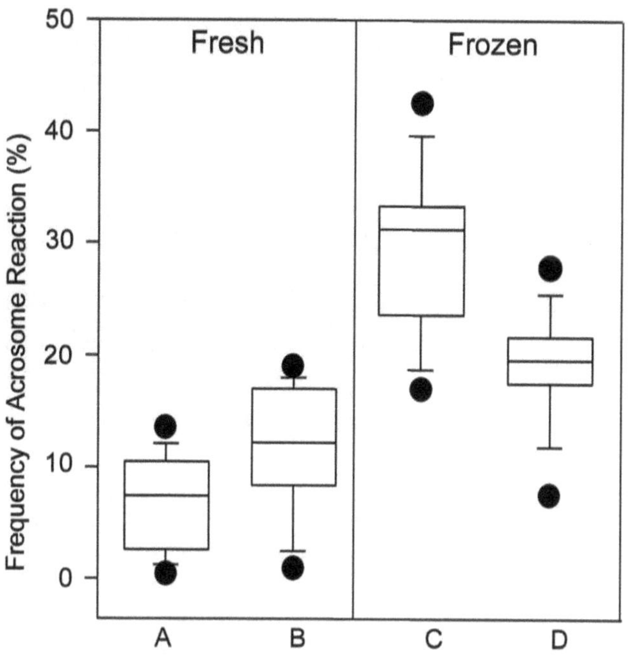

Fig. 11.5 Frequency of acrosome reaction (AR) in live human spermatozoa from 11 samples of fertile donors, as determined by FITC-PNA in conjunction with HOST (**a** and **c**), and FITC-PNA in conjunction with Hoechst-33258 (**b** and **d**), in fresh and post-thaw specimens. AR rates were not different in fresh specimens using either FITC-PNA/HOST or FITC-PNA/Hoechst-33258 ($p=0.07$). In frozen-thawed specimens, the frequencies of AR in viable spermatozoa assessed by the methods were significantly different ($p=0.01$). Box covers the middle 50% of the data values between the lower and upper quartile. The central line is the median and the whiskers extend out to 80 % of the data. Bars represent values between the 5th and 95th percentile. (Reprinted from Esteves SC, Sharma RK, Thomas AJ Jr, Agarwal A. Evaluation of acrosomal status and sperm viability in fresh and cryopreserved specimens by the use of fluorescent peanut agglutinin lectin in conjunction with hypo-osmotic swelling test. Int Braz J Urol 2007; 33:364–74. With permission from International Brazilian Journal of Urology)

The use of FITC-PNA and HOST is our preferred approach to assess the acrosomal status of fresh sperm, and this method can be used in the investigation of men with UI. Briefly, specimens are incubated in hyposmotic conditions and smears are prepared on glass microscope slides. Sperm membranes are then permeabilized in ice-cold methanol and the fixed smears are immersed in a 40-µg/mL FITC-PNA solution. A microscope equipped with phase contrast and fluorescence epi-illumination module is used to examine the slides at 1000× magnification. Each spermatozoon is first examined for tail swelling using phase contrast with halogen illumination. Spermatozoa are classified as viable if tail swelling is observed after exposure to the hyposmotic solution. Then, illumination is changed to the mercury ultraviolet epi-illumination source for assessing FITC-PNA staining.

Alternatively, Hoechst-33258 can be used to monitor viability [79, 80]. In this method, sperm specimens are centrifuged and resuspended in 2 µg/mL Hoechst-33258 solution. The sperm suspension is incubated for 10 min in the dark and then spermatozoa are washed to remove excess stain. Smears are prepared on glass microscope slides and then immersed in ice-cold methanol to permeabilize the sperm membranes. The fixed smears are immersed in a 40-µg/mL FITC-PNA solution, incubated at room temperature, and washed gently in PBS to remove the excess label. A microscope equipped with phase contrast and fluorescence epi-illumination module is used to examine the slides at 1000× magnification. The illumination is selected to the mercury ultraviolet epi-illumination source for assessing FITC-PNA and Hoechst-33258 labeling by using appropriate filter cubes. FITC-PNA and Hoechst-33258 fluoresces "apple-green" and bright medium blue, respectively (Fig. 11.6). Examination of the same spermatozoon for FITC-PNA labeling and for Hoechst-33258 staining is performed by interchanging the fluorescence filter cubes.

To evaluate the enzymatic release from sperm acrosomes, artificial (ionophores) or physiological inducers (progesterone, FF, and ZP) are used. After stimulation by

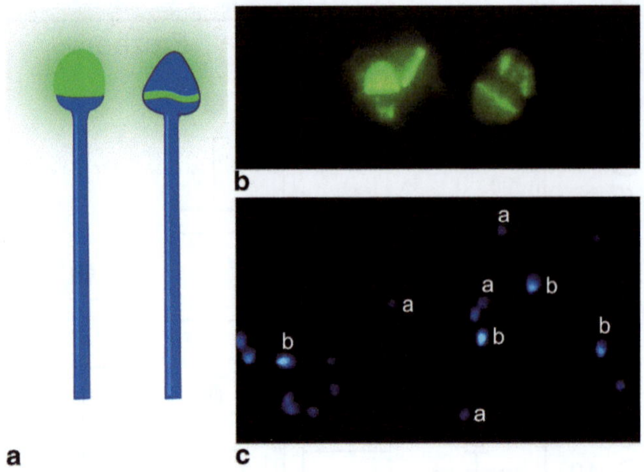

Fig. 11.6 Assessment of acrosome reaction (AR). **a** Illustration of spermatozoa labeled by FITC-PNA: spermatozoa with intact acrosomes show uniform apple-green fluorescence at the acrosomal region of the sperm head (*left*); staining is limited to the equatorial segment of the acrosome in spermatozoa exhibiting AR (*right*). **b** Photomicrographs of spermatozoa labeled by FITC-PNA: only the equatorial segment of the acrosome is stained in spermatozoa exhibiting AR. **c** Photomicrographs of spermatozoa stained with Hoechst-33258: live spermatozoa show pale-blue fluorescence due to the exclusion of the dye (**a**) while dead spermatozoa show bright blue-white fluorescence (**b**). (Adapted from Esteves SC, Sharma RK, Thomas AJ Jr, Agarwal A. Evaluation of acrosomal status and sperm viability in fresh and cryopreserved specimens by the use of fluorescent peanut agglutinin lectin in conjunction with hypo-osmotic swelling test. Int Braz J Urol 2007; 33:364–74. With permission from International Brazilian Journal of Urology)

the aforementioned stimulants, the proportion of reacted spermatozoa is assessed. Our preference is to use calcium ionophore A23187, which exchanges Ca^{2+} for $2H^{+}$. The ionophore-induced AR, also termed "AR to ionophore challenge (ARIC)" has been validated as a sperm function test with high predictive value for the outcomes of assisted reproduction techniques [17, 39, 77, 84–86]. Briefly, motile spermatozoa are first capacitated by incubation in sperm culture medium at 37°C for 3 h. Then, capacitated sperms are divided into two equal aliquots: one is incubated with 2.5 µmol/L calcium ionophore A23187 solution, and the other is treated with dimethylsulfoxide (10%, v/v) as a control [49, 80, 81]. Acrosome status can be determined by FITC-PNA or FITC-PSA in combination with the nuclear stain bis-benzimide or HOST to monitor viability. The ARIC test score is calculated by subtracting the baseline frequency of AR from the values obtained following ionophore challenge. ARIC results have shown to be a reliable indicator of fertility potential in IUI and conventional IVF treatment cycles [86]. The AR threshold values for predicting complete fertilization failure and pregnancy in IVF, as determined by receiver-operating curves (ROC) analysis, were 21 and 26%, respectively [86]. Moreover, no pregnancies were obtained by IUI when ARIC results were below 11% [86]. In ICSI, ZP penetration and oolemmal fusion are bypassed and thus the role of the AR is unclear. In fact, ARIC results do not seem to predict ICSI outcome since injections using sperm from different acrosome reacted sperm populations had no impact on fertilization rates [28, 86]. As an alternative to ionophores, AR can be induced by ZP (ZP-induced AR [ZPIAR]. In one study, defective ZPIAR was found in 25% of normozoospermic subfertile men [65].

Patients with AR defects usually have UI and normal sperm–ZP binding. However, their sperm fail to penetrate the ZP and have zero or low rates of fertilization with conventional IVF [64]. The diagnostic feature is that very low proportions of sperm undergo AR after ionophore or ZP challenge. Nevertheless, these patients achieve normal fertilization and pregnancy rates with ICSI [87].

Interestingly, seminal zinc concentrations were shown to be significantly higher in a group of normozoospermic men with defective ZPIAR. Zinc has a role as a decapacitation factor by binding to the sperm plasma membrane. High seminal zinc concentrations seem to have an adverse effect not only on ZPIAR [88] but also in the AR induced by calcium ionophore [89]. The mechanism of AR induced by ionophores differs from physiological AR induced by the ZP [32]. While the physiological AR involves activation of several signal transduction pathways, the ionophore-induced AR involves mainly a chemical effect on calcium influx that partially reflects the physiological AR process [32].

Assessment of the Fusogenic Ability of the Acrosome-Reacted Sperm with the Oolema (Enhanced Sperm Penetration Assay (SPA))

The ability of the equatorial region of the acrosome-reacted human sperm to fuse with the vitelline membrane of the oocyte is tested using the SPA, also known as the zona-free hamster oocyte penetration test. Although this test does not assess sperm–ZP, it measures the spermatozoon's ability to undergo capacitation, AR, fusion and penetration through the oolema, and decondensation within the cytoplasm of an oocyte [12].

Sperm preparation for the test includes two steps: (i) preparation of a selected motile sperm population free of seminal plasma (e.g., by swim-up or discontinuous gradient technique) and (ii) incubation and treatment of the selected sperm population under conditions that stimulate capacitation and AR. The calcium ionophore (A23187) incubation method is recommended for this step. The final volume should be calculated to obtain a sperm population of about 10 million motile cells per milliliter. Hamster oocytes from which the ZP had been removed are incubated with sperm specimens. A 20-µL oil-covered droplet of the sperm suspension is prepared using a Petri dish, and 10–15 zona-free eggs are transferred into

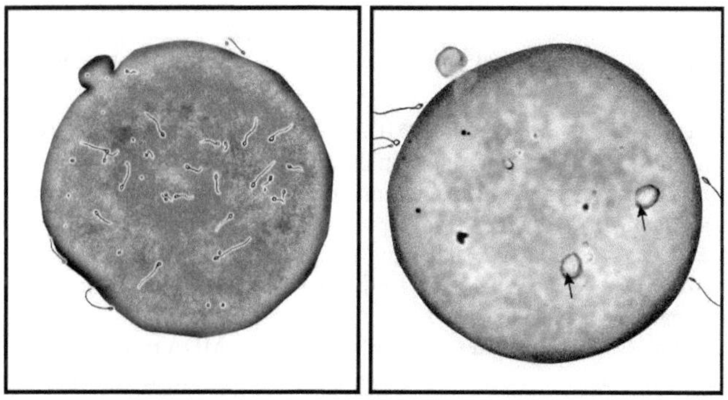

a b

Fig. 11.7 Illustration depicting the sperm penetration assay (SPA). Human spermatozoa are seen into the hamster oocyte cytoplasm **a**. The arrows point to the swollen sperm heads indicative of sperm decondensation within the oocyte's cytoplasm **b**.

the droplet. The dish is incubated under 5–6% CO_2 in the air at 37°C for 3 h. Afterwards, the zona-free eggs are examined using phase-contrast microscopy. The presence of either swollen sperm heads or male pronuclei (slightly larger than the female one and that contains small dark nucleoli), or both, are used to confirm sperm penetration [21] (Fig. 11.7).

The assay is scored by calculating either the percentage of ova that is penetrated by at least one spermatozoon or the average number of sperm penetrations per ovum. Normal sperm are able to penetrate 10–30% of hamster ova [90]. The assay should be run in parallel with a positive control semen specimen exhibiting >50% penetration. Recent refinements of SPA include sperm incubation with more potent capacitating media, which allow the majority of ova to be penetrated; scores are obtained by calculating the number of sperm that penetrate each ovum. Aitken et al. reported that approximately one third of men with UI had less than 10% ova penetration compared to none in the control group of fertile men [66]. The ability of the SPA to predict the success or failure of IVF is debatable. Some investigators have shown no correlation with an abnormal test [91], whereas others have claimed 100% predictability [92]. Taking an average from different studies, a normal SPA seems to have 70% predictability of fertilization in in vitro conditions [93]. Nevertheless, semen samples that fail to fertilize the hamster ova are usually unable to fertilize human ova. Although the SPA is considered a research tool, it may be of clinical value for men with UI with poor fertilization rate in IVF.

Oxidative Stress

ROS are byproducts of oxygen metabolism and energy production that act as regulators of vital physiological intracellular processes. In the male reproductive tract, the primary producers of ROS are the leukocytes and immature spermatozoa. Small quantities of ROS have important roles in sperm function including regulation of capacitation, AR, HA, and the fusion of spermatozoa with the oocyte [94]. In sperm, ROS are generated by two ways, (1) NADPH oxidase system at the level of the sperm plasma membrane [95], and (2) NADH-dependent oxido-reductase system at the mitochondrial level, which is the major source of ROS in sperm of infertile men [96, 97]. When ROS levels disproportionately increase, mainly by the presence of superoxide (O_2^-), hydroxyl radicals (OH), or nitric derivatives (NO), compared with the neutralizing capacity of intracellular and extracellular antioxidants, or when a reduction in the antioxidant capacity occurs, oxidative stress usually follows and target lipids, proteins, sugars, and nucleic acids through a variety of mechanisms.

In sperm, ROS primarily target membranes and DNA. By having an available valence electron, oxidative species interact with the cell membrane and cause lipid peroxidation of which the final product is malondialdehyde (MDA), a measurable compound used to determine the extent of ongoing oxidative modification of membrane-polyunsaturated fatty acids (PFA). The peroxidation of PFAs has detrimental effects on the structure of the sperm head and midpiece membranes, causing changes in the sperm membrane fluidity that ultimately lead to suboptimal sperm motility and fertilization [94]. Oxidative species also target DNA molecules and cause a variety of defects in the cell genetic material. ROS can inflict serious damage to DNA, including point mutations, polymorphisms, deletions, chromosomal rearrangements, frame shifts, and single-stranded or double-stranded breaks [98]. The OS-induced sperm damage has been suggested to be a significant contributing factor in 30–80% of all cases of male infertility [99]. Likewise immunologic infertility and fertilization defects, oxidative stress cannot be detected in the routine semen analysis.

Laboratory Tests to Measure ROS

The methods used for ROS detection are broadly divided into two major categories based on their ability to directly or indirectly measure oxidative radicals (Table 11.4). Indirect measurements involve the assessment of lipid peroxidation products (MDA), protein oxidation products (such as protein carbonyl) and oxidized DNA (8-hydroxy-2′-deoxyguanosine [8-OHdG]) [105] whereas direct oxidative-stress measurements include total or specific ROS level in semen and total antioxidant capacity (TAC).

Table 11.4 Tests for measuring reactive oxygen species in UMI

Assay	Principle	Specimen	How results are expressed	Normal limits	Clinical relevance
Thiobarbituric acid reactive substances (TBARS)	Malondialdehyde (MDA), a byproduct of lipid peroxidation, condense with two equivalents thiobarbituric acid to give a fluorescent red derivative that can be assayed spectrophotometrically	Semen and seminal plasma	Absorbance at 532 nm is recorded and expressed as nmoL MDA/10×10^7 cells, nmoL MDA mL^{-1} seminal plasma, or nmoL MDA/total seminal plasma	Mean ± SD of MDA concentrations in the sperm and seminal plasma of fertile men were reported to be 0.0287 ± 0.0162 nM/10^8 spermatozoa [100] and averaged as 0.65 ± 0.17 nmol/mL^{-1}, respectively [101]	ROS degrade polyunsaturated lipids of sperm membrane forming MDA, which is a reactive aldehyde toxic to sperm MDA reacts with deoxyadenosine and deoxyguanosine DNA, forming DNA adducts, and is therefore potentially mutagenic
Chemiluminescence	Intra- and extracellular ROS levels (mainly H_2O_2, $O_2^{\bullet-}$, and OH^-) react with probes and emit photons that can be measured using a luminometer. The final chemiluminescent signal is the integrated sum of the partial signals generated by every spermatozoon	Semen or sperm fractions	$\times10^6$ counted photons per minute (cpm) per 20×10^6 cells/mL	$\leq 0.0185\times10^6$ cpm/20×10^6 sperm [102]	Men with unexplained infertility generally present with significantly higher seminal ROS levels than healthy controls [103]
Enhanced chemiluminescence	Seminal total antioxidant capacity (TAC) is a measure of the seminal plasma's ability to scavenge ROS and counteract oxidative stress	Seminal plasma	Total antioxidant capacity (TAC) of the seminal plasma is expressed in molar Trolox equivalents	>1420 micromoles of Trolox for seminal plasma TAC [104]	Men with unexplained infertility generally present with significantly lower antioxidant properties than healthy controls [104]
Nitroblue tetrazolium (NBT) reduction test	NBT is a yellow water-soluble nitrosubstituted aromatic tetrazolium compound that reacts with cellular superoxide ions to form a colored intermediate and visible formazan derivative. Depending on the concentration of superoxide anion and the cellular content of various oxidoreductases, a precipitate with a color that vary from a light pink to dark purple or almost black is seen	Semen and seminal plasma	Color intensity of precipitates is compared to a reference card indicating different levels of free superoxide	Light pink or white precipitate compared to reference card	Superoxide anion is the primary form of ROS generated by the addition of an electron to the oxygen molecule. Superoxide anions can be converted into hydrogen peroxide, peroxyl radical, and hydroxyl radical

Indirect Measure of ROS by Thiobarbituric Acid Reactive Substances (TBARS) Assay

MDA is a byproduct of lipid peroxidation that can be easily measured by the TBARS assay. Briefly, semen samples are centrifuged for 7 min at 2000*g*, and then 100 µl of the supernatant seminal plasma is added to 900 µl of distilled water into a glass tube. To each tube, 500 µl of thiobarbituric acid reagent (0.67*g* of 2-thiobarbituric acid dissolved in 100 ml of distilled water with 0.5*g* NaOH and 100 ml glacial acetic acid) is added and then heated for 1 h in a boiling water bath. After cooling, each tube is centrifuged for 10 min at 4000*g* and the supernatant absorbance is read on a spectrophotometer at 534 nm [106].

Direct Measure of ROS Using Chemiluminescence

ROS levels can be measured by the chemiluminescence method using luminol (5-amino-2,3-dihydro-1,4-phthalazinedione) or lucigenin (N, N′-dimethyl-9,9′-biacridinium dinitrate) as the probe. Luminol measures global ROS whereas lucigenin measures specifically the production of superoxide anions. Both H_2O_2 and $O_2^{\bullet-}$ are involved in luminol-dependent chemiluminescence because both catalase and SOD can disrupt the luminol signal very efficiently. Oxidation of luminol (one-electron) leads to the creation of a radical species which interacts with ground state oxygen to produce $O_2^{\bullet-}$, which participates in the oxygenation of luminol radical species to create an unstable endoperoxide, which breaks down and leads to light emission.

Luminol is extremely sensitive and reacts with a variety of ROS at neutral pH. It has the ability to measure both extracellular as well as the intracellular ROS. Free radicals have a very short half-life and are continuously produced. The free-radical combines with luminol to produce a light signal that is then converted to electrical signal (photon) by the instrument called luminometer (Model: LKB Autoplus 953). Lucigenin works through a one-electron reduction unlike luminol, which requires one-electron oxidation, that creates a radical from lucigenin; this radical gives up its electron to the ground state oxygen to create $O_2^{\bullet-}$, thus returning the lucigenin to its parent state. The number of free radicals produced is measured as relative light units/sec/$10\times^{6}$ sperm [107].

A 100 mM stock solution of luminol is prepared by dissolving 177.09 mg of luminol to 10 mL of DMSO solution in a polystyrene tube. The tube is covered in aluminum foil due to the light sensitivity of luminol. A 5 mM working solution is prepared by mixing 20 µL luminol stock solution with 380 µL DMSO in a foil covered polystyrene tube. It is prepared fresh prior to use and is stored at room temperature in the dark until needed. It is stable for 24 h if not exposed to the light. After complete liquefaction, manual semen analysis is performed for assessment of sperm concentration and motility. The instrument is set up for ROS measurement. ROS can be performed in a variety of samples: neat liquefied whole seminal ejaculate, processed sample either by a simple wash and resuspend procedure or by swim-up and density gradient.

The luminometer is attached to the computer and 11 polyestirene tubes (12 × 75 mm) are prepared and labeled as blank (triplicate), negative control (triplicate), test sample (duplicate), and positive control (triplicate) as shown (Figs. 11.2 and 11.3). Four-hundred microliters of PBS or test samples are added. Positive control tubes contain 50 µL of hydrogen peroxide (30 %). To start the reaction, 10 µL of the luminol working solution is added to all tubes except blank. The reaction is started for 15 min using the Berthold tube master program. From the "setup menu" each parameter is defined as: read time (1 s), background read time (0 s), total time (900 s), cycle time (30 s), delay injector "M" read (0 s), injector M (0 s), temperature (37°C), and temperature control (O = Off and 1 ON). A unique assay name is given and the work load file is saved. The assay is started and the tubes are scanned and saved as an excel sheet. Both the average RLU for the negative control, sample and positive control are calculated. The average negative control is subtracted from the test sample. ROS level is calculated by dividing the test sample result by the sperm concentration (Fig. 11.8a). ROS levels <20 RLU/s/$\times 10^6$ sperm are considered normal (Fig. 11.8b). ROS has high sensitivity and therefore can be a useful diagnostic tool in screening infertile men for oxidative stress.

Total Nonenzymatic Antioxidant Capacity (TAC)

The antioxidant system of living organisms includes enzymes such as superoxide dismutase, catalase, and glutathione peroxidase; macromolecules such as albumin, ceruloplasmin, and ferritin; and an array of small molecules, including ascorbic acid, α-tocopherol, β-carotene, reduced glutathione, uric acid, and bilirubin. The sum of endogenous and food-derived antioxidants represents the total antioxidant activity of the extracellular fluid. Thus, the overall antioxidant capacity may give more relevant biological information compared to that obtained by the measurement of individual components, as it considers the cumulative effect of all antioxidants present in plasma and body fluids. The TAC in the seminal plasma can be measured by the colorimetric assay using an antioxidant assay kit (Cat # 709001; Cayman Chemical, Ann Arbor, Michigan) using a 96 well plate and a plate reader (BioTek Instruments, Inc., Winooski, Vermont). Seminal plasma samples are batched

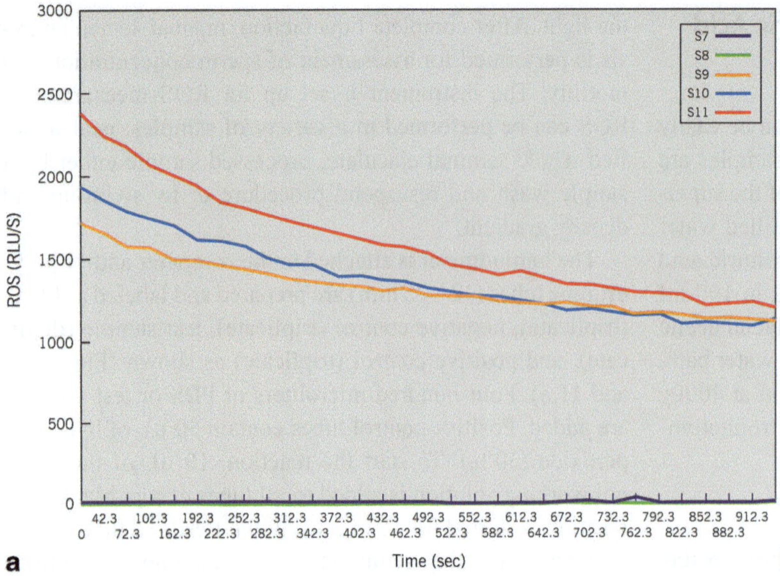

a

Sample	Sample ID	Status	RLU Mean	Read Date	Read Time
1	Blank	Done	6269	11/17/2010	1:35:54 PM
2		Done	6713	11/17/2010	1:35:56 PM
3		Done	6189	11/17/2010	1:35:57 PM
4	Negative Control	Done	8454	11/17/2010	1:35:59 PM
5		Done	8104	11/17/2010	1:36:00 PM
6		Done	9993	11/17/2010	1:36:02 PM
7	Test Sample	Done	12954	11/17/2010	1:36:03 PM
8		Done	11368	11/17/2010	1:36:05 PM
9	Positive Control	Done	1261225	11/17/2010	1:36:06 PM
10		Done	1207794	11/17/2010	1:36:08 PM
11		Done	1458674	11/17/2010	1:36:10 PM

Example

Patient average (P_{av}) = 12161 RLU / sec   Sperm count = 12.6 x 10^6 /mL

Negative Control average (NC_{av}) = 8850.3 RLU / sec

Corrected value = P_{av} - NC_{av}

12161 - 8850.3 RLU / sec = 3310.7 RLU / sec

Corrected ROS = $\frac{3310.7}{12.6}$ = 262.7 RLU / sec / x 10^6 sperms

Result = ROS positive

b

Fig. 11.8 **a** A typical ROS curve showing high ROS levels (tubes 9–11) and low ROS levels (tubes 7 and 8). **b** A representative printout generated after the ROS measurement is complete. The chart shows the 11 tubes (S1–S11), each representative of the type of sample and the mean RLU value for each tube. At the bottom is also an example illustrating how to calculate the final amount of ROS generated in a given test (patient) sample

and frozen till the time of assay [104]. The assay relies on the ability of antioxidants in the sample to inhibit the oxidation of ABTS (2,2′-azino-di-[3-ethylbenzthiazoline sulphonate]) to ABTS·+ by metmyoglobin. Under the reaction conditions used, the antioxidants in the seminal plasma cause suppression of the absorbance at 750 nm to a degree which is proportional to their concentration. The capacity of the antioxidants present in the sample to prevent ABTS oxidation is compared with that of standard Trolox, a water-soluble tocopherol analogue. Results are reported as micromoles of Trolox equivalent. This assay measures the combined antioxidant activities of all its constituents including vitamins, proteins, lipids, glutathione, uric acid, etc.

All the reagents are prepared as per the manufacturer's instructions. The kit contains antioxidant buffer (Vial # 1), Metmyoglobin (Vial # 2), standard Trolox (6-hydroxy-2,5,7,8-tetramethylchroman-2-carboxylic acid) (Vial # 3), hydrogen peroxide (Via; # 4), and Chromogen (Vial # 5). Frozen seminal plasma is brought to room temperature and diluted 1:10 with assay buffer. Standard Trolox is prepared to give seven different concentrations (A–G) ranging from 0 to 0.33 mM trolox). For the assay, a multichannel pipette is used. To each well, 10 μL of trolox standard (tubes A–G) or sample in duplicate + 10 μL of metmyoglobin + 150 μL of chromogen per well. The reaction by adding 40 μL of hydrogen peroxide (441 μM working solution) using a multichannel pipette. The reaction is started for 5 min. The plate is covered and placed on the plate shaker. After 5 min the plate is removed and the absorbance is read at 750 nm using a plate reader. The worksheet for calculating the results is available at www.caymanchem.com.

The normal values are >2000 μM Trolox. In an earlier study, it was demonstrated that combining ROS and TAC results to provide a composite ROS–TAC score was of clinical relevance in a variety of clinical diagnoses. Infertile men with male factor or idiopathic infertility diagnosis were reported to have poor ROS–TAC scores compared to healthy fertile men who are able to initiate a pregnancy [108].

Qualitative Measurement of Superoxide Anion by NBT Reduction Test

Recently, a ready-to-use colorimetric commercial kit has been made available to detect superoxide anion in sperm based on the NBT reduction test (Oxisperm®, Halotech DNA, Madrid, Spain). Superoxide anion, the primary form of ROS, is formed by the addition of an electron to the oxygen molecule. Superoxide anions can be converted into hydrogen peroxide, peroxyl radical, and hydroxyl radical, all of which are secondary ROS [109]. NBT is a yellow water-soluble nitrosubstituted aromatic tetrazolium compound that reacts with cellular superoxide ions to form a colored intermediate and visible formazan derivative [96]. The cytoplasmic NADPH, which is produced by oxidation of glucose through the hexose monophosphate shunt, helps to transfer

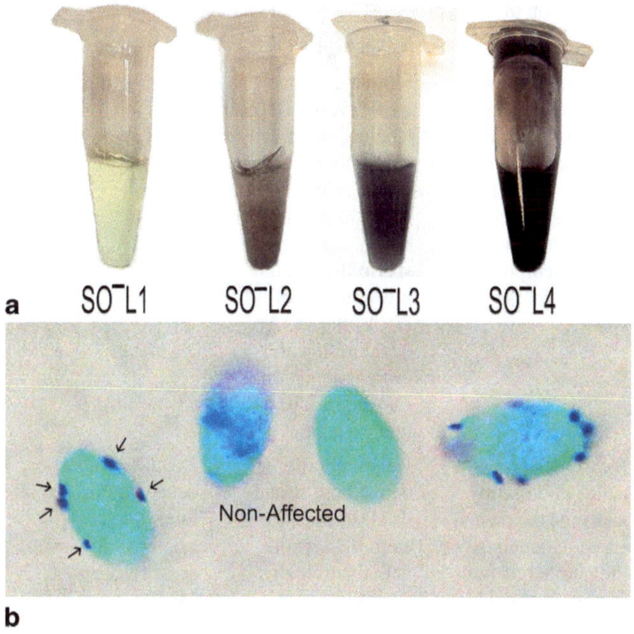

Fig. 11.9 Colorimetric representation of different levels of oxidative stress in the human semen based on the nitroblue tetrazolium reduction test (Oxisperm®, Halotech DNA, Madrid, Spain). The color intensity is related to the levels of superoxide anion in the sample (no color change is indicative of negligible levels; pink and blue are indicative of low and moderate levels, respectively, whereas dark blue represents high levels of superoxide anion (**a**). Affected sperm can be visualized using bright-field microscopy because farmazan precipitates (arrows) on the membrane (**b**). (Courtesy of Altea Gosálbez, Madrid, Spain)

electrons to NBT and reduces NBT into formazan. The NBT reaction represents the ROS-generating activity in the cytoplasm of cells and therefore can help to determine the cellular origin of ROS in a heterogeneous suspension such as the semen. Depending on the concentration of superoxide anion and the cellular content of various oxidoreductases, a precipitate with a color that varies from light pink to dark purple or almost black will form [110]. To perform this assay, a tube containing a reagent gel is placed in a water bath at 90°C for approximately 5 min to allow the gel to liquefy. After gel stabilization at 37°C, liquefied semen is added (1:1, v/v) and the mixture is incubated for 45 min at 37°C. The color of the tested sample is compared with the reference card to determine the level of oxidative stress. Despite not providing a quantitative measure of ROS, the test estimates the level of oxidative stress in the sample based on the intensity of the color (from L1 low to L4 high, Fig. 11.9a) without the need of an expensive equipment such as the luminometer. The method also offers the possibility of analyzing the proportion of affected spermatozoa and the intensity of the reaction on the sperm membrane under bright field microscopy (Fig. 11.9b).

Sperm DNA Integrity Defects

Sperm DNA integrity is characterized by the absence of both single and double DNA strand breaks and nucleotide modifications or base loss thus giving rise to a linear disposition of the nucleotides along each single chromosome. Loss of DNA integrity is termed DNA damage and it may occur at any level during spermatogenesis, spermiogenesis, and epididymal transit [111]. Sperm DNA damage is a broad term that accounts for many defects in the DNA structure including (i) single or double DNA strand breaks, (ii) base deletion or modification, (iii) interstrand or intrastrand cross-linkage, and (iv) DNA-protein cross linkage [112]. Sperm DNA fragmentation refers to the breaks occurring at the DNA strands, and they are termed single (ss) or double strand breaks (ds) depending on the partial (one free 5′-3′ end) or whole (two free 5′-3′ ends) liberation of each DNA strand, respectively. Postmeiotically initiated abortive apoptosis, unresolved strand breaks during spermiogenesis, and oxidative stress have all been implicated as potential sources of this damage [113]. Sperm with damaged DNA are released in the semen, and despite the likely result of infertility, these defective cells may still retain the ability to fertilize. Several studies reported on the increased proportions of sperm with damaged DNA both in men with unexplained and idiopathic infertility compared to fertile controls [114, 115]. In fact, sperm DNA damage has been associated with several infertility phenotypes including UI, idiopathic infertility, repeated IUI and IVF failure, and recurrent miscarriage [116–119]. Also, the birth of offspring generated from such defective sperm is associated with an increased risk of imprinting defects and cancer [120, 121].

DNA damage may be the result of both intrinsic and extrinsic disturbances usually associated with oxidative stress. As such, several researchers consider that sperm DNA damage is a marker of elevated oxidative stress [121–124].

Laboratory Tests to Assess Sperm DNA Integrity

From the laboratory standpoint, different assays have been developed to assess sperm DNA damage. These assays are based on different principles and therefore differ in their ability to detect DNA damage [125]. In general, these methods can be grouped into (i) assays that measure DNA damage directly, by incorporating probes at the site of damage (Table 11.5); (ii) assays that measure the susceptibility of DNA to denaturation, that is, their principle is to first promote DNA denaturation and then measure DNA damage by detecting the formation of single-strand DNA from na-

Table 11.5 Methods for assessing sperm DNA damage based on direct incorporation of DNA probes at the site of damage

Name and acronym	Characteristics	Principle	Test results	Advantages	Disadvantages
In situ nick translation (ISNT) assay	The template-dependent enzyme, DNA polymerase I incorporates fluorescent biotinylated dUTP at free 3′-OH single- or double-strand DNA breaks	Sperm with the incorporation of labeled nucleotides can be detected on examination under fluorescence microscopy; fluorescence increases proportionally with the number of DNA strand breaks	By using fluorescence microscopy analysis, the measured parameter is the number of fluorescent sperm which represent those with dUTP incorporated to DNA breaks	Simple and low cost; level of DNA labeling is typically higher than TUNEL, which is advantageous to assess highly degraded sperm that exhibit low amounts of DNA after DNA denaturation and protein depletion; easy control of polymerase action	Requires fluorescence microscopy; relatively low sensitivity
Terminal deoxy nucleotidyl transferase mediated dUTP nick end labeling (TUNEL) assay	The template-independent enzyme, terminal deoxynucleotidyl transferase, incorporates fluorescent UTP at single and double 3′-OH free ends	Sperm with the incorporation of labeled nucleotides to DNA 3′-OH ends fluoresce and can be identified using fluorescence microscopy; fluorescence increases proportionally with the number of DNA strand breaks; TUNEL can be applied with both fluorescence microscopy and flow cytometry	By using fluorescence microscopy analysis, the measured parameter is the number of fluorescent sperm which represent those with dUTP incorporated to DNA breaks	Relatively simple; detect both ss and ds DNA breaks but cannot discriminate them; high specificity	Requires fluorescence microscopy; labor intensive; relatively low sensitivity. Measurement by flow cytometry is more robust, rapid, and accurate

tive double-strand DNA [111] (Table 11.6); and (iii) assays that indirectly measure the level of chromatin compaction (Table 11.7).

In our laboratories, TUNEL and SCD assays have been implemented as the methods to assess sperm DNA damage, as described below.

Terminal Deoxy Nucleotidyl Transferase Mediated dUTP Nickend Labeling (TUNEL) Assay

This single-step staining method label DNA breaks with FITC-dUTP (APO-DIRECT™ kit; BD Pharmigen, San Diego, CA, Catalog # 556381). TUNEL utilizes a template-independent DNA polymerase called terminal deoxynucleotidyl transferase (TdT) which nonpreferentially adds deoxyribonucleotides to 3′ hydroxyl (OH) single- and double-stranded DNA. Deoxyuridine triphosphate (dUTP) is the substrate that is added by the TdT enzyme to the free 3′-OH break-ends of DNA (Fig. 11.10). The more DNA strand break sites present, the more label is incorporated within a cell. After FITC-dUTP incorporation, these sites are identified using either flow cytometry or fluorescence microscopy.

For this assay, a sperm aliquot containing 1–2 million spermatozoa is washed in phosphate-buffered saline (PBS) and resuspended in ice-cold 3.7 % paraformaldehyde for 2 h. Specimens can be either stored overnight at 4°C or processed immediately. The paraformaldehyde is removed by centrifuging at 300*g* for 7 min and resuspended in 70 % ice-cold ethanol. After this step, sperm can be stored at −20°C until the time of analysis. 2 mL negative (Cat# 6553LZ; white cap) and positive control cells suspensions (Cat# 6552LZ; brown cap) provided in the kit are included in each run; the suspensions are centrifuged as described above. A positive control specimen (treated with DNase I) or any previously run negative- and positive-sperm sample with known DNA damage is included. To all the tubes 1 mL of wash buffer (6548AZ) (blue cap) is added and vortexed. The mixtures are centrifuged as before and the supernatants are discarded. An additional washing step with the buffer is carried out, and the supernatants are discarded. Based on the number of tubes to be run, the staining solution is prepared by mixing the reagents provided in the assay kit. For a single assay, 10 µL of reaction buffer (green cap); 0.75 µL of TdT Enzyme (yellow cap), 8.00 µL of FITC-dUTP (orange cap), and 32.25 µL of distilled H_2O are mixed to give a total volume of 51.00 µL of the stain solution. The pellets (control and test specimens) are resuspended in 50 µL of the staining solution and then incubated for 60 min at 37°C. The tubes are covered with aluminum foil. At the end of the incubation time, 1.0 mL of rinse buffer (Cat# 6550AZ) (red cap) is added to

Table 11.6 Methods for assessing sperm DNA damage based on the susceptibility of DNA to denaturation with formation of single-strand (ss) DNA from native double-strand (ds) or single-strand (ss) DNA*

Name and acronym	Characteristics	Principle	How results are expressed	Advantages	Disadvantages
Acridine orange (AO) test	AO is a fluorescent cationic and metachromatic dye with specificity to nucleic acids. When AO intercalates into double stranded DNA it fluoresces green (525 nm), and when it interacts with RNA or single DNA stretches (by electrostatic attraction) it fluoresces red/orange (>630 nm)	DNA of sperm with a damaged chromatin structure is more prone to denaturation than intact counterparts. After a mild acid treatment, sperm is exposed to AO which binds to ds DNA (nondenatured) and to ss DNA (denatured). The metachromatic shift in fluorescence is used to differentiate sperm with intact (green) and damaged (red) chromatin structure	By using a fluorescence microscopy-based analysis, the measured parameter is the number of cells with red fluorescence which reflects the proportion of sperm with damaged DNA in the sample	Simple and inexpensive	Requires fluorescence microscopy; heterogeneous staining of slides and fast fluorescence fading are usual A series of intermediate colors (between red and green), related to differential sperm susceptibility to sperm denaturation, decreases interobserver reproducibility Overestimate "true" sperm DNA fragmentation; low specificity for DNA breaks compared to Comet and TUNEL
Sperm chromatin structure assay (SCSA)	Identical to AO assay	Variation of AO test using flow cytometry	By using flow cytometry-based analysis and a dedicated software, measurement of fluorescence at both the wavelengths after denaturation is used to assess the percentage of fragmented DNA (DNA fragmentation index: DFI) in the sample	High statistical robustness and inter- and intralaboratory reproducibility; SCSA has been applied extensively in clinical studies of human fertility	Requires flow cytometry and dedicated software; expensive; overestimate "true" sperm DNA fragmentation; lower specificity than alkaline comet assay, ISNT and TUNEL since it detects not only DNA fragmentation but also protamine content, disulphide cross linkage, immature sperm, and traces of RNA
Comet assay	Under electrophoresis, small DNA fragments migrate farther than the large fragments. Migration of these small broken pieces of DNA away from the DNA core of the cell creates a characteristic figure of a "comet" tail. The performance of the test varies according to different pH conditions	Spermatozoa are sandwiched between agarose layers and then lysed and electrophoresed During the lysis step, the sulfhydryl groups in protamines are reduced which eases the movement of fragmented DNA on electrophoresis; fluorochromes such as propium iodide, SYBR-green and YOYO-1 iodide can be used for staining	By using an electrophoresis-basis analysis, the percentage of the DNA in the tail of the comet, as well as the tail length and the intensity of staining, is measured using specific image analysis software	Evaluates DNA strand breaks in a single cell; allows quantification of different degrees of fragmentation by comparing individual sperm; requires few sperm for analysis; can differentiate the nature of DNA break; specific for DNA breaks	Labor intensive; high inter-observer subjectivity; dedicated software is expensive; neutral comet assay evaluates ds breaks only and underestimates the true frequency of DNA breaks; alkaline comet assay evaluates both ds and ss breaks and may overestimate true DNA damage due to artificial damage induced at alkali-labile sites within the DNA strand

Table 11.6 (continued)

Name and acronym	Characteristics	Principle	How results are expressed	Advantages	Disadvantages
Sperm chromatin dispersion (SCD) test	Agarose embedded sperm is subjected to DNA denaturation to remove protamines. As a result, disulfide bonds break in the intact and tightly packed chromatin generating ss DNA from the nicks. Subsequently, cell lysis allows the loops of ss DNA relax, forming halos around the residual nuclear core structure. The characteristic patterns of the loops are assessed after staining	Spermatozoa embedded in agarose are submitted to acid treatment and lysis. After DNA staining, a halo can be seen in nondamaged cells while the cells with more extensive DNA breaks show small or no halo because the "broken" DNA loops do not diffuse; simple dyes or fluorochromes can be used for staining	By using bright-field or fluorescence-based microscopy, the percentage of fragmented DNA (DNA fragmentation index: DFI) in the sample is assessed	Very simple, low cost and does not require expensive equipment; halos can be observed by bright field microscope; requires a low number of sperm for analysis	Interobserver subjectivity to categorize the borderline halos; sperm with similar degrees of fragmentation and different nuclear sizes may show variations in halos' size; it is not a direct measure of DNA breaks but a representation of the overall chromatin structure

*The signals emitted from these probes are used to quantify the DNA fragmentation in the spermatozoa

each tube and centrifuged at 300*g* for 7 min. The supernatants are discarded and rinsing is repeated with 1.0 mL of the rinse buffer. Centrifugation is repeated and the supernatants are discarded. The cell pellets are resuspended in 0.5 mL of the PI/RNase staining buffer (Cat# 6551AZ) and incubated in the dark for 30 min at room temperature. The tubes are then numbered and are ready for flow cytometry. For flow cytometry evaluation, a minimum of 10,000 events is examined for each measurement. The flow rate is set at ~200 events/s. The excitation wavelength is set at 488 nm supplied by an argon laser at 15 mW. Green fluorescence (522–537 nm) is measured in the FL-1 channel and red (PI) fluorescence (575–589 nm) is measured in the FL-2 channel [126]. Raw data from the flow cytometer is imported into the *FlowJo* software (Mac version 8.2.4, FlowJo, LLC, Ashland, OR). After "gating" the samples, the percentage of TUNEL-positive cells is calculated and DNA damage is reported as the percentage of cells exhibiting DNA damage (Figs. 11.4 and 11.11).

The TUNEL protocol for fluorescence microscopy is basically the same [127]. The sperm suspension is counterstained with 4,6 diamidoino-2-phenylindole (DAPI, 2 µg/mL in vecta shield (Vector, Burlingame, CA) or propidium iodide (5 µL). A minimum of 400 spermatozoa per sample is scored under 40× objective of the epifluorescence microscope. For the green signal (FITC), an excitation wavelength in the range of 450–500 nm (e.g., 488 nm) and detection in the range of 525–565 nm is adequate (green). In each field, the number of spermatozoa stained with DAPI (blue) or PI (red) is counted first, and then the number of cells emitting green fluorescence (TUNEL positive) is assessed; the numbers are expressed as percentage of TUNEL-positive spermatozoa. Sperm showing green fluorescence represent damaged cells (TUNEL-positive), in which dUTP was incorporated to DNA breaks, in contrast to nonstained cells representing nondamaged sperm (Fig. 11.12). A minimum of 400 sperm is assessed per specimen.

SCD Test

For the SCD test, we use the Halosperm kit (Halotech DNA, Madrid, Spain) according to the manufacturer's recommended method [128]. In brief, a tube containing agarose is first heated at 100°C for 5 min to allow the agarose to melt. After stabilization at 37°C, 25-µL semen aliquots are added to the tube, and a 15-µL aliquot of the mixture is placed onto a pretreated microscope slide. A coverslip is placed and the slide is kept in the fridge for 5 min in order for the agarose to solidify. Meanwhile, 80 µL of a denaturing solution is added to 10 mL of distilled water to produce a fresh working solution. The slide is then taken from the fridge and the coverslip is removed. Thereafter, the slide is immersed in the denaturation solution and incubated for 7 min. The slide is then transferred to the lysis solution and incubated for 25 min. Finally, the slide is washed by incubation in a Coplin jar containing distilled water for 5 min, followed by incubation in ethanol solutions of 70, 90, and 100% each for 2 min. After air dry at room temperature, slides are stained with Diff-Quick or Wright's stain, and an analysis is carried out using bright-field microscopy. Sperm with intact DNA appear with a characteristic chromatin dispersion halo, whereas

Table 11.7 Methods for assessing sperm chromatin integrity based on direct incorporation of probes to nuclear proteins

Name and acronym	Characteristics	Principle	Test results	Advantages	Disadvantages
Aniline blue staining	Aniline blue is an acidic dye with high affinity for proteins loosely attached to DNA in the sperm nucleus. Increased aniline blue staining indicates loose chromatin packing	The method discriminates between lysine-rich histones and arginine/cysteine-rich protamines. Histone-rich nuclei of immature spermatozoa are rich in lysine and will stain in blue. In contrast, protamine rich nuclei of mature spermatozoa are rich in arginine and cysteine and contain relatively low levels of lysine, and will not be stained	The measured parameter is the presence of sperm heads stained in blue. The percentage of stained spermatozoa is determined by counting 200 spermatozoa per slide under bright field microscopy	Simple and inexpensive	Indirect measure of chromatin packaging; not specific for DNA fragmentation
Toluidine blue	Toluidine blue is a basic dye that stains phosphate residues of sperm DNA with fragmented ends and lysine-rich regions of histones	When the stain attaches it produces violet-bluish intense coloration whereas a pale-blue color is seen with interactions with protamines. Flow cytometer can also be used for evaluation	The measured parameter is the presence of sperm heads stained in violet-bluish. The percentage of stained spermatozoa is determined by counting under bright field microscopy or flow cytometry	Simple and inexpensive (bright-field microscopy); severe DNA damage can be revealed	Indirect measure of chromatin packaging; intermediate colors decreases interobserver reproducibility
Chromomicyn A3 (CMA3)	Chromomycin A3 is a membrane-impermeant glycosidic antibiotic that specifically bind to G/C-enriched DNA sequences. CMA3 binds to accessible sperm DNA stretches and emits fluorescence. DNA stretches are more or less accessible due to protamination differences with respect to AT-enriched DNA stretches	Evaluation of CMA3 staining is done by distinguishing spermatozoa that stain bright yellow (CMA3 positive) from those that stain a dull yellow (CMA3 negative) on examination under fluorescent microscopy	A total of 200 spermatozoa are randomly evaluated on each slide. The percentage of stained spermatozoa is determined	Simple and inexpensive	Intra- and interobserver variability; low specificity. CMA3-positive sperms have been erroneously interpreted as having defective protamination

those with damaged DNA present with no halo (Fig. 11.13). Alternatively, fluorescent DNA specific ligands (e.g., 6-diamino-2-phenylindole [DAPI]) can also be used for staining. This method has the advantage of reducing the staining step considerably. A differential chromatin decondensation pattern can be noted between cells with DNA fragmentation and those with intact DNA (Fig. 11.10). Regardless of the staining method, the sperm DNA fragmentation index (SDFi) is calculated as the percentage of fragmented sperm in the whole analyzed sample (approximately 400 spermatozoa per analysis).

The mechanism for DNA damage assessment in various assays is related to the differential interaction between chromatin proteins and DNA state (supercoiled, relaxed or fragmented) which determines the affinity of probes targeting DNA or proteins [111]. In supercoiled and double-strand DNA, the binding of an intercalating DNA probe is only possible by the interaction of the probe with the minor or major DNA groove, whereas in a fragmented DNA the partial loose interionic interactions between DNA and chromatin proteins allow the external binding of specific dyes to DNA phosphate groups.

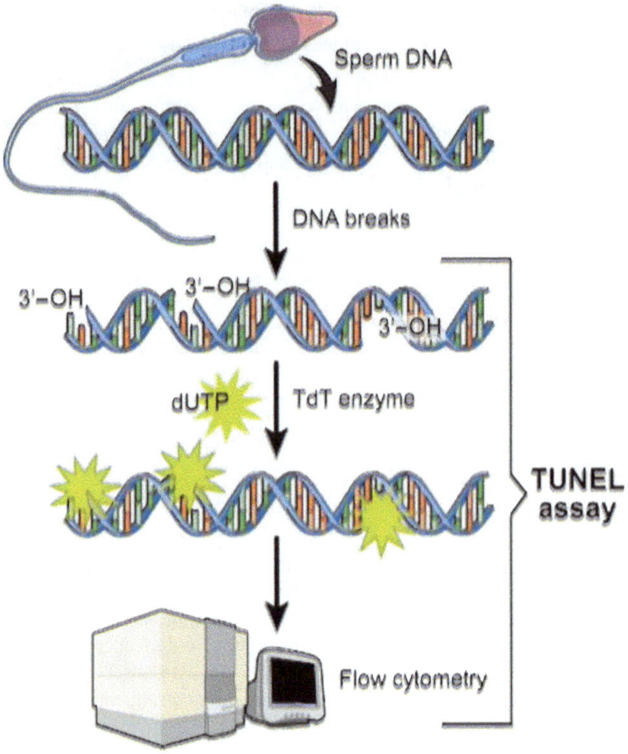

Fig. 11.10 Schematics of the TUNEL staining using flow cytometry. Single- or double-stranded DNA breaks are stained by the TdT enzyme and measured by flow cytometry. Alternatively, measurements can be carried out using fluorescence microscopy

In assays using enzymes to catalyze the probe incorporation, such as ISNT and TUNEL, the type of enzyme (terminal transferase and polymerase) cannot determine the nature of DNA damage being assessed, that is, double- or single-DNA strand breaks. In the comet assay, pH conditions have

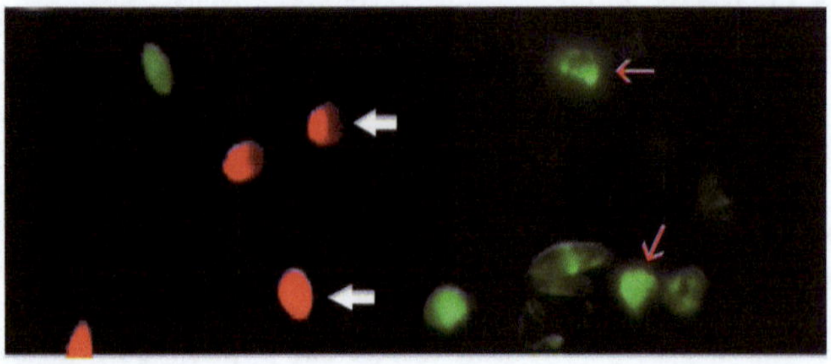

Fig. 11.12 Photomicrographs of spermatozoa assessed by fluorescence microscopy using the terminal uridine nick-end labeling (TUNEL) assay and propidium iodide. Sperm showing green fluorescence represent damaged cells (*red arrows*), in which dUTP is incorporated to DNA breaks, in contrast to nondamaged sperm stained in red (*white arrows*)

a direct influence on assay performance. While the neutral comet assay solely quantifies ds DNA breaks, its alkaline variation assesses the presence of ss and ds DNA breaks as well as alkali labile sites within the DNA strand. However, both experimental strategies can be combined with assessment of both ss and ds DNA breaks in each cell [129, 130] (Fig. 11.14).

Chromomycin A3 is a membrane-impermeant glycosidic antibiotic that specifically bind to G/C-enriched DNA sequences. Fluorometric assays using Chromomycin A3 (CMA3) have been claimed to indirectly measure the amounts of sperm protamines [131]. When used on spermatozoa CMA3 binds to accessible DNA stretches and emits fluorescence [132]. DNA stretches are more or less accessible due to protamination differences with respect to AT-enriched DNA stretches (G-bands in general), and this has been misinterpreted as a marker of defective protamination. Differential sperm protamination can be better assessed using

Fig. 11.11 Receiver operating characteristic curve showing the cutoff value, the area under the curve, the sensitivity, and the specificity of the TUNEL assay to discriminate infertile men from infertile controls with regard to DNA damage

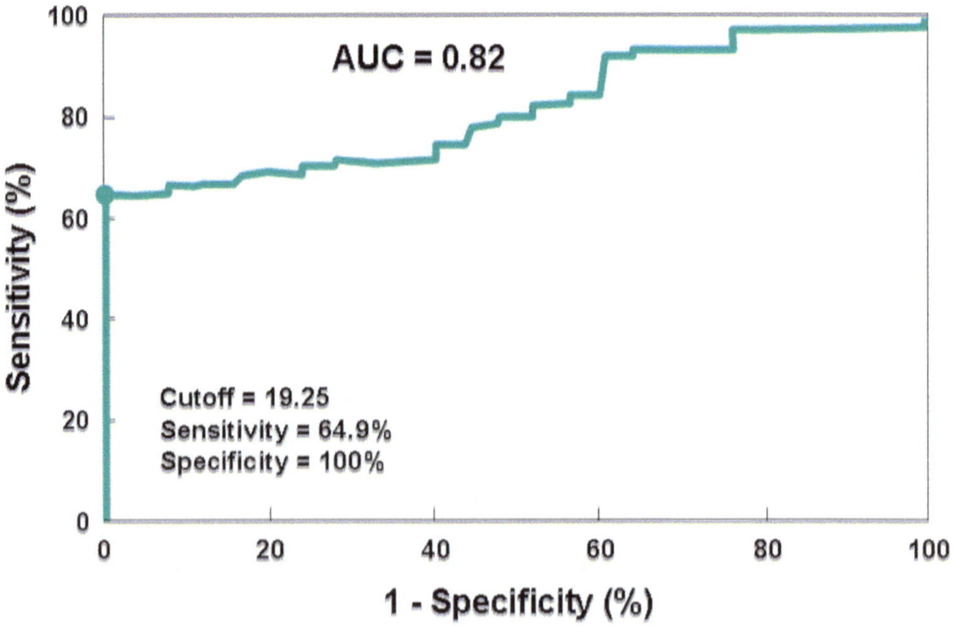

2,7-dibrom-4-hydroxy-mercuri-fluorescein, a specific compound which targets for enriched disulphide bond proteins. Using a solution of 0.05g/mL in phosphate buffered saline for 10 min on partially protein depleted spermatozoa, and in the presence of an appropriate counterstaining for DNA, such as 4′,6-diamidino-2-phenylindole or propidiun iodide, a dual emission for DNA and proteins can be assessed.

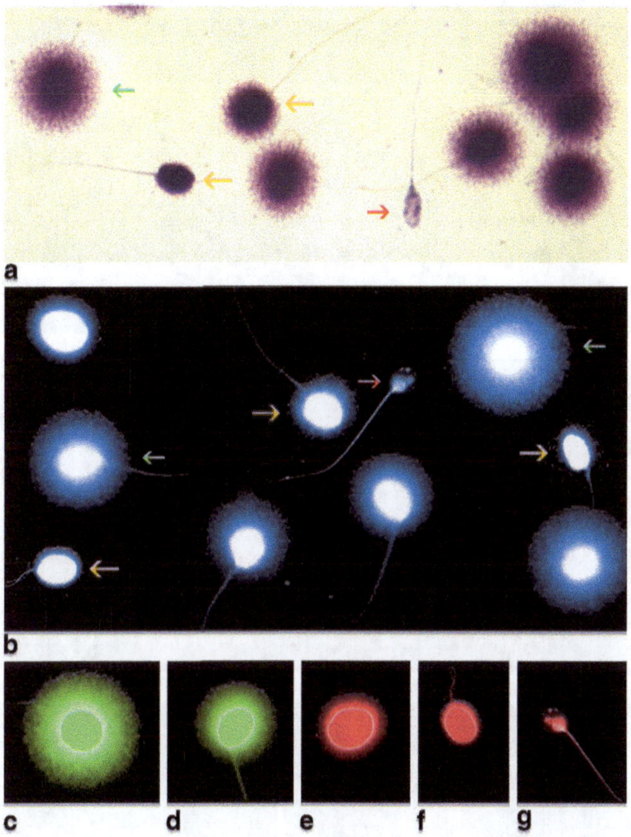

Fig. 11.13 Assessment of sperm DNA fragmentation using the sperm chromatin dispersion (SCD) test. Nucleoids from human spermatozoa obtained with the improved SCD procedure (Halosperm, Halotech DNA, SL, Madrid, Spain) under bright field microscopy and Wright's stain (**a**) and under fluorescence microscopy and DAPI staining (**b**). Green arrows target spermatozoa containing a normal DNA molecule. Yellow arrows target spermatozoa with a fragmented DNA molecule. Red arrows target a highly fragmented spermatozoon (degraded sperm). (**c**–**g**) Electronic filtered images showing a series of nucleoids with different levels of sperm DNA damage. Nucleoids with highlighted core delineation in green correspond to large (**c**) and medium (**d**) halos of dispersed chromatin representing a normal DNA molecule. Nucleoids in red are spermatozoa containing fragmented DNA and are represented by small (**e**) or absence (**f**) halos of dispersed chromatin and degraded spermatozoa (**g**). Bright-field and fluorescence microphotographs were obtained using a motorized fluorescence microscope controlled with software for automatic scanning and image digitization (Leica Microsystems, Barcelona, Spain). The microscope was equipped with a Leica EL6000 metal halide fluorescence light source and Plan-Fluotar 60× objectives with three independent filter blocks (DAPI-5060B; FITC-3540B and TRITC-A; Semrock, Rechestern NY, USA). A charge-coupled device (Leica DFC350 FX, Leica Microsystems, Barcelona, Spain) was used for image capture

Finally, the difference in the pattern of forming a loop around lysed and acid treated nuclear membrane carcass reflects the overall chromatin structure and is used to indirectly measure DNA breaks in the SCD test.

Clinical Utility of Sperm Functional Tests in Unexplained Male Infertility

Nowadays, sperm function tests aimed to assess fertilization defects are rarely used in the clinical work-up of men with UI. Both accuracy, the degree to which the measurement reflects the true value, and precision, the reproducibility of the results, are vitally important for clinicians who rely upon the values provided by the laboratory to direct the further work-up, diagnosis and counseling of the infertile male. Given the complexity to perform some of these tests, the difficulties in interpreting their results, the lack of treatment options for such defects, and in view of the success of assisted reproductive techniques (ART), there is little incentive for infertility clinics to invest in these methods. The clinical validity of assessing sperm-mediated immunity in UI is also uncertain. Sperm-bound antibodies should interfere with sperm function in order to impair fertility, as proposed by Hamada et al. [12]. As such, it is important not only to have 50% or more motile spermatozoa attached to the beads but also an impairment in sperm function caused by these elevated ASA levels, as determined by other sperm function tests such as the sperm–mucus penetration test, zona binding assays, and the AR response to stimulants [12]. ASA alone have a poor correlation with natural, IVF, or ICSI pregnancy rates [7]. Moreover, treatment of immunologic-male infertility with corticosteroids not only controversial but also associated with many side effects. As such, ASA as part of the investigation of males with UI is of limited value.

The diagnostic and prognostic validity of seminal oxidative stress and sperm DNA damage measurements seem to exceed that of conventional semen analysis. An oxidative stress test may accurately discriminate between fertile and infertile men [104, 108, 109]. Moreover, such tests can help to select subgroups of patients with infertility in which oxidative stress is an important factor and those who may benefit from antioxidant supplementation [109, 133]. Although consensus is growing about the clinical utility of seminal oxidative stress testing in the male infertility work-up, standardization of protocols and validation of results in the group of men with UI are still required.

As far as sperm DNA damage is concerned, the current methods have several limitations. First, they do not usually measure the degree of sperm DNA damage in a single sperm. Second, the present assays do not discriminate between physiological and pathological damage. Third, none of them enable us to depict the exact etiology and pathogenesis of DNA dam-

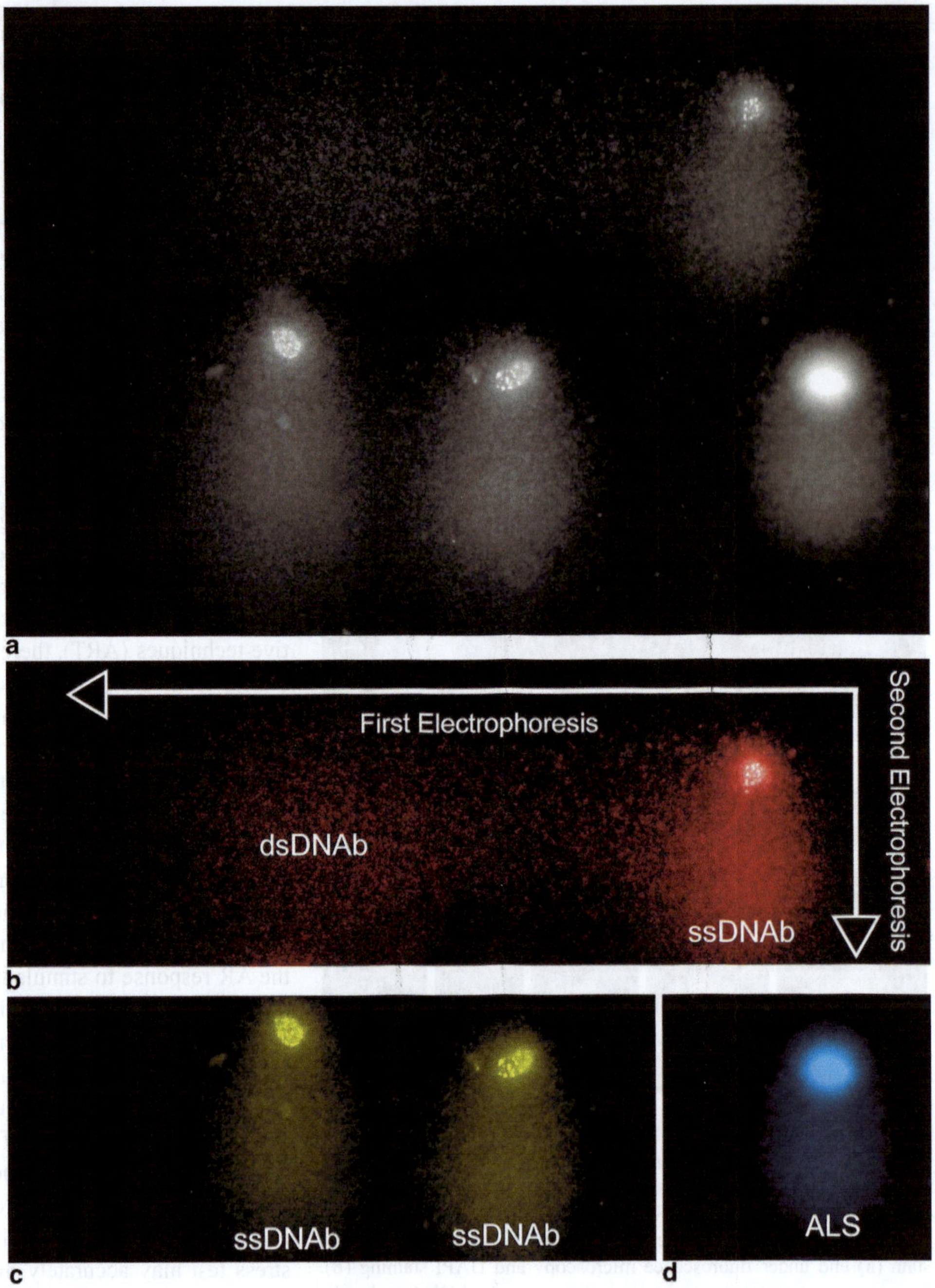

Fig. 11.14 Two-tail comet assay (TT-comet). **a** Original microscope field showing spermatozoa with DNA strand breaks. **b** Spermatozoon in red with both single (ssDNA) and double (dsDNAb) strand breaks. Arrows indicate the perpendicular sense of each electrophoresis. The first electrophoretic run on the *X*-axis was performed using a neutral buffer to identify dsDNAb. The second electrophoretic run was performed on the *Y*-axis using an alkaline buffer to identify ssDNAb. **c** Spermatozoa in yellow showing only ssDNAb. **d** A normal spermatozoon with a comet produced by constitutive alkali labile sites (ALS)

age. Of note, the oocyte cytoplasmic machinery can repair sperm DNA damage to a certain extent [134, 135]. Repair capability is dependent upon oocyte ageing and the type of DNA damage. In general, single-stranded DNA damage is easier to repair than double-stranded DNA damage [136]. In the mouse, it has been shown that embryonic and fetal development were related to the degree of damage, and that the oocytes had the capacity to repair sperm DNA when no more than 8% DNA was damaged [137, 138]. Obviously, assays cannot provide information on the sperm DNA reparability by the oocyte. It is also known that not all DNA damage is detrimental. In fact, few nicks occur as a normal process during winding and unwinding of DNA, which are usually joined by topoisomerase after histone–protamine replacement [111]. If breaks persist, then a detrimental defective protamination takes place. The probability of DNA breaks affecting critical parts of the genome is relatively low. In fact, in mammalian species comprising 3000 to 4000 megabases, about 30% of the genome has DNA related to genes, while the remaining 70% are pseudogenes, spacer sequences, and highly or moderately repetitive DNA sequences. Within the 30% of gene-related sequences, only 3% are DNA sequences directly involved in amino-acid coding sequences while the remaining comprises regulatory sequences, introns and nontranslated sequences, as well as active repetitive DNA sequences such as ribosomal, RNAs, and tRNAs. DNA damage in noncoding regions (close to 97% of the genome) is not expected to be as detrimental as damage occurring in a coding region of the genome (only about 3%).

But even within this scenario of low probabilities, epigenetics effects may negatively impact the reproductive process due to disrupted gene control [121, 139]. Unfortunately, the current assays are incapable of determining which genes are affected by DNA damage; hence, their ability to discriminate pathological from physiological DNA damage is nil. Still, different mechanisms cause sperm DNA damage. Despite being oxidatively induced in the vast majority, sperm DNA damage may also occur as a result of apoptosis during the process of spermatogenesis, alterations in chromatin remodeling during the process of spermiogenesis, as well as exposure to environmental toxicants and gonadotoxins such as chemotherapy and radiotherapy [135]. DNA damage induced by apoptosis usually affects a fraction of the spermatozoa giving rise to double-strand breaks. In contrast, DNA damage induced by oxidative stress and other ionizing stressing agents, such as those used in radiation therapy, leads to a massive production of single-stranded-DNA damage. In general, it is assumed that the amount of single-strand DNA damage generated by these aforementioned stressing factors is three times higher than double-strand DNA damage [140, 141]. 8-OH-2-deoxyguanosine (oxo8dG) type is one of the commonly nucleotide transformation derived from the aforesaid processes. This type of base mutation can be easily detected using specific immunoassaying on spermatozoa and its presence can be directly related to the presence of DNA fragmentation [142]. To explain the decreased reproductive potential of men with elevated levels of sperm DNA damage, it is possible that the remaining spermatozoa with no measurable DNA damage have some type of damage at varying extents [143]. This concept is supported by clinical data showing that sperm injections using testicular sperm samples in which the TUNEL test values were >15% resulted in significantly lower pregnancy rates (5.6%) compared with TUNEL values of <6% (44.4%; $p<0.05$) [144].

The lack of consensus with regard to the best method to assess sperm DNA damage, the normal threshold values of different tests and the correlation among tests in reporting abnormal levels of sperm DNA damage are also important issues limiting its widespread clinical application. Sakkas and Alvarez are in favor of using TUNEL as the preferential method to detect DNA fragmentation, especially if combined with flow cytometry, for its ability to assess "true" sperm DNA fragmentation [136]. In contrast, Evenson et al. claim that only SCSA has been clinically validated to be used in the fertility clinic [143]. Bungum et al., along the same lines, argue that SCSA seems to be the most powerful predictor for in vivo fertility and among the two in vitro methods, SCSA results are more related to the outcome of IVF than ICSI [145]. Also, proposed threshold values vary widely among tests and also by different authors using the same method (Table 11.8). Cutoff points of 10, 12, 19, and 20% have been reported for TUNEL [126, 139, 146–148], 15, 27, and 30% for SCSA [145, 149], and 17% for SCD [148]. SCD test cutoff points have been adapted from those offered by SCSA [128]. In a recent study with SCD specifically conducted in an egg donation program to control oocyte quality, a cutoff point of 17% was found to best discriminate pregnant and nonpregnant couples in IVF with sensitivity and specificity close to 75% [150]. Importantly, values above a given cutoff point do not preclude the achievement of full-term pregnancy [151].

Finally, conflicting data also exist on the correlation among different tests in reporting abnormal levels of sperm DNA fragmentation. In one study, Chohan et al. have shown that SCSA, TUNEL, and SCD techniques had similar predictive

Table 11.8 Cutoff points for sperm DNA assays to predict in vivo and in vitro fertility

Authors, year	Method	Cutoff point (%)	Purpose
Evenson et al. 1999	SCSA	30	Discriminate infertile from fertile males
Giwercman et al. 2010	SCSA	20	Discriminate infertile from fertile males
Spano et al. 2000	SCSA	40	Discriminate infertile from fertile males
Sharma et al. 2010	TUNEL	19	Discriminate infertile from fertile males
Duran et al. 2002	TUNEL	12	Pregnancy prediction in IUI
Bungum et al. 2004	SCSA	27	Pregnancy prediction in IUI, IVF, and ICSI
Bungum et al. 2007	SCSA	30	Pregnancy prediction in IUI, IVF, and ICSI
Seli et al. 2004	TUNEL	20	Pregnancy prediction in IVF and ICSI
Huang et al. 2005	TUNEL	10	Pregnancy prediction in IVF and ICSI
Boe-Hansen et al. 2006	SCSA	27	Pregnancy prediction in IVF and ICSI
Borini et al. 2006	TUNEL	10	Pregnancy prediction in IVF and ICSI
Benchaib et al. 2007	TUNEL	15	Pregnancy prediction in IVF and ICSI
Greco et al. 2005	TUNEL	15	Pregnancy prediction in ICSI
Micinski et al. 2009	SCSA	15	Pregnancy prediciton in ICSI
Simon et al. 2011	Alkaline comet	25	Pregnancy prediction in IVF
Nuñez-Calonge et al. 2012	SCD	17	Pregnancy prediction in ICSI with egg donation

SCSA sperm chromatin structure assay, *TUNEL* terminal deoxynucleotidyl transferase-mediated digoxigenin-dUTP nick-end labeling technique, *SCD* sperm chromatin dispersion test values for detecting DNA fragmentation while AOT consistently overestimated DNA damage [152]. A high correlation between SCSA and TUNEL results ($r=0.859$; $p<0.01$) has also been reported by Gorczyca et al. [153]. In contrast, Henkel et al. could not corroborate the aforesaid findings and concluded that the assays were not comparable [154]. Our own data on TUNEL and SCD to measure sperm DNA fragmentation in a population of men with UI showed that the methods were poorly correlated ($r=0.28$) [127]. However, it should be stressed that TUNEL only works precisely when the chromatin is partially freed from the proteins protecting the DNA. Under this condition, results of SCD and TUNEL are expected to be similar (Fig. 11.15). Moreover, TUNEL is a technically challenging method for a terminal transferase should be used to incorporate modified nucleotides at 3′ ends in a fixed specimen. If nucleotides such as biotin or digoxigenin are used, immulogical revelation needs to be included in the processing step. Finally, counterstaining of nonlabeled cells completes the process. In contrast, the rationale of the SCD technique is very simple and, in fact, represents a combination of the DNA denaturation step used in the SCSA method and the controlled protein depletion used in the comet assay. While the denaturation step result in the production of single-strand DNA motifs from preexisting single- or double-strand breaks, the lysis step differentially remove proteins linked to single- or double-strand DNA stretches. Since the expected amount of DNA damage in each spermatozoon is variable, it is also expected that the sizes of the haloes are also variable due to differential chromatin removal.

Altogether, these considerations may explain the reluctance of clinicians against the introduction of sperm DNA damage assays into the routine work-up of infertile males, and fuel the ongoing debate on the usefulness of sperm DNA utility to predict reproductive outcomes in vivo and in vitro [155–159]. Notwithstanding, there seems to be an association with increased DNA fragmentation and reduced fertility, both in vivo and in vitro, and with pregnancy loss after IVF or ICSI (risk ratio (RR) = 2.16 (95% confidence interval: 1.54 to 3.03), $p<0.00001$) [160]. Yet, at present no single test seems to be reliable enough to detect the pathological DNA damage with high accuracy to predict the reproductive profile of the sperm in natural conception, IUI, IVF, or ICSI, thus preventing recommendation of the routine use of sperm DNA fragmentation tests in the evaluation and treatment of infertile males. Hence, there is an urgent need to refine the methods for assessing the sperm DNA integrity and validate their cutoff points in different subsets of patients, as well as in different interventions, to allow the widespread clinical use of these tests. Despite all that, the results provided by sperm DNA damage assays can be used as additional markers of sperm quality in men with UI for they have been associated with better diagnostic and prognostic value than routine semen analyzes [2, 125, 136, 145].

Future Perspectives

The use of novel genomic, proteomic, and metabolomic techniques may add to the existing tests to more precisely diagnose men with UI.

Genomic techniques include microarray technologies, which assess copy number variations, gene expression levels, and single nucleotide polymorphisms (SNPs) [161] while proteomic analysis involves the use of one- or two-dimensional sodium dodecyl sulfate polyacrylamide gel electrophoresis (SDS-PAGE) coupled with mass spectrometry. Sperm chromatin assessment using the aforesaid tests has already been made clinically available and can be included in this category.

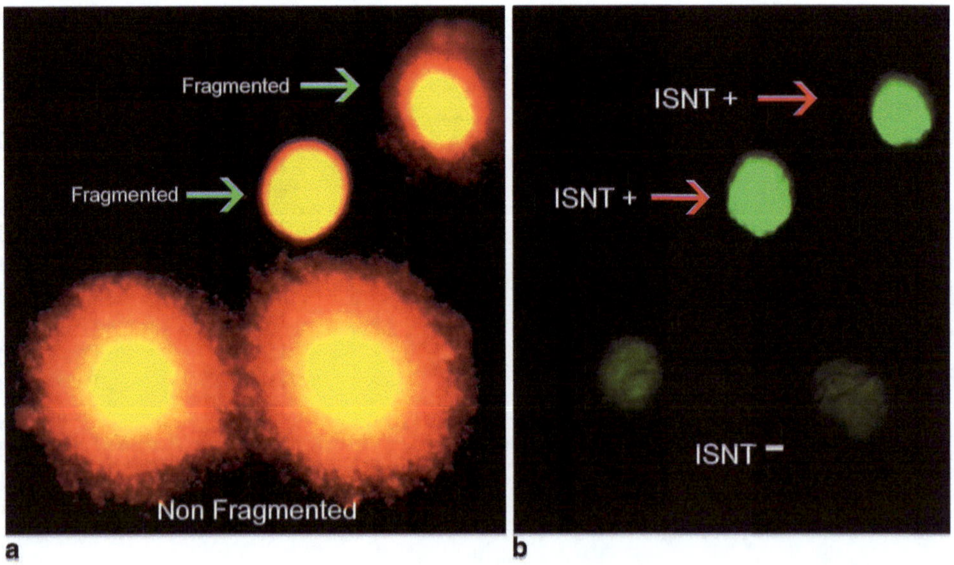

Fig. 11.15 Simultaneous assessment of sperm DNA damage with the sperm chromatin dispersion (SCD) test and in situ nick translation (ISTN). A direct association is demonstrated between spermatozoa with fragmented DNA as detected by SCD (absence of halo or presence of small halo) and ISNT (high nucleotide incorporation). The same cells were assessed by SCD (**a**) and ISNT (**b**). The Klenow fragment was used to expand the DNA nicks and its results are equivalent to those obtained by TUNEL. Spermatozoa with large halos of relaxed chromatin do not incorporate labeled nucleotides ($ISNT^{-}$), while those with small or no halo are highly labeled ($ISNT^{+}$)

Proteomic analysis can not only confirm the presence of a given protein but also measure its quantity in different isoforms. At present, most proteomic investigation focuses on discovering various proteins present in the semen. A database listing thousands of proteins in the semen has been recently reviewed [162]. The most abundant proteins identified so far in the seminal plasma include fibronectin, lactoferrin, laminin, albumin, and semenogelin, whose molecular functions are associated with catalytic enzymatic activity, protein metabolism, RNA processing/transcription, cell transport/structure, and signal transduction [163]. The next step will be the identification of the proteins that can be used as biomarkers of male fertility and infertility. In this sense, Heat shock protein 2 and SPACA1 (sperm acrosome membrane-associated protein) are two examples of proteins with different expression in sperm of fertile and infertile males [164, 165].

Metabolomics, on the other hand, is the study of small molecular metabolites with low molecular weight that are the products of cell metabolism [166, 167]. It has been conceived with an expectation that body-fluid analysis can be optimized to create a low-cost, informative and clinically relevant means of measuring metabolic changes, even when standard clinical chemistry markers are within normal limits [100]. These biomarkers are quantified by various forms of analytical, biochemical, and spectral analysis to establish the quantitative lists or signatures of the metabolites for healthy control population and test subjects with specific illnesses [168]. Measurement of metabolic markers of oxidative stress can be included in this category. Other methods used in metabolomics include gas chromatography, high-performance liquid chromatography (HPLC), and capillary electrophoresis for separation of metabolites, whereas mass spectrometry, Fourier-transform infrared and Raman or near-infrared spectroscopy are used for identification and quantification of the metabolites [167]. Metabolomics testing using the latter in the field of male infertility is just beginning, but preliminary observations are promising.

Acknowledgment The authors are grateful to Fabiola C. Bento for her help in language revision.

References

1. Esteves SC, Zini A, Aziz N, Alvarez JG, Sabanegh ES Jr, Agarwal A. Critical appraisal of World Health Organization's new reference values for human semen characteristics and effect on diagnosis and treatment of subfertile men. Urology. 2012;79:16–22.
2. Samplaski MK, Agarwal A, Sharma R, Sabanegh E. New generation of diagnostic tests for infertility: review of specialized semen tests. Int J Urol. 2010;17:839–47.
3. Hamada A, Esteves SC, Agarwal A. Unexplained male infertility—looking beyond routine semen analysis. Eur Urol Rev. 2012;7:90–6.
4. Kopa Z, Berenyi M. Inflammatory parameters of the ejaculate. In: Bjõrndahl L GA, Tournaye H, Weidner W, editors. Clinical Andrology EAU/ESAU course guidelines. New York: Informa Healthcare; 2010. pp. 301–8.
5. Ayvaliotis B, Rosenfeld D, Cooper G. Conception rates in couples where autoimmunity to sperm is detected. Fertil Steril. 1985;43:739–42.
6. Turek PJ. Immunopathology and infertility. In: Lipshultz LI, Howards SS, editors. Infertility in the male. St. Louis: Mosby-Year Book Inc; 1997. pp. 305–25.
7. Esteves SC, Schneider DT, Verza S Jr. Influence of antisperm antibodies in the semen on intracytoplasmic sperm injection outcome. Int Braz J Urol. 2007;33:795–802.
8. Mortimer D. Practical laboratory andrology. New York: Oxford University Press; 1994. pp. 221–32.
9. Shibahara H, Burkman LJ, Isojima S, Alexander NJ. Effects of sperm—immobilizing antibodies on sperm-zona pellucida tight binding. Fertil Steril. 1993;60:533–9.
10. Bates CA. Antisperm antibodies and male subfertility. Br J Urol. 1997;80:691–7.
11. Bronson RA. Antisperm antibodies: a critical evaluation and clinical guidelines. J Reprod Immunol. 1999;45:159–83.
12. Hamada A, Esteves SC, Agarwal A. Unexplained male infertility: potential causes and management. Hum Androl. 2011;1:2–16.
13. Rajah SV, Parslow JM, Howell RJ, Hendry WF. Comparison of mixed antiglobulin reaction and direct immunobead test for detection of sperm-bound antibodies in subfertile males. Fertil Steril. 1992;57:1300–3.
14. BioRad. Immunobead binding test (IBT) protocol for anti-sperm cell antibody detection. Bulletin. 1987;170:1–4.
15. Chiu WW, Chamley LW. Clinical associations and mechanisms of action of antisperm antibodies. Fertil Steril. 2004;82(2):529–35.
16. WHO. Laboratory manual for the examination and processing of human semen. 5th edn. Switzerland: WHO Press; 2010. pp. 108–13.
17. Henkel R, Muller C, Miska W, Gips H, Schill WB. Determination of the acrosome reaction in human spermatozoa is predictive of fertilization in vitro. Hum Reprod. 1993;8(12):2128–32.
18. Mortimer D. From the semen to oocyte: the long route in vivo and in vitro short cut. In: Testart J, Frydman R, editors. Human in vitro fertilization: actual problems and prospects. Amsterdam: Elsevier Science; 1985. p. 93.
19. Fraser LR. Mechanisms controlling mammalian fertilization. In: Clarke JR, editors. Oxford reviews of reproductive biology. Oxford: Oxford University Press; 1984. p. 173.
20. Cross NL. Effect of cholesterol and other sterols on human sperm acrosomal responsiveness. Mol Reprod Dev. 1996;45(2):212–7.
21. Mortimer D. Practical laboratory andrology. New York: Oxford University Press; 1994. p. 393.
22. Lamirande E, Leclerc P, Gagnon C. Capacitation as a regulatory event that primes spermatozoa for the acrosome reaction and fertilization. Mol Hum Reprod. 1997;3(3):175–94.
23. Lindemann, CB, Kanous, KS. Regulation of mammalian sperm motility. Arch Androl. 1989;23(1):1–22.
24. Matsumura K, Aketa K. Proteasome (multicatalytic proteinase) of sea urchin sperm and its possible participation in the acrosome reaction. Mol Reprod Dev. 1991;29(2):189–99.
25. Inaba K, Akazome Y, Morisawa M. Two high molecular mass proteases from sea urchin sperm. Biochem Biophys Res Commun. 1992;182(2):667–74.
26. Morales P, Kong M, Pizarro E, Pasten C. Participation of the sperm proteasome in human fertilization. Hum Reprod. 2003;18(5):1010–7.
27. Zaneveld LJ, De Jonge CJ, Anderson RA, Mack SR. Human sperm capacitation and the acrosome reaction. Hum Reprod. 1991;6(9):1265–74.
28. Mansour RT, Serour MG, Abbas AM, et al. The impact of spermatozoa preincubation time and spontaneous acrosome reaction in intracytoplasmic sperm injection: a controlled randomized study. Fertil Steril. 2008;90(3):584–91.

29. Yanagimachi R, Bhattacharyya A. Acrosome-reacted guinea pig spermatozoa become fusion competent in the presence of extracellular potassium ions. J Exp Zool. 1988;248(3):354–60.
30. Katz DF, Drobnis EA, Overstreet JW. Factors regulating mammalian sperm migration through the female reproductive tract and oocyte vestments. Gamete Res. 1989;22:443.
31. Nichol R, Hunter RH, Gardner DK, Leese HJ, Cooke GM. Concentrations of energy substrates in oviductal fluid and blood plasma of pigs during the periovulatory period. J Reprod Fertil. 1992;96:699–707.
32. Breitbart H, Spungin B. The biochemistry of the acrosome reaction. Mol Hum Reprod. 1997;3(3):195–202.
33. Kopf GS, Gerton GL. The mammalian sperm acrosome and the acrosome reaction. In: Wasserman PM, editors. Elements of mammalian fertilization. Boston: CRC Press; 1991. pp. 153–203.
34. Chiu PCN, Wong BST, Chung MK, et al. Effects of native human zona pellucida glycoproteins 3 and 4 on acrosome reaction and zona pellucida binding of human spermatozoa. Biol Reprod. 2008;79(5):869–77.
35. Ganguly A, Bukovsky A, Sharma RK, Bansal P, Bhandari B, Gupta SK. In humans, zona pellucida glycoprotein-1 binds to spermatozoa and induces acrosomal exocytosis. Hum Reprod. 2010;25(7):1643–56.
36. Gupta SK, Chakravarty S, Suraj K, et al. Structural and functional attributes of zona pellucida glycoproteins [abstract]. Soc Reprod Fertil. 2007;63(Suppl. 1):203–16.
37. Gupta SK, Bansal P, Ganguly A, Bhandari B, Chakrabarti K. Human zona pellucida glycoproteins: functional relevance during fertilization. J Reprod Immunol. 2009;83(1–2):50–5.
38. Chiu PC, Wong BS, Lee CL, et al. Zona pellucida-induced acrosome reaction in human spermatozoa is potentiated by glycodelin-A via down-regulation of extracellular signal-regulated kinases and up-regulation of zona pellucida-induced calcium influx. Hum Reprod. 2010;25(11):2721–33.
39. Liu DY, Baker HW. Defective sperm-zona pellucida interaction: a major cause of failure of fertilization in clinical in-vitro fertilization. Hum Reprod. 2000;15:702–8.
40. Liu DY, Baker HW. Disordered zona pellucida-induced acrosome reaction and failure of in vitro fertilization in patients with unexplained infertility. Fertil Steril. 2003;79:74–80.
41. Mackenna A, Barratt CL, Kessopoulou E, Cooke I. The contribution of a hidden male factor to unexplained infertility. Fertil Steril. 1993;59:405–411.
42. Yanagimachi, R. Mammalian fertilization. In: Knobil E, Neill JD, Ewing LL, et al., editors. The physiology of reproduction. New York: Raven Press; 1994. p. 189.
43. Brucker C, Lipford GB. The human sperm acrosome reaction: physiology and regulatory mechanisms. An update. Hum Reprod Update. 1995;1(1):51–62.
44. Thomas P, Meizel S. Phosphatidylinositol 4,5-bisphosphate hydrolysis in human sperm stimulated with follicular fluid or progesterone is dependent upon Ca2+ influx. Biochem J. 1989;264(2):539–46.
45. Aquila S, Sisci D, Gentile M, et al. Towards a physiological role for cytochrome P450 aromatase in ejaculated human sperm. Hum Reprod. 2003;18(8):1650–9.
46. Baldi E, Luconi M, Bonaccorsi L, Muratori M, Forti G. Intracellular events and signaling pathways involved in sperm acquisition of fertilizing capacity and acrosome reaction. Front Biosci. 2000;1(5):110–23.
47. Cummins JM, Fleming AD, Crozet N, Kuehl TJ, Kosower NS, Yanagimachi R. Labelling of living mammalian spermatozoa with the fluorescent thiol alkylating agent, monobromobimane (MB): immobilization upon exposure to ultraviolet light and analysis of acrosomal status. J Exp Zool. 1986;237(3):375–82.
48. Esteves SC, Sharma RK, Thomas AJ Jr, Agarwal A. Cryopreservation of human spermatozoa with pentoxifylline improves the post-thaw agonist-induced acrosome reaction rate. Hum Reprod. 1998;13(12):3384–9.
49. Kilani Z, Ismail R, Ghunaim S, et al. Evaluation and treatment of familial globozoospermia in five brothers. Fertil Steril. 2004;82(5):1436–9.
50. Tesarik J, Mendoza C. Alleviation of acrosome reaction prematurity by sperm treatment with egg yolk. Fertil Steril. 1995;63(1):153–7.
51. Esteves SC, Sharma RK, Thomas AJ Jr, Agarwal A. Effect of in vitro incubation on spontaneous acrosome reaction in fresh and cryopreserved human spermatozoa. Int J Fertil Womens Med. 1998;43(5):235–42.
52. Chang TH, Jih MH, Wu TC. Relationship of sperm antibodies in women and men to human in vitro fertilization, cleavage, and pregnancy rate. Am J Reprod Immunol. 1993;30(2–3):108–12.
53. Junk SM, Matson PL, Yovich JM, Bootsma B, Yovich JL. The fertilization of human oocytes by spermatozoa from men with antispermatozoal antibodies in semen. J In Vitro Fert Embryo Transf. 1986;3(6):350–2.
54. Meinertz H, Linnet L, Fogh-Andersen P, Hjort T. Antisperm antibodies and fertility after vasovasostomy: a follow-up study of 216 men. Fertil Steril. 1990;54(2):315–21.
55. De Almeida M, Gazagne I, Jeulin C, et al. In-vitro processing of sperm with autoantibodies and in-vitro fertilization results. Hum Reprod. 1989;4(1):49–53.
56. Matson PL, Junk SM, Spittle JW, Yovich JL. Effect of antispermatozoal antibodies in seminal plasma upon spermatozoal function. Int J Androl. 1988;11(2):101–6.
57. Kumi-Diaka J, Townsend J. Toxic potential of dietary genistein isoflavone and beta-lapachone on capacitation and acrosome reaction of epididymal spermatozoa. J Med Food. 2003;6(3):201–8.
58. Feng HL, Han YB, Hershlag A, Zheng LJ. Impact of Ca 2+ flux inhibitors on acrosome reaction of hamster spermatozoa. J Androl. 2007;28(4):561–4.
59. Whan LB, West M, McClure N, Lewis SEM. The effects of Delta-9-tetrahydrocannabinol, the primary psychoactive cannabinoid in marijuana, on human sperm function in vitro. Fertil Steril. 2006;85:653–60.
60. Falzone N, Huyser C, Becker P, Leszczynski D, Franken DR. The effect of pulsed 900-MHz GSM mobile phone radiation on the acrosome reaction, head morphometry and zona binding of human spermatozoa. Int J Androl. 2011;34(1):20–6.
61. Mukhopadhyay D, Nandi P, Varghese AC, Gutgutia R, Banerjee S, Bhattacharyya AK. The in vitro effect of benzo[a]pyrene on human sperm hyperactivation and acrosome reaction. Fertil Steril. 2010;94(2):595–8.
62. Liu DY, Clarke GN, Lopata A, Johnston WI, Baker HW. A sperm-zona pellucida binding test and in vitro fertilization. Fertil Steril. 1989;52:281–7.
63. Munire M, Shimizu Y, Sakata Y, Minaguchi R, Aso T. Impaired hyperactivation of human sperm in patients with infertility. J Med Dent Sci. 2004;51:99–104.
64. Liu DY, Baker HW. Disordered acrosome reaction of spermatozoa bound to the zona pellucida: a newly discovered sperm defect causing infertility with reduced sperm-zona pellucida penetration and reduced fertilization in vitro. Hum Reprod. 1994;9:1694–700.
65. Liu de Y Liu ML Garrett C Baker HW. Comparison of the frequency of defective sperm-zona pellucida (ZP) binding and the ZP-induced acrosome reaction between subfertile men with normal and abnormal semen. Hum Reprod. 2007;22:1878–84.
66. Aitken RJ, Best FS, Richardson DW, Djahanbakhch O, Mortimer D, Templeton AA, et al. An analysis of sperm function in cases of unexplained infertility: conventional criteria, movement characteristics, and fertilizing capacity. Fertil Steril. 1982;38:212–21.
67. Liu DY, Lopata A, Johnston WI, Baker HW. A human sperm-zona pellucid binding test using oocytes that failed to fertilize in vitro. Fertil Steril. 1988;50:782–88.

68. Mackenna A, Barratt CL, Kessopoulou E, Cooke I. The contribution of a hidden male factor to unexplained infertility. Fertil Steril. 1993;59:405–11.
69. Esteves SC, Sharma RK, Thomas Jr AJ, Agarwal A. Effect of swim-up sperm washing and subsequent capacitation on acrosome status and functional membrane of normal sperm. Int J Fertil. 2000;45:335–41.
70. Kay VJ, Robertson L. Hyperactivated motility of human spermatozoa: a review of physiological function and application in assisted reproduction. Hum Reprod Update. 1998;4:776–86.
71. Burkman LJ. Discrimination between nonhyperactivated and classical hyperactivated motility patterns in human spermatozoa using computerized analysis. Fertil Steril. 1991;55:363–71.
72. Esteves SC, Glina S, Wonchockier R, Correa NR. Sperm kinematics of normozoospermic specimens after stimulation by varying concentrations of a specific inhibitor of cGMP phosphodiesterase type-5 (sildenafil). Fertil Steril. 2003;80(Suppl. 3):236.
73. Garrett C, Liu DY, Clarke GN, Rushford DD, Baker HW. Automated semen analysis: 'zona pellucida preferred' sperm morphometry and straight-line velocity are related to pregnancy rate in subfertile couples. Hum Reprod. 2003;18:1643–9.
74. Mackenna A, Barratt CL, Kessopoulou E, Cooke I. The contribution of a hidden male factor to unexplained infertility. Fertil Steril. 1993;59:405–11.
75. Pacey AA, Ladbrook MB, Barratt CL, Cooke ID. The potential shortcomings of measuring hyperactivated motility by computer-aided sperm analysis when sperm motion is multiphasic. Hum Reprod Update. 1997;3:185–93.
76. Esteves SC, Verza Jr S. Relationship of in vitro acrosome reaction to sperm function: an update. Open Reprod Sci J. 2011;3:72–84.
77. Cummins JM, Pember SM, Jequier AM, Yovich JL, Hartmann PE. A test of the human sperm acrosome reaction following ionophore challenge. Relationship to fertility and other seminal parameters. J Androl. 1991;12:98–103.
78. Cross NL, Morales P, Overstreet JW, Hanson FW. Two simple methods for detecting acrosome-reacted human sperm. Gam Res. 1986;15:213–26.
79. Esteves SC, Sharma RK, Thomas AJ Jr, Agarwal A. Evaluation of acrosomal status and sperm viability in fresh and cryopreserved specimens by the use of fluorescent peanut agglutinin lectin in conjunction with hypo-osmotic swelling test. Int Braz J Urol. 2007;33:364–74.
80. Esteves SC, Sharma RK, Thomas Jr AJ, Agarwal A. Improvement in motion characteristics and acrosome status in cryopreserved human spermatozoa by swim-up processing before freezing. Hum Reprod. 2000;15:2173–9.
81. Esteves SC, Spaine DM, Cedenho AP. Effects of pentoxifylline treatment before freezing on motility, viability and acrosome status of poor quality human spermatozoa cryopreserved by the liquid nitrogen vapor method. Braz J Med Biol Res. 2007;40:985–92.
82. Aitken RJ, Buckingham DW, Fang HG. Analysis of the responses of human spermatozoa to A23187 employing a novel technique for assessing the acrosome reaction. J Androl. 1993;14(2):132–41.
83. Esteves SC, Sharma RK, Thomas AJ Jr, Agarwal A. Suitability of the hypo-osmotic swelling test for assessing the viability of cryopreserved sperm. Fertil Steril. 1996;66(5):798–804.
84. Calvo L, Dennison-Lagos L, Banks SM, et al. Acrosome reaction inducibility predicts fertilization success at in-vitro fertilization. Hum Reprod. 1994;9(10):1880–6.
85. Yovich JM, Edirisinghe WR, Yovich JL. Use of the acrosome reaction to ionophore challenge test in managing patients in an assisted reproduction program: a prospective, double-blind, randomized controlled study. Fertil Steril. 1994;61(5):902–10.
86. Katsuki T, Hara T, Ueda K, Tanaka J, Ohama K. Prediction of outcomes of assisted reproduction treatment using the calcium ionophore-induced acrosome reaction. Hum Reprod. 2005;20(2):469–75.
87. Liu DY, Bourne H, Baker HW. High fertilization and pregnancy rates after intracytoplasmic sperm injection in patients with disordered zona pellucida induced acrosome reaction. Fertil Steril. 1997;67:955–8.
88. Talbot P, Chacon R. A new procedure for rapidly scoring acrosome reactions of human sperm. Gamete Res. 1980;3:211–6.
89. Liu DY, Sie BS, Liu ML, Agresta F, Baker HW. Relationship between seminal plasma zinc concentration and spermatozoa-zona pellucida binding and the ZP-induced acrosome reaction in subfertile men. Asian J Androl. 2009;11:499–507.
90. Zini A, Sigman M. Evaluation of sperm function. In: Lipshultz LI, Howards SS, Craig S, editors. Infertility in the male. Cambridge: Cambridge University Press; 2009. pp. 177–198.
91. Wolf DP, Sokoloski JE, Quigley MM. Correlation of human in vitro fertilization with the hamster egg bioassay. Fertil Steril. 1983;40:53–9.
92. Chan SY, Fox EJ, Chan MM, Tsoi WL, Wang C, Tang LC, et al. The relationship between the human sperm hypoosmotic swelling test, routine semen analysis, and the human sperm zona-free hamster ovum penetration assay. Fertil Steril. 1985;44:668–72.
93. Check JH, Nowroozi K, Lee M, Adelson H, Katsoff D. Evaluation and treatment of a male factor component to unexplained infertility. Arch Androl. 1990;25:199–211.
94. Agarwal A, Hamada A, Esteves SC. Insight into oxidative stress in varicocele-associated male infertility: part 1. Nat Rev Urol. 2012;9:678–90.
95. Aitken RJ, Buckingham D, West K, Wu FC, Zikopoulos K, Richardson DW. Differential contribution of leucocytes and spermatozoa to the generation of reactive oxygen species in the ejaculates of oligozoospermic patients and fertile donors. J Reprod Fertil. 1992;94:451–62.
96. Esfandiari N, Sharma RK, Saleh RA, Thomas Jr AJ, Agarwal A. Utility of the nitroblue tetrazolium reduction test for assessment of reactive oxygen species production by seminal leukocytes and spermatozoa. J Androl. 2003;24:862–70.
97. Gavella M, Lipovac V. NADH-dependent oxido-reductase (diaphorase) activity and isozyme pattern of sperm in infertile men. Arch Androl. 1992;28:135–41.
98. Aitken RJ, Krausz C. Oxidative stress, DNA damage and the Y chromosome. Reproduction. 2001;122:497–506.
99. Lewis SE, Boyle PM, McKinney KA, Young IS, Thompson W. Total antioxidant capacity of seminal plasma is different in fertile and infertile men. Fertil Steril. 1995;64(4):868–70.
100. Pauling L, Robinson AB, Teranishi R, Cary P. Quantitative analysis of urine vapor and breath by gas-liquid partition chromatography. Proc Natl Acad Sci. 1971;68:2374–76.
101. Colagar AH, Pouramir M, Marzony ET, Jorsaraei SGA. Relationship between seminal malondialdehyde levels and sperm quality in fertile and infertile men. Braz Arch Biol Technol. 2009;52(6):1387–92.
102. Desai N, Sharma RK, Makker K, Sabanegh E, Agarwal A. Physiologic and pathologic levels of reactive oxygen species in neat semen of infertile men. Fertil Steril. 2009;92(5):1626–31.
103. Pasqualotto FB, Sharma RK, Kobayashi H, Nelson DR, Thomas Jr AJ, Agarwal A. Oxidative stress in normospermic men undergoing infertility evaluation. J Androl. 2001;22:316–22.
104. Mahfouz R, Sharma R, Sharma D, Sabanegh E, Agarwal A. Diagnostic value of the total antioxidant capacity (TAC) assay in human seminal plasma. Fertil Steril. 2009;91:805–11.
105. Hamada A, Esteves SC, Agarwal A. Insight into oxidative stress invaricocele-associated male infertility: part 2. Nat Rev Urol. 2013;10(1):26–37.

106. Gomez E, Irvine DS, Aitken RJ. Evaluation of a spectrophotometric assay for the measurement of malondialdehyde and 4-hydroxyalkenals in human spermatozoa: relationships with semen quality and sperm function. Int J Androl. 1998;21:81–94.
107. Benjamin D, Sharma RK, Moazzam A, Agarwal A. Method for the detection of ROS in human sperm samples. In: Agarwal A, Robert J, Aitken J, Alvarez G, editors. Studies on men's health and fertility. New York: Springer; 2012. (Chap. 13). pp. 257–73.
108. Sharma RK, Pasqualotto FF, Nelson DR, Thomas AJ Jr, Agarwal A. The reactive oxygen species—total antioxidant capacity score is a new measure of oxidative stress to predict male infertility. Hum Reprod. 1999;14:2801–7.
109. Lampiao F, Opperman CJ, Agarwal A, du Plessis SS. Oxidative stress. In: Parekattil SJ, Agarwal A, editors. Male infertility: contemporary clinical approaches, andrology, ART & antioxidants. 1st edn. New York: Springer; 2012. pp. 225–35.
110. Tunc O, Thompson J, Tremellen K. Development of the NBT assay as a marker of sperm oxidative stress. Int J Androl. 2010;33(1):13–21.
111. Shamsi MB, Imam SN, Dada R. Sperm DNA integrity assays: diagnostic and prognostic challenges and implications in management of infertility. J Assist Reprod Genet. 2011;28(11): 1073–85.
112. Aitken RJ, de Iullis GN, McLachlan RI. Biological and clinical significance of DNA damage in the male germ line. Int J Androl. 2009;32:46–56.
113. Hamada A, Esteves SC, Nizza M, Agarwal A. Unexplained male infertility: diagnosis and management. Int Braz J Urol. 2012;38:576–94.
114. Host E, Lindenberg S, Ernst E, Christensen F. DNA strand breaks in human spermatozoa: a possible factor, to be considered in couples suffering from unexplained infertility. Acta Obstet Gynecol Scand. 1999;78:622–5.
115. Saleh RA, Agarwal A, Nelson DE, Nada EA, El-Tonsy MH, Alvarez JG, et al. Increased sperm nuclear DNA damage in normozoospermic infertile men: a prospective study. Fertil Steril. 2002;78:313–8.
116. Spano M, Bonde JP, Hjollund HI, Kolstad HA, Cordelli E, Leter G. Sperm chromatin damage impairs human fertility. The Danish first pregnancy planner study team. Fertil Steril. 2000;73:43–50.
117. Larson-Cook KL, Brannian JD, Hansen KA, Kasperson KM, Aamold ET, Evenson DP. Relationship between the outcomes of assisted reproductive techniques and sperm DNA fragmentation as measured by the sperm chromatin structure assay. Fertil Steril. 2003;80:895–902.
118. Saleh RA, Agarwal A, Nada ES, El-Tonsy MH, Sharma RK, Meyer A. Negative effects of increased sperm DNA damage in relation to seminal oxidative stress in men with idiopathic and male factor infertility. Fertil Steril. 2003;79(3):1597–605.
119. Check JH, Graziano V, Cohen R, Krotec J, Check ML. Effect of an abnormal sperm chromatin structural assay (SCSA) on pregnancy outcome following (IVF) with ICSI in previous IVF failures. Arch Androl. 2005;51:121–4.
120. Aitken RJ, Koopman P, Lewis SE. Seeds of concern. Nature. 2004;432:48–52.
121. Zini A, Meriano J, Kader K, et al. Potential adverse effect of sperm DNA damage on embryo quality after ICSI. Hum Reprod. 2005;20:3476–80.
122. Aitken RJ, Koppers AJ. Apoptosis and DNA damage in human spermatozoa. Asian J Androl. 2011;13:36–42.
123. Esteves SC, Agarwal A. Novel concepts in male infertility. Int Braz J Urol. 2011;37(1):5–15.
124. Marchetti F, Wyrobek AJ. DNA repair decline during mouse spermiogenesis results in the accumulation of heritable DNA damage. DNA Repair. 2008;7:572–81.
125. Gosálvez J, López-Fernández C, Fernández JL. Sperm Chromatin Dispersion (SCD) test: technical aspects and clinical applications. In: Armand Z, Agarwal A, editors. Sperm DNA damage: biological and clinical applications in male infertility and assisted reproduction. New York: Springer; 2011. pp. 151–170.
126. Sharma RK, Sabanegh E, Mahfouz R, Gupta S, Thiyagarajan A, Agarwal A. TUNEL as a test for sperm DNA damage in the evaluation of male infertility. Urology. 2010;76(6):1380–6.
127. Feijó CM, Esteves SC. Diagnostic accuracy of sperm chromatin dispersion (SCD) test to evaluate sperm DNA damage in men with unexplained infertility. Fertil Steril. 2014;101(1):58-63.
128. Fernández JL, Muriel L, Goyanes V, Segrelles E, Gosálvez J, Enciso M, Lafrombois ME, De Jonge C. Simple determination of human sperm DNA fragmentation with an improved sperm chromatin dispersion (SCD) test. Fertil Steril. 2005;84:833–42.
129. Zee YP, López-Fernández C, Arroyo F, Johnston SD, Holt WV, Gosálvez J. Evidence that single-stranded DNA breaks are a normal feature of koala sperm chromatin, while double-stranded DNA breaks are indicative of DNA damage. Reproduction. 2009;138:267–78.
130. Enciso M, Sarasa J, Agarwal A, Fernández JL, Gosálvez J. A two-tailed Comet assay for assessing DNA damage in spermatozoa. Reprod BioMed Online. 2009;18:609–16.
131. Bianchi PG, Manicardi GC, Bizzaro D, Bianchi U, Sakkas D. Effect of deoxyribonucleic acid protamination on fluorochrome staining and in situ nick-translation of murine and human mature spermatozoa. Biol Reprod. 1993;49(5):1083–8.
132. Hayasaka T, Inoue Y. Chromomycin A3 studies in aqueous solutions. Spectrophotometric evidence for aggregation and interaction with herring sperm deoxyribonucleic acid. Biochemistry. 1969;8(6):2342–7.
133. Deepinder F, Cocuzza M, Agarwal A. Should seminal oxidative stress measurement be offered routinely to men presenting for infertility evaluation? Endocr Pract. 2008;14:484–91.
134. Meseguer M, Santiso R, Garrido N, García-Herrero S, Remohí J, et al. Effect of sperm DNA fragmentation on pregnancy outcome depends on oocyte quality. Fertil Steril. 2011;95:124–8.
135. Ashwood-Smith MJ, Edwards RG. DNA repair by oocytes. Mol Hum Reprod. 1996;2:46–51.
136. Sakkas D, Alvarez JG. Sperm DNA fragmentation: mechanisms of origin, impact on reproductive outcome, and analysis. Fertil Steril. 2010;93(4):1027–36.
137. Ahmadi A, Ng SC. Fertilizing ability of DNA damaged spermatozoa. J Exp Zool. 1999;284:696–704.
138. Ahmadi A, Ng SC. Developmental capacity of damaged spermatozoa. Hum Reprod. 1999;14:2279–85.
139. Borini A, Tarozzi N, Bizzaro D, Bonu MA, Fava L, et al. Sperm DNA fragmentation: paternal effect on early post-implantation embryo development in ART. Hum Reprod. 2006;21:2876–81.
140. Pogozelski WK, Tullius TD. Oxidative strand scission of nucleic acids: routes initiated by hydrogen abstraction from the sugar moiety. Chem Rev. 1998;98:1089–107.
141. Caldecott KW. Single-strand break repair and genetic disease. Nat Rev Genet. 2008;9:619–31.
142. Santiso R, Tamayo M, Gosálvez J, Meseguer M, Garrido N, Fernández JL. Simultaneous determination in situ of DNA fragmentation and 8-oxoguanine in human sperm. Fertil Steril. 2010;93:314–8.
143. Evenson DP, Jost LK, Marshall D, Zinaman MJ, Clegg E, Purvis K, et al. Utility of the sperm chromatin assay as a diagnostic and prognostic tool in the human fertility clinic. Hum Reprod. 1999;14:1039–49.
144. Greco E, Scarselli F, Iacobelli M, Rienzi L, Ubaldi F, Ferrero S, Franco G, Anniballo N, Mendoza C, Tesarik J. Efficient treatment of infertility due to sperm DNA damage by ICSI with testicular spermatozoa. Hum Reprod. 2005;20:226–30.
145. Bungum M, Bungum L, Giwercman A. Sperm chromatin structure assay (SCSA): a tool in diagnosis and treatment of infertility. Asian J Androl. 2011;13:69–75.

146. Benchaib M, Lornage J, Mazoyer C, Lejeune H, Salle B, Francois Guerin J. Sperm deoxyribonucleic acid fragmentation as a prognostic indicator of assisted reproductive technology outcome. Fertil Steril. 2007;87:93–100.
147. Huang CC, Lin DP, Tsao HM, Cheng TC, Liu CH, Lee MS. Sperm DNA fragmentation negatively correlates with velocity and fertilization rates but might not affect pregnancy rates. Fertil Steril. 2005;84:130–40.
148. Seli E, Gardner DK, Schoolcraft WB, Moffatt O, Sakkas D. Extent of nuclear DNA damage in ejaculated spermatozoa impacts on blastocyst development after in vitro fertilization. Fertil Steril. 2004;82:378–83.
149. Boe-Hansen GB, Fedder J, Ersboll AK, Christensen P. The sperm chromatin structure assay as a diagnostic tool in the human fertility clinic. Human Reprod. 2006;21:1576–82.
150. Nuñez-Calonge R, Caballero P, López-Fernández C, Guijarro JA, Fernández JL, Johnston S, Gosálvez J. An improved experimental model for understanding the impact of sperm DNA fragmentation on human pregnancy following ICSI. Reprod Sci. 2012;19:1163–8.
151. Payne JF, Raburn DJ, Couchman GM, Price TM, Jamison MG, et al. Redefining the relationship between sperm deoxyribonucleic acid fragmentation as measured by the sperm chromatin structure assay and outcomes of assisted reproductive techniques. Fertil Steril. 2005;84:356–64.
152. Chohan KR, Griffin JT, Lafromboise M, De Jonge CJ, Carrell DT. Comparison of chromatin assays for DNA fragmentation evaluation in human sperm. J Androl. 2006;27:53–9.
153 Gorczyca W, Traganos F, Jesionowska H, Darzynkiewicz Z. Presence of DNA strandbreaks and increased sensitivity of DNA in situ to denaturation in abnormal human sperm cells: analogy to apoptosis of somatic cells. Exp Cell Res. 1993;207(1):202–5.
154. Henkel R, Hoogendijk CF, Bouic PJ, Kruger TF. TUNEL assay and SCSA determine different aspects of sperm DNA damage. Andrologia. 2010;42:305–13.
155. Collins JA, Barnhart KT, Schlegel PN. Do sperm DNA integrity tests predict pregnancy with in vitro fertilization? Fertil Steril. 2008;89:823–31.
156. Zini A, Boman JM, Belzile E, Ciampi A. Sperm DNA damage is associated with an increased risk of pregnancy loss after IVF and ICSI: systematic review and metaanalysis. Hum Reprod. 2008;23:2663–8.
157. Barratt CL. Male infertility joins the translational medicine revolution. Sperm DNA: from basic science to clinical reality. Mol Hum Reprod. 2010;16:1–2.
158. Lewis SE, Agbaje I, Alvarez J. Sperm DNA tests as useful adjuncts to semen analysis. Syst Biol Reprod Med. 2008;54:111–25.
159. The Practice Committee of the American Society for Reproductive Medicine. The clinical utility of sperm DNA integrity testing: a guideline. Fertil Steril. 2013;99:673–7.
160. Robinson L, Gallos ID, Conner SJ, Rajkhowa M, Miller D, Lewis S, Kirkman-Brown J, Coomarasamy A. The effect of sperm DNA fragmentation on miscarriage rates: a systematic review and meta-analysis. Hum Reprod. 2012;27:2908–17.
161. Kovac JR, Pastuszak AW, Lamb DJ. The use of genomics, proteomics, and metabolomics in identifying biomarkers of male infertility. Fertil Steril. 2013;99:998–1007.
162. Oliva R, de Mateo S, Estanyol JM. Sperm cell proteomics. Proteomics. 2009;9(4):1004–17.
163. Pilch B, Mann M. Large-scale and high-confidence proteomic analysis of human seminal plasma. Genome Biol. 2006;7:R40.
164. Redgrove KA, Nixon B, Baker MA, Hetherington L, Baker G, Liu DY, et al. The molecular chaperone HSPA2 plays a key role in regulating the expression of sperm surface receptors that mediate sperm-egg recognition. PLoS One. 2012;7:e50851.
165. Fujihara Y, Satouh Y, Inoue N, Isotani A, Ikawa M, Okabe M. SPACA1-deficient male mice are infertile with abnormally shaped sperm heads reminiscent of globozoospermia. Development. 2012;139:3583–9.
166. Nicholson JK, Lindon JC. Systems biology: metabonomics. Nature. 2008;455:1054–6.
167. Deepinder F, Chowdary HT, Agarwal A. Role of metabolomic analysis of biomarkers in the management of male infertility. Expert Rev Mol Diagn. 2007;7:351–8.
168. Hollywood K, Brison DR, Goodacre R. Metabolomics: current technologies and futures trends. Proteomics. 2006;6:4716–23.

Role of Environmental Factors and Gonadotoxin Exposure in Unexplained Male Infertility

12

Pieter Johann Maartens, Yapo Guillaume Aboua and Stefan S. Plessis

Introduction: Unexplained Male Infertility

Infertility is a term generally used to reference the reproductive state of a couple who are sexually active without the use of contraceptives and yet are unable to achieve spontaneous natural pregnancy after a year of attempt. Infertility stems from both male and female reproductive impediments. Though the range of diagnostic tools, tests and treatments have developed at an exponential rate over time, it is estimated that 5% of couples, nearly half the number of people seeking fertility treatment, remain unwillingly infertile. *Unexplained male infertility* (*UMI*) is the term used to describe the reproductive state of a couple who are infertile despite displaying normal female fertility parameters as well as male seminal parameters within the expected ranges for successful reproduction. Prevalence is estimated at between 6 and 27%, subject to the comprehensiveness of diagnostic effort [1–4]. The inability of modern medicine to explain the phenomenon of UMI has attracted the interest of many researchers worldwide and several possible causes have been investigated, including morphologic, molecular and genetic defects (male and female), coital difficulties such as erectile dysfunction, autoimmune infertility and sperm dysfunction [5]. However, few of the theories have had concrete results such as successful treatment strategies. Successful reproduction, it seems, remains ever elusive to many hopeful couples presenting with UMI.

Seminal quality has deteriorated rapidly over the past 50 years, making it an increasingly prevalent and relevant issue in UMI. Researchers believe that the ever-changing environmental and lifestyle conditions to which the human body is exposed throughout an entire lifespan contribute greatly to this deterioration. Developments in industry and changes in modern lifestyle give rise to a range of different factors such as exposure to chemicals and toxins, harmful environmental agents and adverse lifestyle factors, all of which the body and, consequently, the reproductive system has to cope with. Environmental insults during maternal and infancy phases of human development can mediate mechanisms disturbing the morphologic, endocrine hormonal or oxidative aspects of testicular tissue and can have severe and irreversible effects on spermatogenesis (sperm production in mature testes) in a subject or its offspring. This will adversely affect seminal parameters.

This chapter aims to identify the most prominent toxins and environmental factors affecting male infertility today, as seen in Table 12.1. Some of the possible effects that the most prevalent of these toxins and environmental factors may have as the result of exposure of the male reproductive system to the adverse elements will be discussed in more detail.

Phases of Male Reproductive Development and Environmental Insult

Male reproductive development starts *in utero* during gestation and starts with the initiation of testes development from the bipotential gonad. The bipotential gonad differentiates from the genital ridge, which forms as a thickening of somatic cells on the surface of the mesonephros from which it originates. After gonadal determination structures develop dependent on hormone regulation and this process is known as sexual differentiation. The gonad gives rise to three bipotential cell lineages responsible for the formation of Sertoli cells, steroidogenic cells and cells responsible for completion of gonadal structural development. The first foetal precursor cell lineage is responsible for the formation of steroidogenic cells responsible for the secretion of sex hormones and secondary sexual characteristics. The second cell lineage gives origin to Sertoli cells and mesenchymal cells.

S. S. duPlessis (✉) · P. J. Maartens
Division of Medical Physiology, Department of Biomedical Sciences, Stellenbosch University, PO Box 19063, Tygerberg, 7505 Cape Town, South Africa
e-mail: ssdp@sun.ac.za

Y. G. Aboua
Department of Biomedical Sciences, Faculty of Health and Wellness Sciences, Cape Peninsula University of Technology, PO Box 1906 Bellville 7535, South Africa

G. L. Schattman et al. (eds.), *Unexplained Infertility,* DOI 10.1007/978-1-4939-2140-9_12,

Table 12.1 List of environmental factors, lifestyle factors and gonadotoxins and their possible mechanism of action and effect on the male reproductive system

Table of toxins and environmental factors affecting male fertility			
Environmental and lifestyle factors	Mechanism of action	Effect	Reference
Agricultural influences			
Fertilizers			
Nitric oxide	Impaired spermatogenesis	Decreased sperm function parameters: motility, viability, acrosome reaction	[26]
Pesticides			
Dichlorodiphenyltrichloroethane (DDT)	Impaired Leydig cell development, decreased testosterone receptors	Decreased testosterone levels, decreased sperm concentration	[27–29]
Ethylenedibromide			
1,2-dibromo-3-chloropropane ethylenedibromide			[30]
Chlorpyrifos	Increased production of reactive oxygen species (ROS)	ROS-induced DNA damage and lipid peroxidation of spermatozoa	[31]
Arsenic	Genetic and epigenetic changes in the genome, carcinogenesis	Subfertility	[38]
Herbicides			
Lindane	Increased production of ROS, damaged Sertoli cell morphology, impeded function of steroidogenic enzymes and proteins	Oxidative stress-induced DNA damage, decreased sperm counts and reduced circulating testosterone levels	[32, 36–37]
Methoxychlor	Increased production of ROS	Oxidative stress-induced DNA damage, decreased sperm counts	[34, 35]
Dioxin-TCDD			[33]
Vinclozolin	Acts as endocrine disruptor and androgen receptor antagonist, impaired embryonic testicular cord formation, increased apoptotic germ cell numbers	Impaired testes development, impaired spermatogenesis later in adult life, reduced sperm function	[39]
Industrial Influences			
Toluene	Increased production of ROS, decreased antioxidant levels	Oxidative damage, reproductive toxicity and decreased sperm count and testosterone levels	[31, 40]
Xylene	Inhibition of mitochondrial respiration and enhanced ROS production	Decreased sperm functional parameters	[40–44]
Acrylamide	Inhibition of sperm maturation and motility and increased inheritable DNA fragmentation	Spontaneous abortion and birth defects in the offspring	[30]
Perchloroethylene (PCE)	Impaired sperm function parameters	Prolonged conception timeframe and spontaneous abortion	[45]
Polychlorinated biphenyl (PCB)	Impaired spermatogenesis, increased gonadotropin-releasing hormone, decreased LH, antiandrogenic and antioestrogenic	Impaired sperm function, decreased testosterone levels	[46]
Epigenetics	Mutations in gametes and gamete production line	Transmission of genetic phenotypes between generations and possible harm to testes and subsequent seminal parameters of progeny	[8, 47–57]
Cigarette smoke			
Nicotine	Disrupted oxygen supply to tissues, induced inflammation and oxidative stress, impaired Leydig cell function	Lowered sperm concentration, declined motility and increased abnormal morphology, lowered male to female ratio of offspring, lowered testosterone levels	[58–70]
Hydroxycotinine			
Nitrosamines			
Carbon monoxide			
Alkaloids			
Polycylic aromatic hydrocarbon (PAH)			[9]

Table 12.1 (continued)

Table of toxins and environmental factors affecting male fertility			
Environmental and lifestyle factors	Mechanism of action	Effect	Reference
Nutrition, Obesity, Exercise			
Vitamin C	Decrease in quality of diet, less intake of key antioxidants	Subfertility	[72, 75]
Vitamin E			[73, 74]
Selenium			[76]
Carbendazim	Inhibited steroidogenic- and anti-oxidant enzymes and increased production of H_2O_2-inducing oxidative stress in Leydig cells	Decreased testes weights, decreased sperm functional parameters, reduced seminiferous tube diameters	[90–93]
Parabens	Lowered oestrogenic activity and mitochondrial interaction	Possible role in unexplained male infertility	[94]
Alcoholism	Increased circulating levels of oestrogens, induced hypoxia, reduced FSH, LH and testos-terone levels, oxidative stress, reduced antioxidants and lipid peroxidation	Impaired spermatogenesis, testicular atrophy, impotence, impaired libido, severely impaired seminal parameters	[97–111]
Radiation			
RF-EMW	Stimulation of NADH oxidase, activation of leukocytes and generation of ROS, decreased melatonin, impaired Leydig cells, increased scrotal temperatures	Lipid peroxidation and oxidative stress, decreased cellular antioxi-dant levels, increased malonyldi-aldehyde (MDA) levels	[112–121, 127]
X-ray radiation	Endocrine disruption and decreased sperm quality	Dose responsive subfertility, high dosages leading to irreversible sterility	[122–126]
Stress			
Scrotal heat stress	Impaired spermatogenesis	Decreased sperm profile param-eters and difficulties in achieving pregnancy	[128–151]
Influenza			
Malaria			
Varicocele			
Cryptorchidism			
Psychological, noise stress	Decreased antioxidants, increased free radical production, induced oxidative stress, increased gluco-corticoids, decreased testosterone, lipofuscin accumulation in Leydig cells, decreased testosterone	Impaired male reproductive func-tion, lowered semen quality	[152–161]
Gonadotoxins, chemicals and male reproductive system			
Plastics			
Plasticizers	Increased ROS production, increased H_2O_2 levels, antioxidant depletion, induced oxidative stress	Impaired sperm parameters and difficulties with reproduction	[30, 95, 164–168, 175]
Bisphenol A (BPA)			
Nonylphenol			
Di (2-ethyhexyl) phthalate [DEHP]	Testicular atrophy, inhibition of spermatogenesis via ROS produc-tion and Zinc depletion		[169–174]
Heavy metals			
Lead	Increased ROS synthesis and induced oxidative stress, inhibi-tion of antioxidant enzymes	Impeded spermatogenesis and decreased sperm concentration	[176–183]
Cadmium	Antisteroidogenic: lowered testosterone secretion. Impaired Leydig cell function. Pro-oxidant: increased free radical production and reduced zinc levels. Disrupts inter-Sertoli cell tight junctions and impairs blood/testes barrier		[183–187]

Table 12.1 (continued)

Table of toxins and environmental factors affecting male fertility			
Environmental and lifestyle factors	Mechanism of action	Effect	Reference
Pharmacological agents			
Sulfa-drugs	Impaired spermatogonia	Impaired spermatogenesis and long-term use can lead to infertility	[189–195]
Tetracyclines			
Finasteride	Impaired spermatogenesis	Decreased sperm function parameters	
Recreational drugs: marijuana, cocaine, methamphetamine	Endocrine disruption	Impaired male reproductive capabilities	[196]
Anabolic steroids	Impaired LH secretion, impaired testosterone production, impaired spermatogenesis	Oligozoospermia, hypogonadotropic hypogonadism	[197, 198]

The Sertoli cells regulate the synthesis of the seminiferous tubes, while the mesenchymal cells differentiate into Leydig cells. The third cell lineage differentiates into the gonad structure. Development of the bipotential gonad is dependent on the anti-Mullerian hormone secreted by the Sertoli cells, testosterone secreted by interstitial cells and the insulin-like 3 hormone. The intermediate mesoderm is homologous for male and female development and gives rise to the Wolffian ducts, Mullerian ducts and the gonad precursors. During male development, the Mullerian duct, under influence of testosterone, dissolves away while the Wolffian duct gives rise to the epididymis, vas deferens, ductus deferens, ejaculatory duct and the seminal vesicle. Thus, the precursor cells and subsequent spermatogonia are of cardinal importance to spermatogenesis in the adult male. It is crucial that precursor cells proliferate unimpeded and give rise to an optimal amount of spermatogonia. The development of the external male genitalia is dependent on dihydrotestosterone. The transfer of the testes from the genital ridge to the scrotum is a process of cardinal importance to sexual differentiation. Testosterone induces the relaxation of the cranial suspensory ligaments allowing the descent of the testes into the scrotum. The increased abdominal pressure due to the viscera growth and the elastic properties of the testes then cause the testes to be forced through the inguinal canal and into the scrotum. After the initial development of the essential male reproductive organs, the reproductive system lies dormant until puberty when the hypothalamic-pituitary gland (HPG) axis becomes active and the process of spermatogenesis can initiate.

With the onset of puberty the hypothalamus secretes gonadotropin releasing hormone (GnRH), which stimulates the anterior pituitary causing the secretion of the gonadotropins: follicle stimulating hormone (FSH) and luteinizing hormone (LH). The LH is responsible for the stimulation of testosterone and thus the onset of secondary sexual characteristics. The FSH is responsible for the stimulation of Sertoli cells responsible for the onset of spermatogenesis [6–8].

Spermatogenesis is the process whereby the mature male reproductive system produces haploid gametes from diploid spermatogonia during a complex and delicate process that initiates in puberty and continues right through a male's lifetime. Spermatogenesis requires a combination of synchronized gene expression and cell division and takes place in the testes over a period of a little more than 2 months.

Of cardinal importance to the normal occurrence of spermatogenesis are the Sertoli cells as they alter rates of sperm production in adult testes and produce factors essential to gamete development [9–11]. Leydig cells are responsible for the secretion of androgenic hormones. These androgens are key to appropriate testicular development, such as urethral groove fusion and descent of the testis [12, 13].

Due to the intricacy of the process, spermatogenesis is totally dependent on the existence of optimal conditions. It is extremely sensitive to changes in the external environmental elements. Therefore, environmental insult that affects gonadal differentiation, Sertoli- or Leydig-cell proliferation or spermatogenesis at any age could affect male reproductive development and thus lead to adverse reproductive pathologies such as oligozoospermia, asthenozoospermia, hypospadias, testicular spermatogonia cancer and cryptorchidism [7–9].

The male reproductive system can be exposed to adverse environmental factors during any of its three stages of development: maternal-dependent (gestation and lactation) development, early-life (prepubertal)—development or sexual maturity (Fig. 12.1). Specifically, the effects of environmental factors during the two developmental stages (maternal/early-life) can be detrimental to testicular development and spermatogenesis. This can result in poor semen parameters later in life, including impaired sperm concentration and motility. There can also be direct exposure to hostile environmental factors during adulthood. Similar to the maternal and infancy stages of development, such factors can have a negative impact on spermatogenesis. However, direct exposure during later life is regarded as reversible while early life exposure is considered to be irreversible [14, 15]. Overall exposure to adverse elements can impair the male reproductive system during any of its stages of maturity and thus affect spermatogenesis through several mechanisms of action:

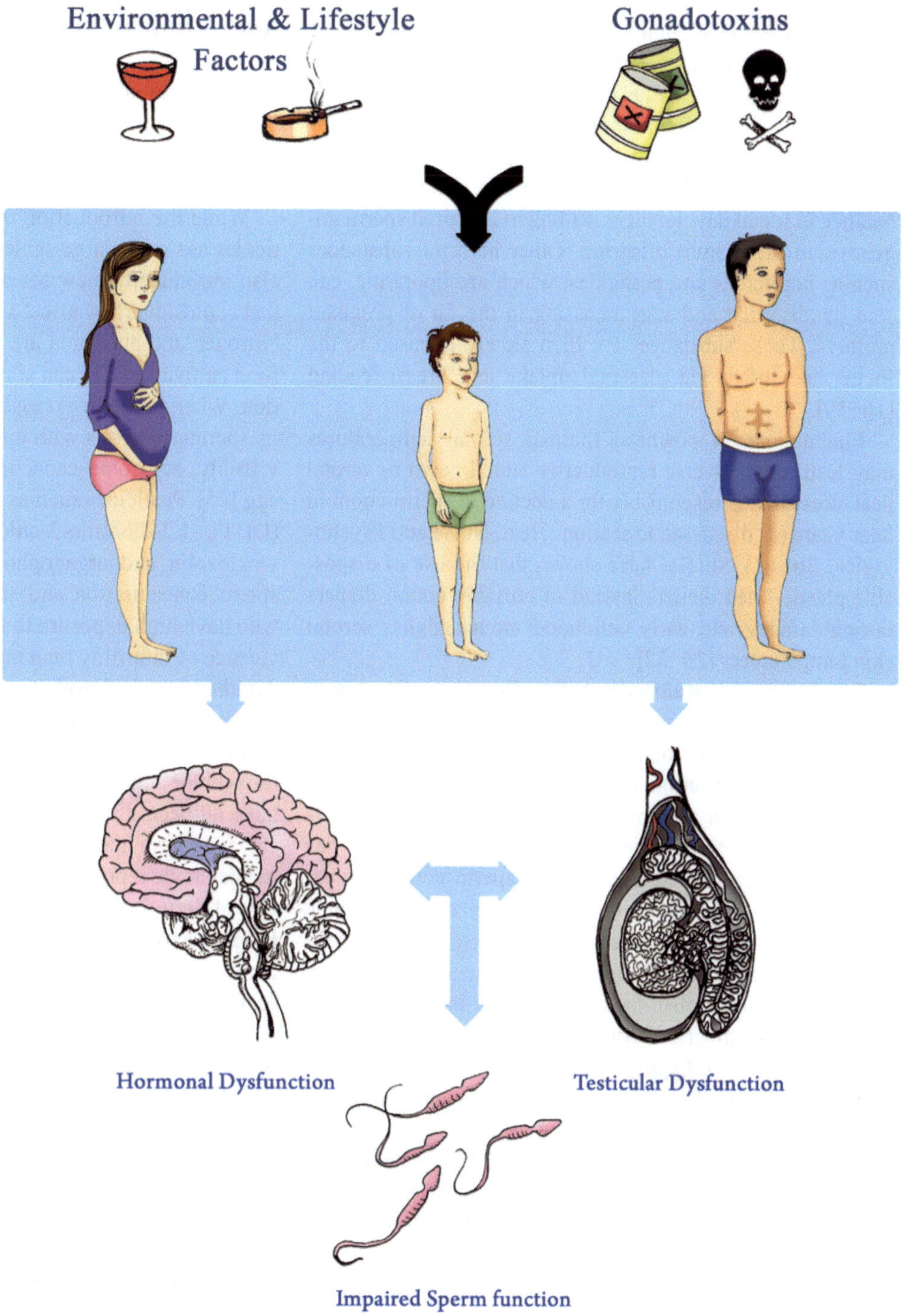

Fig. 12.1 Effects of environmental factors, lifestyle factors and gonadotoxins on male fertility. Exposure of male reproductive system to environmental factors, lifestyle factors and gonadotoxins during gestation, early life and adulthood could affect hormonal and testicular regulation, thus contributing to impaired sperm function and associated male infertility

- Any stage of maturity: Impediment of spermatogenesis and/or Sertoli- and Leydig-cell function can affect spermatogenesis in later life.
- Maternal exposure: Endocrine-inhibiting substances and adverse lifestyle factors can affect reproductive organ development.
- Postnatal exposure: Environmental fluctuations such as changes in scrotal temperatures can affect spermatogenesis in later life.
- Adulthood exposure: Harmful substances such as xenobiotics or adverse lifestyle factors can affect spermatogenesis.

Lifestyle factors, such as cigarette smoking during pregnancy, have proven to reduce sperm concentration in developing males as well as Sertoli cell count. This is because the components in cigarette smoke antagonize androgen receptor-mediated function and thus impede reproductive organ development. Maternal obesity has also been shown to reduce sperm concentration in the male offspring and inhibit testicular development via interference of the foetus' testosterone/oestrogen balance. Diet of the mother can also affect the developing foetus through, for example, ingestion of anabolic steroids found in meat. These anabolic steroids and the oestrogenic substances used to process and cook the meat can act as xenobiotics and impair the critical hormone balance in foetal development leading to impaired spermatogenesis in the mature offspring. Other harmful substances such as herbicides and pesticides, which are lipophilic, can also be absorbed and start amassing in the fat of pregnant mothers. These substances are then slowly released to the foetus and infant via placental uptake and breast-feeding [16–19].

Fluctuations in postnatal thermal scrotal temperatures may lead to an adverse reproductive state known as scrotal heat stress that is responsible for a decline in sperm count in later years (as discussed in section 'Heat, Noise and Psychological Stress'). Studies have shown that the use of disposable plastic-lined diapers instead of reusable cotton diapers during infancy and early childhood induce higher scrotal skin temperatures [20–22].

Environmental insults in the form of oestrogens have been shown to cause responsive changes in the neuroendocrine system of the mature male with effects notable in reproductive function and spermatogenesis [23]. Such environmental oestrogens, known as xenobiotics, can have a negative impact on male fertility as ingestion of these substances has been directly correlated to decreased sperm concentration. Xenobiotics have been found to adversely affect the male reproductive system in the following ways:

- The inhibition of FSH secretion by the foetal pituitary gland and thus a disturbance in the HPG-axis leading to a decreased number of Sertoli cells
- The inhibition of Leydig cell formation and function leading to decreased testosterone production and decreased gamete differentiation
- The inhibition of androgen receptors within foetal testes
- The conversion of xenobiotics to quinones that produce reactive oxygen species (ROS) that, when produced in excess, induce oxidative stress or damage DNA [24].

Environmental Factors, Lifestyle Factors and Male Infertility

As already noted, it is increasingly evident that spermatogenesis is an immensely sensitive and delicate process that is dependent on optimal conditions and severely susceptible to fluctuations in external factors [7]. The rapid expansion of Western lifestyle with its concomitant increase in industry, changes in diet, excessive alcohol consumption, bad smoking habits and high levels of stress may be responsible for the aforementioned decrease in male fertility.

Agricultural Influences

With a world population of just under 7 billion people, sufficient food production has become a major worldwide issue, giving rise to biotechnology and food engineering/modification as a whole new form of industry.

While the introduction of fertilizers, herbicides and pesticides has made large-scale food production possible, it has also introduced a new set of chemicals and possible toxins that could adversely affect a great number of people globally. Nitrogen and ammonia are two currently used fertilizers in food cultivation and can stimulate nitric oxide (NO) production. When found in excessive levels in the body, NO, inhibits spermatogenesis with a resultant drop in sperm motility, viability, acrosome capacitation and ability to fertilize the egg [25]. Pesticides such as dichlorodiphenyltrichloroethane (DDT), 1,2-dibromo-3-chloropropane, ethylenedibromide, vinclozolin and organophosphates have proved to inhibit sperm concentration and studies have shown that farmers who have high exposure to such pesticides have a higher incidence of infertility than men in other occupations [26–29]. Another organophosphate pesticide, chlorpyrifos, has been implicated in ROS-induced DNA damage and lipid peroxidation of spermatozoa [30]. Herbicides such as lindane, methoxychlor and 2,3,7,8-tetrachlorodibenzo-*p*-dioxin (TCDD) have all been directly correlated to oxidative stress and decreased sperm concentration. Lindane exposure is also detrimental to the reproductive system by damaging the morphology of Sertoli cells, resulting in decreased spermatogenesis. Lindane exposure also impedes the function of steroidogenic enzymes, steroidal regulatory and transport proteins and thus reduces circulating testosterone levels [31–36].

The large-scale use of such fertilizers, herbicides and pesticides is proving to be of major concern to fertility specialists. Eradicating the use of these agents is probably not a realistic solution to the problem as the agents address the much more basic human need for food on which millions of lives depend.

Industrial Influences

In industrial environments substances commonly occur that have been found to adversely affect the fertility of males that regularly work in these environments. Examples of such substances are toluene, xylene, acrylamide and perchloroethylene (PCE).

Toluene is an organic solvent found in paint, rubber, glue, gasoline and several cleaning agents. It is ingested through the inhalation of vapour. Studies have shown toluene to decrease epididymal sperm concentration and decrease testosterone levels by inducing a state of oxidative stress through the excess production of ROS or a decrease in the antioxidative capacity of cells [27, 37]. Another substance commonly found in industrial areas, Xylene, has presented in workers' blood and semen where it has been found in the air in excess of the allowable atmospheric amount. Studies have shown xylene to decrease sperm viability, motility and acrosin activity by inducing a total impediment of mitochondrial respiration and stimulating mitochondrial ROS production [37–41]. Acrylamide, known as an intermediate in the production of polyacrylamide, is used in water purification, paper production and mining. Acrylamide has been associated with the inhibition of sperm maturation and motility and increased inheritable DNA fragmentation. PCE is a substance found in the cleaning industry and has been found to prolong conception timeframes and even cause spontaneous abortion in the partners of men exposed to it [42].

As industry expands, better health and safety regulations should be put in place to protect the health of workers. Fertility specialists should do a full history check and test for industrial substances when attempting to treat men working in this sector who are experiencing fertility issues.

Epigenetics

Transgenerational inheritance is a term that refers to the ability of environmental factors to not only promote a pathophysiologic condition in an individual but to promote it in successive generations. Most environmental parameters such as nutrition or toxins do not directly cause DNA mutations or alterations in DNA sequence but do have the ability to alter the epigenome. Mutations in the gametes and gamete production line, which become irreversible, can cause transmission of genetic phenotypes between generations and can cause downstream harm to the testes and subsequent seminal parameters of the progeny. Transgenerational and early life exposure to adverse environmental factors, such as endocrine disruptors, are now considered key factors in the onset of adult reproductive impediment. *Imprinted genes* are specific genetic factors dependent on epigenetic programming that can be influenced by environmental factors such as nutritional factors, inorganic toxins such as arsenic, endocrine interrupters such as bisphenol A (BPA), phytoestrogens and chemicals used as fungicides and pesticides [43–54].

Cigarette Smoke

The adverse effects of smoking on the body and on male fertility are well-established—yet cigarettes remain one of the world's top selling commodities. Smoke inhalation has been correlated to lower sperm concentration, declined motility and increased abnormal morphology in sperm. Smoking disrupts the oxygen supply to tissues and the reproductive system as well as exposing the reproductive system to more than 2000 substances that have the potential to harm, such as nicotine, carbon monoxide, nitrosamines, alkaloids and hydroxycotinine. These substances can increase the production of free radicals such as ROS and reactive nitrogen species (RNS), which when produced at pathophysiologic levels, can lead to oxidative stress and ultimately to infertility [55–58]. Studies have found a direct correlation between cigarette smoke intake, increased ROS levels and decreased levels of antioxidants. Studies have also correlated smoking with an increase in cadmium levels. Cadmium is a heavy metal known for its detrimental effects on reproduction [56, 58]. It is understood that metabolites that enter the circulation as a result of smoking act as chemotactic stimuli-inducing inflammation and attract leukocytes that produce ROS and induce oxidative stress [56, 59]. Smoking has proved to decrease seminal levels of antioxidants such as vitamins C and E [60, 61] and has been associated with higher levels of tetrazoospermia [62].

Tobacco smoking has also been shown to reduce the ratio of male to female offspring, even if only the father smokes [63]. The nicotine and cotinine found in smoke either inhibit the intracellular calcium content or completely block the effects of calcium on steroidogenesis in Leydig cells, resulting in a decline in circulating testosterone levels [64]. In addition, nicotine intake results in increased blood cholesterol levels causing atherosclerosis in arteries supplying blood to the reproductive system and thus resulting in lowered blood [65]. Chronic exposure of the male reproductive system to nicotine leads to a state of vasoconstriction or vasospasm within the penile arteries and smooth muscle leading to an impairment of Leydig cell function [66, 67].

Nutrition and Exercise

When assessing nutritional factors and their effects on the male reproductive system, there are three factors to take into account:

- Diet and malnutrition
- Obesity
- Ingestion of preservatives

With the spread of Westernized lifestyle in modern times, many cultures have moved away from their traditional diets and conform to new eating habits by consuming more refined carbohydrates and less fresh fruit and vegetables. Fruits and vegetables contain essential nutrients such as antioxidants, vitamins and folate that play key roles in DNA and RNA synthesis during spermatogenesis. Many of these nutritional elements are also antioxidants of paramount importance. Vitamins C and E are both antioxidants that neutralize ROS and prevent oxidative stress. Vitamin C protects the sperm DNA in the seminal fluid and Vitamin E protects the spermatozoa membranes. Selenium is a mineral that also functions as an antioxidant. Studies have reported that these antioxidants improve male fertility parameters when either used alone or in combination. Studies have shown that a decrease in ingestion of these nutritional substances is correlated to subfertility [27, 68–73].

With an increased intake of refined carbohydrates, lipids and proteins as associated with increased global Westernization; overweight and obese individuals have become an ever-growing issue affecting the health and economic status of many countries. Men with a body mass index (BMI) of over 25 are up to three times more at risk to be classified as infertile due to reduced sperm concentration and increased sperm DNA fragmentation.

There are three main theories that attempt to explain the link between obesity and infertility. First, studies have shown a direct correlation between change in BMI trends and changes in endocrine and exocrine functions of the testes. The prevalence of excess adipose tissue leads to the conversion of testosterone to oestrogen, thereby decreasing the levels of circulating testosterone and increasing the levels of estradiol. These changes are accompanied by decreases in LH and FSH, leading to impaired spermatogenesis. Second, accumulation of inner thigh, pubic and abdominal fat could cause infertility through increased scrotal temperatures. Third, obesity and many of its associated conditions such as dyslipidemia and insulin resistance, which all form part of the broader condition known as metabolic syndrome, are associated with induced states of systemic proinflammation. Systemic proinflammation is accompanied by increased activation of leukocytes, production of ROS and subsequent onset of oxidative stress and lipid peroxidation, which severely impair sperm parameters [74–85].

Preservatives found in food and other consumer products as broad spectrum antifungal agents (such as fruit, paint and textiles) can be harmful to male reproductive parameters. Studies have correlated carbendazim (methyl-2-benzimidazole carbamate) intake to decreased testes weight, low sperm concentration and motility, reduced seminiferous tube diameters and increased incidence of abnormal sperm. Researchers postulate that carbendazim adversely affects reproductive systems by inhibiting steroidogenic and antioxidant enzymes and increasing production of hydrogen peroxide (H_2O_2) radicals. These changes then induce oxidative stress and cause lipid peroxidation in Leydig cells [86–89]. Recent research done on preservatives that have been commonly used and regarded as safe for many years, such as parabens (alkyl esters of *p*-hydroxybenzoic acid), has concluded that these substances may not be as safe as previously thought. Such substances may interact with mitochondria and so play a role in unexplained infertility [90–92].

Alcohol

Evidence suggests that moderate alcohol consumption does not have any effect on male reproductive function. Excessive chronic alcohol use, however, does harm spermatogenesis and male fertility. Alcoholism has been associated with testicular atrophy, impotence, impaired libido, reduced FSH, LH and testosterone levels, oxidative stress, reduced antioxidants and lipid peroxidation and severely impaired seminal parameters. Studies suggest that alcohol adversely affects the reproductive system by promoting the overproduction of free radicals such as ROS, and inducing a state of oxidative stress in the testes as well as inducing hypoxia and causing tissue damage in a system already very sensitive to changes in oxygen supply. Alcoholics often follow diets that deprive them of antioxidants [93–99].

Excessive alcohol intake also causes an increase in circulating levels of oestrogens in males. The increased oestrogen levels disrupt the normal production of testosterone and cause saturation of testosterone receptors in the hypothalamus in the brain. This in turn leads to a reduced signal sent to the pituitary gland, which in turn reduces the secretion of luteinizing hormone (LH). Ultimately, this results in reduced testosterone production in the gonads. An increase in circulating oestrogen also increases the production of sex hormone-binding globulin (SHBG). The SHBG binds testosterone and reduces the plasma levels of testosterone. Testosterone levels in plasma are key to the homeostasis of the gonadotropins (LH and FSH), which regulate spermatogenesis and the maturation of sperm cells [100, 101].

Cell Phone, Laptop and Ionizing Radiation

With the increasing modern day usage of electronics that transmit electromagnetic waves, much attention has been drawn to the possible effects of such devices on the human body. Studies have shown that cell phone usage directly correlates to a decline in male fertility parameters. Cell phones transmit via radiofrequency electromagnetic waves (RF-EMW) that significantly increase malonyldialdehyde (MDA) levels (a lipid product of lipid peroxidation and oxidative stress) and decrease cellular antioxidant levels. Researchers postulate that cell phone-associated radiation can lead to the induction of oxidative stress through either

- the stimulation of the sperm plasma membrane redox system, which entails activation of NADH oxidase, or
- the activation of leukocytes and the subsequent generation of ROS.

Cell phone-associated radiation also seems to decrease melatonin, which acts as an antioxidant in the body. Other morphological research reports that RF-EMW emitted from cell phones adversely affects Leydig cells via a thermal molecular mechanism resulting in impaired spermatogenesis. Electromagnetic field (EMF) exposure was directly correlated to a decline in seminiferous tubular diameter and epithelium thickness [102–110].

Exposure of ionizing radiation in chronic doses has also been associated with endocrine disruption and decreased sperm quality. Studies done on cooperating prisoners opting for testicle X-ray irradiation, as well as men exposed to radiation after the Chernobyl nuclear tragedy, reported a direct correlation between dose of ionizing radiation and increasing infertile parameters with high dosages of exposure even leading to irreversible sterility [111–115].

Laptops wirelessly connected to the Internet through Wi-Fi, transmit via RF-EMW radiation and, when used on a person's lap, increase scrotal temperatures. A recent pilot study shows that ex vivo exposure of human spermatozoa to RF-EMW via an Internet-connected laptop decreases motility and increases DNA fragmentation. This suggests that laptops connected to the Internet, used on the lap in close proximity to the testes, could impede male infertility, but here more research is needed [116].

Heat, Noise and Psychological Stress

Exteriorization (descending) of the testes is unique to mammals. It is an evolutionary adaptation to keep the testes at a core temperature of 3–4 °C cooler than the normal 37 °C internal abdominal temperature. Keeping the testes cool reduces rates of DNA damage and resulting sperm mutations. Any fluctuations in the testes temperature, caused for, e.g. by occupations, lifestyle choices or disease, can disrupt this susceptible system of homeostasis and impair spermatogenesis [117–119].

Occupational chronic exposure of the body to raised temperatures has been correlated to decreased sperm profile parameters and difficulties in achieving pregnancy. This problem is especially prevalent in people with occupations that entail working in close proximity to a furnace, for example welders, bakers and stokers. Some studies, however, still contest these findings and thus the effect of chronic heat exposure remains a somewhat controversial subject. Prolonged periods of sitting and inactivity associated with office jobs have been shown to correlate with high scrotal temperatures and decreased sperm concentration. Sperm density has been directly correlated to a decrease by 40 % per 1 °C change in the daytime scrotal temperature. Professional drivers have also been associated with reduced seminal quality and difficulties in achieving pregnancy [120–129].

Lifestyle choices can have an effect on scrotal heat temperatures and subsequent infertility. Wearing tight fitting underclothing such as briefs as opposed to wearing looser fitting boxers can cause increased scrotal temperatures. Prolonged hot baths, steam rooms and saunas increase scrotal temperature to such an extent as to inhibit spermatogenesis. As previously mentioned, dietary choices leading to obesity can increase scrotal temperature and thus impede spermatogenesis [130–137].

Illnesses such as influenza or malaria and conditions such as varicocele or cryptorchidism could also lead to heightened scrotal temperatures. Studies have shown a decrease in seminal quality after the onset of fever caused by influenza or malaria [138–140].

Situations causing a subject to experience mental stress have been associated with impaired male reproductive function. Mental stress has been associated with lower levels of antioxidant enzymes and higher levels of oxidants possibly leading to an induced state of oxidative stress. Studies have also shown a correlation between mental stress and lowered semen quality. For example, a study done on students showed that semen quality was severely affected by stress caused by exams. It is well-established that stress leads to increased levels of glucocorticoids, but it is also associated with decreased levels of testosterone [141–145]. Corticosterone administration is known to stimulate free radical production and lipofuscin formation in the mitochondria of Leydig cells. Similarly, studies show that chronic noise stress can lead to lipofuscin accumulation in testes and decreased testosterone levels. This means that chronic noise stress could prove to be detrimental to male reproductive systems [146–148].

Studies that provide a good example of the effect of both mental and noise stress on the male reproductive system examine the effect of war on the reproductive system. Studies on the 15-year Lebanese civil war have reported that infertile males had a 57 % correlation to civil war-related trauma (residence in bombing areas, participation in combat, injuries, kidnapping and displacement from home). There was also a significant association between war involvement and decreased sperm concentration and increased abnormal sperm morphology [149, 150].

Gonadotoxins and Male Infertility

It is inevitable that, with spermatogenesis proving to be such a susceptible process, chemical exposure as a result of environmental pollution will lead to adverse sperm parameters and difficulties with reproduction [111]. Over the past 50 years, average sperm concentrations in the general population have decreased by 50 %. During this same period extensive environmental and lifestyle changes have occurred in both First and Third World Countries. There has been astronomic growth in the chemical industry, with an ever-increasing market for new products leading to ever-increasing masses of product waste [151, 152]. Studies in this field battle with the immense difficult of identifying and analysing the effect of a single external factor such as environmental pollution on a complex organism which is constantly exposed to a mixture of toxins and environmental insults.

Plastics

Plastic has become a very common substance in consumer products found in most households all over the world. Plastic suppliers often add substances when producing plastics to make them more functional and useful. Many of these added substances are, however, quite toxic to the reproductive system. Plasticizers are polyphenolic chemical substances used to prolong the elasticity and durability of plastics and are common in clear, heat-resilient and indestructible plastics. Plasticizers have been found to be harmful to the male reproductive system. Another chemical commonly found in plastics is bisphenol A (BPA). BPA is an additive to disposable plastics used to improve polycarbonate plastics; it is also used in dental materials. BPA has been found to have the ability to migrate from the plastic of food containers into food and from dental sealants and fillings into circulation in the human body. BPA has been found to be present in the blood of 90% of Americans. BPA has proved to inhibit sperm concentration, motility and viability. Studies have shown that BPA generates ROS in several tissues, including the reproductive tissues, and causes an increase in the levels of H_2O_2 in testicular tissue. This increase in free radicals ultimately leads to a depletion in cellular antioxidant defences, an imbalance in oxidant–antioxidant production and a subsequent induced state of oxidative stress [153–157]. Phthalate esters have been used to increase the elasticity of plastics in bags, toys, clothing and pharmaceutical products such as soaps and shampoos. Animal studies report that a specific phthalate ester, Di(2-ethyhexyl) phthalate (DEHP), causes testicular atrophy and inhibition of spermatogenesis via ROS production and zinc depletion, but the effects in humans are still in dispute [158–163]. Nonylphenol is a synthetic constituent of plastic that has oestrogen-like properties and is lipophilic and is therefore capable of crossing cell membranes and concentrating in tissue. Nonylphenol is often found in cleaning chemicals, paints, pharmaceutical products, foods and in certain forms of packaging materials. Adult exposure to nonylphenol has been correlated to decreased sperm concentration [91, 164].

Heavy Metals

Studies show a direct correlation between heavy metal exposure and fertility implications such as impeded spermatogenesis and decreased sperm concentration [165–168]. Lead and cadmium are two key metals of concern to male infertility. Lead has been banned from most products by governmental legislation but was previously found in products such as lead paint and gasoline leading to occupational overexposure. Lead can also accumulate in fish and be ingested when eating fish. Inorganic lead can disturb the oxidant–antioxidant balance and induce a state of oxidative stress. Lead inhibits the delta amino levulanic acid synthase enzyme and thus promotes ROS synthesis and induces oxidative stress. Lead has also been associated with inhibited antioxidant enzyme activity through the impediment of superoxide dismutase, catalase and glutathione peroxidase activity [169–172].

Cadmium has been found to be directly connected to male fertility problems. Cadmium levels are higher in the seminal plasma and blood of infertile men than that of fertile men. Cadmium affects the male reproductive system in several ways. It directly inhibits sperm concentration due to its antisteroidogenic properties that lead to a lowered testosterone secretion. It directly impedes the function of Leydig cells and thus the testosterone levels. It has been found to have pro-oxidant properties and may mediate generation of free radicals and reduction in zinc levels, zinc being crucial to spermatogenesis. Finally, cadmium may disrupt inter-Sertoli cell tight junctions and thus disrupt the blood/testes barrier and consequently inhibit spermatogenesis. Chronic smoking has been associated with significantly increased cadmium levels [173–176].

Other metals such as zinc, copper, aluminium, mercury and vanadium are under scrutiny for their possible adverse effects on male fertility [177]. More research is of paramount importance, but there is sufficient evidence that heavy metal exposure is harmful to the male reproductive system. Metal workers and other men who are occupationally exposed or exposed through lifestyle choices that seek infertility treatment should have a full heavy metal assessment as part of their diagnosis and treatment course.

Pharmacological Agents

Since pharmacological agents have become more readily available on mainstream markets the human body has been bombarded by a whole range of pharmacological agents. These agents have often not been properly investigated as to their effects of long-term use on reproductive and other tissues. Drugs in long-term use whether prescription, recreational or muscle enhancing have been associated with possible adverse effects on the male reproductive system. Therapeutic drugs such as antibiotics and chemotherapy can impede the function of spermatogonia. Antibacterial drugs such as sulfa-drugs and tetracyclines can impair spermatogenesis and long-term use can lead to infertility. Studies have shown that men that ceased use of common chronic drugs such as allergy, epilepsy and bacterial infection treatment drugs showed a 93 % improvement in semen profile. Drugs used to treat reproductive conditions such as androgenic alopecia and benign prostatic hyperplasia such as finasteride, impede spermatogenesis and further decrease sperm function parameters. Such studies all state that the type of drug, dosage and duration of use are factors that contribute to the effect on the male reproductive system. All studies, however, conclude that such drugs affect the male reproductive capabilities [178–184].

Use of recreational drugs such as marijuana, cocaine and methamphetamine and their effect on the male reproductive status is still under investigation, but studies have shown a strong link between excessive recreational drug use and endocrine disruption and thus many believe that more research is bound to prove adverse effects to male reproductive capabilities [185].

The use of anabolic steroids for athletic performance enhancement or body enhancement has become very popular worldwide. Anabolic steroids can impede spermatogenesis by suppressing LH secretion and thus inhibiting testosterone production with possible oligozoospermic consequences. Hypogonadotropic hypogonadism is the main cause of impaired spermatogenesis in people using anabolic steroids. These effects have however been found to be reversible after discontinuation in use of steroids for a couple of months [186–187].

Possible Treatment Solutions for Male Infertility Caused by Environmental Insults

The treatment of unexplained male infertility does not allow for the protocol of standard clinical practice decision making. Such circumstances call for a specific scientific plan to identify and correct a known defect and the risk and treatment management [1]. There are two forms of UMI management that can be followed: expectant management and interventional management. Expectant management entails the regulation of environmental and lifestyle factors to such an extent as to better sperm function parameters and thus better chances for successful conception. Interventional management entails any form of assistance to conception whether invasive such as surgical or pharmacological via the use of oral medication.

Expectant management is to be recommended if the woman is less than or between 28–30 years of age and the duration of unsuccessful infertility is less than 2–3 years [188]. Lifestyle factors that are addressed and managed are chemicals, smoking, nutrition, exercise and environmental pollution.

The children of smokers are subject to a bombardment of tobacco combustion products causing an enormous developmental risk of genetic defects. The consequences may not be apparent immediately at birth but can manifest later in life. It is therefore imperative that antismoking measures continue to be implemented; that prospective parents be strongly encouraged to give up smoking and be supported in their efforts to do so.

The amount of evidence on the known health benefits of regular exercise and balanced nutritious diets as well as the detrimental effect of obesity on the reproductive system is overwhelming. Fertility is decreased by being either overweight or underweight. Studies have proved fertility treatment to be less successful in overweight women. More research into the effect of diet and exercise on fertility is needed. In the meanwhile people trying to conceive should be advised to exercise moderately and aim to have a BMI between 20 and 25 kg/m^2.

Environmental pollutants may have a negative effect on fertility and foetal development. People planning pregnancy should have a detailed history checkup and advisement on reducing their home, environment and occupational exposure to pollutants [189–190].

Interventional management which includes medication, surgery or assisted conception is justified in cases of unexplained infertility of long duration and/or advanced maternal and paternal age. In recent times managements have been solely based on surgical treatments or antioxidant-based treatments.

Spermatozoa are particularly vulnerable to oxidative stress not only because of their high polyunsaturated fatty acid content but also because of inherent deficiencies in their intracellular antioxidant enzyme protection and their limited capacity for DNA repair. Fortunately, the reproductive tract contains a powerful array of enzymatic and nonenzymatic antioxidant molecules in the epididymal and seminal plasmas that act in coordinated manner to protect spermatozoa against a barrage of toxic oxygen metabolites [191]. The scavenger enzymes superoxide dismutase, catalase and glutathione peroxidase that are found in the seminal fluid are the primary defence mechanism against ROS. Studies found that impediment of these enzymes caused a state of oxidative stress that influences the incidence of miscarriage and birth defects in mated wild-type female mice, thus demonstrating the protection that these enzymes normally provide [192].

A decrease in levels of reduced glutathione (GSH) during sperm production has been correlated with disruptions in the membrane integrity of spermatozoa as a consequence of induced oxidative stress. Intracellular glutathione levels of spermatozoa are shown to be decreased in certain populations of infertile men. Glutathione is not only vital to sperm antioxidant defences but is also essential for the formation of phospholipid hydroperoxide glutathione peroxidase—an enzyme which forms an integral part of a structural protein in the mid-piece of mature spermatozoa. Deficiencies in either substance can lead to instability of the mid-piece resulting in defective motility of the spermatozoa. Scavengers such as glutathione can be used to treat these cases as they can restore the physiological constitution of polyunsaturated fatty acids in the cell membrane [193–199].

In general terms, antioxidants are compounds which scavenge, suppress and dispose of ROS. Major antioxidants are vitamins A, E and C, beta-carotene and the trace mineral selenium. A number of nutritional therapies have been shown to improve sperm counts and sperm motility, including carnitine, arginine, zinc and vitamin B_{12}. Folic acid and zinc supplements have, when used in combination, been shown to increase sperm counts in a placebo-controlled trial. Antioxidants, such as glutathione and coenzyme Q10, have also proven beneficial in treating male infertility [200–206]. Coenzyme Q10 (CoQ10) is a component of the mitochondrial respiratory chain and plays a crucial role in energy metabolism. Furthermore, it is an important antioxidant associated with membranes and lipoproteins. It has long been known that CoQ10 biosynthesis is markedly active in testes and high levels of its reduced form QH2 (ubiquinol) are present in semen; this suggests a protective role as a scavenger in this biological system. There is evidence that sperm cells with reduced motility also have a significant reduction in the phospholipid pool as well as phosphatidylethanolamine and phosphatidylcholine content probably related to a reduction in the antioxidant capacity of spermatozoa and seminal plasma. It has been demonstrated that reduced levels of CoQ10 in the seminal plasma and sperm cells of infertile men with idiopathic and varicocele were associated with asthenospermia. On the basis of these findings CoQ10 has been identified as one of the key compounds contributing to the total antioxidant buffer capacity of semen and loss of its function leads to an impairment of the system. Whether the exogenous administration of CoQ10 could lead to any modification of its content in semen or to any benefit on sperm cell function still remains an interesting future research topic [201, 207–214].

Many plant-derived substances collectively termed “phytonutrients” or “phytochemicals” are becoming increasingly known for their antioxidant activity. Phenolic compounds such as flavonoids are ubiquitous within the plant kingdom: approximately 3000 flavonoid substances have been described. In plants, flavonoids serve as protectors against a wide variety of environmental stresses while in humans flavonoids appear to function as biological response modifiers. The broad therapeutic effects of flavonoids can be largely attributed to their antioxidant properties [204, 215].

Surgical treatment can be an effective approach in the treatment of male infertility of defective morphologic origin such as obstructive azoospermia. Accurate identification of the cause of infertility and microsurgical approaches will often provide effective treatment with low morbidity rates. Appropriate training in microsurgery and overall experience with surgical techniques will produce the most effective treatment of the infertile man.

Shortcomings/Constraints of Current Research on UMI and Environmental Influences

The diagnosis, evaluation and treatment recommendations for male infertility are normally based on a standard semen analysis even though diagnostic tools, tests and parameter guidelines are limited and vary between urologic societies, fertility clinics and the World Health Organization laboratory manual for the processing of human semen editions [216–219]. The parameters for which guidelines are laid out (sperm concentration, motility and morphology) also vary between different ejaculates collected from the same individual. This variation in samples is attributed to sexual activity and abstinence, function of accessory reproductive glands and environmental exposures and thus cannot be regarded as accurate and finitely representative of an individual’s fertility profile.

Analyses of the results of studies evaluating effects of environmental factors on the male reproductive system are limited in the sense that they are inconsistent in the use of biological analytical techniques, controlling for variance in factors and weakness of study design. *In vivo* studies done on animals may also prove to have limited applicability to human conditions such as gestation and lactation. Developmental periods in animals are much shorter than in humans. Treatment with a factor and the cessation and measurement of its effect is much easier in the controlled environment under which such experiments are conducted on animals than in the complex, uncontrolled and chaotic conditions under which humans live. Animals, as opposed to humans, vary much less between subjects in terms of their spermatogenesis profile. Humans are exposed to a mixture of environmental chemicals, toxins and other factors so that isolating and interpreting the effect of a single factor without interference by other parameters is near impossible [111, 219].

Diagnostics such as comprehensive history investigation, and molecular and genetic inquiry should be employed and should be complemented with an all-inclusive physical examination before conclusions are drawn and treatment plans are based on fertility status. The use of the most recent updated World Health Organization (WHO) reference values in clinical practice will likely change the classification of infertility for many couples. Rapidly developing technology and constant change in seminal parameter baselines emphasize the need for clinicians to consider a much more diverse variety of parameters than just sperm concentration and motility when assessing male subfertility.

Assisted reproductive technologies (ARTs) might be an interim solution to the problem of unexplained male infertility—but as a technique it is not without its difficulties and shortcomings and refinement through research is required [1]. ART has allowed a large proportion of men experiencing fertility problems to procreate. As amazing as this technology is, it is a mere treatment of the symptom and not of the actual causal problem and thus is counterproductive, in a sense, to understanding the causes, effects and possible treatments of male infertility.

Conclusion

Seminal quality has deteriorated rapidly in the past 50 years making it an increasingly prevalent and relevant issue to UMI. Researchers believe that the ever-changing environmental and lifestyle conditions to which the human body is exposed throughout an entire lifespan are of paramount importance in this occurrence. Modern day developments in industry and changes in lifestyle have led to a range of negative factors that the body and reproductive system have to cope with, such as exposure to chemicals and toxins, harmful environmental agents and adverse lifestyle factors. Environmental insults during the maternal, infancy and adult phases of human development can mediate mechanisms disturbing morphologic aspects, endocrine hormonal aspects or oxidative aspects of testicular tissue and can have severe and irreversible effects on spermatogenesis in a subject or its offspring.

Ultimately UMI could be caused by any number or combination of effects such as morphologic, molecular and genetic defects. Nevertheless, as the prevalence of UMI has been rapidly increasing in recent times and environmental and lifestyle factors have been drastically changing in recent years, it is not an unwarranted assumption to conclude that environmental and lifestyle factors play at least some, if not a definitive, role in the development of UMI.

Diagnoses, evaluations and treatment recommendations for male infertility and analyses of the results of studies evaluating the effects of environmental factors on the male reproductive system are, however, not without their constraints and weaknesses. ART is not the beginning and end to male infertility. It is merely a backroad around the real issue. It is thus of cardinal importance that research be done on UMI and the effects of environmental exposure on the reproductive system so that we may better our understanding of and eventually hope for solutions to the prevention and cure of this growing and topical problem.

References

1. Hamada A, Esteves S, Agarwal A. Unexplained male infertility—looking beyond routine semen analysis. Androl Fertil. 2012;5:90–6.
2. World Health Organization. WHO manual for the standardized investigation and diagnosis of the infertile couple. Cambridge: Cambridge University Press; 2000.
3. Moghissi K, Wallach E. Unexplained infertility. Fertil Steril. 1983;39(1):5–21.
4. Dohle G, Diemer T, Giwercman A, Jungwirth A, Kopa Z, Krausz C. Guidelines of male infertility. In: European Association of Urology. 2010. http://www.uroweb.org. Accessed on 13 Dec 2012.
5. Lipshultz L, Sigman M. Office evaluation of the subfertile male. In: Howards S, Lipshultz L, Niederberger C, editors. Infertility in the male. Cambridge: Cambridge University Press; 2009. p. 153–76.
6. Orth J, Jester W, Li L, Laslett A. Gonocyte-Sertoli cell interactions during development of the neonatal rodent testis. Curr Top Dev Biol. 2000;50:103.
7. Moffett D, Moffett S, Schauf C. Reproduction and its endocrine control. In: Moffett D, Moffett S, Schauf C, editors. Human physiology: foundations & frontiers. St. Louis: Mosby; 1993. p. 684–724.
8. Rajalakshmi M, Sharma R, Pal P. Structure and physiology of mammalian testis. In Kumar S, Tiwari R, editors. Environmental and occupational exposures. Reproductive impairment. New Delhi: Daya Publishing House; 2010. p. 1–44.
9. Mocarelli P, Gerthoux P, Patterson D, Milani S, Limonta G, Bertona M, et al. Dioxin exposure, from infancy through puberty, produces endocrine disruption and affects human semen quality. Environ Health Perspect. 2008;116(1):70–7.
10. Nef S, Parada L. Cryptorchidism in mice mutant for Insl3. Nat Genet. 1999;22:295–9.
11. Amann, R. The male rabbit. IV. Quantitative testicular histology and comparisons between daily sperm production as determined histologically and daily sperm output. Fertil Steril. 1970;21:662–72.
12. Zimmermann S, Steding G, Emmen J, Brinkmann A, Nayernia K, Holstein A, Engel W, Adham I. Targeted disruption of the Insl3 gene causes bilateral cryptorchidism. Mol Endocrinol. 1999;13:681–91.
13. Calzolari E, Contiero M, Roncarati E, Mattiuz P, Volpato S. Aetiological factors in hypospadias. J Med Genet. 1986;23(4):333–7.
14. Aitken R, Desai N, Ruffoli R, Carpi A. Lifestyle and testicular dysfunction: a brief update. Biomed Pharmacother. 2008;62(8):550–3.
15. Mann D, Gould K, Collins D, Wallen K. Blockade of neonatal activation of the pituitary-testicular axis: effect on prepubertal luteinizing hormone and testosterone secretion and on testicular development in male monkeys. J Clin Endocrinol Metab. 1989;68(3):600–7.
16. Storgaard L, Bonde J, Ernst E, Spano M, Andersen C, Frydenberg M, et al. Does smoking during pregnancy affect son's sperm counts? Epidemiol. 2003;14(3):278–86.
17. Jensen M, Mabeck L, Toft G, Thulstrup A, Bonde J. Lower sperm counts following prenatal tobacco exposure. Hum Reprod. 2005;20(9):2559–66.
18. Kizu R, Okamura K, Toriba A, Kakishima H, Mizokami A, Burnstein K, et al. A role of aryl hydrocarbon receptor in the antiandrogenic effects of polycylic aromatic hydrocarbons in LNCap human prostate carcinoma cells. Arch Toxicol. 2003;77(6):335–43.
19. Barnes-Ellerbe S, Knudsen K, Puga A. 2,3,7,8-Tetrachlorodibenzo-p-dioxin blocks androgen-dependent cell proliferation of LNCaP cells through modulation of pRB phosphorylation. Mol Pharmacol. 2004;66(3):502–11.
20. Brown-Woodman P, Post E, Gass G, White I. The effect of a single sauna exposure on spermatozoa. Arch Androl. 1984;12:9–15.
21. Rock J, Robinson D. Effect of induced intrascrotal hyperthermia on testicular function in man. Am J Obstet Gynecol. 1965;93:793–801.

22. Partsch C, Aukamp M, Sippell W. Scrotal temperature is increased in disposable plastic lined nappies. Arch Dis Child. 2000;83(4):364–8.
23. Thomas K, Colborn T. Organochlorine endocrine disruptors in human tissue. In: Colborn T, Ckement C, Herausgeber. Chemically-induced alterations in sexual and functional development: the wildlife/human connection. Adv Mod Environ Toxicol. 1992;21:365–94.
24. Sharpe R. The 'oestrogen hypothesis'—where do we stand now? Int J Androl. 2003;26(1):2–15.
25. Wu T, Huang B, Tsai H, Lui M, Liu M. Effects of nitric oxide on human spermatozoa activity, fertilization and mouse embryonic development. Arch Androl. 2004;50(3)173–9.
26. Guillette L, Gross T, Gross D, Rooney A, Percival H. Gonadal steroidogenesis in vitro from juvenile alligators obtained from contaminated or control lakes. Environ Health Persp. 1995;103(Suppl 4):31.
27. Wong W, Zielhuis G, Thomas C, Merkus H, Steegers-Theunissen R. New evidence of the influence of exogenous and endogenous factors on sperm count in man. Eur J Obset Gynecol Reprod Biol. 2003;110(1):49–54.
28. Olivia A, Spira A, Multigner L. Contribution of environmental factors to the risk of male infertility. Hum Reprod. 2001;16(8):1762–76.
29. Uzumcu M, Suzuki H, Skinner M. Effect of the anti-androgenic endocrine disruptor vinclozolin on embryonic testis cord formation and postnatal testis development and function. Reprod Toxicol. 2004;18(6):765–74.
30. Kovacic P. Mechanism of organophosphates (nerve gases and pesticides) and antidotes: electron transfer and oxidative stress. Curr Med Chem. 10:2705–10.
31. Chitra K, Sujatha R, Latchoumycandane C, Mathur P. Effect of lindane on antioxidant enzymes in epididymis and epididymal sperm of adult rats. Asian J Androl. 2001;3(3):205–8.
32. Latchoumycandane C, Chitra K, Mathur P. 2,3,7,8-Tetrachlorodibenzo-p-dioxin (TCDD) induces oxidative stress in the epididymis and epididymal sperm of adult rats. Arch Toxicol. 2003;77(5):280–4.
33. Latchoumycandane C, Mathur P. Induction of oxidative stress in the rat testis after short-term exposure to the organochlorine pesticide methoxychlor. Arch Toxicol. 2002;76(12):692–8.
34. Vaithinathan S, Saradha B, Mathur P. Transient inhibitory effect of methoxychlor on testicular steroidogenesis in rat: an in vivo study. Arch Toxicol. 2008;82(11):833–9.
35. Defamie N, Mograbi B, Roger C, Cronier L, Malassine A, Brucker-Davis F, et al. Disruption of gap junctional intercellular communication by lindane is associated with aberrant localization of connexin43 and zonula occludens-1 in 42GPA9 Sertoli cells. Carcinogen. 2001;22(9):1537–42.
36. Saradha B, Vaithinathan S, Mathur P. Single exposure to low dose of lindane causes transient decrease in testicular steroidogenesis in adult male Wistar rats. Toxicol. 2008;244(2–3):190–7.
37. Edelfors S, Hass U, Hougaard K. Changes in markers of oxidative stress and membrane properties in synaptosomes from rats exposed prenatally to toluene. Pharmacol Toxicol. 2002;90(1):26–31.
38. Nakai N, Murata M, Nagahama M, Hirase T, Tanaka M, Fujikawa T, et al. Oxidative DNA damage induced by toluene is involved in its male reproductive toxicity. Free Radic Res. 2003;37(1):69–76.
39. Xiao G, Pan C, Cai Y, Lin H, Fu Z. Effect of benzene, toluene, xylene on the semen quality of exposed workers. Chin Med J. 1999;112(8):709–12.
40. Chen Q, Vazquez E, Moghaddas S, Hoppel C, Lesnefsky EJ. Production of reactive oxygen species by mitochondria: central role of complex III. J Biol Chem. 2003;278(38):36027–31.
41. Adam-Vizi V. Production of reactive oxygen species in brain mitochondria: contribution by electron transport chain and non-electron transport chain sources. Antioxid Redox Signal. 2005;7(9–10):1140–9.
42. Hruska K, Furth P, Seifer D, Sharara F, Flaws J. Environmental factors in infertility. Clinical Obstet Gynaecol. 2000;43(4):821–9.
43. Andersen H, Schmidt I, Grandjean P, Jensen T, Budtz-Jorgensen E, Kjaerstad M, et al. Impaired reproductive development in sons of women occupationally exposed to pesticides during pregnancy. Environ Health Perspect. 2008;116(4):566–72.
44. Skinner M, Manikkam M, Guerrero-Bosagna C. Epigenetic transgenerational actions of environmental factors in disease etiology. Trends Endocrinol Metab. 2010;21(4):214–22.
45. Wu Q, Ohsako S, Ishimura R, Suzuki J, Tohyama C. Exposure of mouse preimplantation embryos to 2,3,7,8-tetrachlorodibenzo-p-dioxin (TCDD) alters the methylation status of imprinted genes H19 and Igf2. Biol Reprod. 2004;70(6):1790–7.
46. Waalkes M, Liu J, Chen H, Xie Y, Achanzar W, Zhou Y, et al. Estrogen signalling in livers of male mice with hepatocellular carcinoma induced by exposure to arsenic in utero. J Natl Cancer Inst. 2004;96(6):466–74.
47. Yaoi T, Itoh K, Nakamura K, Ogi H, Fujiwara Y, Fushiki S. Genome-wide analysis of epigenomic alterations in fetal mouse forebrain after exposure to low doses of bisphenol A. Biochem Biophys Res Commun. 2008;376(3):563–7.
48. Dolinoy D, Huang D, Jirtle R. Maternal nutrient supplementation counteracts bisphenol A-induced DNA hypomethylation in early development. Proc Natl Acad Sci U S A. 2007;104(32):13056–61.
49. Ho S, Tang W, Belmonte de Frausto J, Prins G. Developmental exposure to estradiol and bisphenol A increases susceptibility to prostate carcinogenesis and epigenetically regulates phosphodiesterase type 4 variant 4. Cancer Res. 2006;66(11):5624–32.
50. Guerrero-Bosagna C, Sabat P, Valdovinos F, Valladares L, Clark S. Epigenetic and phenotypic changes result from a continuous pre and post natal dietary exposure to phytoestrogens in an experimental population of mice. BMC Physiol. 2008;8:17.
51. Dolinoy D, Weidman J, Waterland R, Jirtle R. Maternal genistein alters coat color and protects Avy mouse offspring from obesity by modifying the fetal epigenome. Environ Health Perspect. 2006;114(4):567–72.
52. Anway M, Cupp A, Uzumcu M, Skinner M. Epigenetic transgenerational actions of endocrine disruptors and male fertility. Science. 2005;308(5727):1466–9.
53. Anway M, Rekow S, Skinner M. Transgenerational epigenetic programming of the embryonic testis transcriptome. Genomics. 2008;91(1):30–40.
54. Singh K, DuMond J. Genetic and epigenetic changes induced by chronic low dose exposure to arsenic of mouse testicular Leydig cells. Int J Oncol. 2007;30(1):253–60.
55. Kunzle R, Mueller M, Hanggi W, Birkhauser M, Drescher H, Bersinger N. Semen quality of male smokers and nonsmokers in infertile couples. Fertil Steril. 2003;79(2):287–91.
56. Saleh R, Agarwal A, Sharma R, Nelson D, Thomas A. Effect of cigarette smoking on levels of seminal oxidative stress in infertile men: a prospective study. Fertil Steril. 2002;78(3):491–9.
57. Vine M, Tse C, Hu P, Truong K. Cigarette smoking and semen quality. Fertil Steril. 1996;65(4):835–42.
58. Saleh R, Agarwal A. Oxidative stress and male infertility: from research bench to clinical practice. J Androl. 2002;23(6):737–52.
59. Richthoff J, Elzanaty S, Rylander L, Hagmar L, Giwercman A. Association between tobacco exposure and reproductive parameters in adolescent males. Int J Androl. 2008;31(1):31–9.
60. Mostafa T, Anis T, El-Nashar A, Imam H, Othman I. Varicocelectomy reduces reactive oxygen species levels and increases antioxidant activity of seminal plasma from infertile men with varicocele. Int J Androl. 2001;24(5):261–5.
61. Fraga C, Motchnik P, Wyrobek A, Rempel D, Ames B. Smoking and low antioxidant levels increase oxidative damage to sperm DNA. Mutat Res. 1996;351(2):199–203.
62. Gaur D, Talekar M, Pathak V. Effect of cigarette smoking on semen quality of infertile men. Singapore Med J. 2007;48(2):119–23.

63. Fukuda M, Fukuda K, Shimizu T, Andersen C, Byskov A. Parental peri-conceptional smoking and male: female ratio of newborn infants. Lancet. 2002;359:1407–8.
64. Patterson T, Stringham J, Meikle A. Nicotine and cotinine inhibit steroidogenesis in mouse Leydig cells. Life Sci. 1990;46:265–72.
65. Zgliczynski J, Ossowski M, Slowinska S, Brzezinska A, Zgliczynski W, Soszynski P, et al. Effect of testosterone replacement therapy on lipids and lipoproteins in hypogonadal and elderly men. Atherosclerosis. 1996;121(1):35–43.
66. Yamamoto Y, Isoyama E, Sofikitis N, Miyagawa I. Effects of smoking on testicular function and fertilizing potential in rats. Urol Res. 1998;26:45–8.
67. Rosen M, Greenfield A, Walker T, Grant P, Dubrow J, Bettmann M, et al. Cigarette smoking: an independent risk factor for atherosclerosis in the hypogastric-cavernous arterial bed of men with arteriogenic impotence. J Urol. 1991;145(1):759–63.
68. Du Plessis S Cabler S McAlister D Sabanegh E Agarwal A. The effect of obesity on sperm disorders and male infertility. Nat Rev Urol. 2010;7(3):153–61.
69. Song G, Norkus E, Lewis V. Relationship between seminal ascorbic acid and sperm DNA integrity in infertile men. Int J Androl. 2006;29(6):569–75.
70. Eskenazi B, Kidd S, Marks A, Sloter E, Block G, Wyrobek A. Antioxidant intake is associated with semen quality in healthy men. Hum Reprod. 2005;20(4):1006–12.
71. Therond P, Auger J, Legrand A, Jouannet P. Alpha-Tocopherol in human spermatozoa and seminal plasma: relationships with motility, antioxidant enzymes and leukocytes. Mol Hum Reprod. 1996;2(10):739–44.
72. Fraga C, Motchnik P, Shigenaga M, Helbock H, Jacob R, Ames B. Ascorbic acid protects against endogenous oxidative DNA damage in human sperm. Proc Natl Acad Sci U S A. 1991;88(24):11003–6.
73. Hawkes W, Turek P. Effects of dietary selenium on sperm motility in healthy men. J Androl. 2001;22(5):764–72.
74. Hammoud A, Gibson M, Peterson C, Hamilton B, Carrell D. Obesity and male reproductive potential. J Androl. 2006;27(5):619–26.
75. Nielsen T, Hagen C, Wraae K, Brixen K, Petersen P, Haug E, et al. Visceral and subcutaneous adipose tissue assessed by magnetic resonance imaging in relation to circulating androgens, sex hormone-binding globulin, and luteinizing hormone in young men. J Clin Endocrinol Metab. 2007;92(7):2696–705.
76. Fejes I, Koloszar S, Zavaczki Z, Daru J, Szollosi J, Pal A. Effect of body weight on testosterone/estradiol ratio in oligozoospermic patients. Arch Androl. 2006;52(2):97–102.
77. Kort H, Massey J, Elsner C, Mitchell-Leef D, Shapiro D, Witt M, et al. Impact of body mass index values on sperm quantity and quality. J Androl. 2006;27(3):450–2.
78. Nguyen R, Wilcox A, Skjaerven R, Baird D. Men's body mass index and infertility. Hum Reprod. 2007;22(9):2488–93.
79. Koloszar S, Fejes I, Zavaczki Z, Daru J, Szollosi J, Pal A. Effect of body weight on sperm concentration in normozoospermic males. Arch Androl. 2005;51(4):299–304.
80. Cabler S, Agarwal A, Flint M, Du Plessis S. Obesity: modern man's fertility nemesis. Asian J Androl. 2010;12(4):480–9.
81. Shafik A, Olfat S. Scrotal lipomatosis. Br J Urol. 1981;53(1):50–4.
82. Mohamed-Ali V, Goodrick S, Rawesh A, Katz D, Miles J, Yudkin J, Coppack S. Human subcutaneous adipose tissue secretes interleukin-6, but not tumor necrosis factor-alpha, in vivo. J Clin Endocrinol Metab.1997;82:4196–200.
83. Davì G, Guagnano M, Ciabattoni G, Basili S, Falco A, Marinopiccoli M, Patrono C. Platelet activation in obese women. J Am Med Assoc. 2002;288(16):2008–14.
84. Kodama H, Yamaguchi R, Fukuda J, Kasai H, Tanaka T. Increased oxidative deoxyribonucleic acid damage in the spermatozoa of infertile male patients. Fertil Steril. 1997;68(3):519–24.
85. Twigg J, Fulton N, Gomez E, Irvine DS, Aitken RJ. Analysis of the impact of intracellular reactive oxygen species generation on the structural and functional integrity of human spermatozoa: lipid peroxidation, DNA fragmentation and effectiveness of antioxidants. Hum Reprod. 1998;13(6):1429–36.
86. Selmanoglu G, Barlas N, Songur S, Kockaya EA. Carbendazim-induced haematological, biochemical and histopathological changes to the liver and kidney of male rats. Hum Exp Toxicol. 2001;20(12):625–30.
87. Carter S, Hess R, Laskey J. The fungicide methyl 2-benzimidazole carbamate causes infertility in male Sprague-Dawley rats. Biol Reprod. 1987;37(3):709–17.
88. Akbarsha M, Kadalmani B, Girija R, Faridha A, Hamid K. Spermatotoxic effect of carbendazim. Indian J Exp Biol. 2001;39(9):921–4.
89. Rajeswary S, Kumaran B, Ilangovan R, Yuvaraj S, Sridhar M, Venkataraman P, Aruldhas M. Modulation of antioxidant defense system by the environmental fungicide carbendazim in Leydig cells of rats. Reprod Toxicol. 2007;24(3–4):371–80.
90. Prusakiewicz J, Harville H, Zhang Y, Ackermann C, Voorman R. Parabens inhibit human skin estrogen sulfotransferase activity: possible link to paraben estrogenic effects. Toxicology. 2007;232(3):248–56.
91. Chitra K, Mathur P. Vitamin E prevents nonylphenol-induced oxidative stress in testis of rats. Indian J Exp Biol. 2004;42(2):220–3.
92. Moutsatsou P. The spectrum of phytoestrogens in nature: our knowledge is expanding. Horm. 2007;6(3):173–93.
93. Martini A, Molina R, Estofan D, Senestrari D, Fiol de Cuneo M, Ruiz R. Effects of alcohol and cigarette consumption on human seminal quality. Fertil Steril. 2004;82(2):374–7.
94. Villalta J, Ballesca J, Nicolas J, Martinez de Osaba M, Antunez E, Pimentel C. Testicular function in asymptomatic chronic alcoholics: relation to ethanol intake. Alcohol Clin Exp Res. 1997;21(1): 128–33.
95. Boyden T, Pamenter R. Effects of ethanol on the male hypothalamic-pituitary-gonadal axis. Endocr Rev Fall. 1983;4(4):389–95.
96. Muthusami K, Chinnaswamy P. Effect of chronic alcoholism on male fertility hormones and semen quality. Fertil Steril. 2005;84(4):919–24.
97. Goverde H, Dekker H, Janssen H, Bastiaans B, Rolland R, Zielhuis G. Semen quality and frequency of smoking and alcohol consumption—an explorative study. Int J Fertil Menopausal Stud. 1995;40(3):135–8.
98. Maneesh M, Dutta S, Chakrabarti A, Vasudevan D. Alcohol abuse-duration dependent decrease in plasma testosterone and antioxidants in males. Indian J Physiol Pharmacol. 2006;50(3):291–6.
99. Dahchour A, Lallemand F, Ward R, De Witte P. Production of reactive oxygen species following acute ethanol or acetaldehyde and its reduction by acamprosate in chronically alcoholized rats. Eur J Pharmacol. 2005;520(1–3):51–8.
100. Crémoux P. Aromatase inhibitors: pharmacological aspects. Bulletin Cancer. 2000;87(1):23–30.
101. Sharpe RM. Natural and anthropogenic environmental oestrogens: the scientific basis for risk assessment—Environmental oestrogens and male infertility. Pure App Chem. 1998;70(1):1685–701.
102. Stopczyk D, Gnitecki W, Buczynski A, Kowalski W, Buczynska M, Kroc A. Effect of electromagnetic field produced by mobile phones on the activity of superoxide dismutase (SOD-1)—in vitro researches. Ann Acad Med Stetin. 2005;51(Suppl 1):125–8.
103. Agarwal A, Deepinder F, Sharma R, Ranga G, Li J. Effect of cell phone usage on semen analysis in men attending infertility clinic: an observational study. Fertil Steril. 2008;89(1):124–8.
104. Kilgallon S, Simmons L. Image content influences men's semen quality. Biol Lett. 2005;1(3):253–5.
105. Fejes I, Zavaczki Z, Szollosi J, Koloszar S, Daru J, Kovacs L, et al. Is there a relationship between cell phone use and semen quality? Arch Androl. 2005;51(5):385–93.
106. Baste V, Riise T, Moen BE. Radiofrequency electromagnetic fields; male infertility and sex ratio of offspring. Eur J Epidemiol. 2008;23(5):369–77.

107. Agarwal A, Desai N, Makker K, Varghese A, Mouradi R, Sabanegh E, et al. Effects of radiofrequency electromagnetic waves (RF-EMW) from cellular phones on human ejaculated semen: an in vitro pilot study. Fertil Steril. 2009;92(4):1318–25.
108. Friedman J, Kraus S, Hauptman Y, Schiff Y, Seger R. Mechanism of short-term ERK activation by electromagnetic fields at mobile phone frequencies. Biochem J. 2007;405(3):559–68.
109. Burch J, Reif J, Yost M, Keefe T, Pitrat C. Nocturnal excretion of a urinary melatonin metabolite among electric utility workers. Scand J Work Environ Health. 1998;24(3):183–9.
110. Ozguner M, Koyu A, Cesur G, Ural M, Ozguner F, Gokcimen A, et al. Biological and morphological effects on the reproductive organ of rats after exposure to electromagnetic field. Saudi Med J. 2005;26(3):405–10.
111. Lahdetie J. Occupation- and exposure-related studies on human sperm. J Occup Environ Med. 1995;37(8):922–30.
112. Ash P. The influence of radiation on fertility in man. Br J Radiol. 1980;53(628):271–8.
113. Clifton D, Bremner W. The effect of testicular x-irradiation on spermatogenesis in man. A comparison with the mouse. J Androl. 1983;4(6):387–92.
114. Popescu H, Lancranjan I. Spermatogenesis alterations during protracted irradiation in man. Health Phys. 1975;28(5):567–73.
115. Cheburakov I, Cheburakova O. Disorders of spermatogenesis in people working at the clean-up of the Chernobyl nuclear power plant accident. Radiats Biol Radioecol. 1993;33(6):771–4.
116. Avendano C, Mata A, Sarmiento C, Doncel G. Use of laptop computers connected to internet through Wi-Fi decreases human sperm motility and increases sperm DNA fragmentation. Fertil Steril. 2012;97(1):39–45.
117. Yaeram J, Setchell B, Maddocks S. Effect of heat stress on the fertility of male mice in vivo and in vitro. Reprod Fertil Dev. 2006;18:647–53.
118. Werdelin L, Nilsonne A. The evolution of the scrotum and testicular descent in mammals: a phylogenetic view. J Theor Biol. 1999;196(1):61–72.
119. Ali J, Weaver D, Weinstein S, Grimes E. Scrotal temperature and semen quality in men with and without varicocele. Arch Androl. 1990;24:215–9.
120. Thonneau P, Ducot B, Bujan L, Mieusset R, Spira A. Effect of male occupational heat exposure on time to pregnancy. Int J Androl. 1997;20(5):274–8.
121. Brun B, Clavert A. Modifications morphologiques de l'acrosome chez un homme exposé Ã la chaleur. J Gyn Obstet Reprod. 1977;6:907–8.
122. Bonde J. Semen quality in welders exposed to radiant heat. Br J Ind Med. 1992;49(1):5–10.
123. Mur J, Wild P, Rapp R, Vautrin J, Coulon J. Demographic evaluation of the fertility of aluminium industry workers: influence of exposure to heat and static magnetic fields. Hum Reprod. 1998;13(7):2016–9.
124. Figa-Talamanca I, Dell'Orco V, Pupi A, Dondero F, Gandini L, Lenzi A, et al. Fertility and semen quality of workers exposed to high temperatures in the ceramics industry. Reprod Toxicol.1992;6(6):517–23.
125. Hjollund N, Bonde J, Jensen T, Olsen J. Diurnal scrotal skin temperature and semen quality. The Danish first pregnancy planner study team. Int J Androl. 2000;23(5):309–18.
126. Hjollund N, Storgaard L, Ernst E, Bonde J, Olsen J. The relation between daily activities and scrotal temperature. Reprod Toxicol. 2002;16(3):209–14.
127. Magnusdottir E, Thorsteinsson T, Thorsteinsdottir S, Heimisdottir M, Olafsdottir K. Persistent organochlorines, sedentary occupation, obesity and human male subfertility. Hum Reprod. 2005;20(1):208–15.
128. Sas M, Szollosi J. Impaired spermiogenesis as a common finding among professional drivers. Arch Androl. 1979;3(1):57–60.
129. Rubben H, Recker F, Lutzeyer W. Exogene warm Exposure—eine Ursahe der Subfertilitat. Urologe. 1988;25:67–68.
130. Yamaguchi M, Sakatoku J, Takihara H. The application of intrascrotal deep body temperature measurement for the noninvasive diagnosis of varicoceles. Fertil Steril. 1989;52(2):295–301.
131. Jockenhovel F, Grawe A, Nieschlag E. A portable digital data recorder for long-term monitoring of scrotal temperatures. Fertil Steril. 1990;54(4):694–700.
132. Parazzini F, Marchini M, Luchini L, Tozzi L, Mezzopane R, Fedele L. Tight underpants and trousers and risk of dyspermia. Int J Androl. 1995;18(3):137–40.
133. Oldereid N, Rui H, Purvis K. Life styles of men in barren couples and their relationship to sperm quality. Int J Fertil. 1992;37:343–9.
134. Jung A, Leonhardt F, Schill W, Schuppe H. Influence of the type of undertrousers and physical activity on scrotal temperature. Hum Reprod. 2005;20(4):1022–7.
135. Procope B. Effect of repeated increase of body temperature on human sperm cells. Int J Fertil. 1965;10(4):333–9.
136. Brown-Woodman P, Post E, Gass G, White I. The effect of a single sauna exposure on spermatozoa. Arch Androl. 1984;12(1):9–15.
137. Setchell B. The Parkes Lecture. Heat and the testis. J Reprod Fertil. 1998;114(2):179–94.
138. Jung A, Schuppe H, Schill W. Fever as etiology of temporary infertility in the man. Hautarzt. 2001;52(12):1090–3.
139. Carlsen E, Andersson A, Petersen J, Skakkebaek N. History of febrile illness and variation in semen quality. Hum Reprod. 2003;18(10):2089–92.
140. Evenson D, Jost L, Corzett M, Balhorn R. Characteristics of human sperm chromatin structure following an episode of influenza and high fever: a case study. J Androl. 2000;21(5):739–46.
141. Eskiocak S, Gozen A, Kilic A, Molla S. Association between mental stress & some antioxidant enzymes of seminal plasma. Indian J Med Res. 2005;122(6):491–6.
142. Eskiocak S, Gozen A, Yapar S, Tavas F, Kilic A, Eskiocak M. Glutathione and free sulphydryl content of seminal plasma in healthy medical students during and after exam stress. Hum Reprod. 2005;20(9):2595–600.
143. Eskiocak S, Gozen A, Taskiran A, Kilic A, Eskiocak M, Gulen S. Effect of psychological stress on the L-arginine-nitric oxide pathway and semen quality. Braz J Med Biol Res. 2006;39(5):581–8.
144. Fenster L, Katz D, Wyrobek A, Pieper C, Rempel D, Oman D, Swan S. Effects of psychological stress on human semen quality. J Androl. 1997;18:194–202.
145. Monder C, Miroff Y, Marandici A, Hardy MP. 11 beta-Hydroxysteroid dehydrogenase alleviates glucocorticoid- mediated inhibition of steroidogenesis in rat Leydig cells. Endocrinology. 1994;134(3):1199–204.
146. Ruffoli R, Carpi A, Giambelluca M, Grasso L, Scavuzzo M, Giannessi F. Diazepam administration prevents testosterone decrease and lipofuscin accumulation in testis of mouse exposed to chronic noise stress. Andrologia. 2006;38(5):159–65.
147. Terman A, Brunk U. Lipofuscin. Int J Biochem Cell Biol. 2004;36(8):1400–4.
148. Gao H, Tong M, Hu Y, You H, Guo Q, Ge R, et al. Mechanisms of glucocorticoid-induced Leydig cell apoptosis. Mol Cell Endocrinol. 2003;199(1–2):153–63.
149. Kobeissi L, Inhorn M, Hannoun A, Hammoud N, Awwad J, Abu-Musa A. Civil war and male infertility in Lebanon. Fertil Steril. 2008;90(2):340–5.
150. Abu-Musa A, Nassar A, Hannoun A, Usta I. Effect of the Lebanese civil war on sperm parameters. Fertil Steril. 2007;88(6):1579–82.
151. de Krester D. Declining sperm counts. Environmental chemicals may be to blame. Brit Med J. 1996;312:458–547.
152. Swan S, Liu F, Overstreet J, Brazil C, Skakkebaek N. Semen quality of fertile US males in relation to their mother's beef consumption during pregnancy. Hum Reprod. 2007;22(6):1497–502.

153. Le H, Carlson E, Chua J, Belcher S. Bisphenol A is released from polycarbonate drinking bottles and mimics the neurotoxic actions of estrogen in developing cerebellar neurons. Toxicol Lett. 2008;176(2):149–56.
154. Korasli D, Ziraman F, Ozyurt P, Cehreli S. Microleakage of self-etch primer/adhesives in endodontically treated teeth. J Am Dent Assoc. 2007;138(5):634–40.
155. Chitra K, Latchoumycandane C, Mathur P. Induction of oxidative stress by bisphenol A in the epididymal sperm of rats. Toxicology. 2003;185(1–2):119–27.
156. Kabuto H, Amakawa M, Shishibori T. Exposure to bisphenol A during embryonic/fetal life and infancy increases oxidative injury and causes underdevelopment of the brain and testis in mice. Life Sci. 2004;74(24):2931–40.
157. Obata T, Kubota S. Formation of hydroxy radicals by environmental estrogen-like chemicals in rat striatum. Neurosci Lett. 2000;296(1):41–4.
158. Gesler R. Toxicology of di-2-ethylhexyl phthalate and other phthalic acid ester plasticizers. Environ Health Perspect. 1973;3:73–9.
159. Peakall D. Phthalate esters: occurrence and biological effects. Residue Rev. 1975;54:1–41.
160. Ishihara M, Itoh M, Miyamoto K, Suna S, Takeuchi Y, Takenaka I, et al. Spermatogenic disturbance induced by di-(2-ethylhexyl) phthalate is significantly prevented by treatment with antioxidant vitamins in the rat. Int J Androl. 2000;23(2):85–94.
161. Lee E, Ahn M, Kim H, Kim I, Han S, Kang T, et al. Effect of di(n-butyl) phthalate on testicular oxidative damage and antioxidant enzymes in hyperthyroid rats. Environ Toxicol. 2007;22(3):245–55.
162. Kasahara E, Sato E, Miyoshi M, Konaka R, Hiramoto K, Sasaki J, et al. Role of oxidative stress in germ cell apoptosis induced by di (2-ethylhexyl)phthalate. Biochem J. 2002;365(Pt 3):849–56.
163. Park J, Habeebu S, Klaassen C. Testicular toxicity of di-(2-ethylhexyl)phthalate in young Sprague-Dawley rats. Toxicol. 2002;171(2–3):105–15.
164. Hayashi K, Nakae A, Fukushima Y, Sakamoto K, Furuichi T, Kitahara K, et al. Contamination of rice by etofenprox, diethyl phthalate and alkylphenols: effects on first delivery and sperm count in mice. J Toxicol Sci. 2010;35(1):49–55.
165. Hsu P, Liu M, Hsu C, Chen L, Guo Y. Lead exposure causes generation of reactive oxygen species and functional impairment in rat sperm. Toxicology. 1997;122:133–43.
166. Acharya U, Acharya S, Mishra M. Lead acetate induced cytotoxicity in male germinal cells of Swiss mice. Ind Health. 2003;41(3):291–4.
167. Xu D, Shen H, Zhu Q, Chua L, Wang Q, Chia S, et al. The associations among semen quality, oxidative DNA damage in human spermatozoa and concentrations of cadmium, lead and selenium in seminal plasma. Mutat Res. 2003;534(1–2):155–63.
168. Naha N, Chowdhury A. Inorganic lead exposure in battery and paint factory: effect on human sperm structure and functional activity. J UOEH. 2006;28(2):157–71.
169. Courtois E, Marques M, Barrientos A. Lead-induced down-regulation of soluble guanylate cyclase in isolated rat aortic segments mediated by reactive oxygen species and cyclo-oxygenase-2. J Am Soc Nephrol. 2003;14:1464–70.
170. Ercal N, Neal R, Treeratphan P, Lutz P, Hammond T, Dennery P, Spitz D. A role for oxidative stress in suppressing serum immunoglobulin levels in lead-exposed Fisher 344 rats. Arch Environ Contam Toxicol. 2000;39:251–6.
171. Farmand F, Ehdaie A, Roberts C, Sindhu R. Lead-induced dysregulation of superoxide dismutase, catalase, glutathione peroxidase, and guanylate cyclase. Environ Res. 2005;98:33–9.
172. Gunnarsson D, Svensson M, Selstam G, Nordberg G. Pronounced induction of testicular PGF(2 alpha) and suppression of testosterone by cadmium-prevention by zinc. Toxicology. 2004;200(1):49–58.
173. Yang J, Arnush M, Chen Q, Wu X, Pang B, Jiang X. Cadmium-induced damage to primary cultures of rat Leydig cells. Reprod Toxicol. 2003;17(5):553–60.
174. Benoff S, Auborn K, Marmar J, Hurley I. Link between low-dose environmentally relevant cadmium exposures and asthenozoospermia in a rat model. Fertil Steril. 2008;89(Suppl 2):e73–9.
175. Agency for Toxic Substances and Disease Registry (ATSDR). Cadmium toxicity—case studies in environmental medicine. Atlanta: U.S. Department of Health and Human Services; 2008.
176. Yuyan L, Junqing W, Wei Y, Weijin Z, Ersheng G. Are serum zinc and copper levels related to semen quality? Fertil Steril. 2008;89(4):1008–11.
177. Shalet S. Effects of cancer chemotherapy on gonadal function of patients. Cancer Treat Rev. 1980;7(3):141–52.
178. Schlegel P, Chang T, Marshall F. Antibiotics: potential hazards to male fertility. Fertil Steril. 1991;55(2):235–42.
179. Ericsson R, Baker V. Binding of tetracycline to mammalian spermatozoa. Nature. 1967;214(5086):403–4.
180. O'Morain C, Smethurst P, Dore C, Levi A. Reversible male infertility due to sulphasalazine: studies in man and rat. Gut. 1984;25(10):1078–84.
181. Hayashi T, Miyata A, Yamada T. The impact of commonly prescribed drugs on male fertility. Hum Fertil. 2008;11(3):191–6.
182. Sikka S, Wang R. Endocrine disruptors and estrogenic effects on male reproductive axis. Asian J Androl. 2008;10(1):134–45.
183. Chiba K, Yamaguchi K, Li F, Ando M, Fujisawa M. Finasteride-associated male infertility. Fertil Steril. 2011;95(5):1786e9–11.
184. Rubin J, Ferencz C, Loffredo C. Use of prescription and non-prescription drugs in pregnancy. J Clin Epidem. 1993;46(6):581–9.
185. Bellis M, Hughes K, Calafat A, Juan M, Ramon A, Rodriguez J, Phillips-Howard P. Sexual uses of alcohol and drugs and the associated health risks: a cross sectional study of young people in nine European cities. BMC Public Health. 2009;8(1):155.
186. Knuth UA, Maniera H, Nieschlag E. Anabolic steroids and semen parameters in bodybuilders. Fertil Steril. 1989;52(6):1041–7.
187. Sahakyan M, Harlow L, Hornstein M. Influence of age, diagnosis, and cycle number on pregnancy rates with gonadotropin-induced controlled ovarian hyperstimulation and intrauterine insemination. Fertil Steril. 1999;72:500–4.
188. Sklar C, Kaplan S, Grumbach M. Evidence for dissociation between adrenarche and gonadarche: studies in patients with idiopathic precocious puberty, gonadal dysgenesis, isolated gonadotropin deficiency, and constitutionally delayed growth and adolescence. J Clin Endocrinol Metab. 1980;51(3):548–56.
189. Whorton D, Milby T, Krauss R, Stubbs H. Testicular function in DBCP exposed pesticide workers. J Occup Environ Med. 1979;21(3):161–6.
190. De Iuliis G Thomson L Mitchell L Finnie J Koppers A Hedges A Nixon B Aitken R. DNA damage in human spermatozoa is highly correlated with the efficiency of chromatin remodelling and the formation of 8-hydroxy-2'-deoxyguanosine, a marker of oxidative stress. Biol Reprod. 2009b;81:517–24.
191. Chabory E, Damon C, Lenoir A, Kauselmann G, Kern H, Zevnik B, et al. Epididymis seleno-independent glutathione peroxidase 5 maintains sperm DNA integrity in mice. J Clin Invest. 2009;119:2074–85.
192. Bhardwaj A, Verma A, Majumdar S, Khanduja K. Status of vitamin E and reduced glutathione in semen of oligozoospermic and azoospermic patients. Asian J Androl. 2000;2(3):225–8.
193. Ochseedorf F, Buhl R, Bästlein A, Beschmann H. Glutathione le spermatozoa and seminal plasma of infertile men. Hum Reprod. 2008;13(2):353–9.
194. Ota H, Igarashi S, Kato N, Tanaka T. Aberrant expression of glutathione peroxidase in eutopic and ectopic endometrium in endometriosis and adenomyosis. Fertil Steril. 2000;74:313–8.
195. Ursini F, Heim S, Kiess M, Maiorino M, Roveri A, Wissing J, et al. Dual function of the selenoprotein PHGPx during sperm maturation. Science. 1999;285(5432):1393–6.

196. Noack-Füller G, Beer C, Seibert H. Cadmium, lead, selenium, and zinc in semen of occupationally unexposed men. Andrologia. 1993;25(1):7–12.
197. Lenzi A, Picardo M, Gandini L, Lombardo F, Terminali O, Passi S, Dondero F. Glutathione treatment of dyspermia: effect on the lipoperoxidation process. Hum Reprod. 1994;9:2044–50.
198. Lenzi A, Culasso F, Gandini L, Lombardo F, Dondero F. Placebo controlled, double-blind, cross-over trial of glutathione therapy in male infertility. Hum Reprod. 1993;8:1657–62.
199. Balercia G, Mosca F, Mantero F, Boscaro M, Mancini A, Ricciardo- Lamonica G, et al. Coenzyme Q(10) supplementation in infertile men with idiopathic asthenozoospermia: an open, uncontrolled pilot study. Fertil Steril. 2004;81(1):93–8.
200. Suzuki M, Kurabayashi T, Yamamoto Y, Fujita K, Tanaka K. Effects of antioxidant treatment in oligozoospermic and asthenozoospermic men. J Reprod Med. 2006;48(9):707–12.
201. Henmi H, Endo T, Kitajima Y, Manase K, Hata H, Kudo R. Effects of ascorbic acid supplementation on serum progesterone levels in patients with a luteal phase defect. Fertil Steril. 2003;80(2):459–61.
202. Zuskin E, Lewis A, Bouhuys A. Inhibition of histamine induced airway constriction by ascorbic acid. J Allergy Clin Immunol. 1973;51:218–26.
203. Crha I, Hruba D, Ventruba P, Fiala J, Totusek J, Visnova H. Ascorbic acid and infertility treatment. Cent Eur J Public Health. 2003;11(2):63–7.
204. Wong W, Merkus H, Thomas C, Menkveld R, Zielhuis G, Steegers-Theunissen R. Effects of folic acid and zinc sulfate on male factor subfertility: a double-blind, randomized, placebo-controlled trial. Fertil Steril. 2002;77(3):491–8.
205. Kaliszuk S, Borzecki Z, Swies Z. The influence of bromocriptine on sexual activity in ethanol-exposed male rats. Annales Universitatis Mariae Curie-Sklodowska Sectio D Med. 1989;44:109–14.
206. Rosen M, Greenfield A, Walker T, Grant P, Dubrow J, Bettmann M, et al. Cigarette smoking: an independent risk factor for atherosclerosis in the hypogastric-cavernous arterial bed of men with arteriogenic impotence. J Urol. 1991;145(1):759–63.
207. Mancini A, Conte G, Milardi D, Marinis L, Littarru G. Relationship between sperm cell ubiquinone and seminal parameters in subjects with and without varicocele. Androl. 1998;30(1):1–4.
208. Alleva R, Tomasetti M, Battino M, Curatola G, Littarru G, Folkers K. The roles of coenzyme Q10 and vitamin E on the peroxidation of human low density lipoprotein subfractions. Proc Nat Acad Sc U S A. 1995;92(20):9388–91.
209. Mancini A, De Marinis L, Oradei A, Hallgass M, Conte G, Pozza D, Dittarru G. Coenzyme Q10 concentrations in normal and pathological human seminal fluid. J Androl. 1994;15(6):591.
210. Kelso K, Redpath A, Noble R, Speake B. Lipid and antioxidant changes in spermatozoa and seminal plasma throughout the reproductive period of bulls. J Reprod Fertil. 1997;109(1):1–6.
211. Balercia G, Arnaldi G, Fazioli F, Serresi M, Alleva R, Mancini A, et al. Coenzyme Q10 levels in idiopathic and varicocele-associated asthenozoospermia. Andrologia. 2002;34(2):107–11.
212. Balercia G, Regoli F, Armeni T, Koverech A, Mantero F, Boscaro M. Placebo-controlled double-blind randomized trial on the use of L-carnitine, L-acetylcarnitine, or combined L-carnitine and L-acetylcarnitine in men with idiopathic asthenozoospermia. Fertil Steril. 2005;84(3):662–71.
213. Bendich A. Role of antioxidants in the maintenance of immune functions. In Frei B, editor. Natural antioxidants in human health and disease. San Diego: Academic; 1994. p. 447–467.
214. Esteves S, Zini A, Aziz N, Alvarez J, Sabanegh E, Agarwal A. Critical appraisal of World Health Organization's new reference values for human semen characteristics and effect on diagnosis and treatment of subfertile men. Urol. 2011;79(1):16–22.
215. Cooper T, Noonan E, Von Eckardstein S, Auger J, Baker H, Behre H, et al. World Health Organization reference values for human semen characteristics. Hum Reprod Update. 2010;16(3):231–45.
216. World Health Organization. WHO laboratory manual for the examination of human semen and sperm-cervical mucus interaction. 2nd ed. Cambridge: Cambridge University Press; 1987.
217. World Health Organization. WHO laboratory manual for the examination and processing of human semen. 5th ed. Geneva: WHO Press; 2010.
218. World Health Organization. WHO laboratory manual for the examination of human semen and sperm-cervical mucus interaction. 4th ed. Cambridge: Cambridge University Press; 1999.
219. Sharpe R. Lifestyle and environmental contribution to male infertility. Br Med Bull. 2000;56(3):630–42.

Part III
Pathophysiology: Female

Potential Etiologies of Unexplained Infertility in Females

13

Daniela Galliano and Antonio Pellicer

Introduction

Infertility is defined as a failure to conceive after an interval of approximately 12 months of regular and unprotected intercourse [1]. An estimated 4–17% of couples seek medical treatment to resolve their infertility, but it is generally accepted that there are more cases unreported [2]. Therefore, infertility remains both prevalent and problematic among couples worldwide [3].

Unexplained infertility (UI) is said to be unexplained when a couple fails to conceive after 12 months of regular and unprotected intercourse and in the absence of any identified abnormalities with an incidence of approximately 15–30% [1, 4, 5]. This incidence may vary depending on the population studied and the criteria used to make the diagnosis. UI has no identified pathophysiologic basis and, as such, is a diagnosis of exclusion that should be made after a thorough but time-efficient investigation of the couple is performed, [6] including a semen analysis, assessment of ovulation, evaluation of tubal patency by hysterosalpingogram (HSG), or laparoscopy (LPS) [7] and, if indicated, tests for ovarian reserve.

UI may be a multifactorial disorder of reproduction [8] and if so, it is unlikely that all the etiologies involved could be diagnosed even after a meticulous evaluation [9], with many suspected etiologies without definitive diagnostic methods or criteria. However, significant improvements in diagnostic tools and assisted reproductive technology (ART) treatments have led to the finding of many causes of infertility that in the past have only been suspected, but now are well known. Poor embryo development and quality may be identified in the ART lab or if further testing is performed, chromosomal aneuploidies may be revealed by preimplantation genetic screening (PGS).

On these grounds, the validity of the term "unexplained infertility" has been doubted by some authors and they propose to substitute the term "unexplained" with "undiagnosed" [10], since UI seems to be sensitive to the number and quality of the tests performed. Indeed, data from a study by Taylor and Collins showed that the percentage of couple with UI decreases as the number of diagnostic tests increases, from 22% in studies published prior to 1960 to 14% in studies published after 1980 [11]. Additionally, the difference in diagnosis may be related to the duration of infertility prior to seeking treatment (which may have been longer in the earlier studies as there was little intervention possible), and just on the number of diagnostic tests used.

Nonetheless, despite improvements in the diagnosis and treatment of reproductive disorders, at the present time many couples still have no explanation for their infertility [12], as posed by Southam in 1960 [13].

UI should not be regarded as a permanent condition but rather a relative incapacity to conceive, and as such, it would be better considered as subfertility [1], since time may lead these couples to achieve pregnancy without treatment. In fact, it has been estimated that approximately 40–60% of couples with UI will spontaneously conceive within 3 years [14], with the duration of infertility and the age of the female partner being the most important prognostic factors [15]. Furthermore, the outcomes of ART treatment for idiopathic infertility are promising [6–8, 16].

Possible Etiologies of UI in Females

As far as is known and after a thorough evaluation, the etiologies below appear to be potential causes of UI. These include ovarian, tuboperitoneal, uterine, and embryonic factors (Fig. 13.1).

D. Galliano (✉) · A. Pellicer
Department of Reproduction, Instituto Valenciano Iinfertilidad (IVI), Ronda General Mitre (Pza. Belianes), 14, 08017 Barcelona, Spain
e-mail: Daniela.Galliano@ivi.es

G. L. Schattman et al. (eds.), *Unexplained Infertility,* DOI 10.1007/978-1-4939-2140-9_13,

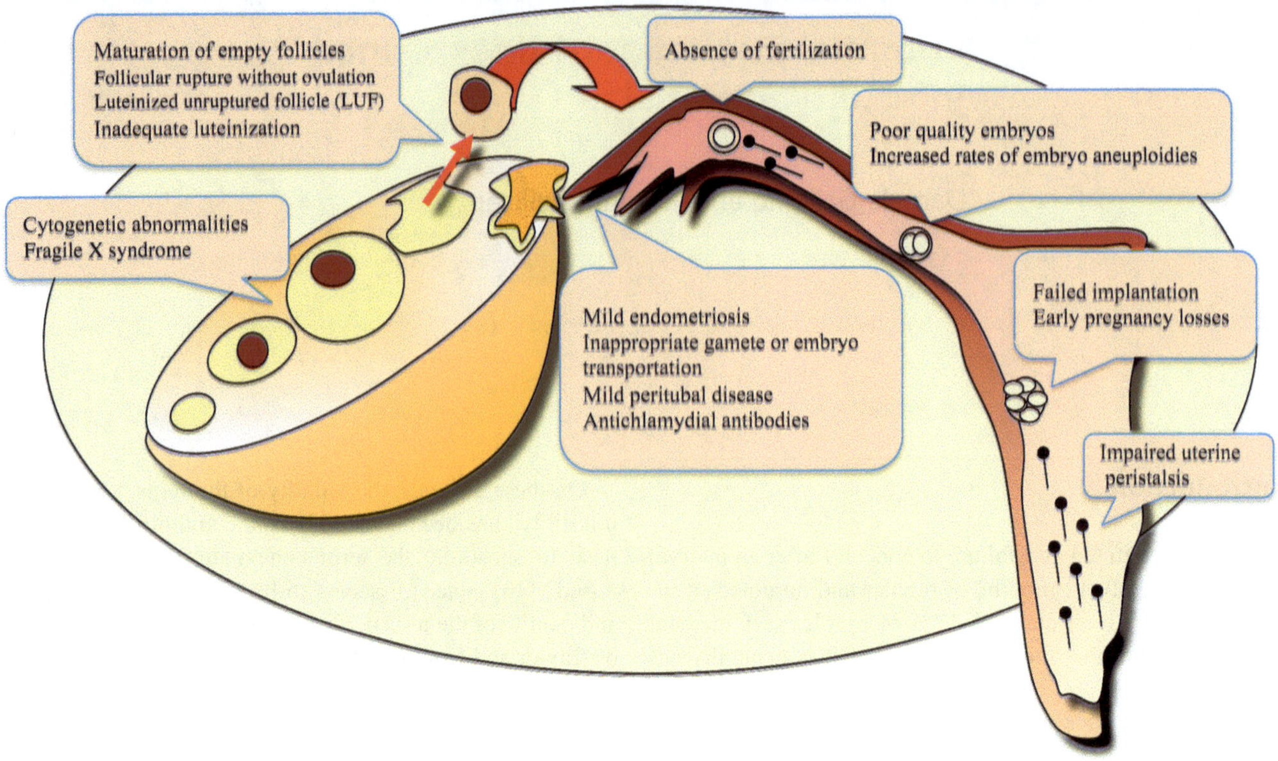

Fig. 13.1 Possible etiologies of UI in females: abnormal ovarian folliculogenesis, ovulatory dysfunction, tuboperitoneal disorders, impaired fertilization, abnormal embryo development, abnormal endometrial receptivity, and altered sperm transport due to impaired uterine peristalsis

Abnormal Ovarian Folliculogenesis

UI can occur, even in the presence of regular menstrual cycles, as a result of diminished ovarian reserve, defined as a reduced quantity and quality of the remaining population of primordial follicles within the ovary than would be expected for a given chronological age. Even though chronological age is the most important determinant of ovarian reserve, evidence has shown great variability in the rate of ovarian ageing [17]. Therefore, women with prematurely ageing ovaries (PAO) [18] may be mistakenly diagnosed with UI, since nobody would expect such fertility decline be based on their age alone.

In this setting, female fertility loss may be assessed by tests of ovarian reserve, such as day 3 serum follicle stimulating hormone (FSH), anti-Müllerian hormone (AMH) levels, and antral follicle count (AFC) [19]. FSH and AMH do not measure the same ovarian reserve parameters. Indeed, FSH is mostly representative of the last 2 weeks of follicular maturation when follicles come to be gonadotropin-sensitive [20], while AMH, exclusively produced by the granulosa cells of early antral and preantral follicles, mainly reflects the earlier stages of folliculogenesis [21, 22, 23]. AFC, visualized by transvaginal ultrasound, is considered the best predictor of ovarian response to stimulation [24], since it correlates with the number of oocytes retrieved and ART outcomes in terms of ongoing pregnancy [25, 26].

In this context, ovarian reserve testing and genetic screening could be of great importance, especially in women <35 years old, to reveal cytogenetic abnormalities, as in the case of the Fragile X syndrome (FXS), that is caused by an increased number of trinucleotide (CGG) repeats on the fragile X (FMR1) gene and linked to premature ovarian failure [27].

Such genetic and ovarian reserve screening may help women potentially have some knowledge about the duration of their own reproductive window and help clinicians counsel patients and direct them to an appropriate treatment option, which in some cases may include gamete donation [19].

Ovulatory Dysfunction

Several abnormalities of ovulation can occur at the gonadal level, such as rupture of the follicle without release of the oocyte, maturation of an empty follicle that does not contain an oocyte, ovulation with inadequate luteinization, incomplete maturation of a follicle resulting in atresia, and finally luteinization of a follicle, under the action of luteinizing hormone (LH), without its rupture and with entrapment of the oocyte, which is also called the luteinized unruptured follicle (LUF) syndrome [28]. This ovulatory dysfunction is considered as a potential cause of female UI [29, 30] and has been linked to endometriosis and pelvic adhesions [31]. Many publications have appeared since 1978 to describe this syndrome, but the exact mechanism by which the ovulatory follicle fails to rupture is not clearly known. Different mechanisms have been suggested for this syndrome, such as a chronic follicular inflammatory-like reaction involving inhibition of synthesis of prostaglandins [32], luteal phase defect [33] or a primary granulosa cell defect [34].

LUF is characterized by normal endocrine signs of ovulation, such as secretory endometrium, normal production of progesterone, and duration of the luteal phase [20], and is usually diagnosed by ultrasound demonstration of a follicle that does not change in size or consistency after ovulation should have occurred [35]. LUF has been demonstrated in both spontaneous and stimulated cycles [36] and it is estimated to be present in 6–12% of cases of female subfertility and in 20–25% of cases when ovarian stimulation is used [37], but the incidence varies depending on the methods of diagnosis such as LPS or ultrasound or steroid hormone concentrations in peritoneal fluid [38]. Qublan et al. found the recurrence rate of LUF increased from 25% in the first cycle of intrauterine insemination (IU) to 78 and 90% in the second and third cycle, respectively [25]. These data are consistent with those reported by others [23–26], but in contrast to previous studies in which LUF was associated with no recurrence rate in subsequent cycles [39, 40].

Tuboperitoneal Disorders

It has been shown that mild endometriosis can affect normal tubal function, as well as other reproductive processes and since this diagnosis is clinically frequently missed, it may represent a possible etiology of UI. For this reason, diagnostic LPS could be considered as an integral part of the evaluation, and the role of tubal function, not just patency should not be underestimated [41].

The prevalence of endometriosis among women who underwent LPS for an infertility evaluation has been reported to be in the range of 10 [10]–50% [42]. Even if performed by experienced laparoscopists, the diagnosis of subtle endometriosis can be hard to make because the disease is often microscopic and presents with atypical lesions [43, 44], and as such may be underdiagnosed.

Evidence shows that endometriosis may also affect IVF outcomes [45, 46] interfering with many aspects of the process, including follicular development, oocyte retrieval, fertilization and embryo development [47, 48], distortion of adnexal anatomy and creating an adverse peritoneal environment characterized by increased inflammatory cytokines, oxidative stress [22, 49, 50, 51], and augmented number of peritoneal fluid macrophages [52–54]. If endometriosis does so in vitro, it can be expected to have similar effects in vivo leading to impaired conception [5]. Studies have demonstrated that, even in mild cases of endometriosis, pregnancy outcomes may have been affected by subtle tubal abnormalities [55, 56], thus reflecting microscopic endometriosis in the fallopian tubes, which can never be totally excluded, even by LPS [19–20]. Furthermore, data on patients undergoing LPS for infertility indicate that of those who have no macroscopic endometriosis at LPS, at least 6% have microscopic lesions [57, 58] and thus confirms how this diagnosis, especially in patients with infertility may be underestimated [59].

The fallopian tubes play an important role in sperm transport, oocyte capture and transport, fertilization, and early embryo development [60]. Abnormalities in any one of these functions cause defective transport of the oocyte and impaired fertilization, through alterations in tubal peristaltic or ciliary activity [61], which may affect one or both fallopian tubes.

Tubal function can be abnormal despite documentation of tubal patency [62, 63], but HSG has limited value in evaluating tubal function and peritubal disease [64, 65] and may be less accurate in detecting tubal disease than LPS [66, 67]. Moreover, a study performed in an infertile population showed that HSG missed at least one tubal abnormality in 84% of the cases [68]. Despite all these limitations, HSG represents the first line tool to evaluate tubal status, because of its safety and low cost. LPS remains the gold standard for the evaluation of mechanical factors affecting the fallopian tubes, but it can miss proximal disease [65] and cannot be used to directly observe the ampulla, where the fertilization between oocyte and sperm occurs. This may be explored by salpingoscopy. Some researchers think that salpingoscopy could be informative in patients with UI, since it can identify nonobstructive tubal diseases such as fibrosis, adhesions, debris, and foreign bodies [69].

Furthermore, the impact of chlamydial infection in the etiology of tubal pathology secondary to salpingitis [70–72] on female fertility is well documented. Although neither HSG or LPS may identify tubal pathology secondary to chlamydial infections in the absence of overt occlusion or peritubal adhesions, subfertile women with a positive Chlamydia trachomatis antibody have lower chances for pregnancy than seronegative women [73]. This evidence confirms the validity of assessment for chlamydial serology in women under fertility investigation [74, 75].

Impaired Fertilization

A decrease in fertilization has been documented in IVF cycles performed in couple with UI, suggesting gamete defects as potential causes of UI.

Absence of fertilization has been shown in a prospective study from Ruiz et al. [76], in couples with UI and mild endometriosis undergoing IVF/ICSI after four failed intrauterine insemination cycles. It has been found that 11.4% of these couples suffered fertilization failure with standard IVF, and if ICSI would not have been employed, they might have had no embryos available for transfer. In this study, ICSI did not increase fertilization rates over standard IVF in case of UI, but avoided complete fertilization failure in those patients.

Alboughar et al. [77] reached similar conclusions with regards to gamete dysfunction in couples with UI, in which the rate of fertilization failure was 22.7%, very similar to those observed in other studies in couples with UI [78, 79].

Abnormal Embryo Development

The use of assisted reproductive techniques has been important not only for therapeutic reasons, but also because it helps to understand the complex process that leads to conception in a given couple. Indeed, it is noteworthy that there is a high incidence of chromosomal abnormalities in human embryos cultured in vitro [80] and that many repetitive implantation failure (RIF) cases are due to embryonic defects, including chromosomal aneuploidy, which increase with maternal age [81] and with the number of previous failed IVF cycles [82, 83]. Different therapeutic options have been proposed to improve the outcome of these patients, including assisted zona hatching [84] and coculturing embryos to the blastocyst stage [85]. However, other studies have found dramatic declines in implantation and pregnancy rates using blastocyst culture in RIF patients due to the limited development of these embryos in extended culture [86].

In a randomized controlled trial of infertile couples with RIF and prior transfers of good-quality embryos, Rubio et al. reported a trend towards an increased incidence of genetic abnormalities in embryos from these couples and an improvement in live-birth rates per transfer by selection of the healthiest embryos with PGS, highlighting the mechanisms of action by which chromosomal abnormalities can have an impact on UI.

Abnormal Endometrial Receptivity

An altered endometrial receptivity may interfere with apposition, adhesion, or penetration of the embryo and results in a failed implantation [87].

Since the 1950s, traditional histologic evaluation of the endometrium performed by pathologists, has been used as a predictor of endometrial receptivity [88, 89], the clinical relevance and reproducibility of which has been questioned in randomized studies [90, 91]. The development of microarray technology [92] helped to analyze the expression of thousands of genes at the same time in an endometrial sample of development in the peri-implantation period. On those grounds, and consistent with the findings that endometrial receptivity may be related to its transcriptomic profile, molecular assessment of endometrial receptivity has been developed [93, 94], a molecular diagnostic tool that contains 238 expressed genes coupled to a computational predictor, which is able to identify endometrial samples within the window of implantation, independent of their histological appearance. The endometrial receptivity array (ERA) test may help to identify patients with implantation failure caused by a nonreceptive endometrium, improving the ability to control the endometrial environment for implantation. Moreover, an endometrial database (EDB) (http://www.endometrialdatabase.com) has been created to facilitate the exchange of information on the genomics of endometrial receptivity, for the improvement of knowledge in this field worldwide [95].

UI may reflect a malfunction of the endometrial-embryo "dialogue" in the early phases of implantation that leads to early pregnancy loss (EPL), or biochemical pregnancy (BP) which could be erroneously interpreted as a failure to conceive. EPL or BP are defined as increases in beta-human chorionic gonadotropin (B-hCG) at the end of the luteal phase due to embryonic implantation that does not result in a clinical pregnancy. The development of sensitive immunoassays for the detection of urinary B-hCG has allowed for detection of a pregnancy within a few days of embryo implantation, which shows high rates of BP in spontaneous conception [96]. Moreover, data from patients who have undergone ART and PGS show that many preclinical implantation failures are due to chromosomal alterations and are found in high rates in natural (25%) [97] and ART conceptions (40%) [98]. Chromosomal aberrations are probably not the only cause of EPL. Indeed, an altered endometrial receptivity due to environmental factors, such as age and excessive ovarian stimulation in IVF cycles, may also play an important role in the etiologies of this disorder, as shown by Troncoso et al. [99].

Altered Sperm Transport due to Impaired Uterine Peristalsis

There is clear evidence that sperm transport through the female genital tract from the cervix into the tubes, assisted by cervico-fundal uterine peristaltic contractions [100, 101], is altered in patients with UI and endometriosis which results in impaired uterine contractility, documented by hysterosalpingoscintigraphy (HSSG) [102]. Data have shown that endometriosis is associated with uterine hyperperistalsis and dysperistalsis, which may cause impaired or total failure in sperm transport capacity respectively, especially when diffuse adenomyosis is also detected [103]. Dysperistalsis is associated with reduced natural conception rates [104, 105] and consequently IVF/ICSI may be required even in couples with otherwise patent fallopian tubes and normal semen parameters.

Conclusions

Infertility is unexplained after thorough evaluation in about 15–30 % of cases and constitutes a multifactorial disorder of reproduction, as discussed in this chapter. Many potential etiologies of UI have been proposed here, including ovarian factors, fertilization failure, failure of the embryo to develop, failure of implantation and impaired or total failure in oocyte and sperm transport due to altered tubal and uterine function.

Increasingly, complex ART options have led to the finding of many causes of infertility that in the past have only been suspected, but can now be diagnosed, as in the case of chromosomal aneuploidies identified with PGS. However, multiple potential etiologies of UI could coexist with identified causes for infertility and therefore many couples with identified factors may fail to conceive despite receiving appropriate treatment for the identified causes. It is, therefore, imperative to perform a complete and thorough evaluation of the infertile couple, including evaluation for these subtle etiologies, even in couples whose infertility evaluation has revealed a potential etiology.

References

1. Evers JL. Female subfertility. Lancet. 2002;360:151–9.
2. Gnoth C, Godehardt E, Frank-Herrmann P, Friol K, Tigges J, Freundl G. Definition and prevalence of subfertility and infertility. Hum Reprod. 2005;20:1144–7.
3. Hamada A, Esteves SC, Nizza M, Agarwal A. Unexplained male infertility: diagnosis and management. Int Braz J Urol. 2012;38(5):576–94
4. The Practice Committee of the American Society for Reproductive Medicine, authors. Effectiveness and treatment for unexplained infertility. Fertil Steril. 2006;86(5 suppl):S111–S4.
5. Smith S, Pfiefer SM, Collins J. Diagnosis and management of female infertility. JAMA. 2003;290:17.
6. Quaas A, Dokras A. Diagnosis and treatment of unexplained infertility. Rev Obstet Gynecol. 2008;1(2):69–76.
7. The Practice Committee of the American Society for Reproductive Medicine, authors. Optimal evaluation of the infertile female. Fertil Steril. 2006;86(5 suppl):S264–S7.
8. Marrero MA, Ory SJ. Unexplained infertility. Curr Opin Obstet Gynecol. 1991;3(2):211–8.
9. Collins JA, Crosignani PG. Unexplained infertility: a review of diagnosis, prognosis, treatment efficacy and management. Int J Gynaecol Obstet. 1992;39:267.
10. Gleicher N, Barad D. Unexplained infertility: does it really exist? Hum Reprod. 2006;21:1951–1955.
11. Taylor PJ, Collins JA. Unexplained infertility. New York: Oxford University Press; 1992. p. 153–69.
12. Isaksson R, Tiitinen A. Present concept of unexplained infertility. Gynecol Endocrinol. 2004;18(5):278–90.
13. Southam A. What to do with the "normal" infertile couple. Fertil Steril. 1960;11:543–9.
14. Collins JA, Burrows EA, Willan AR. The prognosis for live birth among untreated infertile couples. Fertil Steril. 1995;64:22.
15. Collins J, Rowe T. Age of the female partner is a prognostic factor in prolonged unexplained infertility: a multicenter study. Fertil Steril. 1989;52:15.
16. Templeton AA, Penney GC. The incidence, characteristics and prognosis of patients whose infertility is unexplained. Fertil Steril. 1982;37:175–82.
17. te Velde ER Pearson PL. The variability of female reproductive ageing. Hum Reprod Update. 2002;8:141–54.
18. Gleicher N, Weghofer A, Oktay K, Barad D. Do etiologies of premature ovarian aging (POA) mimic those of premature ovarian failure (POF)? Hum Reprod. 2009;24(10):2395–400.
19. Broekmans FJ, Kwee J, Hendriks DJ, Mol BW, Lambalk CB. A systematic review of tests predicting ovarian reserve and IVF outcome. Hum Reprod Update. 2006;12(6):685–718.
20. Wolff E, Taylor H. Value of the day 3 follicle-stimulating hormone measurement. Fertil Steril. 2004;81:1486–8.
21. Feyereisen E, Mèndez Lozano DH, Taieb J, Hesters L, Frydman R, Fanchin R. Anti-Müllerian hormone: clinical insights into a promising biomarker of ovarian follicular status. Reprod Biomed Online. 2006;12:695–703. doi:10.1016/S1472–6483(10)61081-4.
22. Gleicher N, Weghofer A, Barad DH. Discordances between follicle stimulating hormone (FSH) and anti-Müllerian hormone (AMH) in female infertility. Reprod Biol Endocrinol. 2010;8:64. doi:10.1186/1477-7827-8-64.
23. Visser JA, de Jong F, Laven J, Themmen A. Anti-Müllerian hormone: a new marker for ovarian function. Reproduction. 2006;131:1–9.
24. Hendriks DJ, Kwee J, Mol BW, te Velde ER, Broekmans FJ. Ultrasonography as a tool for the prediction of outcome in IVF patients: a comparative meta-analysis of ovarian volume and antral follicle count. Fertil Steril. 2007;87(4):764–75.
25. Frattarelli JL, Levi AJ, Miller BT, Segars JH. A prospective assessment of the predictive value of basal antral follicles in in vitro fertilization cycles. Fertil Steril. 2003;80(2):350–5.
26. Devroey P, Fauser B, Diedrich K. Approaches to improve the diagnosis and management of infertility. Hum Reprod Update. 2009;15(4):391–408.
27. Wittenberger MD, Hagerman RJ, Sherman SL et al. The FMR1 premutation and reproduction. Fertil Steril. 2007;87:456–65.
28. Katz E. The luteinized unruptured follicle and other ovulatory dysfunctions (Review). Fertil Steril. 1998;50(6):839–50.
29. Hamilton CJ, Wetzels LC, Evers JL, Hoogland HJ, Muitjens A, De Haan J. Follicle growth curves and hormonal patterns in patients with the luteinized unruptured follicle syndrome. Fertil Steril. 1985;43:541–8.
30. Koninckx PR, Brosens IA. Clinical significance of the luteinized unruptured follicle syndrome as a cause of infertility. Eur J Obstet Gynecol Reprod Biol. 1982;13:355–68.
31. Marik J, Hulka J. Luteinized unruptured follicle syndrome: a subtle cause of infertility. Fertil Steril. 1978;29:270–4.
32. Murdoch WJ, Cavender JL. Effect of indomethacin on the vascular architecture of preovulatory ovine follicle: possible implication in the luteinized unruptured follicle syndrome. Fertil Steril. 1989;51:153–5.
33. Kugu K, Taketani Y, Kohda K, Mizuno M. Exaggerated prolactin response to thyrotopin-releasing hormone in infertile women with the luteinized unruptured follicle syndrome. Arch Gynecol Obstet. 1991;249:27–31.
34. Zaidi J, Jurkovic D, Campbell S, Collins W, McGregor A, Tan SL. Luteinized unruptured follicle: morphology, endocrine function and blood flow changes during the menstrual cycle. Hum Reprod. 1995;10:44–9.

35. Liukkonen S, Koskimies AI, Tenhunen A, Ylöstalo P. Diagnosis of luteinized unruptured follicle (LUF) syndrome by ultrasound. Fertil Steril. 1984;41(1):26–30.
36. Craft I, Shelton K, Yovich L, Smith D. Ovum retention in the human. Fertil Steril. 1980;34:537–41.
37. Qublan H, Amarin Z, Nawasreh M, Diab F, Malkawi S, Al-Ahmad N, Balawneh M. Luteinized unruptured follicle syndrome: incidence and recurrence rate in infertile women with unexplained infertility undergoing intrauterine insemination. Hum Reprod. 2006;21(8):2110–3. (Epub 2006 Apr 13).
38. Temmerman M, Devroey P, Naaktgeboren N, Amy JJ, Van Steirteghem AC. Incidence, recurrence and treatment of the luteinized unruptured follicle syndrome. Acta Eur Fertil. 1984;15:179–83.
39. Aksel S. Thou shall not luteinize nor rupture. Fertil Steril. 1987;47:762–4.
40. Luciano AA, Peluso J, Koch E, Maier D, Kuslis S, Davison E. Temporal relationship and reliability of the clinical, hormonal, and ultrasonographic indices of ovulation in infertile women. Obstet Gynecol. 1990;75:412–6.
41. Bérubé S, Marcoux S, Langevin S, Maheux R. Canadian Collaborative Group on Endometriosis. Fecundity of infertile women with minimal or mild endometriosis and women with unexplained infertility. Fertil Steril. 1998;69:1034–41.
42. Endometriosis and infertility: a committee opinion. Fertil Steril. 2012;98 (3):591–8.
43. Olive DL, Schwartz LB. Endometriosis. N Engl J Med. 1993;328:1759–69.
44. Cook AS, Rock JA. The role of laparoscopy in the treatment of endometriosis. Fertil Steril. 1995;55:663–80.
45. Guidice LC, Kao LC. Endometriosis. Lancet. 2004;364:1789–99.
46. Huang JY, Rosenwaks Z. In vitro fertilisation treatment and factors affecting success. Best Pract Res Clin Obstet Gynaecol. 2012;26(6):777–88.
47. Toya M, Saito H, Ohta N, et al. Moderate and severe endometriosis is associated with alterations in the cell cycle of granulosa cells in patients undergoing in vitro fertilization and embryo transfer. Fertil Steril. 2000;73:344–50.
48. Pellicer A, Oliveira N, Ruiz A, Remohi J, Simon C. Exploring the mechanism(s) of endometriosis-related infertilityan analysis of embryo development and implantation in assissted reproduction. Hum Reprod. 1995;10(2):91–97.
49. Harada T, Iwabe T, Terakawa N. Role of cytokines in endometriosis. Fertil Steril. 2001;76(1):1–10.
50. Tsudo T, Harada T, Iwabe T, Tanikawa M, Nagano Y, Ito M, et al. Altered gene expresion and secretion of interleukin-6 in stromal cells derived from endometriotic tissues. Fertil Steril. 2000;73:205–11.
51. Pellicer A, Albert C, Mercader A, Bonilla-Musoles F, Remohi J, Simon C. The follicular and endocrine environment in women with endometriosis: local and systemic cytokine production. Fertil Steril 1998;70:425–31.
52. Halme J., Becker S., Hammond MG, et al. Increased activation of pelvic macrophages in infertile women with mild endometriosis. Am J Obstet Gynecol. 1983;145:333–7.
53. Halme J, Becker S, Haskill S. Altered maturation and function macrophages. Thus cells with the appropriate receptors could of peritoneal macrophages: possible role in pathogenesis of endometriosis. Am J Obstet Gynecol. 1987;156:783–9.
54. McLaren J, Dealtry G, Prentice A, Charnock-Jones D, Smith S. Decreased levels of the potent regulator of monocyte/macrophage activation, interleukin-13, in the peritoneal fluid of patients with endometriosis. Hum Reprod. 1997;12(6):1307–10.
55. Fakih H, Marshall J. Subtle tubal abnormalities adversely affect gamete intrafallopian transfer outcome in women with endometriosis. Fertil Steril. 1994;62:799–801.
56. Guzick DS, Grefenstette I, Baffone K, et al. Infertility evaluation in infertile women: a model for answering the efficacy of infertility testing. Hum Reprod. 1994a;9:2306–10.
57. Nisolle M, Berlière M, Paindaveine B, Casanas-Roux F, Bourdon A, Donnez J. Histologic study of peritoneal endometriosis in infertile women. Fertil Steril. 1990;53:984–8.
58. Balasch J, Creus M, Fabregues F, Carmona F, Ordi J, Martinez-Roman S, et al. Visible and non-visible endometriosis at laparoscopy in fertile and infertile women and in patients with chronic pelvic paina prospective study. Hum Reprod. 1996;11:387–91.
59. Bérubé S, Marcoux S, Langevin S, Maheux R. Canadian collaborative group on endometriosis. Fecundity of infertile women with minimal or mild endometriosis and women with unexplained infertility. Fertil Steril. 1998;69:1034–1041.
60. Nakagawa K, Inoue M, Nishi Y, Sugiyama R, Motoyama K, Kuribayashi Y, Akira S, Sugiyama R. A new evaluation score that uses salpingoscopy to reflect fallopian tube function in infertile women. Fertil Steril. 2010;94(7):2753–57.
61. Jansen RP. Endocrine response in the Fallopian tube. Endocr Rev. 1984;5:525–51.
62. Karande VC, Pratt DE, Gleicher N. The assessment of tubal functional status by tubal perfusion pressure measurements. Hum Reprod. 1996;2:429–33.
63. Papaioannou S, Afnan M, Girling AJ, Cooarasamy A, McHugo JM, Sharif K. The potential value of tubal perfusion pressure measured during selective salpingography in predicting fertility. Hum Reprod. 2003;18:358–63.
64. Mol BWJ, Swant P, Bossuyt PMM, van Beurden M, van der Veen F. Reproducibility of the interpretation of hysterosalpingography in the diagnosis of tubal pathology. Hum Reprod. 1996;11:1204–08.
65. Glatstein IZ, Sleeper LA, Lavy Y, Simon A, Adoni A, Palti Z, Hurwitz A, Laufer N. Observer variability in the diagnosis and management of the hysterosalpingogram. Fertil Steril. 1997;67:233–7.
66. Mol BW, Collins JA, Burrows EA, van der Veen F, Bossuyt PM. Comparison of hysterosalpingography and laparoscopy in predicting infertility outcome. Hum Reprod. 1999;14:1237–42.
67. Tanahatoe S, Hompes PG, Lambalk CB. Accuracy of diagnostic laparoscopy in the infertility wash-ups before intrauterine insemination. Fertil Steril. 2003;79:361–6.
68. Karande V, Pratt D, Rabin DS, Gleicher N. The limited value of hysterosalpingography in answering tubal status and fertility potential. Fertil Steril. 1995a;63:1167–71.
69. Nakawaga K, Inoue M, Nishi Y, Sugiyama R, Motoyama K, Kuribayashi Y, Akira S, Sugiyama R. A new evaluation score that uses salpingoscopy to reflect fallopian tube function in infertile women. Fertil Steril. 2010;94(7):2753–57.
70. Arrestad G. Lunde 0, Moen M, Dalaker K. Infertility and chlamydial infection. Fertil Steril. 1987;58:787–90.
71. Akande VA, Hunt LP, Cahill DJ, Caul EO., Ford WC, Jenkins JM. Tubal damage in infertile women: prediction using chlamydia serology. Hum Reprod. 2003;18(9):1841–47.
72. Broeze KA, Opmeer BC, Coppus SFPJ., Van Geloven N, Alves MFC., Ånestad G, Bhattacharya S, Mol BW. Chlamydia antibody testing and diagnosing tubal pathology in subfertile women: an individual patient data meta-analysis. Hum Reprod Update. 2011;17(3):301–10.
73. Coppus SFPJ, Land JA, Opmeer BC, Teures P, Eijkemans MJC, Hompes PGA, Bossuyt PMM, van der Veen F, Mol BWJ, van der Steeg JW. Chlamydia trachomatis IgG seropositivity is associated with lower natural conception rates in ovulatory subfetile women without visible pathology. Hum Reprod. 2011;26(11):3061–7.
74. Bjercke, S., Purvis, K. Characteristics of women under fertility investigation with IgA/IgG seropositivity for Chlamydia trachomatis. European J Obstet Gynecol Reprod Biol. 1993;51(2):157–61.

75. Thomas K, Coughlin L, Mannion PT, Haddad NG. The value of Chlamydia trachomatis antibody testing as part of routine infertility investigations. Hum Reprod. 2000;15(5):1079–82.
76. Ruiz A, Guanes PP, Remohi J, Simon C, Minguez Y, Pellicer A. The role of in vitro fertilization and intracytoplasmic sperm injection in couples with unexplained infertility after failed intrauterine insemination. Fertil Steril. 1997;68:171–3.
77. Alboughar MA, Mansour RT, Serour GI, et al. Intracytoplasmatic sperm injection and conventional in vitro fertilization for sibling oocytes in cases of unexplained infertility and borderline semen. J Assist Reprod Genet. 1996;13:38–42.
78. Gurgan T, Urman B, Yarali H, Kisnisci HA. The results of in vitro fertilization-embryo transfer in couples with unexplained infertility failing to conceive with superovulation and intrauterine insemination. Fertil Steril. 1995;64:93.
79. Takeuchi S, Minoura H, Shibahara T, Shen X, Futamura N, Toyoda N. In vitro fertilization and intracytoplasmic sperm injection for couples with unexplained infertility after failed direct intraperitoneal insemination. J Assist Reprod Genet. 2000;17:515.
80. Munné S. Chromosome abnormalities and their relationship to morphology and development of human embryos. Reprod Biomed Online. 2006;12(2):234–53.
81. Munné S, Alikani M, Tomkin G, Grifo J, Cohen J. Embryo morphology, developmental rates, and maternal age are correlated with chromosome abnormalities. Fertil Steril. 1995;64(2):382–91.
82. Gianaroli L, Magli MC, Munné S, Fiorentino A, Montanaro N, Ferraretti AP. Will preimplantation genetic diagnosis assist patients with a poor prognosis to achieve pregnancy? Hum Reprod. 1997;12:1762–7.
83. Pehlivan T, Rubio C, Rodrigo L, Romero J, Remohi J, Simón C, Pellicer A. Impact of preimplantation genetic diagnosis on IVF outcome in implantation failure patients. Reprod Biomed Online. 2003;6(2):232–7.
84. Stein A, Rufas O, Amit S, Avrech O, Pinkas H, Ovadia J, Fisch B. Assisted hatching by partial zona dissection of human pre-embryos in patients with recurrent implantation failure after in vitro fertilization. Fertil Steril. 1995;63(4):838–41.
85. Simón C, Mercader A, Garcia-Velasco J, Nikas G, Moreno C, Remohí J, Pellicer A. Coculture of human embryos with autologous human endometrial epithelial cells in patients with implantation failure. J Clin Endocrinol Metab. 1999;84(8):2638–46.
86. ShapiroBS, Richter KS, Harris DC, Daneshmand ST. Dramatic declines in implantation and pregnancy rates in patients who undergo repeated cycles of in vitro fertilization with blastocyst transfer after one or more failed attempts. Fertil Steril. 2001;76(3):538–42.
87. Tapia A, Gangi LM, Zegers-Hochschild F, Balmaceda J, Pommer R, Trejo L, Pacheco IM, Salvatierra AM, Henriquez S, Quezada M, Vargas M, Rios M, Munroe DJ, Croxatto HB, Velasquez L. Differences in the endometrial transcript profile during the receptive period between women who were refractory to implantation and those who achieved pregnancy. Hum Reprod. 2008; 23:340.
88. Noyes RW, Hertig AT, Rock J. Dating the endometrial biopsy. Fertil Steril. 1950;1:3–25.
89. Noyes RW, Hertig AT, Rock J. Dating the endometrial biopsy. Am J Obstet Gynecol. 1975;122:262–3.
90. Coutifaris C, Myers ER, Guzick DS, Diamond MP, Carson SA, Legro RS, et al. Histological dating of timed endometrial biopsy tissue is not related to fertility status. Fertil Steril. 2004;82:1264–72.
91. Murray MJ, Meyer WR, Zaino RJ, Lessey BA, Novotny DB, Ireland K, et al. A critical analysis of the accuracy, reproducibility, and clinical utility of histologic endometrial dating in fertile women. Fertil Steril. 2004;81:1333–43.
92. Schena M, Shalon D, Davis RW, Brown PO. Quantitative monitoring of gene expression patterns with a complementary DNA microarray. Science. 1995; 270:467–70.
93. Díaz-Gimeno P., Horcajadas JA, Martínez-Conejero JA. A genomic diagnostic tool for human endometrial receptivity based on the transcriptomic signature. Fertil Steril. 2011;95(1):50–60.
94. Díaz-Gimeno P, Ruiz-Alonso M, Blesa D, Bosch N, Martínez-Conejero J, Alamá P, Garrido N, Pellicer A, Simón C. The accuracy and reproducibility of the endometrial receptivity array is superior to histology as a diagnostic method for endometrial receptivity. Fertil Steril. 2013;99(2):508–17.
95. Horcajadas JA, Pellicer A, Simón C. Wide genomic analysis of human endometrial receptivity: new times, new opportunities. Hum Reprod Update. 2007;13(1):77–86.
96. Macklon NS, Geraedts JP, Fauser BC. Conception to ongoing pregnancy: the 'black box' of early pregnancy loss. Hum Reprod Update. 2002;8:333–43.
97. Wilcox AJ, Weinberg CR, O'Connor JF, Baird DD, Schlatterer JP, Canfield RE, et al. Incidence of early loss of pregnancy. N Eng J Med. 1988;319:189–94.
98. Simon C, Landeras J, Zuzuarregui J, Martin J, Remohi J, Pellicer A. Early pregnancy losses in in vitro fertilization and oocyte donation. Fertil Steril. 1999;72:1061–5.
99. Troncoso C, Bosch E, Rubio C, Remohí J, Simón C, Pellicer A. The origin of biochemical pregnancies: lessons learned from preimplantation genetic diagnosis. Fertil Steril. 2003;79(2):449–50.
100. Kunz G, Beil D, Deiniger H, Einspanier A, Mall G, Leyendecker G. The uterine peristaltic pump. Normal and impeded sperm transport within the female genital tract. Adv Exp Med Biol. 1997;424:267–77.
101. Kunz G, Beil D, Deininger H, Wildt L, Leyendecker G. The dynamics of rapid sperm transport through the female genital tract: evidence from vaginal sonography of uterine peristalsis and hysterosalpingoscintigraphy. Hum Reprod. 1996;11(3):627–32.
102. Leyendecker G, Kunz G, Wildt L, Beil D, Deininger H. Uterine hyperperistalsis and dysperistalsis as dysfunctions of the mechanism of rapid sperm transport in patients with endometriosis and infertility. Hum Reprod. 1996;11(7):1542–51.
103. Kissler S, Zangos S, Wiegratz I, Kohl J, Rody A, Gaetje R, Doebert N, Wildt L, Kunz G, Leyendecker G, Kaufmann M. Uterotubal sperm transport and its impairment in endometriosis and adenomyosis. Ann N Y Acad Sci. 2007;1101:38–48.
104. Kissler S, Hamscho N, Zangos S, Gätje R, Müller A, Rody A, Döbert N, Menzel C, Grünwald F, Siebzehnrübl E, et al. Diminished pregnancy rates in endometriosis due to impaired uterotubal transport assessed by hysterosalpingoscintigraphy. BJOG. 2005;112(10):1391–6.
105. Kissler S, Wildt L, Schmiedehausen K, et al. Predictive value of impaired uterine transport function assessed by negative hysterosalpingoscintigraphy (HSSG). Eur J Obstet Gynecol Reprod Biol. 2004;113:204–208.

Oxidative Stress in Unexplained Female Infertility

14

Fatma Ferda Verit

Introduction

Unexplained infertility is one of the controversial subjects in infertility on which agreement is rarely found among practitioners. It is a term used to define 30–40% of couples in whom standard investigations including semen analysis, tests of ovulation and tubal patency have failed to detect any gross abnormality [1]. Couples with unexplained infertility suffer from both diminished and delayed fecundity. The possible underlying etiologies are defective endometrial receptivity, impaired oocyte quality, premature ovarian failure, minimal and mild endometriosis, tubal disease, pelvic adhesions, immunological and endocrinological abnormalities, and oxidative stress [2].

A couple is referred for infertility investigation if they are not able to conceive within a year. The diagnosis of unexplained infertility may be frustrating because if there is no explanation for infertility, there is no effective treatment. The prognosis is worse if the duration of infertility exceeds 3 years and female partner is >35 years of age [3]. Treatment has been indicated if the duration is more than 2 years or the female partner is >35 years [3, 4] of age.

Oxidative stress has been known to play a key role in the pathogenesis of subfertility in both males and females [5]. The adverse effects of oxidative stress on sperm quality and functions have been studied in detail [6]. Although it has been associated with female reproductive disorders such as endometriosis and polycystic ovarian syndrome (PCOS), the impact of oxidative stress on unexplained female infertility has not been adequately studied. The aim of the review is to investigate the possible relationship between underlying mechanisms that may be associated with unexplained infertility and oxidative stress by using the currently available literature.

F. F. Verit (✉)
Department of Obstetrics & Gynecology, Infertility Research & Treatment Center, Suleymaniye Maternity, Research &Training Hospital, Zeytinburnu, Istanbul, Turkey
email: fverit@gmail.com

What Is Oxidative Stress?

Biological systems contain an abundant amount of O_2. Free radicals are often generated from O_2 and partially from normal metabolic processes in the body. They are unstable and highly reactive due to unpaired electrons that are capable of initiating an uncontrolled cascade of chain reactions, resulting in cellular damage and disease [7]. There are two major types of free radical species: reactive oxygen species (ROS) and reactive nitrogen species (RNS).The three major types of ROS are superoxide (O_2^-), which are formed when electrons leak from the electron transport chain; hydrogen peroxide (H_2O_2), resulting from the dismutation of superoxide or directly from the action of oxidase enzymes, and hydroxyl ($HO^\bullet$), a highly reactive species that can modify purines and pyrimidines and cause strand breaks that result in DNA damage.

The controlled production of ROS plays a role in the production of physiological reproductive processes such as hormone signaling, oocyte maturation, folliculogenesis, tubal function, ovarian steroidogenesis, cyclical endometrial changes, and germ cell function. Oxidative stress occurs when ROS overwhelm antioxidant capacity. ROS extensively damage cellular organelles, including mitochondria, nuclear and mitochondrial DNA, and cell membrane, leading to cellular demise [8, 9]. ROS may also impact signaling pathways, transcription factors, and epigenetic mechanisms and cause a reduction in oocyte, embryo quality and implantation [6, 10].

Energy from adenine triphosphate (ATP) is essential for gamete functions and any disturbance in mitochondrial functions can lead to altered generation of ATP. Mitochondria are major sites of ROS production and increased generation of ROS can affect functions of the mitochondria in oocytes and embryos.

RNS include nitric oxide (NO) and nitrogen dioxide as well as nonreactive species such as peroxynitrite, nitrosamines, and others. NO, an important RNS that is present in the body, is specifically synthesized by nitric oxide synthase

G. L. Schattman et al. (eds.), *Unexplained Infertility*, DOI 10.1007/978-1-4939-2140-9_14,

(NOS) during the conversion of L-arginine to L-citrulline. Excess NO is toxic and has an unpaired electron, making it a highly reactive free radical that can damage proteins, carbohydrates, nucleotides, and lipids. It contributes to cell and tissue damage, low grade, sterile inflammation, and adhesions with other inflammatory mediators [11]. NOS have been known to generate H_2O_2, superoxide, and NO. Superoxide reacts with NO, resulting in increased generation of peroxynitrite and cell toxicity. The effects of NO are proposed to be mediated through cyclic guanosine monophosphate (cGMP) as a second messenger or by generation of ROS resulting from interaction of NO with superoxide radicals [12].

Intracellular hemostasis is maintained by a balance between pro-oxidant compounds and antioxidants. Antioxidants have the ability to oppose the effects of pro-oxidants by hindering ROS production, scavenging ROS, and repairing cell damage caused by ROS. Enzymatic antioxidants include superoxide dismutase, catalase, and glutathione peroxidase. Nonenzymatic antioxidants are vitamins C and E, taurine, hypotaurine, cysteamine, and glutathione. Some agents such as lycopene, metallothionein, and bilirubin also have antioxidant properties.

Antioxidants can be found in various cell compartments. For example, Mn–SOD is localized in the mitochondria, whereas Cu–Zn–SOD is mainly localized in the cytoplasm. Enzymatic antioxidant defenses have been found in mammalian embryos and oocytes [13, 14], and nonenzymatic defenses in tubal [14] and follicular fluids [15]. Increased levels of antioxidants have been shown in normal pregnancy [16, 17], whereas loss of antioxidant defenses have been observed in patients with recurrent abortion as a result of their increased consumption [18, 19]. The lower antioxidant levels could aggravate pro-oxidant injury in endothelial cells, altering prostacyclin–thromboxane balance and may contribute to preeclampsia or abortion [20]. Glutathione peroxidase expression was increased and selenium levels were reduced in patients with diabetes and spontaneous abortion [16].

Redox Cell Signaling

Redox reactions can be defined as oxidation or reduction of oocyte and embryo metabolism by electron transfer mechanisms [6]. Oocytes are protected from oxidative damage by antioxidants such as catalase, SOD, glutathione transferase, paraoxanase, and heat shock proteins [21].

The deleterious effects of ROS are summarized as follows:

1. Opening of ion channels: Elevated levels of ROS release Ca^{+2} from endoplasmic reticulum resulting in mitochondrial permeability, so the mitochondrial membrane potential becomes unstable and ATP production ceases.
2. Lipid peroxidation: It occurs in polyunsaturated fatty acid side chains. These chains react with O_2 creating the peroxyl radical, which can obtain H^+ from another fatty acid, creating a continuous reaction. Vitamin E can break this chain reaction due to its lipid solubility and hydrophobic tail.
3. Protein modifications: Amino acids are targets for oxidative damage. Direct oxidation of side chains can lead to the formation of carbonyl groups.
4. DNA oxidation: Mitochondrial DNA is susceptible to ROS due to the presence of O_2^- in the electron transport chain, lack of histone protection, and absence of repair mechanisms.

ROS may react with other molecules to disrupt many cellular components and processes. ROS target the pathway and also act as second messengers in some reactions [22]. ROS are known to effect ovulation and implantation [23].

Nuclear factor-kappa B (NF-KB) is a transcription factor that plays a crucial role in inflammation, immunity, cell adhesion, invasion, cellular proliferation, apoptosis and angiogenesis [24]. Oxidative stress is known to be a potent activator of NF-KB [24]. Induced NF-KB activation then leads to expression of numerous proinflammatory genes such as cytokines, which may provide positive feedback to the pathway [25].

One of the most signaling pathways in the body is mitogen-activated protein kinases (MAPK). MAPK pathways are important in gene transcription mechanisms in response to oxidative stress. Their signaling cascades are controlled by phosphorylation and dephosphorylation of serine and/or threonine residues. It contributes to increased actions of receptors of tyrosine kinases, protein tyrosine kinases, cytokines, and growth factors [26, 27]. c-jun N-terminal kinases (JNK) and p38 pathways can also be activated by ROS. The addition of H_2O_2 to this cascade can disrupt the complex and promote phosphorylation [28, 29].

Oxidative Stress and the Ovary

ROS are a double-edged sword; they not only serve as key signal molecules in physiological processes but also have a role in pathological situations involving female reproductive tract. Oxidative stress is important in ovarian germ cell and stromal cell physiology. A cohort of oocytes begins to grow and develop in the ovary each month. Hypoxia of the granulosa cells is a normal event during the growth of ovarian follicles [30]. Hypoxic or anoxic conditions reduce ROS and increase antioxidant activity [31]. Oxygen deprivation stimulates follicular angiogenesis, which is important for growth and development of the ovarian follicle. Impairment of angiogenesis within ovarian follicles contributes to follicular atresia. Meiosis I resumes in the dominant follicle that is regulated by ROS. Antioxidants positively affect dominant follicle selection [32].

It has been found that cyclical ROS production and diminished antioxidant activity may contribute to oophoritis associated with autoimmune premature ovarian failure [33].

Meiosis II is promoted by antioxidants [33]. Granulosa and luteal cells respond negatively to ROS and affect MII progression, leading to diminished gonadotropin, and antisteriodogenic actions, DNA damage, and inhibited ATP progression in both humans and rats [33]. Glutathione, an antioxidant has been identified as critical for oocyte maturation, particularly in cytoplasmic maturation required for preimplantation development and formation of male sperm pronucleus [34, 35]. Beta carotene, another antioxidant, has been also recognized to enhance cytoplasmic maturation [36].

The steroid production in the leading follicle causes an increase in P450. Overexposure of the ovary to H_2O_2 causes the LH receptor to uncouple from adenylate cyclase, impairing protein synthesis and cholesterol utilization by mitochondrial P450 side chain cleavage, most likely because of impaired production of steroidogenic acute regulatory protein (StAR) [33]. StAR is responsible for moving cholesterol to the inner mitochondrial membrane where $P450_{scc}$ converts cholesterol to pregnenolone [37]. Lecithin-cholesterol acyltransferase (LCAT) plays an important role in cholesterol transport and follicular synthesis to estrogen. High follicular fluid LCAT is positively associated with ascorbate and alpha tocopherol accumulation and the presence of antioxidants in follicular fluid protect LCAT from oxidative damage and steroidogenesis [38].

Oxidative stress is important in ovulation [39]. LH surge is essential for ovulation that is triggered by oxidative stress [40]. Follicular ROS promote apoptosis and glutathione and FSH counterbalance its action. Estrogen increases in response to FSH, triggering the generation of catalase in the dominant follicle, thus avoiding apoptosis [33].

Corpus luteum is produced after ovulation and ROS are also produced in the corpus luteum. Cu, Zn-SOD decreases and ROS increases during the regression of corpus luteum. This activity parallels the change in progesterone levels. Complete disruption of the corpus luteum causes a substantial decrease of Mn-SOD in the regressed cell and cell death is imminent [40]. Cu, Zn-SOD is related to progesterone production and Mn-SOD protects luteal cells from oxidative stress [33]. There are also some other oxidative stress markers such as superoxide dismutase, Cu–Zn superoxide dismutase, Mn superoxide dismutase, glutathione peroxidase, γ glutamyl synthetase, and lipid peroxides ovarian physiology [41–43].

Glutathione concentrations are higher in mature, metaphase hamster and mouse oocytes [44]. Antioxidants aid in meiotic spindle formation in mature MII oocytes [44]. Exposure to oxidative stress before fertilization disrupts the meiotic spindle and increases the risk of abnormal zygote formation. If there is an adequate antioxidant defense, O_2^- does not affect gamete fusion [45].

Oxidative Stress and Oocyte and Embryo Quality

Oxidative stress was increased in repeated ovarian stimulation that leads to mitochondrial DNA mutation and decreased oocyte quality [46]. Lipid peroxides and 8-hydroxydeoxyguanine, a marker of DNA damage, were increased between the first and sixth cycles [46]. It has been suggested that timing antioxidant administration may have an effect on the number and quality of ovulated oocytes as assessed by morphological appearance and chromosomal distribution in female mice [47, 48]. Animals receiving antioxidant supplements showed an increased number of normal MII oocytes compared with the control group and decreased percentage of apoptotic oocytes [48]. Low intrafollicular oxygenation has been associated with decreased oocyte developmental potential as shown by increasing frequency of oocyte cytoplasmic defects, alterations in spindle morphology, impaired cleavage, and abnormal chromosomal segregation in oocytes [49]. It has been reported that high ROS follicular fluid concentrations were correlated with poor oocyte quality and diminished embryo quality [50]. High concentrations of follicular ROS are associated with compromised IVF outcomes [51, 52]. Moreover, selenium-dependent glutathione peroxidase activity and total antioxidant capacity (TAC) in follicular fluid were positively associated with fertilization rates [53, 54].

Oxidative stress is also associated with decreased embryo quality, increased embryo fragmentation, resulting from increasing apoptosis [55]. Melatonin, another antioxidant, has positive effects on oocyte quality and embryo development [56]. High levels of ROS may impair intracellular milieu and lead to disturbed metabolism [15, 57]. Oxidative stress-mediated damage of macromolecules plays a role in fetal embryopathies. Folate deficiency may lead to elevated homocysteine levels. Homocysteine was negatively associated with embryo quality on culture day 3 [58] and homocysteine-induced oxidative stress may cause some fetal abnormalities such as neural tube defects and cleft palate [59]. Higher day 1 ROS levels in culture media were associated with delayed embryonic development, high fragmentation, and development of morphologically abnormal blastocysts after prolonged culture. A significant correlation was reported between elevated ROS levels in day 1 culture media and lower fertilization rates in patients undergoing intracytoplasmic sperm injection (ICSI) [60]. Lower ROS levels were associated with higher fertilization rates, indicating the physiological relevance of low levels of ROS. Clinical pregnancy rates were also higher when antioxidant supplements were added to culture media [61].

Oxidative Stress and Aging Oocyte

ROS increase with age that may contribute to follicular atresia and decline in the number and quality of oocytes [62, 63]. It has been reported that prolonged exposure of aged oocytes to ROS negatively affects calcium hemostasis and impairs Ca^{+2} oscillation-dependent signaling and causes decline in oocyte developmental ability [64]. Oxidative stress damages telomeres and accelerates telomere shortening [65, 66]. Telomere shortening and dysfunction may lead to defects in meiosis, fertilization, and embryo development [67]. In another study, it has been found that follicular fluid catalase and glutathione transferase were lower in older women compared with young ones [68]. Studies have demonstrated that N-acetyl-L-cysteine and vitamin E protect the ovary from aging [69, 70].

Oxidative Stress and Endometrium

ROS are also found in endometrium. They are produced in stromal cells as byproducts of normal metabolism [71]. Intracellular sources of ROS are mitochondrial electron transport system, endoplasmic reticulum, nuclear membrane electron transport systems, and plasma membrane [71]. SOD is highly expressed in glandular epithelial cells and stromal cells in endometrium that plays an important role in regulation of endometrial function [72].

There is a close relationship between SOD, ROS, and PGF2α in the regulation of menstruation. In human endometrium, SOD activities decrease and ROS increase in late secretory phase, just before menstruation [72]. ROS trigger the release of PGF2α production and COX-2 mRNA expression and Cu, Zn-SOD activities decline by withdrawal of ovarian steroids in human endometrial cells [73]. The increases of PGF2α production and COX-2 mRNA expression were completely suppressed by N-acetyl-L-cysteine [74].

Withdrawal of ovarian steroids activates NF-KB via ROS which stimulate the COX-2 and PGF2α in human endometrial stromal cells [74]. NF-KB signaling pathway is present in human endometrium [74]. The gene promoter human COX-2 has a binding site for NF-KB and it has been reported that COX-2 expression is regulated by NF-KB [75, 76].

When implantation is successful and progesterone levels and Cu, Zn-SOD activities are high, ROS generation and PGF2α production is suppressed. In early pregnancy, ROS are low and Cu, Zn-SOD activities are high in the decidua [72]. On the other hand when pregnancy does not occur, the decline of ovarian steroid levels induces the decrease in Cu, Zn-SOD expression in endometrial stromal cells which stimulate PGF2α production by ROS. PGF2α causes endometrial shedding via vasoconstriction.

Decidualization of stromal cell is necessary for successful implantation. Cu, Zn-SOD, and Mn-SOD were found in decidualized stromal cells and in the endometrium of the patient [72]. Decidualization promotes production of many bioactive substances such as growth factors, cytokines, and adhesion molecules. This increase in metabolism stimulates generation of superoxide radicals in the mitochondria. Antioxidants are crucial in eliminating superoxide radicals. Blockage of Mn-SOD induction causes oxidative stress-induced cell death in human endometrial stromal cells [77]. PGF2α were lower and Cu, Zn-SOD activities were higher in the decidua of normal pregnancies compared with failed pregnancies that are accompanied with uterine bleeding and contractions [78]. Cu, Zn-SOD may contribute to uterine quiescence by preventing the accumulation of ROS leading to PGF2α synthesis and uterine contraction.

Oxidative Stress and Tubal Disease

The diagnostic accuracy of hysterosalpingography (HSG) in defining normal tubal physiology and anatomy has been questioned [79]. Consensus stated that HSG is less accurate in detecting and evaluating tubal disease than laparoscopy [80, 81] and is especially poorly suited to assess distal tubal disease and peritubal disease [82, 83]. Routine HSG misses at least one anatomical or physiological tubal abnormality in 84% of the cases [84]. Thus, undiagnosed tubal disease may be associated with unexplained infertility.

The oviduct is the first site contact with the early embryo and has the potential to contribute important factors that affect fertility. Oviduct provides an optimal environment for gamete maturation, fertilization and early embryonic development. It is an active organ that maintains and modulates the fluidic milieu for sperm capacitation, fertilization, and early embryonic development [85–87]. The environmental and metabolic stimuli from the oviduct may have a significant effect on embryonic development. Some growth factors such as insulin-like growth factor, vascular endothelial growth factor, and nitric oxide synthase have been identified as important regulatory factors of oviductal motility and embryo transport [88–91]. NO plays a role as a mediator of PGF2a-induced contractility and is important for secretory functions in the oviduct [92]. It has been reported that *Chlamydia trachomatis* induces an inflammatory response and leads to tubal epithelial destruction and functional impairment caused by high NO output mediated by inducible NOS (iNOS) [93]. Oxidative stress causes infection-induced immune reaction and inflammation-induced tissue lesions [94, 95]. Heat shock proteins (HSPs) are stress proteins that are closely associated with oxidative stress and inflammation [96]. It has been suggested that HSP60 may be involved in the pathogenesis of tubal factor infertility following *C. trachomatis* infection [97]. HSP 60 and 70 contribute to inflammation via anti-inflammatory cytokines such as IL-10 and IL-12 in the fallopian tube resulting in chronic salpingitis with tubal occlusion [98, 99].

Oxidative Stress and Pelvic Adhesions

Adhesions may be one of the etiologic factors in unexplained infertility. Pelvic pathology was found during laparoscopy in 83.4 % patients with unexplained infertility in a study [100]. Adhesions were found in 48.4 % of them [100]. Moreover, the sensitivity of HSG in detecting peritubal adhesions has been reported to be 34–75 % [101]. Twenty-one percent of adnexal adhesions and pelvic endometriosis were identified during surgery in spite of normal HSG [102]. The prevalence of peritubal adhesions was suggested to range from 8.8 to 29 % [103, 104].

Adhesiogenesis is a complex interaction of cellular components involved in inflammation and wound repair. It has been reported that ROS are associated with adhesion formation [105]. Acute oxidative stress in the peritoneum subsequently induces mesothelial cell loss or dysfunction, peritoneal fibrosis, and intra-abdominal adhesion formation [106]. Accumulation of free radicals may result in more collagen synthesis through fibrogenic processes such as transforming growth factor beta (TGF-β) activation and lipid peroxidation [107]. A positive correlation between oxidative stress and the severity of peritoneal adhesions has been demonstrated [108]. It has been also known that endometriosis, another risk factor for pelvic adhesion, is closely associated with endometriosis [6].

It has been reported that antioxidants such as methylene blue, melatonin, vitamin E, and alpha lipoic acid were able to decrease peritoneal adhesions [108, 109]. Peritoneal TAC scavenges free radicals and protects peritoneal tissue from oxidative damage. Furthermore, antioxidants have been shown to increase tissue plasminogen activator gene expression in endothelial cell cultures and to increase plasma fibrinolytic activity in humans [110–112].

Oxidative Stress and Endometriosis

Oxidative stress has been implicated in pathophysiology and progression of endometriosis [113–115]. There are several hypotheses that may explain the relationship between oxidative stress and endometriosis. Erythrocytes yield pro-inflammatory factors hemoglobin and heme, containing the redox generating iron molecule [116]. Oxidative stress precipitates endometriosis and tissue growth may result from iron, macrophages, and environmental contaminants such as polychlorinated biphenyls [117]. The peritoneal fluid of the patients have been found to contain high concentrations of malondialdehyde (MDA), proinflammatory cytokines (IL-6, TNF-alpha, and IL-beta), angiogenic factors (IL-8, VEGF), monocyte chemoattractant protein-1 [118] and oxidized LDL (ox-LDL) [119] and reduced levels of antioxidants such as total antioxidant capacity (TAC) and SOD [114, 120]. Pro-inflammatory and chemotactic cytokines play an important role in the recruitment and activation of phagocytic cells, which produce ROS and RNS [118].

Lipid peroxidation and oxidative stress have been demonstrated by increased levels of 8-iso-prostaglandin F2-alpha (8-iso-PGF2-alpha) [121, 122]. It has been reported that 8-iso-PGF2-alpha in both urine and peritoneal fluid of patients was significantly elevated [123].

Circulating levels of oxidative stress from other sources such as endometrium and ectopic endometrial implants may also contribute to the pathogenesis of endometriosis. Increased lipid–protein modification that contributes to high lipid peroxide concentrations has been shown in the endometrium of the patients with endometriosis [114, 120]. Lipid peroxidation was present in macrophage-enriched areas of both the endometrium and endometriosis implants [124]. High levels of antioxidants inhibit the proliferation of endometrial stromal cells and moderate levels of oxidative stress promote endometrial stromal cell proliferation [125].

NO was also increased in peritoneal fluid and the endometrium of the women with endometriosis [12]. Elevated levels of NO, as generated by activated macrophages, can disrupt fertility in variable ways, including altering the composition of the peritoneal fluid environment that affects ovulation, gamete transport, sperm oocyte interaction, fertilization, and early embryonic development [12]. Increased NO and NOS expression may lead to endometrial receptivity defects and hinder embryo implantation. Elevated levels of oxidative stress in oviductal fluid might have adverse effects, impairing oocyte and spermatozoa viability, fertilization, and embryo transport in women with endometriosis [105]. Oxidative stress may lead to damage to sperm plasma and acrosomal membranes, impairs motility, and hinders the ability of spermatozoa to bind to and penetrate the oocyte. DNA damage as the result of oxidative stress may contribute to failed fertilization, reduced embryo quality, failure of pregnancy and spontaneous abortion.

Immunological Infertility and Oxidative Stress

Many types of antibodies have been implicated in the pathophysiology of unexplained infertility. Antiovarian, antispermatozoal, and anticardiolipin antibodies were demonstrated in women with unexplained infertility [126, 127]. It has been reported that inadequate maternal immunosuppression might cause embryo rejection in that group [128]. The prevalence of celiac disease is also higher in these women compared with fertile women [129]. Elevated anti-*C. trachomatis* antibodies can be detected in more than 70 % of women with tubal occlusion [130]. *C. trachomatis* has a direct cytotoxic effect on the mucosa of the fallopian tube, resulting in loss of microvilli [131]. Permanent tubal damage is predominantly a consequence of a host immune response to persistent or repeated infection. Antiphospholipid antibodies are associated with thrombosis and infarction in the placenta. They inhibit the release of hCG from human placental explants, block in vitro trophoblast migration, invasion, and multinucleated cell formation, inhibit trophoblast cell adhesion molecules, and activate the complement on the trophoblast surface inducing an inflammatory response [132]. Antisperm and antiovarian antibodies may have an adverse effect on fertilization, early embryonic development, and implantation [132]. Between 10 and 30 % of women with premature ovarian failure have a concurrent autoimmune disease; the most commonly reported one is hypothyroidism. It also has a close relationship between myasthenia gravis, systemic lupus erythematosus, rheumatoid arthritis, and Crohn's disease.

It has been shown that anticardiolipin antibodies were positively correlated to plasma levels of F2-isoprostanes, sensitive markers of lipid peroxidation [133]. Paraoxonase-1 (PON-1), an antioxidant, has been found to be reduced and inversely correlated with anticardiolipin antibodies and directly with total antioxidant status [134]. Increased oxidative stress may be involved in early phases of antiphosholipid syndrome. There is also a close relationship between oxidative stress and autoimmune diseases [135]. MDA is increased and sulfhydryl groups were decreased in patients with systemic lupus erythematosus [136]. PON-1 activity and vitamin E was lower in patients with other autoimmune diseases such as psoriasis, vitiligo, and alopecia [135]. Oxidative stress is associated with autoimmune thyroid destruction and N-acetyl-L-cysteine reduces ROS and restores thyroid morphology [137].

Oxidative Stress and Endocrinological Abnormalities

Five percent of women with unexplained infertility have elevated levels of FSH in the early follicular phase which suggests diminished ovarian reserve [138, 139]. FSH and LH abnormalities may reflect a dysfunction in the pituitary-ovarian axis [140]. Furthermore, serum estradiol levels in the follicular phase and the estradiol/progesterone ratio have been shown to be elevated in that group [138, 141]. An absent midcycle elevation of prolactin has been demonstrated in women with unexplained infertility [142]. The luteal phase was impaired in 30 % of women with the presence of shorter luteal phase or decreased peak serum estradiol [138, 141]. Abnormal follicular LH pulse frequency or decreased midfollicular FSH level have been reported to induce an impaired luteal phase which may be related to functional imbalance in the hypothalamus [143]. Decreased inhibin-B and increased FSH concentrations may reflect a poor ovarian reserve [138, 144]. AMH and AMHRII polymorphisms were also associated with unexplained infertility [145].

Oxidative stress may have a close relationship with these endocrinologic abnormalities. It has been demonstrated that there is a positive association between oxidative stress and high FSH levels [146]. Exposure to supraphysiological levels of ROS is detrimental to oogonia [147]. ROS may contribute to mitochondrial dysfunction, low production of ATP due to impaired oxidative phosphorylation and impaired oogenesis, low oocyte number, and result in increased FSH and LH levels. LH surge is maintained by the oxidant/antioxidant balance [40]. Antioxidants have a positive effect in dominant follicle selection and also modulate the daily rhythm of LH and prolactin secretion and excess ROS may have a detrimental effect on these actions [32, 148]. Serum lipoperoxide levels were increased in women with luteal phase defects [149]. Antioxidants prevent luteal phase defects, they maintain progesterone production and protect corpus luteum against regression [33]. Another study demonstrated that elevated serum levels of advanced glycosylated end products (AGEs), markers of oxidative stress, have been positively correlated with serum AMH levels that may be another etiologic factor in unexplained infertility [150].

Oxidative Stress and Unexplained Infertility

Oxidative stress has been implicated in the pathophysiology of the disease. Lipid peroxidation marker, MDA, was increased and TAC was decreased in the peritoneal fluid of women with unexplained infertility [151]. It has been hypothesized that peritoneal fluid diffuses into the fallopian tube where it may cause damage to sperm.

Folate is a B9 vitamin that plays a role in amino acid metabolism, and the methylation of proteins, lipids, and nucleic acids. Acquired or hereditary folate deficiency results in homocysteine accumulation. Polymorphisms in folate-metabolizing pathways of genes may be responsible for unexplained infertility in this group [152]. Hyperhomocysteinemia may activate apoptosis leading to follicular atresia [153]. Pregnancy and implantation rates were lower and abortion rates were higher in women elevated homocysteine [154]. It disturbs the endometrium and contributes to poor oocyte quality [152]. eNOS mRNA in the endometrium of the women with unexplained infertility was significantly higher compared with controls [155]. Its increased expression suggests the detrimental effect of NO in endometrial receptivity and implantation [155]. Excess NO could impair implantation through several mechanisms. NO has been found to induce endometrial epithelial apoptosis [156, 157]. Increased eNOS expression at luminal surface could induce epithelial apoptosis and implantation failure. The second mechanism is that NO may impair implantation through localized nitrosative stress. It is suggested that excess eNOS expression can create local oxidative stress which could impair implantation [11, 158].

Increased ROS in patients with unexplained infertility suggest reduced levels of antioxidants such as vitamin E and GSH would reduce ROS scavenging ability and prevent the neutralization of toxic ROS effects [159]; however, the use of antioxidants in women with unexplained infertility is unclear. Studies are needed to explore the efficacy of antioxidant therapy in these patients.

Conclusion

Oxidative stress is an imbalance between ROS and antioxidants. There seems to be a close relationship between oxidative stress and the underlying etiologic factors that may contribute to unexplained infertility such as defective endometrial receptivity, impaired oocyte quality, premature ovarian failure, minimal and mild endometriosis, tubal disease, pelvic adhesions, and immunological and endocrinological abnormalities. Moreover, it has been demonstrated that ROS can also negatively affect ovulation, fertilization, implantation, embryo quality, and pregnancy rates. Although oxidative stress may contribute to unexplained infertility, the role of antioxidant therapy in that group remains unclear. Further studies are needed to show the effectiveness of antioxidants in that group.

References

1. Crosignani PC, Collins J, Cooke ID, Diczfalusy E, Rubin B. Unexplained infertility (recommendations of ESHRE workshop). Hum Reprod. 1993;8:977–80.
2. Siristatidis C, Bhattacharya S. Unexplained infertility: does it really exist? Does it matter? Hum Reprod. 2007;22:2084–7.
3. Collins JA, Burrows EA, Wilan AR. The prognosis for live birth among untreated infertile couples. Fertil Steril. 1995;64:22–8.
4. Bhattacharya S, Harrild K, Mollison J, Wordsworth S, Tay C, Harrold A, et al. Clomifene citrate or unstimulated intrauterine insemination compared with expectant management for unexplained infertility: pragmatic randomised controlled trial. BMJ. 2008;337:a716.
5. Agarwal A, Gupta S, Sikka S. The role of free radicals and antioxidants in reproduction. Curr Opin Obstet Gynecol. 2006;18:325–32.
6. Agarwal A, Gupta S, Sekhon L, Shah R. Redox considerations in female reproductive function and assisted reproduction: from molecular mechanisms to health implications. Antioxid Redox Signal. 2008;10:1375–403.
7. Sikka SC. Role of oxidative stress and antioxidants in andrology and assisted reproductive technology. J Androl. 2004;25:5–18.
8. Kowaltowski AJ, Vercesi AE. Mitochondrial damage induced by conditions of oxidative stress. Free Radic Biol Med. 1999;26:463–71.
9. Pierce GB, Parchment RE, Lewellyn AL. Hydrogen peroxide as a mediator of programmed cell death in the blastocyst. Differentiation. 1991;46:181–6.
10. Sugino N, Takiguchi S, Umekawa T, Heazell A, Caniggia I Oxidative stress and pregnancy outcome: a workshop report. Placenta. 2007;28(Suppl A): S48–50.
11. Dong M, Shi Y, Cheng Q, Hao M. Increased nitric oxide in peritoneal fluid from women with idiopathic infertility and endometriosis. J Reprod Med. 2001;46:887–91.
12. Gupta S, Agarwal A, Krajcir N, Alvarez JG. Role of oxidative stress in endometriosis. Reprod Biomed Online. 2006;13:126–34.
13. El Mouatassim S, Guérin P, Ménézo Y. Expression of genes encoding antioxidant enzymes in human and mouse oocytes during the final stages of maturation. Mol Hum Reprod. 1999;5:720–5.
14. Gardiner CS, Salmen JJ, Brandt CJ, Stover SK. Glutathione is present in reproductive tract secretions and improves development of mouse embryos after chemically induced glutathione depletion. Biol Reprod. 1998;59:431–6.
15. Guérin P, El Mouatassim S, Ménézo Y. Oxidative stress and protection against reactive oxygen species in the pre-implantation embryo and its surroundings. Hum Reprod Update. 2001;7:175–89.
16. Gupta S, Agarwal A, Banerjee J, Alvarez JG. The role of oxidative stress in spontaneous abortion and recurrent pregnancy loss: a systematic review. Obstet Gynecol Surv. 2007;62:335–47.
17. Behne D, Wolters W. Selenium content and glutathione peroxidase activity in the plasma and erythrocytes of non-pregnant and pregnant women. J Clin Chem Clin Biochem. 1979;17:133–5.
18. Simşek M, Naziroğlu M, Simşek H, Cay M, Aksakal M, Kumru S. Blood plasma levels of lipoperoxides, glutathione peroxidase, beta carotene, vitamin A and E in women with habitual abortion. Cell Biochem Funct. 1998;16:227–31.
19. Vural P, Akgül C, Yildirim A, Canbaz M. Antioxidant defence in recurrent abortion. Clin Chim Acta. 2000;295:169–77.
20. Wang YP, Walsh SW, Guo JD, Zhang JY. Maternal levels of prostacyclin, thromboxane, vitamin E, and lipid peroxides throughout normal pregnancy. Am J Obstet Gynecol. 1991;165:1690–4.
21. Angelucci S, Ciavardelli D, Di Giuseppe F, Eleuterio E, Sulpizio M, Tiboni GM, et al. Proteome analysis of human follicular fluid. Biochim Biophys Acta. 2006;1764:1775–85.
22. Irani K. Oxidant signaling in vascular cell growth, death, and survival: a review of the roles of reactive oxygen species in smooth muscle and endothelial cell mitogenic and apoptotic signaling. Circ Res. 2000;87:179–83.
23. Al-Gubory KH, Garrel C, Faure P, Sugino N. Roles of antioxidant enzymes in corpus luteum rescue from reactive oxygen species-induced oxidative stress. Reprod Biomed Online. 2012;25:551–60.
24. Defrère S, González-Ramos R, Lousse JC, Colette S, Donnez O, Donnez J, et al. Insights into iron and nuclear factor-kappa B (NF-kappaB) involvement in chronic inflammatory processes in peritoneal endometriosis. Histol Histopathol. 2011;26:1083–92.
25. González-Ramos R, Van Langendonckt A, Defrère S, Lousse JC, Colette S, Devoto L, et al. Involvement of the nuclear factor-κB pathway in the pathogenesis of endometriosis. Fertil Steril. 2010;94:1985–94.
26. Boutros T, Chevet E, Metrakos P. Mitogen-activated protein (MAP) kinase/MAP kinase phosphatase regulation: roles in cell growth, death, and cancer. Pharmacol Rev. 2008;60:261–310.
27. Brown MD, Sacks DB. Protein scaffolds in MAP kinase signalling. Cell Signal. 2009;21:462–9.
28. Nagai H, Noguchi T, Takeda K, Ichijo H. Pathophysiological roles of ASK1-MAP kinase signaling pathways. J Biochem Mol Biol. 2007;40:1–6.

29. Kamata H, Honda S, Maeda S, Chang L, Hirata H, Karin M. Reactive oxygen species promote TNFalpha-induced death and sustained JNK activation by inhibiting MAP kinase phosphatases. Cell. 2005;120:649–61.
30. Tropea A, Miceli F, Minici F, Tiberi F, Orlando M, Gangale MF, et al. Regulation of vascular endothelial growth factor synthesis and release by human luteal cells in vitro. J Clin Endocrinol Metab. 2006;91:2303–9.
31. Basini G, Grasselli F, Bianco F, Tirelli M, Tamanini C. Effect of reduced oxygen tension on reactive oxygen species production and activity of antioxidant enzymes in swine granulosa cells. Biofactors. 2004;20:61–9.
32. Behl R, Pandey RS. FSH induced stimulation of catalase activity in goat granulosa cells in vitro. Anim Reprod Sci. 2002;70:215–21.
33. Behrman HR, Kodaman PH, Preston SL, Gao S. Oxidative stress and the ovary. J Soc Gynecol Investig. 2001;8:S40–2.
34. Yoshida M, Ishigaki K, Nagai T, Chikyu M, Pursel VG. Glutathione concentration during maturation and after fertilization in pig oocytes: relevance to the ability of oocytes to form male pronucleus. Biol Reprod. 1993;49:89–94.
35. Eppig JJ. Coordination of nuclear and cytoplasmic oocyte maturation in eutherian mammals. Reprod Fertil Dev. 1996;8:485–9.
36. Ikeda S, Kitagawa M, Imai H, Yamada M. The roles of vitamin A for cytoplasmic maturation of bovine oocytes. J Reprod Dev. 2005;51:23–35.
37. Behrman HR, Aten RF. Evidence that hydrogen peroxide blocks hormone-sensitive cholesterol transport into mitochondria of rat luteal cells. Endocrinology. 1991;128:2958–66.
38. Cigliano L, Balestrieri M, Spagnuolo MS, Dale B, Abrescia P. Lecithin-cholesterol acyltransferase activity during maturation of human preovulatory follicles with different concentrations of ascorbate, alpha-tocopherol and nitrotyrosine. Reprod Fertil Dev. 2002;14:15–21.
39. Ruder EH, Hartman TJ, Goldman MB. Impact of oxidative stress on female fertility. Curr Opin Obstet Gynecol. 2009;21:219–22.
40. Shkolnik K, Tadmor A, Ben-Dor S, Nevo N, Galiani D, Dekel N. Reactive oxygen species are indispensable in ovulation. Proc Natl Acad Sci U S A. 2011;108:1462–7.
41. Attaran M, Pasqualotto E, Falcone T, Goldberg JM, Miller KF, Agarwal A, et al. The effect of follicular fluid reactive oxygen species on the outcome of in vitro fertilization. Int J Fertil Womens Med. 2000;45:314–20.
42. Suzuki T, Sugino N, Fukaya T, Sugiyama S, Uda T, Takaya R, et al. Superoxide dismutase in normal cycling human ovaries: immunohistochemical localization and characterization. Fertil Steril. 1999;72:720–6.
43. Sugino N, Takiguchi S, Kashida S, Karube A, Nakamura Y, Kato H. Superoxide dismutase expression in the human corpus luteum during the menstrual cycle and in early pregnancy. Mol Hum Reprod. 2000;6:19–25.
44. Zuelke KA, Jones DP, Perreault SD. Glutathione oxidation is associated with altered microtubule function and disrupted fertilization in mature hamster oocytes. Biol Reprod. 1997;57:1413–9.
45. Miesel R, Drzejczak PJ, Kurpisz M. Oxidative stress during the interaction of gametes. Biol Reprod. 1993;49:918–23.
46. Chao HT, Lee SY, Lee HM, Liao TL, Wei YH, Kao SH. Repeated ovarian stimulations induce oxidative damage and mitochondrial DNA mutations in mouse ovaries. Ann N Y Acad Sci. 2005;1042:148–56.
47. Tarin J, Ten J, Vendrell FJ, de Oliveira MN, Cano A. Effects of maternal ageing and dietary antioxidant supplementation on ovulation, fertilisation and embryo development in vitro in the mouse. Reprod Nutr Dev. 1998;38:499–508.
48. Tarin JJ, Perez-Albala S, Cano A. Oral antioxidants counteract the negative effects of female aging on oocyte quantity and quality in the mouse. Mol Reprod Dev. 2002;61:385–97.
49. Van Blerkom J, Antczak M, Schrader R. The developmental potential of the human oocyte is related to the dissolved oxygen content of follicular fluid: association with vascular endothelial growth factor levels and perifollicular blood flow characteristics. Hum Reprod. 1997;12:1047–55.
50. Das S, Chattopadhyay R, Ghosh S, Ghosh S, Goswami SK, Chakravarty BN, et al. Reactive oxygen species level in follicular fluid-embryo quality marker in IVF? Hum Reprod. 2006;21:2403–7.
51. Agarwal A, Allamaneni SS. Role of free radicals in female reproductive diseases and assisted reproduction. Reprod Biomed Online. 2004;9:338–47.
52. Pasqualotto EB, Agarwal A, Sharma RK, Izzo VM, Pinotti JA, Joshi NJ, et al. Effect of oxidative stress in follicular fluid on the outcome of assisted reproductive procedures. Fertil Steril. 2004;81:973–6.
53. Paszkowski T, Traub AI, Robinson SY, McMaster D. Selenium dependent glutathione peroxidase activity in human follicular fluid. Clin Chim Acta. 1995;236:173–80.
54. Oyawoye O, Abdel Gadir A, Garner A, Constantinovici N, Perrett C, Hardiman P. Antioxidants and reactive oxygen species in follicular fluid of women undergoing IVF: relationship to outcome. Hum Reprod. 2003;18:2270–4.
55. Yang HW, Hwang KJ, Kwon HC, Kim HS, Choi KW, Oh KS. Detection of reactive oxygen species (ROS) and apoptosis in human fragmented embryos. Hum Reprod. 1998;13:998–1002.
56. Tamura H, Takasaki A, Taketani T, Tanabe M, Kizuka F, Lee L, et al. The role of melatonin as an antioxidant in the follicle. J Ovarian Res. 2012;5:5.
57. Harvey AJ, Kind KL, Thompson JG. REDOX regulation of early embryo development. Reproduction. 2002;123:479–86.
58. Ebisch IM, Peters WH, Thomas CM, Wetzels AM, Peer PG, Steegers-Theunissen RP. Homocysteine, glutathione and related thiols affect fertility parameters in the (sub)fertile couple. Hum Reprod. 2006;21:1725–33.
59. Knott L, Hartridge T, Brown NL, Mansell JP, Sandy JR. Homocysteine oxidation and apoptosis: a potential cause of cleft palate. In Vitro Cell Dev Biol Anim. 2003;39:98–105.
60. Bedaiwy MA, Falcone T, Mohamed MS, Aleem AA, Sharma RK, Worley SE, et al. Differential growth of human embryos in vitro: role of reactive oxygen species. Fertil Steril. 2004;82:593–600.
61. Catt JW, Henman M. Toxic effects of oxygen on human embryo development. Hum Reprod. 2000;15(Suppl 2):199–206.
62. Wiener-Megnazi Z, Vardi L, Lissak A, Shnizer S, Reznick AZ, Ishai D, et al. Oxidative stress indices in follicular fluid as measured by the thermochemiluminescence assay correlate with outcome parameters in in vitro fertilization. Fertil Steril. 2004;82(Suppl 3):1171–6.
63. Tatone C, Amicarelli F, Carbone MC, Monteleone P, Caserta D, Marci R, et al. Cellular and molecular aspects of ovarian follicle ageing. Hum Reprod Update. 2008;14:131–42.
64. Takahashi T, Takahashi E, Igarashi H, Tezuka N, Kurachi H. Impact of oxidative stress in aged mouse oocytes on calcium oscillations at fertilization. Mol Reprod Dev. 2003;66:143–52.
65. Liu L, Trimarchi JR, Navarro P, Blasco MA, Keefe DL. Oxidative stress contributes to arsenic-induced telomere attrition, chromosome instability, and apoptosis. J Biol Chem. 2003;278:31998–2004.
66. Richter T, von Zglinicki T. A continuous correlation between oxidative stress and telomere shortening in fibroblasts. Exp Gerontol. 2007;42:1039–42.
67. Liu L, Franco S, Spyropoulos B, Moens PB, Blasco MA, Keefe DL. Irregular telomeres impair meiotic synapsis and recombination in mice. Proc Natl Acad Sci U S A. 2004;101:6496–501.
68. Carbone MC, Tatone C, Delle Monache S, Marci R, Caserta D, Colonna R, et al. Antioxidant enzymatic defences in human fol-

licular fluid: characterization and age-dependent changes. Mol Hum Reprod. 2003;9:639–43.
69. Yeh J, Bowman MJ, Browne RW, Chen N. Reproductive aging results in a reconfigured ovarian antioxidant defense profile in rats. Fertil Steril. 2005;84(Suppl 2):1109–13.
70. Liu J, Liu M, Ye X, Liu K, Huang J, Wang L, et al. Delay in oocyte aging in mice by the antioxidant N-acetyl-L-cysteine (NAC). Hum Reprod. 2012;27:1411–20.
71. Sugino N. The role of oxygen radical-mediated signaling pathways in endometrial function. Placenta. 2007;28(Suppl A):S133–6.
72. Sugino N, Shimamura K, Takiguchi S, Tamura H, Ono M, Nakata M, et al. Changes in activity of superoxide dismutase in the human endometrium throughout the menstrual cycle and in early pregnancy. Hum Reprod. 1996;11:1073–8.
73. Sugino N, Karube-Harada A, Kashida S, Takiguchi S, Kato H. Differential regulation of copper-zinc superoxide dismutase and manganese superoxide dismutase by progesterone withdrawal in human endometrial stromal cells. Mol Hum Reprod. 2002;8:68–74.
74. Sugino N, Karube-Harada A, Taketani T, Sakata A, Nakamura Y. Withdrawal of ovarian steroids stimulates prostaglandin F2alpha production through nuclear factor-kappaB activation via oxygen radicals in human endometrial stromal cells: potential relevance to menstruation. J Reprod Dev. 2004;50:215–25.
75. Newton R, Kuitert LM, Bergmann M, Adcock IM, Barnes PJ. Evidence for involvement of NF-kappaB in the transcriptional control of COX-2 gene expression by IL-1beta. Biochem Biophys Res Commun. 1997;237:28–32.
76. Allport VC, Slater DM, Newton R, Bennett PR. NF-kappaB and AP-1 are required for cyclo-oxygenase 2 gene expression in amnion epithelial cell line (WISH). Mol Hum Reprod. 2000;6:561–5.
77. Sugino N, Karube-Harada A, Sakata A, Takiguchi S, Kato H. Nuclear factor-kappa B is required for tumor necrosis factor-alpha-induced manganese superoxide dismutase expression in human endometrial stromal cells. J Clin Endocrinol Metab. 2002;87:3845–50.
78. Sugino N, Nakata M, Kashida S, Karube A, Takiguchi S, Kato H. Decreased superoxide dismutase expression and increased concentrations of lipid peroxide and prostaglandin F(2alpha) in the decidua of failed pregnancy. Mol Hum Reprod. 2000;6:642–7.
79. Gleicher N, Parrilli M, Redding L, Pratt D, Karande V. Standardization of hysterosalpingography and selective salpingography: a valuable adjunct to simple opacification studies. Fertil Steril. 1992;58:1136–41.
80. Opsahl MS, Miller B, Klein TA. The predictive value of hysterosalpingography for tubal and peritoneal infertility factors. Fertil Steril. 1993;60:444–8.
81. Mol BW, Collins JA, Burrows EA, van der Veen F, Bossuyt PM. Comparison of hysterosalpingography and laparoscopy in predicting fertility outcome. Hum Reprod. 1999;14:1237–42.
82. Mol BW, Swart P, Bossuyt PM, van Beurden M, van der Veen F. Reproducibility of the interpretation of hysterosalpingography in the diagnosis of tubal pathology. Hum Reprod. 1996;11:1204–8.
83. Glatstein IZ, Sleeper LA, Lavy Y, Simon A, Adoni A, Palti Z, et al. Observer variability in the diagnosis and management of the hysterosalpingogram. Fertil Steril. 1997;67:233–7.
84. Karande VC, Pratt DE, Rabin DS, Gleicher N. The limited value of hysterosalpingography in assessing tubal status and fertility potential. Fertil Steril. 1995;63:1167–71.
85. Leese HJ, Hugentobler SA, Gray SM, Morris DG, Sturmey RG, Whitear SL, et al. Female reproductive tract fluids: composition, mechanism of formation and potential role in the developmental origins of health and disease. Reprod Fertil Dev. 2008;20:1–8.
86. Rodriguez-Martinez H. Role of the oviduct in sperm capacitation. Theriogenology. 2007;68(Suppl 1):S138–46.
87. Lloyd RE, Romar R, Matás C, Gutiérrez-Adán A, Holt WV, Coy P. Effects of oviductal fluid on the development, quality, and gene expression of porcine blastocysts produced in vitro. Reproduction. 2009;137:679–87.
88. Winger QA, de los RP, Han VK, Armstrong DT, Hill DJ, Watson AJ. Bovine oviductal and embryonic insulin-like growth factor binding proteins: possible regulators of "embryotrophic" insulin-like growth factor circuits. Biol Reprod. 1997;56:1415–23.
89. Xia P, Han VK, Viuff D, Armstrong DT, Watson AJ. Expression of insulin-like growth factors in two bovine oviductal cultures employed for embryo co-culture. J Endocrinol. 1996;149:41–53.
90. Rosselli M, Dubey RK, Rosselli MA, Macas E, Fink D, Lauper U, et al. Identification of nitric oxide synthase in human and bovine oviduct. Mol Hum Reprod. 1996;2:607–12.
91. Wijayagunawardane MP, Kodithuwakku SP, Yamamoto D, Miyamoto A. Vascular endothelial growth factor system in the cow oviduct: a possible involvement in the regulation of oviductal motility and embryo transport. Mol Reprod Dev. 2005;72:511–20.
92. Perez Martinez S, Franchi AM, Viggiano JM, Herrero MB, Gimeno M. Effect of prostaglandin F2 alpha (PGF2 alpha) on oviductal nitric oxide synthase (NOS) activity: possible role of endogenous NO on PGF2 alpha-induced contractions in rat oviduct. Prostaglandins Other Lipid Mediat. 1998;56:155–66.
93. Shao R, Zhang SX, Weijdegård B, Zou S, Egecioglu E, Norström A, et al. Nitric oxide synthases and tubal ectopic pregnancies induced by Chlamydia infection: basic and clinical insights. Mol Hum Reprod. 2010;16:907–15.
94. Moncada S, Higgs EA. Endogenous nitric oxide: physiology, pathology and clinical relevance. Eur J Clin Invest. 1991;21:361–74.
95. Rosselli M, Keller PJ, Dubey RK. Role of nitric oxide in the biology, physiology and pathophysiology of reproduction. Hum Reprod Update. 1998;4:3–24.
96. Zügel U, Kaufmann SH. Role of heat shock proteins in protection from and pathogenesis of infectious diseases. Clin Microbiol Rev. 1999;12:19–39.
97. Hjelholt A, Christiansen G, Johannesson TG, Ingerslev HJ, Birkelund S. Tubal factor infertility is associated with antibodies against Chlamydia trachomatis heat shock protein 60 (HSP60) but not human HSP60. Hum Reprod. 2011;26:2069–76.
98. Dieterle S, Wollenhaupt J. Humoral immune response to the chlamydial heat shock proteins hsp60 and hsp70 in Chlamydia-associated chronic salpingitis with tubal occlusion. Hum Reprod. 1996;11:1352–6.
99. Kinnunen A, Surcel HM, Halttunen M, Tiitinen A, Morrison RP, Morrison SG, et al. Chlamydia trachomatis heat shock protein-60 induced interferon-gamma and interleukin-10 production in infertile women. Clin Exp Immunol. 2003;131:299–303.
100. Bonneau C, Chanelles O, Sifer C, Poncelet C. Use of laparoscopy in unexplained infertility. Eur J Obstet Gynecol Reprod Biol. 2012;163:57–61.
101. Rice JP, London SN, Olive DL. Reevaluation of hysterosalpingography in infertility investigation. Obstet Gynecol. 1986;67:718–21.
102. Henig I, Prough SG, Cheatwood M, DeLong E. Hysterosalpingography, laparoscopy and hysteroscopy in infertility: a comparative study. J Reprod Med. 1991;36:573–5.
103. Tsuji I, Ami K, Miyazaki A, Hujinami N, Hoshiai H. Benefit of diagnostic laparoscopy for patients with unexplained infertility and normal hysterosalpingography findings. Tohoku J Exp Med. 2009;219:39–42.
104. Fatum M, Laufer N, Simon A. Investigation of the infertile couple: should diagnostic laparoscopy be performed after normal hysterosalpingography in treating infertility suspected to be of unknown origin? Hum Reprod. 2002;17:1–3.

105. Alpay Z, Saed GM, Diamond MP. Female infertility and free radicals: potential role in adhesions and endometriosis. J Soc Gynecol Investig. 2006;13:390–8.
106. Gotloib L, Wajsbrot V, Cuperman Y, Shostak A. Acute oxidative stress induces peritoneal hyperpermeability, mesothelial loss, and fibrosis. J Lab Clin Med. 2004;143:31–40.
107. Muriel P. Nitric oxide protection of rat liver from lipid peroxidation, collagen accumulation, and liver damage induced by carbon tetrachloride. Biochem Pharmacol. 1998;56:773–9.
108. Ara C, Kirimlioglu H, Karabulut AB, Coban S, Hascalik S, Celik O, et al. Protective effect of melatonin against oxidative stress on adhesion formation in the rat cecum and uterine horn model. Life Sci. 2005;77:1341–50.
109. Galili Y, Ben-Abraham R, Rabau M, Klausner J, Kluger Y. Reduction of surgery-induced peritoneal adhesions by methylene blue. Am J Surg. 1998;175:30–2.
110. Chen PR, Lee CC, Chang H, Tsai CE. Sesamol regulates plasminogen activator gene expression in cultured endothelial cells: a potential effect on the fibrinolytic system. J Nutr Biochem. 2005;16:59–64.
111. Miyamoto S, Kawano H, Takazoe K, Soejima H, Sakamoto T, HokamakiJ, et al. Vitamin E improves fibrinolytic activity in patients with coronary spastic angina. Thromb Res. 2004;113:345–51.
112. Yoshino A, Suzuki K, Urano T, Aoki K, Takada Y, Kazui T, et al. Enhanced secretion of tissue plasminogen activator by simultaneous use of retinoic acid and ascorbic acid from tissue cultured gastroepiploic artery. Life Sci. 2002;70:1461–70.
113. Van Langendonckt A, Casanas-Roux F, Donnez J. Oxidative stress and peritoneal endometriosis. Fertil Steril. 2002;77:861–70.
114. Szczepańska M, Koźlik J, Skrzypczak J, Mikołajczyk M. Oxidative stress may be a piece in the endometriosis puzzle. Fertil Steril. 2003;79:1288–93.
115. Kao LC, Germeyer A, Tulac S, Lobo S, Yang JP, Taylor RN, et al. Expression profiling of endometrium from women with endometriosis reveals candidate genes for disease-based implantation failure and infertility. Endocrinology. 2003;144:2870–81.
116. ReubinoffBE, Har-El R, Kitrossky N, Friedler S, Levi R, Lewin A, et al. Increased levels of redox-active iron in follicular fluid: a possible cause of free radical-mediated infertility in beta-thalassemia major. Am J Obstet Gynecol. 1996;174:914–8.
117. Donnez J, Van Langendonckt A, Casanas-Roux F, Van Gossum JP, Pirard C, Jadoul P, et al. Current thinking on the pathogenesis of endometriosis. Gynecol Obstet Invest. 2002;54(Suppl 1):52–8.
118. Mier-Cabrera J, Jiménez-Zamudio L, García-Latorre E, Cruz-Orozco O, Hernández-Guerrero C. Quantitative and qualitative peritoneal immune profiles, T-cell apoptosis and oxidative stress-associated characteristics in women with minimal and mild endometriosis. BJOG. 2011;118:6–16.
119. Rong R, Ramachandran S, Santanam N, Murphy AA, Parthasarathy S. Induction of monocyte chemotactic protein-1 in peritoneal mesothelial and endometrial cells by oxidized low-density lipoprotein and peritoneal fluid from women with endometriosis. Fertil Steril. 2002;78:843–8.
120. Polak G, Kozioł-Montewka M, Gogacz M, Błaszkowska I, Kotarski J. Total antioxidant status of peritoneal fluid in infertile women. Eur J Obstet Gynecol Reprod Biol. 2001;94:261–3.
121. Montuschi P, Barnes PJ, Roberts LJ 2nd. Isoprostanes: markers and mediators of oxidative stress. FASEB J. 2004;18:1791–800.
122. Morrow JD, Awad JA, Boss HJ, Blair IA, Roberts LJ. 2nd. Non-cyclooxygenase-derived prostanoids (F2-isoprostanes) are formed in situ on phospholipids. Proc Natl Acad Sci USA. 1992;89:10721–5.
123. Sharma I, Dhaliwal LK, Saha SC, Sangwan S, Dhawan V. Role of 8-iso-prostaglandin F2alpha and 25-hydroxycholesterol in the pathophysiology of endometriosis. Fertil Steril. 2010;94:63–70.
124. Murphy AA, Palinski W, Rankin S, Morales AJ, Parthasarathy S. Evidence for oxidatively modified lipid-protein complexes in endometrium and endometriosis. Fertil Steril. 1998;69:1092–4.
125. Foyouzi N, Berkkanoglu M, Arici A, Kwintkiewicz J, Izquierdo D, Duleba AJ, et al. Effects of oxidants and antioxidants on proliferation of endometrial stromal cells. Fertil Steril. 2004;82(Suppl 3):1019–22.
126. Luborsky J, Llanes B, Roussev R, Coulam C. Ovarian antibodies, FSH and inhibin B: independent markers associated with unexplained infertility. Hum Reprod. 2000;15:1046–51.
127. Szczepańska M, Skrzypczak J, Kamieniczna M, Kurpisz M. Antizona and antisperm antibodies in women with endometriosis and/or infertility. Fertil Steril. 2001;75:97–105.
128. Klentzeris LD. The role of endometrium in implantation. Hum Reprod. 1997;12:170–5.
129. Meloni GF, Dessole S, Vargiu N, Tomasi PA, Musumeci S. The prevalence of coeliac disease in infertility. Hum Reprod. 1999;14:2759–61.
130. Rodgers AK, Wang J, Zhang Y, Holden A, Berryhill B, Budrys NM, et al. Association of tubal factor infertility with elevated antibodies to Chlamydia trachomatis caseinolytic protease P. Am J Obstet Gynecol. 2010;203(494):e7–e494.e14.
131. Cooper MD, Rapp J, Jeffery-Wiseman C, Barnes RC, Stephens DS. Chlamydia trachomatis infection of human fallopian tube organ cultures. J Gen Microbiol. 1990;136:1109–15.
132. Cline AM, Kutteh WH. Is there a role of autoimmunity in implantation failure after in-vitro fertilization? Curr Opin Obstet Gynecol. 2009;21:291–5.
133. Morrow JD, Roberts LJ 2nd. The isoprostanes. Current knowledge and directions for future research. Biochem Pharmacol. 1996;51:1–9.
134. Delgado Alves J, Ames PR, Donohue S, Stanyer L, Nourooz-Zadeh J, Ravirajan C, et al. Antibodies to high-density lipoprotein and beta2-glycoprotein I are inversely correlated with paraoxonase activity in systemic lupus erythematosus and primary antiphospholipid syndrome. Arthritis Rheum. 2002;46:2686–94.
135. Ramadan R, Tawdy A, Abdel Hay R, Rashed L, Tawfik D. The antioxidant role of paraoxonase 1 and vitamin e in three autoimmune diseases. Skin Pharmacol Physiol. 2013;26:2–7.
136. Pérez YG, Pérez LC, Netto Rde C, Lima DS, Lima ES. Malondialdehyde and sulfhydryl groups as biomarkers of oxidative stress in patients with systemic lupus erythematosus. Rev Bras Reumatol. 2012;52:658–60.
137. Poncin S, Colin IM, Decallonne B, Clinckspooor I, Many MC, Denef JF, et al. N-acetylcysteine and 15 deoxy-{delta}12,14-prostaglandin J2 exert a protective effect against autoimmune thyroid destruction in vivo but not against interleukin-1{alpha}/interferon {gamma}-induced inhibitory effects in thyrocytes in vitro. Am J Pathol. 2010;177:219–28.
138. Blacker CM, Ginsburg KA, Leach RE, Randolph J, Moghissi KS. Unexplained infertility: evaluation of the luteal phase; results of the National Center for Infertility Research at Michigan. Fertil Steril. 1997;67:437–42.
139. Luborsky J, Llanes B, Roussev R, Coulam C. Ovarian antibodies, FSH and inhibin B: independent markers associated with unexplained infertility. Hum Reprod. 2000;15:1046–51.
140. Omland AK, Fedorcsák P, Storeng R, Dale PO, Abyholm T, Tanbo T. Natural cycle IVF in unexplained, endometriosis-associated and tubal factor infertility. Hum Reprod. 2001;16:2587–92.
141. Leach RE, Moghissi KS, Randolph JF, Reame NE, Blacker CM, Ginsburg KA, et al. Intensive hormone monitoring in women with unexplained infertility: evidence for subtle abnormalities suggestive of diminished ovarian reserve. Fertil Steril. 1997;68:413–20.

142. Subramanian MG, Kowalczyk CL, Leach RE, Lawson DM, Blacker CM, Ginsburg KA, et al. Midcycle increase of prolactin seen in normal women is absent in subjects with unexplained infertility. Fertil Steril. 1997;67:644–7.
143. Nakajima ST, Gibson M. Pathophysiology of luteal-phase deficiency in human reproduction. Clin Obstet Gynecol. 1991;34:167–79.
144. van Rooij IA, Broekmans FJ, te Velde ER, Fauser BC, Bancsi LF, de Jong FH, et al. Serum anti-Müllerian hormone levels: a novel measure of ovarian reserve. Hum Reprod. 2002;17:3065–71.
145. Rigon C, Andrisani A, Forzan M, D'Antona D, Bruson A, Cosmi E, et al. Association study of AMH and AMHRII polymorphisms with unexplained infertility. Fertil Steril. 2010;94:1244–8.
146. Venkatesh S, Kumar M, Sharma A, Kriplani A, Ammini AC, Talwar P, et al. Oxidative stress and ATPase6 mutation is associated with primary ovarian insufficiency. Arch Gynecol Obstet. 2010;282:313–8.
147. Coulam CB, Adamson SC, Annegers JF. Incidence of premature ovarian failure. Obstet Gynecol. 1986;67:604–6.
148. Misztal T, Romanowicz K. Effective stimulation of daily LH secretion by the combined treatment with melatonin and naloxone in luteal-phase ewes. Acta Neurobiol Exp (Wars). 2005;65:1–9.
149. Scarpellini F, Mastrone M, Sbracia M, Scarpellini L. Serum lipoperoxide level variations in normal and luteal phase defect cycles. Gynecol Obstet Invest. 1996;42:28–30.
150. Diamanti-Kandarakis E, Piouka A, Livadas S, Piperi C, Katsikis I, Papavassiliou AG, et al. Anti-mullerian hormone is associated with advanced glycosylated end products in lean women with polycystic ovary syndrome. Eur J Endocrinol. 2009;160: 847–53.
151. Polak G, Kozioł-Montewka M, Tarkowski R, Kotarski J. Peritoneal fluid and plasma 4-hydroxynonenal and malonyldialdehyde concentrations in infertile women. Ginekol Pol. 2001;72:1316–20.
152. Altmäe S, Stavreus-Evers A, Ruiz JR, Laanpere M, Syvänen T, Yngve A, et al. Variations in folate pathway genes are associated with unexplained female infertility. Fertil Steril. 2010;94:130–7.
153. Forges T, Monnier-Barbarino P, Alberto JM, Guéant-Rodriguez RM, Daval JL, Guéant JL. Impact of folate and homocysteine metabolism on human reproductive health. Hum Reprod Update. 2007;13:225–38.
154. Pacchiarotti A, Mohamed MA, Micara G, Linari A, Tranquilli D, Espinola SB, et al. The possible role of hyperhomocysteinemia on IVF outcome. J Assist Reprod Genet. 2007;24:459–62.
155. Najafi T, Novin MG, Ghazi R, Khorram O. Altered endometrial expression of endothelial nitric oxide synthase in women with unexplained recurrent miscarriage and infertility. Reprod Biomed Online. 2012;25:408–14.
156. Castro A, Johnson MC, Anido M, Cortinez A, Gabler F, Vega M. Role of nitric oxide and bcl-2 family genes in the regulation of human endometrial apoptosis. Fertil Steril. 2002;78:587–95.
157. Johnson MC, Maliqueo M, Boric MA, Villavicencio A, Vantman D, Vega M. Differential in vitro actions of nitric oxide on human endometrial cell survival. Fertil Steril. 2004;81:176–84.
158. Wu MY, Chao KH, Yang JH, Lee TH, Yang YS, Ho HN. Nitric oxide synthesis is increased in the endometrial tissue of women with endometriosis. Hum Reprod. 2003;18:2668–71.
159. Wang Y, Sharma RK, Falcone T, Goldberg J, Agarwal A. Importance of reactive oxygen species in the peritoneal fluid of women with endometriosis or idiopathic infertility. Fertil Steril. 1997;68:826–30.

Role of Environmental Factors and Gonadotoxin Exposure in Unexplained Female Infertility

15

Victor Y. Fujimoto and Michael S. Bloom

Introduction

Information continues to emerge regarding the important roles played by environmental contaminants with respect to female reproductive health, and their impact on treatment outcomes associated with this condition [1]. Reproductive environmental health is steadily gaining global attention as study after study describe adverse effects of environmental exposures on human and mammalian reproduction [2, 3]. Unexplained female infertility, in particular, appears to have great relevance, as commonly recognized etiologies are ruled out by definition. Many environmental agents are known to display endocrine-disrupting potential, especially on reproductive tract development and function [4]. Humans are inconspicuously exposed through normal daily living activities. Some agents bioaccumulate such as the polychlorinated biphenyls (PCBs) [5] and methyl mercury [6], while others are believed to have limited half-lives within humans, such as bisphenol A (BPA) [7]. The common thread between all of these agents is that human exposure is nearly ubiquitous [8].

In this chapter, we summarize the current understanding of the role that environmental contaminants may play in unexplained female infertility. More specifically, we address infertile populations comprising eumenorrheic women without a diagnosis of polycystic ovarian syndrome (PCOS) or endometriosis. While there are many classes of environmental contaminants for which investigators express concern with respect to reproductive toxicity, herein we focus on the effects of cigarette smoke, bisphenol A, polychlorinated biphenyls, polychlorinated diphenyl ethers, perfluorinated compounds, and selected toxic elements on mammalian gametogenesis and embryogenesis, as well as human clinical/epidemiologic reproductive outcomes, including fertility therapy, and, where possible, biologic mechanisms regulating these effects. There is broad literature detailing environmental contamination and reproduction in nonmammalian vertebrates which are not necessarily included in this chapter but are available for review [9, 10]. Essentially, we aim to provide a better appreciation for the effects of various toxic substances on the health and well-being of the female gamete, the human oocyte, and by doing so shed some light on potential etiologies for unexplained female infertility.

V. Y. Fujimoto (✉) · M. S. Bloom
Obstetrics, Gynecology and Reproductive Sciences,
University of California at San Francisco, 2356 Sutter Street, 7th floor, San Francisco, CA 94115-0916, USA
e-mail: fujimotov@obgyn.ucsf.edu

Exposure to Cigarette Smoke

According to the World Bank, approximately 8 % of women and 39 % of men were identified as tobacco smokers in 2006 [11]. The highest percentage of female cigarette smokers existed in Europe and Central Asia although 19 and 25 % of US women and men, respectively, reported active smoking. There are approximately 4000 chemical compounds identified in cigarette smoke, many that are potentially hazardous to reproductive health [12]. Cigarette smoking has long been known to have negative effects on both oocytes and embryos [13]. Many epidemiologic studies have demonstrated a clear association between smoking and reduced fecundity [14, 15]. The time to pregnancy (TTP), in which longer times are associated with compromised fecundity, is consistently delayed in smokers compared to nonsmokers, among populations conceiving unassisted and among those employing in vitro fertilization (IVF) [14, 16, 17]. Van Voorhis et al. found a 50 % reduction in implantation rate in smokers undergoing IVF [18]. A recent study demonstrated a delay in implantation from spontaneous conception in smokers compared to nonsmokers, suggesting impaired reproductive processes [19] and smoking was associated with an increased risk for early pregnancy loss [20]. Studies among women undergoing IVF suggest the deleterious impact is not limited to direct exposure, in that adverse IVF outcomes were increased among women exposed only to second-hand smoke as well [21, 22]. While cigarette smoking is generally avoided following recognition of pregnancy, many women and their

G. L. Schattman et al. (eds.), *Unexplained Infertility*, DOI 10.1007/978-1-4939-2140-9_15,

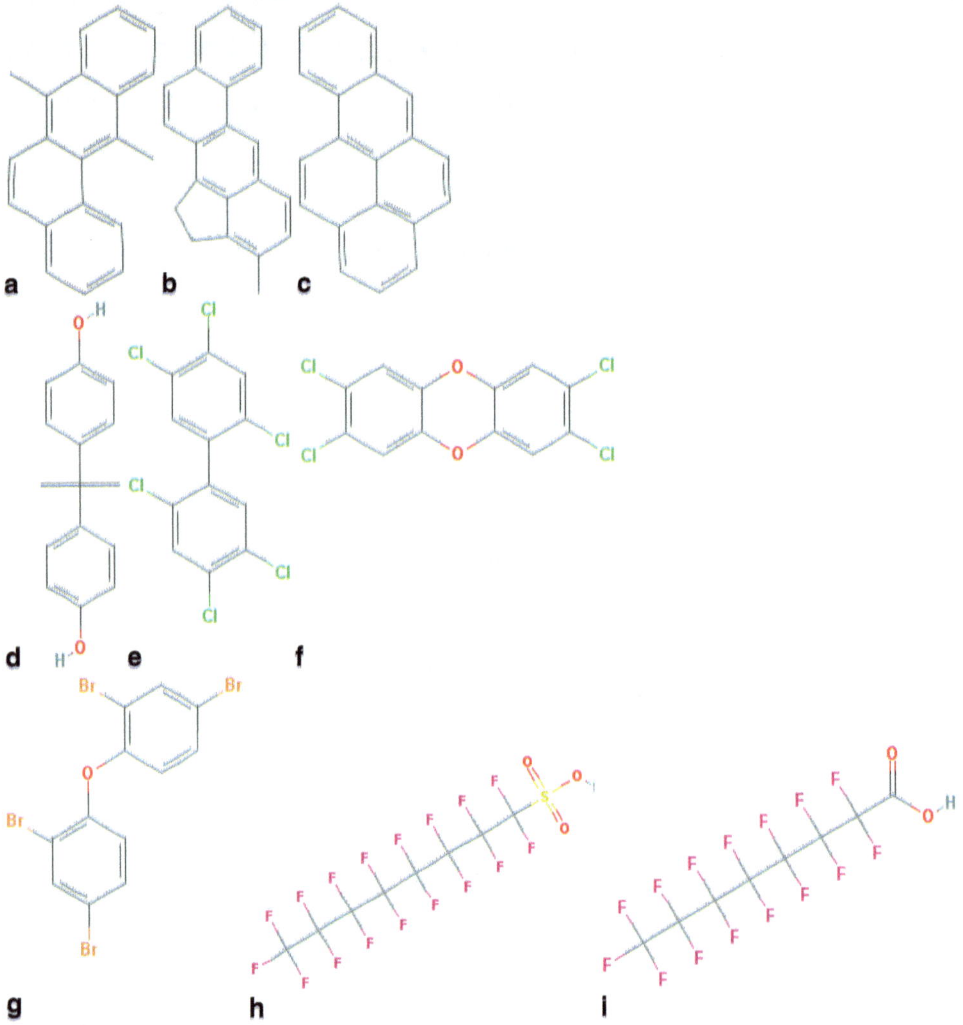

Fig. 15.1 Two-dimensional structures for selected environmental organic pollutants with recognized potential for human reproductive toxicity. **a** 9,10-dimethylbenzanthracene (DMBA). **b** 3-methylcholanthrene (3-MC). **c** Benzo[*a*]pyrene (BaP). **d** 2,2-bis(4-hydroxyphenyl) propane (Bisphenol A, BPA). **e** 2,2'4,4',5,5'-hexachlorobiphenyl (PCB #153). **f** 2,3,7,8-tetrachlorodibenzodioxin (2,3,7,8-TCDD). **g** 2,2',4,4'-tetrabromodiphenyl ether (PBDE #47). **h** Perfluorooctane sulfonate (PFOS). **i** Perfluorooctanoic acid (PFOA). (Source: Reprinted from the National Center for Biotechnology, US National Library of Medicine, PubChem Compound Database, http://pubchem.ncbi.nlm.nih.gov/. Accessed April 21, 2013)

physicians are relatively unaware of the negative impact that cigarette smoking can have on their own as well as their offspring's reproductive health. In fact, the American Society for Reproductive Medicine (ASRM) has produced practice guidelines with a position statement on smoking and reduced fecundity to educate infertile patients who smoke on the potential adverse effects of smoking [23].

There is increasing evidence to suggest multiple mechanisms underlying the effect of cigarette smoke. The adverse actions of chemicals in cigarette smoke may act at the levels of ovarian, tubal, and endometrial function. Concentrations of cotinine, a stable metabolite of nicotine with a half-life of approximately 18–20 h in humans, correlate strongly with tobacco consumption [24]. Cadmium, a potent reproductive toxicant [25], is selectively bioaccumulated by the tobacco plant and levels also correlate to tobacco consumption [26]. Both cotinine and cadmium are present in human follicular fluid, with higher levels in smokers than nonsmokers [27, 28], and have been associated with compromised oocyte quality [29]. Additional toxins recognized in cigarette smoke include the class of compounds known as polycyclic aromatic hydrocarbons (PAHs) [30]. PAHs comprise a family of > 100 related chemical structures consisting of fused aromatic carbon and hydrogen rings and formed as byproducts of incomplete combustion. Specific PAH compounds of interest include 9,10-dimethylbenzanthracene (DMBA), 3-methylcholanthrene (3-MC), and benzo[*a*]pyrene (BaP) (see Fig. 15.1a–c). PAHs, including BaP, have been detected in the follicular fluid of women using IVF [31]. A highly reactive intermediary diol epoxide metabolite of BaP has also been detected in human follicular fluid, and was associated with increased DNA adduct formation in luteinized granulosa cells recovered during IVF, and also correlated with cotinine levels, suggesting an increased risk for granulosa cell DNA damage with cigarette smoking [32]. PAH compounds compromise granulosa cell function, have been indirectly associated with the development of ovarian tumors [33–35], and are linked to an increased risk for mucinous ovarian carcinoma in epidemiologic studies [36, 37].

The most concerning impact of cigarette smoke on female reproduction may be the decline in ovarian reserve associated with chronic exposure. This effect on the "biological clock" is supported by the association of cigarette smoking with an earlier age at menopause [38–40]. Sharara et al. described increased abnormal clomiphene challenge testing in women who smoked cigarettes [41]. While other studies have confirmed an association between cigarette smoking and elevated basal FSH levels [42–44], DMBA, 3-MC, and BaP are known to be ovotoxins, resulting in significant destruction of primordial and primary follicles in mice and rats [45, 46]. There is evidence that PAH-induced reduction of primordial follicles operates via aryl hydrocarbon receptor (AhR)-regulated Bax expression [47, 48]. Furthermore, meiotic spindle disruption is a probable sequelae to cigarette smoke exposure, an increased likelihood for the recovery of diploid oocytes, and a reduced proportion of mature oocytes was reported for cigarette smoking IVF patients [49, 50]. That noted, it is not fully established whether human ovarian antral follicle pools are diminished in response to cigarette smoking when adjusted for maternal age [44, 51]. In a retrospective epidemiologic study, ovarian response during IVF, defined by the number of mature oocytes retrieved following controlled ovarian stimulation, was less in 40 cigarette smokers than in 71 nonsmokers, although correlations were not adjusted for age [52]. A more recent epidemiologic study describes an increased age-related rate of ovarian follicle decline in smokers compared to nonsmokers, suggestive of a negative impact on ovarian reserve [53].

Interestingly, ex-smokers appear to have a similar fecundity rate, compared with nonsmokers implying that active exposure to chemicals in cigarette smoke during the follicular phase and/or luteal phase of the menstrual cycle inhibits normal reproductive processes [54]. There may also be contributing endometrial dysfunction as demonstrated in a large retrospective epidemiologic study in which lower pregnancy rates, and higher rates of multiplicity, were associated with heavy cigarette smoking in an oocyte donation-recipient model [55]. Mechanistically, tubal motility and ciliary function have been implicated as targets of cigarette contaminant exposures [56–58]. Evidence from human fetal ovaries also suggests that somatic cells comprising the ovarian follicle may be influenced by cigarette smoke, which may have profound long-term effects on oocyte development [59]. In a recent epidemiologic study, first trimester maternal smoking was linked to an earlier age of onset of menarche, underscoring the likelihood for developmental programming effects that may later compromise fertility [60]. There is also evidence that women who smoke cigarettes have an increased risk of spontaneous fetal loss [14, 61, 62], and that the risk extends to women exposed as children through smoking parents [63]. However, other studies have not clearly demonstrated an association between maternal cigarette smoking and risk of spontaneous abortion, and so a causal association remains questionable [64–68]. In addition to the risk of spontaneous miscarriage, multiple studies have demonstrated an increased risk of ectopic pregnancy associated with active cigarette smoking [69, 70].

Collectively, the literature points towards a negative impact of cigarette smoking on ovarian aging as well as compromised oocyte function and embryo development. Furthermore, these effects do not only appear to be limited to the smoker herself but are also elicited by second-hand exposure to sidestream smoke in the environment. For women achieving pregnancy, cigarette smoke exposure is also associated with an increased risk for an ectopic implantation as well as spontaneous loss. For those women with live births, gestational exposure to maternal smoking may compromise future reproductive development leading to infertility in the offspring of smokers.

Exposure to Bisphenol A

Bisphenol A (BPA) has gained considerable attention as an environmental chemical with multiple adverse effects on human health and disease. The chemical composition of bisphenol A is 2,2-bis(4-hydroxyphenyl)propane (see Fig. 15.1d). BPA is produced in large quantities (greater than 6 billion pounds per year) as it is incorporated into various resins and plastics (e.g., polycarbonate). Hence, the exposure to BPA is ubiquitous in the USA, frequenting many aspects of daily living primarily through dietary consumption [8]. The Chapel Hill Bisphenol A expert panel issued a consensus statement in 2007 on the relationship between BPA and human health effects [71]. BPA appears to have endocrine disrupting effects through steroid receptor binding. BPA binds to the nuclear estrogen receptor with weak affinity. Recent evidence suggests it may act to induce physiologic responses through cell membrane estrogen receptors in low pg/mL concentrations [72]. BPA levels in humans have been measured in the parts per billion range in serum [73, 74] and urine [75, 76]. The relevance of low levels of BPA exposure in humans remains in question pertaining to significant reproductive biologic effects [77–80].

Adverse female reproductive effects of BPA exposure have been described with respect to meiotic aberrations in the oocyte. In 2000, Takai et al. published their work on the effects of BPA on early embryo development [81]. Two-cell mouse embryos were cultured with BPA at low, environmentally relevant doses in the presence or absence of Tamoxifen, a selective estrogen receptor modulator; blastocyst advancement was adversely affected. A direct link between BPA and murine aneuploidy was first reported by Hunt and colleagues, in which a dramatic increase from 1–2% to 40% was observed in chromosomal alignment defects in the first meiotic spindle [82]. This observation was ultimately traced and attributed to the leaching of BPA from damaged polycarbonate cages and water bottles in which the female mice were housed during the final stages of oocyte maturation. The effects of in utero BPA exposure may also be transgenerational. In 2007, Susiarjo et al. reported abnormal pachytene associations and abnormalities in synaptonemal complex structures of BPA-exposed murine fetuses with higher rates of aneuploidy [83]. A similar meiotic phenotype in prophase fetal oocytes of ßERKO −/− mice with similar rates of synaptonemal aberrations (57 %), compared to those of the BPA-exposed female murine fetuses (52 %), supports the estrogen receptor ß as a potential site of interaction with BPA as a pathway for meiotic disruption.

The clinical relevance of BPA is emerging. A study from Japan was published in which 45 patients with a history of three or more first trimester miscarriages without uterine anomaly or blood karyotype abnormality (study group) and 32 healthy nonpregnant women without prior pregnancy loss (control group) underwent serum BPA testing [84]. Mean serum BPA levels were significantly higher in the study group compared to the control group (2.59 vs. 0.77 ng/mL), concluding that serum BPA is associated with recurrent miscarriage. Yet, methods employed in this study introduced several limitations, including the use of an enzyme-linked immunosorbent assay (ELISA) to assess BPA exposure [85], the cross-sectional assessment of BPA which has a half-life of only several hours, a lack of consideration for "critical" biologic windows in timing the exposure assessment (such as during the LH surge when BPA exposure is most likely to affect the meiotic transition from metaphase I to metaphase II), and the different demographics utilized for recruitment of patients and control subjects. However, additional clinical studies have recently been published with respect to BPA. Serum unconjugated and urinary conjugated BPA levels both inversely correlate with fertilization rates of exposed human oocytes [86, 87]. Additionally, BPA appears to influence estradiol production by inhibiting aromatase activity in vitro [88]. Clinical evidence supporting reduced estradiol secretion exists based on lower peak estradiol responses to gonadotropin stimulation during IVF with increasing BPA exposures [73, 89]. Another study by Hanna et al. explored the potential role of BPA in altering methylation sites in women undergoing IVF [90]. They found BPA to be associated with lower methylation of the promoter region of the TSP (testes-specific protease) 50 gene. However, no evidence has been published to date, to indicate that BPA exposure is associated with increased rates of human embryonic aneuploidy.

Exposure to Polychlorinated Biphenyls

Polychlorinated biphenyls comprise a family of 209 structurally related compounds, or congeners, consisting of two carbon–hydrogen phenyl rings, with a spectrum of chlorine substituents that determine activity. The PCB congener 2,2',4,4',5,5'-hexachlorobiphenyl (PCB #153, see Fig. 15.1e) tends to be found most frequently in US biospecimens, although the relative contributions of various congeners to total PCB body burdens vary. PCBs were originally manufactured as chemical mixtures, variously composed to suit a wide range of industrial applications. These chemicals are ubiquitous and persistent in the environment due to their chemical stability, lipophilic character, and low water solubility [5]. While banned from production in most countries in the 1970s, the persistence of PCBs makes them relevant as environmental contaminants potentially influencing reproductive outcomes. The food chain is the primary source of human exposure, as PCBs bioaccumulate in animal fats leading to biomagnification. PCB congeners were recently classified as carcinogenic to humans by the World Health Organization's International Agency for Research on Cancer (IARC) [91], and variously possess estrogenic and antiestrogenic properties [92]. Congeners absent a chlorine (Cl) substituent at three or four of the ortho-carbon positions can assume a "coplanar" configuration and interact with the AhR, eliciting dioxin-like effects [93], including proinflammatory properties that increase oxidative stress [94].

The first report of PCBs causing reproductive harm came from a 1980s study based in the Netherlands. A decline in the Wassen Sea seal population was traced to reduced litters associated with PCB and DDE contamination [95]. Consumption of sport-caught fish fosters increased exposure to PCBs [96], reflected in higher levels in the serum of sport fish consumers [97, 98]. Several epidemiologic studies have reported associations between PCB body burden and outcomes related to female fertility. A recent prospective cohort study of women, exposed through the consumption of Great Lakes sport fish, reported increased time to pregnancy in association with exposure to estrogenic and antiestrogenic PCB congeners [99]. An association between estrogenic PCBs and increased menstrual cycle length was reported from the same study [100]. Another, larger prospective cohort study with preconception participant enrollment also reported associations between pregnancy delays and PCB congeners [101]. Similar results have been reported by European investigators [102, 103]. Maternal serum PCB concentrations have been documented during critical windows of development, including the periconception interval and early pregnancy [104], and PCB levels are detectable within human follicular fluid [105, 106]. More recently, follicular fluid and serum PCBs have been associated with reduced oocyte fertilization [107] and with reduced embryo implantation during IVF [108], although a systematic review concluded that the epidemiologic evidence to date is insufficient to support a causal association [109].

A substantial number of studies in mammalian models demonstrate the effects of PCBs on ovarian function, oogenesis, and embryogenesis, corroborating positive results reported from epidemiologic investigations in women. In vitro experiments report disrupted oocyte maturation, impaired fertilization, and compromised bovine embryo growth in a dose-dependent manner [110, 111]. Earlier studies demonstrated disruption of estrus and menstrual cycles in rats and primates [112–115], and the negative effects of several PCB mixtures on the fertilizability of murine oocytes [116–118]. More recently, altered synthesis of estradiol, testosterone and progesterone by human cell cultures was reported following treatment with individual PCB congeners [119]. The "dioxin-like" PCB congener #77 was also found to decrease fertilization potential in murine oocytes when female mice were fed a contaminated diet [120]. In another study, a mix of PCBs and related compounds reduced porcine oocyte cumulus expansion in a dose-dependent manner and decreased blastocyst formation [121]. Female rabbits also experienced reduced blastocyst formation following treatment three times a week with a PCB mixture [122].

Investigation has suggested a role for the AhR, as a mechanism to explain murine ovarian weight and cyclicity effects reported following experimental PCB exposure [123, 124]. However, contradictory evidence identified AhR −/− mice to be fertile without compromised reproduction, raising the question of whether PCB effects on reproduction are mediated via other mechanisms [125]. Further evidence against an exclusive role for AhR mediated embryo-toxic effects by PCBs is provided by post-exposure AhR independent changes in rabbit blastocyst gene expression [126]. Though at higher concentrations than typically experienced by human populations, there is clear evidence in various mammalian models that oocyte competence and early embryo development can be compromised by exposures to PCBs.

Exposure to Dioxins

Dioxins represent a class of organic chemicals that are structurally related to PCBs, typically including polychlorinated dibenzodioxins (PCDDs), polychlorinated dibenzofurans (PCDFs), and coplanar polychlorinated biphenyls (co-PCBs). Dioxins are formed primarily as a byproduct of the incomplete combustion of chlorine-containing materials, or as inadvertent contaminants in chemical synthesis; they tend to bioaccumulate and to have very long in vivo half-lives [127]. The most potent dioxin is 2,3,7,8-tetrachlorodibenzodioxin (2,3,7,8-TCDD; see Fig. 15.1f), to which humans are generally exposed via consumption of contaminated food products and inhalation around municipal waste incinerators. TCDD has been classified as a human carcinogen by the IARC [128] and displays antiestrogenic endocrine-disrupting properties [129]. Furthermore, detectable concentrations have been reported in human follicular fluid [130]. Similar to PAHs, dioxins bind as AhR ligands with downstream gene activation and expression [131]. Though the antiestrogenic effects of dioxins are primarily attributed to an increased rate of hepatic estradiol metabolism, there is also evidence that TCDD acts as an endocrine disruptor to reduce estrogen biosynthesis within the ovarian follicle via actions on 17,20-lyase activity of the P450c17 enzyme complex [132]. TCDD may influence ovarian reserve via the AhR activation pathway, similar to PAHs [133, 134].

The clinical evidence for dioxin exposure and impaired fertility among women comes mainly from the Seveso Women's Health Study, which studied an Italian village population north of Milan, exposed to high levels of 2,3,7,8-TCDD from a 1976 chemical plant explosion that released ~30 kg into the atmosphere [135, 136]. Measurable serum levels of TCDD in Seveso residents ranged from 2.5–56,000 parts per trillion (ppt), with a background of 20 ppt among members of a nonexposed reference group [137]. The evidence that dioxins adversely affect female infertility is sparse however and further studies need to be performed to clearly define the risk at more commonly encountered levels in the environment and the potential impact on unexplained female infertility.

Exposure to Polybrominated Diphenyl Ethers

Polybrominated diphenyl ethers (PBDEs) comprise a family of 209 closely related lipophilic chemicals, structurally analogous to PCBs, with the exceptions of bromine substituents and an ether bond. The PBDE congener 2,2',4,4'-tetrabromodiphenyl ether (PBDE #47, see Fig. 15.1g) tends to be found most frequently in US biospecimens, although the relative contributions of various congeners to total PBDE body burdens vary. Like PCBs, these compounds were variously manufactured as mixtures to suit particular purposes, primarily blended into commercial products as flame-retardants [138]. However, their appearance in the environment is more recent, having been introduced in the early 1970s, but now distributed to humans and biota worldwide in near ubiquitous fashion [139]. Given their environmental persistence and lipophilic nature, PBDEs tend to bioaccumulate in animal fats with long half-lives [140], raising concerns with respect to human health. Exposure is likely through inhalation and ingestion of contaminated dust, and through consumption of contaminated food products. Use of the most common PBDE mixtures are being phased out (i.e., deca-BDE) or eliminated in the USA (penta-BDE and octa-BDE), but concerns remain due to the persistence of PBDE congeners in the environment and their widespread presence in commercial products.

There have been few epidemiologic studies of human fertility and PBDE exposures published to date. An increased risk for early onset of menarche in US adolescents was recently reported from a cross-sectional investigation [141]. No association between breast milk PBDE concentrations and menstrual cycle length was reported from a small cross-sectional study conducted among pregnant women in Taiwan [142]. An increased time to pregnancy was reported in association with higher serum PBDE levels among pregnant members of a Mexican-immigrant community in California, at concentrations higher than those measured in the Taiwan study, yet no association was detected for menstrual cycle parameters [143]. In a very large French cohort study, no association was reported for time to pregnancy in association with serum concentrations of a single PBDE congener; however, the latter was infrequently detected among members of the study sample [103]. A more recent prospective study of women undergoing IVF reported an increased implantation failure rate associated with increased follicular fluid PBDE concentrations [144]. In contrast, the recent prospective study with preconception enrollment of women conceiving unassisted reported no associations with PBDEs, following adjustment for confounding variables [101].

Endocrine disruptive effects have been reported for PBDEs and their OH-PBDE metabolites using experimental models [145]. Estrogen and progesterone receptor binding with agonistic or antagonistic effects have been demonstrated using in vitro systems and in vivo using rodents systems [146, 147], as has binding to the androgen receptor, also with antagonistic effects in vitro and in vivo [146, 148]. Furthermore, OH-PBDE metabolites inhibit aromatase activity in vitro [149]. Gestational exposure at environmentally relevant doses elicited structural changes in ovaries, and altered folliculogenesis at higher concentrations [150, 151]. Changes to uterine estrogen-mediated gene expression and the distribution of uterine progesterone receptors was also reported in association with nontoxic PBDE exposures [152]. While many experimental effects have been reported at doses exceeding those usually experienced by humans, differential sensitivities between women and model organisms, and long-term human exposures complicate extrapolation of these data. Moreover, additive or synergistic effects between PBDEs and related compounds such as PCBs may potentiate the impact of low doses [153], and in doing so play an important role in unexplained female infertility.

Exposure to Perfluorinated Compounds

Fluorotelomer and sulfonamide alcohols are widely employed for industrial and commercial applications, including use as surfactants and chemical intermediates, and integrated into food packaging, stain resistant and "non-stick" coatings, and "breathable" waterproof fabrics [154]. Though first used in the 1950s, only recently did the widespread distribution of their breakdown products, the most prevalent of which are perfluoroctane sulfonate (PFOS) and perfluorooctanoic acid (PFOA) (see Fig. 15.1h–i), become widely appreciated by the scientific community [155]. Due to a highly stable carbon-fluorine backbone, environmental persistence is essentially indefinite and their tendency to bind serum proteins and to undergo enterohepatic circulation results in human bioaccumulation. People are generally thought to be exposed through drinking water contamination and use of relevant products. Concerns have led to a voluntary reduction and phase out of PFOS and PFOA by leading US manufacturers.

Similar to PBDEs, human investigation into potential effects on female fertility has been sparse to date. A large prospective epidemiologic study recently reported an increased time to pregnancy in association with higher maternal PFOS and PFOA measured early in gestation [156]. Yet, questions with respect to the temporal nature of the association in that study have been raised by a more recent retrospective investigation [157, 158], complicating the interpretation of these data. Two additional prospective studies recently reported no associations for PFOS or PFOA with conception [101, 159]. Experimental studies in mice have reported altered estrous cyclicity following PFOS treatment [160], and dose-dependent increases in total litter resorption following PFOA treatment [161], albeit at levels exceeding those typically experienced by women. Additional studies suggest PFOS and PFOA possess estrogenic and antiestrogenic activities [162, 163]. No adverse reproductive effects were detected at non-toxic PFOS doses in an earlier two-generation rat study [164] although these results were limited by rapid metabolism and elimination of perfluorinated compounds by the female rat, whereas the elimination half-life in humans is measured in years. Given the widespread distribution and persistence of these compounds, additional investigation is necessary to more conclusively evaluate the potential for reproductive toxicity and possible contributions to unexplained female infertility.

Exposure to Toxic Elements

Another area of emerging interest is the potential effect of toxic elements on female reproductive potential, including arsenic (As), cadmium (Cd), lead (Pb), and mercury (Hg). Though nonessential, toxic elements are distributed in ubiquitous fashion, with detectable levels reported for the vast majority of the US population [8], and investigators have reported accumulation of these agents in female reproductive tissues [165]. There are several environmental sources of exposure, including inhalation of polluted air and consumption of contaminated water and food. Seafood is an important exposure source due to bioaccumulation, and in some cases biomagnification, in the aquatic food chain [166, 167]. Consumption of shellfish, especially bivalves, has been shown to increase exposure to Cd [168]. As mentioned previously, though cigarette smoke is a potent source of Cd exposure, it also contributes to Pb and As exposure. Consumption of predatory fish species has been shown to contribute to the bodily accumulation of the organic species of Hg in particular (methyl-Hg), exposure to which is considered a modifiable health risk. The US National Research Council (NRC) recommends dietary exposure to no more than 0.1 μg/kg per day methyl-Hg, approximately equivalent to a blood Hg level of <5.8 μg/L [169]. Recently published data from the US National Health and Nutrition Examination Survey (NHANES) reveal that Asian women have significantly higher blood Hg than other races surveyed [170], indicating that they are potentially at greater risk for reproductive toxicity from methyl-Hg. For many, consumption of As contaminated drinking water is an important source of exposure to the highly toxic inorganic As species as well as to Pb [171]. Whereas seafood exposes consumers mostly to the relatively innocuous organic species of As [172]. In addition, the widespread use of herbal health and complementary therapies in the USA [173] and elsewhere may also place some groups at an increased risk for reproductive toxicity [174, 175]. A recent case of Pb intoxication resulting from the use of a contaminated herbal infertility treatment underscores the potential significance of this source [176].

Amassing evidence in vitro and in vivo demonstrates adverse reproductive outcomes associated with environmental exposures to toxic elements, including early pregnancy loss and decreased fecundity associated with Hg, Cd, Pb, and As exposures in women [3, 177]. Adverse female reproductive effects have been demonstrated rather clearly at high levels of exposure, such as those encountered in the workplace [178]. For example, Rowland et al. found reduced fertility outcomes among female dental assistants exposed to Hg vapor [179]. However, the effects of the lower, or "trace" doses frequently encountered in the environment are more controversial. Epidemiologic studies of populations lacking occupational exposure reported altered sex-steroid hormone economy [180], and have been associated with clinical female infertility [181–183], increased time to pregnancy [184, 185], and altered oocyte maturation [186, 187], oocyte fertilization [188], embryo development [189], and embryo implantation [190, 191] during IVF. In contrast, other studies do not support an association between pregnancy and female exposures to environmental levels of toxic elements [192–195]. These studies are preliminary though intriguing and warrant further investigation to better understand the potential harm on female reproductive potential caused by exposures to toxic elements widespread throughout the environment.

Using experimental systems in vitro and in vivo, investigators have identified several potential biologic mechanisms by which toxic elements might contribute to unexplained female infertility. Elements including As, Cd, Pb, and Hg enter eukaryotic cells [196] and in doing so can disrupt cytoskeletal function [197, 198], and increase oxidative damage by depletion of protective antioxidant molecules [199] and generation of reactive oxygen species [200]. Investigators also report estrogen-receptor interaction for each As, Cd, Pb, and Hg at concentrations similar to those to which humans are exposed through background sources and with physiologic effects downstream [201–204]. In addition, altered progesterone synthesis has been reported in association with Cd exposure by several studies employing in vitro granulosa cell culture models or in vivo murine models [205]. Disrupted progesterone synthesis has also been demonstrated in association with Hg treatment in vitro and in vivo, using fish oocytes [206]. Potentially inheritable genetic modifications involving gene regulation, rather than nucleic acid substitutions, or "epigenetic" changes have also been linked to toxic element exposure in experimental studies [207, 208] as well as in human observational studies [90]. Alterations in the expression of genes involved in cell replication, or the synthesis of factors required by an early embryo for navigating the early stages of uterine invasion and placentation could feasibly contribute to unexplained female infertility. While many potential biologic mechanisms exist, harmonization of the experimental and epidemiologic literature at environmentally relevant doses will require additional investigation so that the risk to female unexplained infertility can be more definitively assessed.

Summary

There is ever increasing evidence that environmental contaminant exposures may adversely affect human reproduction through effects on female reproductive potential. While cigarette smoking and its component chemicals are known toxic agents affecting the quality and quantity of oocytes, other toxic substances ubiquitous in our environment such as BPA, PCBs, dioxins, PBDEs, perfluorinated compounds, and toxic elements appear to have reproductive toxic effects at environmentally relevant levels as well. That said further studies are clearly needed to fully understand the impact of these various toxic environmental exposures on female as well as male infertility. Large, prospective epidemiologic-based studies are needed to address potentially subtle effects of various environmental contaminants on reproductive health. Within the framework of such studies, we can realize and appropriately counsel the infertile female patient on best practices regarding environmental and lifestyle exposures to toxic substances.

References

1. Sutton P, Giudice LC, Woodruff TJ. Reproductive environmental health. Curr Opin Obstet Gynecol. 2010;22(6):517–24.
2. Caserta D, Mantovani A, Marci R, Fazi A, Ciardo F, La Rocca C, et al. Environment and women's reproductive health. Hum Reprod Update. 2011;17(3):418–33.
3. Mendola P, Messer LC, Rappazzo K. Science linking environmental contaminant exposures with fertility and reproductive health impacts in the adult female. Fertil Steril. 2008;89(2, Suppl. 1):e81-e94.
4. Sanderson JT. The steroid hormone biosynthesis pathway as a target for endocrine-disrupting chemicals. Toxicol Sci. 2006;94(1):3–21.
5. Safe SH. Polychlorinated biphenyls (PCBs): environmental impact, biochemical and toxic responses, and implications for risk assessment. Crit Rev Toxicol. 1994;24(2):87–149.
6. Clarkson TW. The three modern faces of mercury. Environ Health Perspect. 2002;110(Suppl. 1):11–23.
7. Volkel W, Colnot T, Csanady GA, Filser JG, Dekant W. Metabolism and kinetics of bisphenol A in humans at low doses following oral administration. Chem Res Toxicol. 2002;15(10):1281–7.
8. Centers for Disease Control (CDC). Fourth National Report on Human Exposure to Environmental Chemicals. Report. Atlanta, GA; 2009.
9. De Luca-Abbott SB, Wong BSF, Peakall DB, Lam PKS, Young L, Lam MHW, et al. Review of effects of water pollution on the breeding success of waterbirds, with particular reference to ardeids in Hong Kong. Ecotoxicology. 2001;10(6):327–49.
10. Guillette Jr LJ Moore BC. Environmental contaminants, fertility, and multioocytic follicles: a lesson from wildlife? Semin Reprod Med. 2006;24(3):134–41.
11. The World Bank. World development indicators 2010. Washington, D.C.: International Bank for Reconstruction and Development; 2010.
12. Hoffmann D, Hoffmann I. The changing cigarette, 1950–1995. J Toxicol Environ Health. 1997;50(4):307–64.
13. Neal MS, Foster WG, Younglai EV. The detrimental effect of smoking on female fertility and IVF success. Curr Womens Health Rev. 2008;4(1):16–24.
14. Augood C, Duckitt K, Templeton AA. Smoking and female infertility: a systematic review and meta-analysis. Hum Reprod. 1998;13(6):1532–9.
15. Hull MGR, North K, Taylorb H, Farrow A, Christopher L, Ford W. Delayed conception and active and passive smoking. Fertil Steril. 2000;74(4):725–33.
16. Hughes EG, Brennan BG. Does cigarette smoking impair natural or assisted fecundity? Fertil Steril. 1996;66(5):679–89.
17. Klonoff-Cohen H. Female and male lifestyle habits and IVF: what is known and unknown. Hum Reprod Update. 2005;11(2):179–203.
18. Van Voorhis BJ Dawson JD Stovall DW Sparks AET Syrop CH. The effects of smoking on ovarian function and fertility during assisted reproduction cycles. Obstet Gynecol. 1996;88(5):785–91.
19. Jukic AMZ, Weinberg CR, Baird DD, Wilcox AJ. The association of maternal factors with delayed implantation and the initial rise of urinary human chorionic gonadotrophin. Hum Reprod. 2011;26(4):920–6.
20. Wilcox AJ, Weinberg CR, Baird DD. Post-ovulatory ageing of the human oocyte and embryo failure. Hum Reprod. 1998;13(2):394–7.
21. Neal MS, Hughes EG, Holloway AC, Foster WG. Sidestream smoking is equally as damaging as mainstream smoking on IVF outcomes. Hum Reprod. 2005;20(9):2531–5.
22. Benedict MD, Missmer SA, Vahratian A, Berry KF, Vitonis AF, Cramer DW, et al. Secondhand tobacco smoke exposure is associated with increased risk of failed implantation and reduced IVF success. Hum Reprod. 2011;26(9):2525–31.
23. American Society for Reproductive Medicine. Smoking and infertility: a committee opinion. Fertil Steril. 2012;98(6):1400–6.
24. Benowltz NL, Kuyt F, Jacob Iii P, Jones RT, Osman AL. Cotinine disposition and effects. Clin Pharmacol Ther. 1983;34(5):604–11.
25. Thompson J, Bannigan J. Cadmium: toxic effects on the reproductive system and the embryo. Reprod Toxicol. 2008;25(3):304–15.
26. McElroy JA, Shafer MM, Hampton JM, Newcomb PA. Predictors of urinary cadmium levels in adult females. Sci Total Environ. 2007;382(2–3):214–23.
27. Weiss T, Eckert A. Cotinine levels in follicular fluid and serum of IVF patients: effect on granulose-luteal cell function in vitro. Hum Reprod. 1989;4(5):482–5.
28. Zenzes MT, Krishnan S, Krishnan B, Zhang H, Casper RF. Cadmium accumulation in follicular fluid of women in in vitro fertilization-embryo transfer is higher in smokers. Fertil Steril. 1995;64(3):599–603.
29. Zenzes MT. Smoking and reproduction: gene damage to human gametes and embryos. Hum Reprod Update. 2000;6(2):122–31.
30. Bartsch H, Nair U, Risch A, Rojas M, Wikman H, Alexandrov K. Genetic polymorphism of CYP genes, alone or in combination, as a risk modifier of tobacco-related cancers. Cancer Epidemiol Biomarkers Prevent. 2000;9(1):3–28.
31. Neal MS, Zhu J, Foster WG. Quantification of benzo[a]pyrene and other PAHs in the serum and follicular fluid of smokers versus non-smokers. Reprod Toxicol. 2008;25(1):100–6.
32. Zenzes MT, Puy LA, Bielecki R. Immunodetection of benzo[a] pyrene adducts in ovarian cells of women exposed to cigarette smoke. Mol Hum Reprod. 1998;4(2):159–65.
33. Buters J, Quintanilla-Martinez L, Schober W, Soballa VJ, Hintermair J, Wolff T, et al. CYP1B1 determines susceptibility to low doses of 7,12-dimethylbenz[a]anthracene-induced ovarian cancers in mice: correlation of CYP1B1-mediated DNA adducts with carcinogenicity. Carcinogenesis. 2003;24(2):327–34.
34. Goodman MT, McDuffie K, Kolonel LN, Terada K, Donlon TA, Wilkens LR, et al. Case-control study of ovarian cancer and polymorphisms in genes involved in catecholestrogen formation and metabolism. Cancer Epidemiol Biomarkers Prevent. 2001;10(3):209–16.
35. Vidal JD, VandeVoort CA, Marcus CB, Lazarewicz NR, Conley AJ. In vitro exposure to environmental tobacco smoke induces CYP1B1 expression in human luteinized granulosa cells. Reprod Toxicol. 2006;22(4):731–7.
36. Collaborative Group on Epidemiological Studies of Ovarian Cancer. Ovarian cancer and smoking: individual participant meta-analysis including 28 114 women with ovarian cancer from 51 epidemiological studies. Lancet Oncol. 2012;13(9):946–56.
37. Pan SY, Ugnat AM, Mao Y, Wen SW, Johnson KC. Association of cigarette smoking with the risk of ovarian cancer. Int J Cancer. 2004;111(1):124–30.
38. Harlow BL, Signorello LB. Factors associated with early menopause. Maturitas. 2000;35(1):3–9.
39. Mikkelsen TF, Graff-Iversen S, Sundby J, Bjertness E. Early menopause, association with tobacco smoking, coffee consumption and other lifestyle factors: a cross-sectional study. BMC Public Health. 2007;7: 149.
40. Kinney A, Kline J, Levin B. Alcohol, caffeine and smoking in relation to age at menopause. Maturitas. 2006;54(1):27–38.
41. Sharara FJ, Beatse SN, Leonardi MR, Navot D, Scott Jr RT. Cigarette smoking accelerates the development of diminished ovarian reserve as evidenced by the clomiphene citrate challenge test. Fertil Steril. 1994;62(2):257–62.
42. Backer LC. Serum follicle-stimulating hormone and luteinizing hormone levels in women aged 35–60 in the U.S. population: the third National Health and Nutrition Examination Survey (NHANES III, 1988–1994). Menopause. 1999;6(1):29–35.
43. Cramer DW, Barbieri RL, Fraer AR, Harlow BL. Determinants of early follicular phase gonadotrophin and estradiol concentrations in women of late reproductive age. Hum Reprod. 2002;17(1):221–7.

44. Kinney A, Kline J, Kelly A, Reuss ML, Levin B. Smoking, alcohol and caffeine in relation to ovarian age during the reproductive years. Hum Reprod. 2007;22(4):1175–85.
45. Hoyer PB, Sipes IG. Assessment of follicle destruction in chemical-induced ovarian toxicity. Annu Rev Pharmacol Toxicol. 1996;36:307–31.
46. Neal MS, Zhu J, Holloway AC, Foster WG. Follicle growth is inhibited by benzo-[a]-pyrene, at concentrations representative of human exposure, in an isolated rat follicle culture assay. Hum Reprod. 2007;22(4):961–7.
47. Matikainen T, Perez GI, Jurisicova A, Pru JK, Schlezinger JJ, Ryu HY, et al. Aromatic hydrocarbon receptor-driven Bax gene expression is required for premature ovarian failure caused by biohazardous environmental chemicals. Nat Genet. 2001;28(4):355–60.
48. Neal MS, Mulligan Tuttle AM, Casper RF, Lagunov A, Foster WG. Aryl hydrocarbon receptor antagonists attenuate the deleterious effects of benzo[a]pyrene on isolated rat follicle development. Reprod Biomed Online. 2010;21(1):100–8.
49. Zenzes MT, Edward Reed T, Casper RF. Effects of cigarette smoking and age on the maturation of human oocytes. Hum Reprod. 1997;12(8):1736–41.
50. Zenzes MT, Wang P, Casper RF. Cigarette smoking may affect meiotic maturation of human oocytes. Hum Reprod. 1995;10(12):3213–7.
51. Nardo LG, Christodoulou D, Gould D, Roberts SA, Fitzgerald CT, Laing I. Anti-Müllerian hormone levels and antral follicle count in women enrolled in in vitro fertilization cycles: relationship to lifestyle factors, chronological age and reproductive history. Gynecol Endocrinol. 2007;23(8):486–93.
52. Freour T, Masson D, Mirallie S, Jean M, Bach K, Dejoie T, et al. Active smoking compromises IVF outcome and affects ovarian reserve. Reprod Biomed Online. 2008;16(1):96–102.
53. Schuh-Huerta SM, Johnson NA, Rosen MP, Sternfeld B, Cedars MI, Reijo Pera RA. Genetic variants and environmental factors associated with hormonal markers of ovarian reserve in Caucasian and African American women. Hum Reprod. 2012;27(2):594–608.
54. Curtis KM, Savitz DA, Arbuckle TE. Effects of cigarette smoking, caffeine consumption, and alcohol intake on fecundability. Am J Epidemiol. 1997;146(1):32–41.
55. Soares SR, Simon C, Remohí J, Pellicer A. Cigarette smoking affects uterine receptiveness. Hum Reprod. 2007;22(2):543–7.
56. Knoll M, Shaoulian R, Magers T, Talbot P. Ciliary beat frequency of hamster oviducts is decreased in vitro by exposure to solutions of mainstream and sidestream cigarette smoke. Biol Reprod. 1995;53(1):29–37.
57. Knoll M, Talbot P. Cigarette smoke inhibits oocyte cumulus complex pick-up by the oviduct in vitro independent of ciliary beat frequency. Reprod Toxicol. 1998;12(1):57–68.
58. Riveles K, Iv M, Arey J, Talbot P. Pyridines in cigarette smoke inhibit hamster oviductal functioning in picomolar doses. Reprod Toxicol. 2003;17(2):191–202.
59. Lutterodt MC, Sørensen KP, Larsen KB, Skouby SO, Andersen CY, Byskov AG. The number of oogonia and somatic cells in the human female embryo and fetus in relation to whether or not exposed to maternal cigarette smoking. Hum Reprod. 2009;24(10):2558–66.
60. Ernst A, Kristensen SL, Toft G, Thulstrup AM, Håkonsen LB, Olsen SF, et al. Maternal smoking during pregnancy and reproductive health of daughters: a follow-up study spanning two decades. Hum Reprod. 2012;27(12):3593–600.
61. Ness RB, Grisso JA, Hirschinger N, Markovic N, Shaw LM, Day NL, et al. Cocaine and tobacco use and the risk of spontaneous abortion. N Engl J Med. 1999;340(5):333–9.
62. Winter E, Wang J, Davies MJ, Norman R. Early pregnancy loss following assisted reproductive technology treatment. Hum Reprod. 2002;17(12):3220–3.
63. Meeker JD, Missmer SA, Vitonis AF, Cramer DW, Hauser R. Risk of spontaneous abortion in women with childhood exposure to parental cigarette smoke. Am J Epidemiol. 2007;166(5):571–5.
64. Chatenoud L, Parazzini F, Di Cintio E, Zanconato G, Benzi G, Bortolus R, et al. Paternal and maternal smoking habits before conception and during the first trimester: relation to spontaneous abortion. Ann Epidemiol. 1998;8(8):520–6.
65. Maconochie N, Doyle P, Prior S, Simmons R. Risk factors for first trimester miscarriage—results from a UK-population-based case-control study. BJOG. 2007;114(2):170–86.
66. Nielsen A, Hannibal CG, Lindekilde BE, Tolstrup J, Frederiksen K, Munk C, et al. Maternal smoking predicts the risk of spontaneous abortion. Acta Obstet Gynecol Scand. 2006;85(9):1057–65.
67. Windham GC, Swan SH, Fenster L. Parental cigarette smoking and the risk of spontaneous abortion. Am J Epidemiol. 1992;135(12):1394–403.
68. Rasch V. Cigarette, alcohol, and caffeine consumption: risk factors for spontaneous abortion. Acta Obstet Gynecol Scand. 2003;82(2):182–8.
69. Coste J, Job-Spira N, Fernandez H, Papiernik E, Spira A. Risk factors for ectopic pregnancy: a case-control study in France, with special focus on infectious factors. Am J Epidemiol. 1991;133(9):839–49.
70. Karaer A, Avsar FA, Batioglu S. Risk factors for ectopic pregnancy: a case-control study. Aust N Z J Obstet Gynaecol. 2006;46(6): 521–7.
71. vom Saal FS, Akingbemi BT, Belcher SM, Birnbaum LS, Crain DA, Eriksen M, et al. Chapel Hill bisphenol A expert panel consensus statement: Integration of mechanisms, effects in animals and potential to impact human health at current levels of exposure. Reprod Toxicol. 2007;24(2):131–8.
72. Welshons WV, Nagel SC, Vom Saal FS. Large effects from small exposures. III. Endocrine mechanisms mediating effects of bisphenol A at levels of human exposure. Endocrinology. 2006;147(Suppl. 6):56–69
73. Bloom MS, Kim D, Vom Saal FS, Taylor JA, Cheng G, Lamb JD, et al. Bisphenol A exposure reduces the estradiol response to gonadotropin stimulation during in vitro fertilization. Fertil Steril. 2011;96(3):672–7.e2.
74. Ikezuki Y, Tsutsumi O, Takai Y, Kamei Y, Taketani Y. Determination of bisphenol A concentrations in human biological fluids reveals significant early prenatal exposure. Hum Reprod. 2002;17(11):2839–41.
75. Calafat AM, Kuklenyik Z, Reidy JA, Caudill SP, Ekong J, Needham LL. Urinary concentrations of bisphenol A and 4-nonylphenol in a human reference population. Environ Health Perspect. 2005;113(4):391–5.
76. Calafat AM, Ye X, Wong LY, Reidy JA, Needham LL. Exposure of the U.S. population to bisphenol A and 4-tertiary-octylphenol: 2003–2004. Environ Health Perspect. 2008;116(1):39–44.
77. Goodman JE, Witorsch RJ, McConnell EE, Sipes IG, Slayton TM, Yu CJ, et al. Weight-of-evidence evaluation of reproductive and developmental effects of low doses of bisphenol A. Crit Rev Toxicol. 2009;39(1):1–75.
78. Hengstler JG, Foth H, Gebel T, Kramer P-J, Lilienblum W, Schweinfurth H, et al. Critical evaluation of key evidence on the human health hazards of exposure to bisphenol A. Crit Rev Toxicol. 2011;41(4):263–91.
79. Vandenberg LN, Colborn T, Hayes TB, Heindel JJ, Jacobs Jr DR, Lee D-H, et al. Regulatory decisions on endocrine disrupting chemicals should be based on the principles of endocrinology. Reprod Toxicol. 2013;38(0):1–15.
80. Vandenberg LN, Maffini MV, Sonnenschein C, Rubin BS, Soto AM. Bisphenol-A and the great divide: a review of controversies in the field of endocrine disruption. Endocr Rev. 2009;30(1):75–95.
81. Takai Y, Tsutsumi O, Ikezuki Y, Hiroi H, Osuga Y, Momoeda M, et al. Estrogen receptor-mediated effects of a xenoestrogen, bisphenol A, on preimplantation mouse embryos. Biochem Biophys Res Commun. 2000;270(3):918–21.
82. Hunt PA, Koehler KE, Susiarjo M, Hodges CA, Ilagan A, Voigt RC, et al. Bisphenol A exposure causes meiotic aneuploidy in the female mouse. Curr Biol. 2003;13(7):546–53.

83. Susiarjo M, Hassold TJ, Freeman E, Hunt PA. Bisphenol A exposure in utero disrupts early oogenesis in the mouse. PLoS Genet. 2007;3(1):0063–70.
84. Sugiura-Ogasawara M, Ozaki Y, Sonta SI, Makino T, Suzumori K. Exposure to bisphenol A is associated with recurrent miscarriage. Hum Reprod. 2005;20(8):2325–9.
85. Dekant W, Volkel W. Human exposure to bisphenol A by biomonitoring: methods, results and assessment of environmental exposures. Toxicol Appl Pharmacol. 2008;228(1):114–34.
86. Fujimoto VY, Kim D, Vom Saal FS, Lamb JD, Taylor JA, Bloom MS. Serum unconjugated bisphenol A concentrations in women may adversely influence oocyte quality during in vitro fertilization. Fertil Steril. 2011;95(5):1816–9.
87. Ehrlich S, Williams PL, Missmer SA, Flaws JA, Ye X, Calafat AM, et al. Urinary bisphenol A concentrations and early reproductive health outcomes among women undergoing IVF. Hum Reprod. 2012;27(12):3583–92.
88. Kwintkiewicz J, Nishi Y, Yanase T, Giudice LC. Peroxisome proliferator-activated receptor-γ mediates bisphenol A inhibition of FSH-stimulated IGF-1, aromatase, and estradiol in human granulosa cells. Environ Health Perspect. 2010;118(3):400–6.
89. Mok-Lin E, Ehrlich S, Williams PL, Petrozza J, Wright DL, Calafat AM, et al. Urinary bisphenol A concentrations and ovarian response among women undergoing IVF. Int J Androl. 2010;33(2):385–93.
90. Hanna CW, Bloom MS, Robinson WP, Kim D, Parsons PJ, Vom Saal FS, et al. DNA methylation changes in whole blood is associated with exposure to the environmental contaminants, mercury, lead, cadmium and bisphenol A, in women undergoing ovarian stimulation for IVF. Hum Reprod. 2012;27(5):1401–10.
91. Lauby-Secretan B, Loomis D, Grosse Y, El Ghissassi F, Bouvard V, Benbrahim-Tallaa L, et al. Carcinogenicity of polychlorinated biphenyls and polybrominated biphenyls. Lancet Oncol. 2013;14(4):287–8.
92. Cooke PS, Sato T, Buchanan DL. Disruption of steroid hormone signaling by PCBs. In: Robertson LS, Hansen LG, editors. PCBs: Recent advances in environmental toxicology and health effects. Lexington: University Press of Kentucky; 2001. p. 257–63.
93. Van den Berg M, Birnbaum LS, Denison M, De Vito M, Farland W, Feeley M, et al. The 2005 World Health Organization reevaluation of human and mammalian toxic equivalency factors for dioxins and dioxin-like compounds. Toxicol Sci. 2006;93(2):223–41.
94. Hennig B, Meerarani P, Slim R, Toborek M, Daugherty A, Silverstone AE, et al. Proinflammatory properties of coplanar PCBs: in vitro and in vivo evidence. Toxicol Appl Pharmacol. 2002;181(3):174–83.
95. Reijnders PJH. Reproductive failure in common seals feeding on fish from polluted coastal waters. Nature. 1986;324(6096):456–7.
96. Turyk ME, Bhavsar SP, Bowerman W, Boysen E, Clark M, Diamond M, et al. Risks and benefits of consumption of great lakes fish. Environ Health Perspect. 2012;120(1):11–8.
97. Bloom MS, Vena JE, Swanson MK, Moysich KB, Olson JR. Profiles of ortho-polychlorinated biphenyl congeners, dichlorodiphenyldichloroethylene, hexachlorobenzene, and Mirex among male Lake Ontario sportfish consumers: The New York State Angler Cohort Study. Environ Res. 2005;97(2):178–94.
98. Humphrey HEB, Joseph JC, Pandya JR, Sweeney AM, Gasior DM, McCaffrey RJ, et al. PCB congener profile in the serum of humans consuming Great Lakes fish. Environ Health Perspect. 2000;108(2):167–72.
99. Buck Louis GM Dmochowski J Lynch C Kostyniak P McGuinness BM Vena JE. Polychlorinated biphenyl serum concentrations, lifestyle and time-to-pregnancy. Hum Reprod. 2009;24(2):451–8.
100. Buck Louis GM Rios LI McLain A Cooney MA Kostyniak PJ Sundaram R. Persistent organochlorine pollutants and menstrual cycle characteristics. Chemosphere. 2011;85(11):1742–8.
101. Buck Louis GM, Sundaram R, Schisterman EF, Sweeney AM, Lynch CD, Gore-Langton RE, et al. Persistent environmental pollutants and couple fecundity: the LIFE study. Environ Health Perspect. 2013;121(2):231–6.
102. Axmon A, Thulstrup AM, Rignell-Hydbom A, Pedersen HS, Zvyezday V, Ludwicki JK, et al. Time to pregnancy as a function of male and female serum concentrations of 2,2′4,4′5,5′-hexachlorobiphenyl (CB-153) and 1,1-dichloro-2,2-bis (p-chlorophenyl)-ethylene (p, p′-DDE). Hum Reprod. 2006;21(3):657–65.
103. Chevrier C, Warembourg C, Gaudreau E, Monfort C, Le Blanc A, Guldner L, et al. Organochlorine pesticides, polychlorinated biphenyls, seafood consumption, and time-to-pregnancy. Epidemiology. 2013;24(2):251–60.
104. Bloom MS, Buck Louis GM, Schisterman EF, Liu A, Kostyniak PJ. Maternal serum polychlorinated biphenyl concentrations across critical windows of human development. Environ Health Perspect. 2007;115(9):1320–4.
105. Meeker JD, Missmer SA, Altshul L, Vitonis AF, Ryan L, Cramer DW, et al. Serum and follicular fluid organochlorine concentrations among women undergoing assisted reproduction technologies. Environ Health. 2009;8:32.
106. Younglai EV, Foster WG, Hughes EG, Trim K, Jarrell JF. Levels of environmental contaminants in human follicular fluid, serum, and seminal plasma of couples undergoing in vitro fertilization. Arch Environ Contam Toxicol. 2002;43(1):121–6.
107. Petro EML, Leroy JLMR, Covaci A, Fransen E, De Neubourg D, Dirtu AC, et al. Endocrine-disrupting chemicals in human follicular fluid impair in vitro oocyte developmental competence. Hum Reprod. 2012;27(4):1025–33.
108. Meeker JD, Maity A, Missmer SA, Williams PL, Mahalingaiah S, Ehrlich S, et al. Serum concentrations of polychlorinated biphenyls in relation to in vitro fertilization outcomes. Environ Health Perspect. 2011;119(7):1010–6.
109. Kadhel P, Monnier P, Boucoiran I, Chaillet N, Fraser WD. Organochlorine pollutants and female fertility: a systematic review focusing on in vitro fertilization studies. Reprod Sci. 2012;19(12):1246–59.
110. Krogenæs AK, Nafstad I, Skåre JU, Farstad W, Hafne AL. In vitro reproductive toxicity of polychlorinated biphenyl congeners 153 and 126. Reprod Toxicol. 1998;12(6):575–80.
111. Pocar P, Perazzoli F, Luciano AM, Gandolfi F. In vitro reproductive toxicity of polychlorinated biphenyls: effects on oocyte maturation and developmental competence in cattle. Mol Reprod Dev. 2001;58(4):411–6.
112. Barsotti DA, Marlar RJ, Allen JR. Reproductive dysfunction in rhesus monkeys exposed to low levels of polychlorinated biphenyls (Aroclor 1248). Food Cosmet Toxicol. 1976;14(2):99–103.
113. Brezner E, Terkel J, Perry AS. The effect of Aroclor 1254 (PCB) on the physiology of reproduction in the female rat—I. Comp Biochem Physiol C. 1984;77(1):65–70.
114. Jonsson Jr HT Keil JE Gaddy RG Loadholt CB Hennigar GR Walker Jr EM. Prolonged ingestion of commercial DDT and PCB; effects on progesterone levels and reproduction in the mature female rat. Arch Environ Contam Toxicol. 1976;3(4):479–90.
115. Müller WF, Hobson W, Fuller GB, Knauf W, Coulston F, Korte F. Endocrine effects of chlorinated hydrocarbons in rhesus monkeys. Ecotoxicol Environ Saf. 1978;2(2):161–72.
116. Kholkute SD, Dukelow WR. Effects of polychlorinated biphenyl (PCB) mixtures on in vitro fertilization in the mouse. Bull Environ Contam Toxicol. 1997;59(4):531–6.
117. Kholkute SD, Rodriguez J, Richard Dukelow W. Reproductive toxicity of Aroclor-1254: effects on oocyte, spermatozoa, in vitro fertilization, and embryo development in the mouse. Reprod Toxicol. 1994;8(6):487–93.
118. Kholkute SD, Rodriguez J, Richard Dukelow W. Effects of polychlorinated biphenyls (PCBs) on in vitro fertilization in the mouse. Reprod Toxicol. 1994;8(1):69–73.

119. Kraugerud M, Zimmer KE, Dahl E, Berg V, Olsaker I, Farstad W, et al. Three structurally different polychlorinated biphenyl congeners (PCB 118, 153, and 126) affect hormone production and gene expression in the human H295R in vitro model. J Toxicol Environ Health A. 2010;73(16):1122–32.
120. Huang A, Lin S, Inglis R, Powell D, Chou K. Pre- and postnatal exposure to 3,3',4,4'-tetrachlorobiphenyl: II. Effects on the reproductive capacity and fertilizing ability of eggs in female mice. Arch Environ Contam Toxicol. 1998;34(2):209–14.
121. Campagna C, Sirard MA, Ayotte P, Bailey JL. Impaired maturation, fertilization, and embryonic development of porcine oocytes following exposure to an environmentally relevant organochlorine mixture. Biol Reprod. 2001;65(2):554–60.
122. Seiler P, Fischer B, Lindenau A, Beier HM. Effects of persistent chlorinated hydrocarbons on fertility and embryonic development in the rabbit. Hum Reprod. 1994;9(10):1920–6.
123. Son DS, Ushinohama K, Gao X, Taylor CC, Roby KF, Rozman KK, et al. 2,3,7,8-Tetrachlorodibenzo-p-dioxin (TCDD) blocks ovulation by a direct action on the ovary without alteration of ovarian steroidogenesis: lack of a direct effect on ovarian granulosa and thecal-interstitial cell steroidogenesis in vitro. Reprod Toxicol. 1999;13(6):521–30.
124. Gao X, Son DS, Terranova PF, Rozman KK. Toxic equivalency factors of polychlorinated dibenzo-p-dioxins in an ovulation model: validation of the toxic equivalency concept for one aspect of endocrine disruption. Toxicol Appl Pharmacol. 1999;157(2):107–16.
125. Schmidt JV, Su GHT, Reddy JK, Simon MC, Bradfield CA. Characterization of a murine Ahr null allele: involvement of the Ah receptor in hepatic growth and development. Proc Natl Acad Sci U S A. 1996;93(13):6731–6.
126. Kietz S, Fischer B. Polychlorinated biphenyls affect gene expression in the rabbit preimplantation embryo. Mol Reprod Dev. 2003;64(3):251–60.
127. Schecter A, Birnbaum L, Ryan JJ, Constable JD. Dioxins: an overview. Environ Res. 2006;101(3):419–28.
128. International Agency for Research on Cancer (IARC). IARC Working Group on the evaluation of carcinogenic risks to humans: polychlorinated dibenzo-para-dioxins and polychlorinated dibenzofurans. Lyon, France, 4–11 February 1997. IARC Monogr Eval Carcinog Risks Hum. 1997;69:1–631.
129. Heiden TCK, Struble CA, Rise ML, Hessner MJ, Hutz RJ, Carvan Iii MJ. Molecular targets of 2,3,7,8-tetrachlorodibenzo-p-dioxin (TCDD) within the zebrafish ovary: insights into TCDD-induced endocrine disruption and reproductive toxicity. Reprod Toxicol. 2008;25(1):47–57.
130. Tsutsumi O, Uechi H, Sone H, Yonemoto J, Takai Y, Momoeda M, et al. Presence of dioxins in human follicular fluid: their possible stage-specific action on the development of preimplantation mouse embryos. Biochem Biophys Res Commun. 1998;250(2):498–501.
131. Bock KW, Köhle C. Ah receptor: dioxin-mediated toxic responses as hints to deregulated physiologic functions. Biochem Pharmacol. 2006;72(4):393–404.
132. Morán FM, Vandevoort CA, Overstreet JW, Lasley BL, Conley AJ. Molecular target of endocrine disruption in human luteinizing granulosa cells by 2,3,7,8-tetrachlorodibenzo-p-dioxin: inhibition of estradiol secretion due to decreased 17α-hydroxylase/17,20-lyase cytochrome p450 expression. Endocrinology. 2003;144(2):467–73.
133. Abbott BD, Schmid JE, Pitt JA, Buckalew AR, Wood CR, Held GA, et al. Adverse reproductive outcomes in the transgenic Ah receptor-deficient mouse. Toxicol Appl Pharmacol. 1999;155(1):62–70.
134. Benedict JC, Lin TM, Loeffler IK, Peterson RE, Flaws JA. Physiological role of the aryl hydrocarbon receptor in mouse ovary development. Toxicol Sci. 2000;56(2):382–8.
135. Eskenazi B, Warner M, Marks AR, Samuels S, Needham L, Brambilla P, et al. Serum dioxin concentrations and time to pregnancy. Epidemiology. 2010;21(2):224–31.
136. Eskenazi B, Warner M, Mocarelli P, Samuels S, Needham LL, Patterson Jr DG, et al. Serum dioxin concentrations and menstrual cycle characteristics. Am J Epidemiol. 2002;156(4):383–92.
137. Eskenazi B, Mocarelli P, Warner M, Needham L, Patterson Jr DG, Samuels S, et al. Relationship of serum TCDD concentrations and age at exposure of female residents of Seveso, Italy. Environ Health Perspect. 2004;112(1):22–7.
138. Birnbaum LS, Cohen Hubal EA. Polybrominated diphenyl ethers: a case study for using biomonitoring data to address risk assessment questions. Environ Health Perspect. 2006 Nov;114(11):1770–5.
139. Hites RA. Polybrominated diphenyl ethers in the environment and in people: a meta-analysis of concentrations. Environ Sci Technol. 2004;38(4):945–56.
140. Geyer HJ, Schramm K, Darnerud PO, Aune M, Feicht EA, Fried KW, et al. Terminal elimination half-lives of the brominated flame retardants TBBPA, HBCD, and lower brominated PBDEs in humans. Organohalogen Compd. 2004;66:3867–72.
141. Chen A, Chung E, DeFranco EA, Pinney SM, Dietrich KN. Serum PBDEs and age at menarche in adolescent girls: analysis of the national health and nutrition examination survey 2003–2004. Environ Res. 2011;111(6):831–7.
142. Chao HR, Wang SL, Lee WJ, Wang YF, Päpke O. Levels of polybrominated diphenyl ethers (PBDEs) in breast milk from central Taiwan and their relation to infant birth outcome and maternal menstruation effects. Environ Int. 2007;33(2):239–45.
143. Harley KG, Marks AR, Chevrier J, Bradman A, Sjödin A, Eskenazi B. PBDE concentrations in women's serum and fecundability. Environ Health Perspect. 2010;118(5):699–704.
144. Johnson PI, Altshul L, Cramer DW, Missmer SA, Hauser R, Meeker JD. Serum and follicular fluid concentrations of polybrominated diphenyl ethers and in-vitro fertilization outcome. Environ Int. 2012;45(1):9–14.
145. Legler J. New insights into the endocrine disrupting effects of brominated flame retardants. Chemosphere. 2008;73(2):216–22.
146. Hamers T, Kamstra JH, Sonneveld E, Murk AJ, Kester MHA, Andersson PL, et al. In vitro profiling of the endocrine-disrupting potency of brominated flame retardants. Toxicol Sci. 2006;92(1):157–73.
147. Mercado-Feliciano M, Bigsby RM. The polybrominated diphenyl ether mixture DE-71 is mildly estrogenic. Environ Health Perspect. 2008;116(5):605–11.
148. Stoker TE, Cooper RL, Lambright CS, Wilson VS, Furr J, Gray LE. In vivo and in vitro anti-androgenic effects of DE-71, a commercial polybrominated diphenyl ether (PBDE) mixture. Toxicol Appl Pharmacol. 2005;207(1):78–88.
149. Cantón RF, Scholten DEA, Marsh G, de Jong PC, van den Berg M. Inhibition of human placental aromatase activity by hydroxylated polybrominated diphenyl ethers (OH-PBDEs). Toxicol Appl Pharmacol. 2008;227(1):68–75.
150. Talsness CE, Kuriyama SN, Sterner-Kock A, Schnitker P, Grande SW, Shakibaei M, et al. In utero and lactational exposures to low doses of polybrominated diphenyl ether-47 alter the reproductive system and thyroid gland of female rat offspring. Environ Health Perspect. 2008;116(3):308–14.
151. Talsness CE, Shakibaei M, Kuriyama SN, Grande SW, Sterner-Kock A, Schnitker P, et al. Ultrastructural changes observed in rat ovaries following in utero and lactational exposure to low doses of a polybrominated flame retardant. Toxicol Lett. 2005;157(3):189–202.
152. Ceccatelli R, Faass O, Schlumpf M, Lichtensteiger W. Gene expression and estrogen sensitivity in rat uterus after developmental exposure to the polybrominated diphenylether PBDE 99 and PCB. Toxicology. 2006;220(2–3):104–16.
153. Pellacani C, Tagliaferri S, Caglieri A, Goldoni M, Giordano G, Mutti A, et al. Synergistic interactions between PBDEs and PCBs in human neuroblastoma cells. Environ Toxicol. 2014;13(4).

154. Kissa E. Fluorinated surfactants and repellents. New York: Marcel Dekker; 2001.
155. Giesy JP, Kannan K. Global distribution of perfluorooctane sulfonate in wildlife. Environ Sci Technol. 2001;35(7):1339–42.
156. Fei C, McLaughlin JK, Lipworth L, Olsen J. Maternal levels of perfluorinated chemicals and subfecundity. Hum Reprod. 2009;24(5):1200–5.
157. Whitworth KW, Haug LS, Baird DD, Becher G, Hoppin JA, Skjaerven R, et al. Perfluorinated compounds and subfecundity in pregnant women. Epidemiology. 2012;23(2):257–63.
158. Fei C, Weinberg CR, Olsen J. Commentary: perfluorinated chemicals and time to pregnancy: a link based on reverse causation? Epidemiology. 2012;23(2):264–6.
159. Vestergaard S, Nielsen F, Andersson AM, Hjøllund NH, Grandjean P, Andersen HR, et al. Association between perfluorinated compounds and time to pregnancy in a prospective cohort of Danish couples attempting to conceive. Hum Reprod. 2012;27(3):873–80.
160. Austin ME, Kasturi BS, Barber M, Kannan K, MohanKumar PS, MohanKumar SMJ. Neuroendocrine effects of perfluorooctane sulfonate in rats. Environ Health Perspect. 2003;111(12):1485–9.
161. Lau C, Thibodeaux JR, Hanson RG, Narotsky MG, Rogers JM, Lindstrom AB, et al. Effects of perfluorooctanoic acid exposure during pregnancy in the mouse. Toxicol Sci. 2006;90(2):510–8.
162. Dixon D, Reed CE, Moore AB, Gibbs-Flournoy EA, Hines EP, Wallace EA, et al. Histopathologic changes in the uterus, cervix and vagina of immature CD-1 mice exposed to low doses of perfluorooctanoic acid (PFOA) in a uterotrophic assay. Reprod Toxicol. 2012;33(4):506–12.
163. Henry ND, Fair PA. Comparison of in vitro cytotoxicity, estrogenicity and anti-estrogenicity of triclosan, perfluorooctane sulfonate and perfluorooctanoic acid. J Appl Toxicol. 2013;33(4): 265–72.
164. Luebker DJ, Case MT, York RG, Moore JA, Hansen KJ, Butenhoff JL. Two-generation reproduction and cross-foster studies of perfluorooctanesulfonate (PFOS) in rats. Toxicology. 2005;215(1–2):126–48.
165. Kruger PC, Bloom MS, Arnason JG, Palmer CD, Fujimoto VY, Parsons PJ. Trace elements in human follicular fluid: development of a sensitive multielement ICP-MS method for use in biomonitoring studies. J Anal At Spectrom. 2012;27(8):1245–53.
166. Hightower JM, Moore D. Mercury levels in high-end consumers of fish. Environ Health Perspect. 2003;111(4):604–8.
167. MacIntosh DL, Spengler JD, Ozkaynak H, Tsai LH, Barry Ryan P. Dietary exposures to selected metals and pesticides. Environ Health Perspect. 1996;104(2):202–9.
168. Satarug S, Garrett SH, Sens MA, Sens DA. Cadmium, environmental exposure, and health outcomes. Environ Health Perspect. 2010;118(2):182–90.
169. National Research Council (U.S.). Committee on the Toxicological Effects of Methylmercury. Toxicological effects of methyl mercury. Washington, DC: National Academy Press; 2000.
170. Mahaffey KR, Clickner RP, Jeffries RA. Adult women's blood mercury concentrations vary regionally in the United States: association with patterns of fish consumption (NHANES 1999–2004). Environ Health Perspect. 2009;117(1):47–53.
171. Ayotte JD, Gronberg JM, Apodaca LE. trace elements and radon in groundwater across the United States: U.S. Geological Survey Scientific Investigations Report 2011–5059; 2011.
172. Navas-Acien A, Francesconi KA, Silbergeld EK, Guallar E. Seafood intake and urine concentrations of total arsenic, dimethylarsinate and arsenobetaine in the US population. Environ Res. 2011;111(1):110–8.
173. Nahin RL, Barnes PM, Stussman BJ, Bloom B. Costs of complementary and alternative medicine (CAM) and frequency of visits to CAM practitioners: United States, 2007. Nati Health Stat Reports. 2009;(18):1–14.
174. Garvey GJ, Hahn G, Lee RV, Harbison RD. Heavy metal hazards of Asian traditional remedies. Int J Environ Health Res. 2001;11(1):63–71.
175. Saper RB, Phillips RS, Sehgal A, Khouri N, Davis RB, Paquin J, et al. Lead, mercury, and arsenic in US- and Indian-manufactured ayurvedic medicines sold via the internet. J Amer Med Assoc. 2008;300(8):915–23.
176. Geraldine M, Herman DS, Venkatesh T. Lead poisoning as a result of infertility treatment using herbal remedies. Arch Gynecol Obstet. 2007;275(4):279–81.
177. Bloom MS, Fitzgerald EF, Kim K, Neamtiu I, Gurzau ES. Spontaneous pregnancy loss in humans and exposure to arsenic in drinking water. Int J Hyg Environ Health. 2010;213(6):401–13.
178. Figà-Talamanca I. Occupational risk factors and reproductive health of women. Occup Med. 2006;56(8):521–31.
179. Rowland AS, Baird DD, Weinberg CR, Shore DL, Shy CM, Wilcox AJ. The effect of occupational exposure to mercury vapour on the fertility of female dental assistants. Occup Environ Med. 1994;51(1):28–34.
180. Pollack AZ, Schisterman EF, Goldman LR, Mumford SL, Albert PS, Jones RL, et al. Cadmium, lead, and mercury in relation to reproductive hormones and anovulation in premenopausal women. Environ Health Perspect. 2011;119(8):1156–61.
181. Choy CMY, Lam CWK, Cheung LTF, Briton-Jones CM, Cheung LP, Haines CJ. Infertility, blood mercury concentrations and dietary seafood consumption: a case-control study. Br J Obstet Gynaecol. 2002;109(10):1121–5.
182. Gerhard I, Monga B, Waldbrenner A, Runnebaum B. Heavy metals and fertility. J Toxicol Env Health Part A. 1998;54(8):593–611.
183. Chang S-H, Cheng B-H, Lee S-L, Chuang H-Y, Yang C-Y, Sung F-C, et al. Low blood lead concentration in association with infertility in women. Environ Res. 2006;101(3):380–6.
184. Cole DC, Wainman B, Sanin LH, Weber JP, Muggah H, Ibrahim S. Environmental contaminant levels and fecundability among non-smoking couples. Reprod Toxicol. 2006;22(1):13–9.
185. Buck Louis GM, Sundaram R, Schisterman EF, Sweeney AM, Lynch CD, Gore-Langton RE, et al. Heavy metals and couple fecundity, the LIFE Study. Chemosphere. 2012;87(11):1201–7.
186. Bloom MS. Concerning "Toxic trace metals and human oocytes during in vitro fertilization (IVF)" by M.S. Bloom, P.J. Parsons, A.J. Steuerwald, E.F. Schisterman, R.W. Browne, K. Kim, G.A. Coccaro, N. Narayan, V.Y. Fujimoto [Reprod. Toxicol. 29 (2010) 298–305]. Reprod Toxicol. 2012;33(1):126.
187. Bloom MS, Parsons PJ, Steuerwald AJ, Schisterman EF, Browne RW, Kim K, et al. Toxic trace metals and human oocytes during in vitro fertilization (IVF). Reprod Toxicol. 2010;29(3):298–305.
188. Al-Saleh I, Coskun S, Mashhour A, Shinwari N, El-Doush I, Billedo G, et al. Exposure to heavy metals (lead, cadmium and mercury) and its effect on the outcome of in-vitro fertilization treatment. Int J Hyg Environ Health. 2008;211(5–6):560–79.
189. Bloom MS, Parsons PJ, Kim D, Steuerwald AJ, Vaccari S, Cheng G, et al. Toxic trace metals and embryo quality indicators during in vitro fertilization (IVF). Reprod Toxicol. 2011;31(2):164–70.
190. Bloom MS, Fujimoto VY, Steuerwald AJ, Cheng G, Browne RW, Parsons PJ. Background exposure to toxic metals in women adversely influences pregnancy during in vitro fertilization (IVF). Reproductive Toxicology. 2012;34(3):471–81.
191. Silberstein T, Saphier O, Paz-Tal O, Trimarchi JR, Gonzalez L, Keefe DL. Lead concentrates in ovarian follicle compromises pregnancy. J Trace Elem Med Biol. 2006;20(3):205–7.
192. Bloom MS, Buck Louis GM, Sundaram R, Kostyniak PJ, Jain J. Associations between blood metals and fecundity among women residing in New York State. Reprod Toxicol. 2011;31(2):158–63.
193. Arakawa C, Yoshinaga J, Okamura K, Nakai K, Satoh H. Fish consumption and time to pregnancy in Japanese women. Int J Hyg Environ Health. 2006;209(4):337–44.

194. Jain RB. Effect of pregnancy on the levels of blood cadmium, lead, and mercury for females aged 17–39 years old: data from national health and nutrition examination survey 2003–2010. J Toxicol Environ Health A. 2013;76(1):58–69.
195. Jain RB. Effect of pregnancy on the levels of urinary metals for females aged 17–39 years old: data from national health and nutrition examination survey 2003–2010. J Toxicol Environ Health A. 2013;76(2):86–97.
196. Bridges CC, Zalups RK. Molecular and ionic mimicry and the transport of toxic metals. Toxicol Appl Pharmacol. 2005;204(3):274–308.
197. DalleDonne I, Milzani A, Colombo R. Actin assembly by cadmium ions. BBA-Mol Cell Res. 1997;1357(1):5–17.
198. Philbert MA, Billingsley ML, Reuhl KR. Mechanisms of injury in the central nervous system. Toxicol Pathol. 2000;28(1):43–53.
199. Ercal N, Gurer-Orhan H, Aykin-Burns N. Toxic metals and oxidative stress part I: mechanisms involved in metal-induced oxidative damage. Curr Top Med Chem. 2001;1(6):529–39.
200. Chattopadhyay S, Bhaumik S, Purkayastha M, Basu S, Nag Chaudhuri A, Das Gupta S. Apoptosis and necrosis in developing brain cells due to arsenic toxicity and protection with antioxidants. Toxicol Lett. 2002;136(1):65–76.
201. Johnson MD, Kenney N, Stoica A, Hilakivi-Clarke L, Singh B, Chepko G, et al. Cadmium mimics the in vivo effects of estrogen in the uterus and mammary gland. Nat Med. 2003;9(8):1081–4.
202. Martin MB, Reiter R, Pham T, Avellanet YR, Camara J, Lahm M, et al. Estrogen-like activity of metals in MCF-7 breast cancer cells. Endocrinology. 2003;144(6):2425–36.
203. Iavicoli I, Fontana L, Bergamaschi A. The effects of metals as endocrine disruptors. J Toxicol Environ Health Part B, Crit Rev. 2009;12(3):206–23.
204. Waalkes MP, Keefer LK, Diwan BA. Induction of proliferative lesions of the uterus, testes, and liver in Swiss mice given repeated injections of sodium arsenate: possible estrogenic mode of action. Toxicol Appl Pharmacol. 2000;166(1):24–35.
205. Henson MC, Chedrese PJ. Endocrine disruption by cadmium, a common environmental toxicant with paradoxical effects on reproduction. Exp Biol Med. 2004;229(5):383–92.
206. Mondal S, Mukhopadhyay B, Bhattacharya S. Inorganic mercury binding to fish oocyte plasma membrane induces steroidogenesis and translatable messenger RNA synthesis. Biometals. 1997;10(4):285–90.
207. Dolinoy DC, Weidman JR, Jirtle RL. Epigenetic gene regulation: linking early developmental environment to adult disease. Reprod Toxicol. 2007;23(3):297–307.
208. Arita A, Costa M. Epigenetics in metal carcinogenesis: nickel, arsenic, chromium and cadmium. Metallomics. 2009;1(3):222–8.

Cervical Hostility and Vaginal pH in Females with Unexplained Infertility

16

Fabiana Y. Nakano, Rogério B. F. Leão and Sandro C. Esteves

Introduction

The vaginal pH fluctuates between 3.8 and 4.5 [1]. While protecting the vagina from most pathogenic bacteria, this slightly acidic pH is toxic to sperm. The optimal pH to maintain sperm viability and motility ranges from 7.0 to 8.5 [2]. In fact, a reduction in sperm motility is seen at vaginal pH of less than 6.0 [2–5]. The alkaline pH of semen protects sperm temporarily. However, reduction in semen volume and/or decreased alkaline seminal vesicular secretion may negatively impact fertility since semen buffering capacity against vaginal acidity becomes inadequate [6].

The cervix generally functions as an effective barrier to sperm [7]. On the other hand, an adequate production of cervical mucus is essential to transport sperm from the vagina to the uterine cavity [2, 7]. Surgeries, birth defects, and infections can cause cervical constriction or stenosis, and may impair mucus production by the endocervical canal [8–12]. Chronic cervicitis, acute inflammation, and congenital diseases, such as cystic fibrosis (CF), are among the conditions that can reduce cervical mucus receptivity [12–14]. As a result, fertility is impaired due to alterations in cervical anatomy and function [9]. Hormonal fluctuations during the menstrual cycle also impact the production, composition, and ultrastructure of mucus, which ultimately affect sperm penetrability [12, 15]. Hormonal dysfunctions, mainly characterized by inadequate estrogen production and/or premature progesterone elevation, may render cervical mucus inadequate for sperm penetration, and may result in infertility [9]. Medication (e.g., clomiphene citrate (CC) and propranolol) and smoking can also have detrimental effects on mucus receptivity to sperm [16–20]. Lastly, sperm abnormalities affecting motility and/or morphology, as well as elevated levels of antisperm antibodies in the semen and/or female serum may impact sperm ability to transpose the cervical mucus [21–23].

Altogether, these aforementioned factors highlight the importance of both vaginal pH and cervical mucus as the first barrier to sperm penetration into the uterine cavity. In this chapter, we first describe the vaginal physiology. Then, we characterize the cervical mucus, its production, structure, and composition. Finally, we explain how spermatozoa are transported into the cervical mucus and outline several conditions that can interfere with sperm movement through the vagina and cervical mucus and, therefore, be implicated in the pathophysiology of unexplained infertility.

Vaginal Physiology

Vaginal pH

Potential of hydrogen, or pH, is a measure of hydrogen ion concentration, that is, an appraisal of the acidity or alkalinity of a solution. Numerically, it is equal to 7.0 for neutral solutions. Levels of pH less than 7.0 characterize acidic solutions, while levels greater than 7.0 characterize basic (or alkaline) solutions. The vaginal pH fluctuates from 3.8 to 4.5, and is classified as slightly acidic [1].

The fluid content of the vagina is derived from:

1. Mucus secretions of the cervical columnar cells
2. Transudation through the vaginal walls
3. Vulvar secretions originated from sebaceous and sweat glands
4. Mucus secretion of Bartholin's glands
5. Substances produced by microorganisms present in the vagina [24–26]

The vagina is a genital canal that extends from the vulva to the cervix. Its walls consist of noncornified stratified squamous epithelium, a smooth muscle layer, and a prominent connective tissue rich in elastic fibers [27]. The epithelial cells are rich in glycogen. Vaginal cells are stimulated by estrogen to both synthetize and accumulate increased amounts of glycogen. Due to cell shed and desquamation, glycogen accumulates in the vaginal lumen. Glycogen can be metabolized

F. Y. Nakano (✉) · R. B. F. Leão · S. C. Esteves
Androfert, Av. Doutor Heitor Penteado,
1464, Campinas, SP 13075-460, Brazil
e-mail: dra.fabiana@medreprudutiva.com.br

G. L. Schattman et al. (eds.), *Unexplained Infertility*, DOI 10.1007/978-1-4939-2140-9_16,

in a process called glycogenolysis to pyruvic acid, which is converted in lactic acid and water by anaerobic metabolism. This process is carried out by Doderlein's lactobacillus, the predominant vaginal microorganism, thus decreasing the vaginal pH. As such, both epithelium cells rich in glycogen and the presence of lactobacillus are essential to maintain vaginal acidity [24, 25]. This acid environment protects the vagina from pathogenic microorganisms because most bacteria grow best at a pH of about 7.5 [24].

Lactobacilli also protect the vagina by competing with other bacteria for adherence to the vaginal epithelium, thus forming a biofilm on cervical and vaginal mucosa. Furthermore, lactobacilli produce antimicrobial substances such as hydrogen peroxide, bacteriocins, and biosurfactants [26]. Many factors can interfere on the number of Doderlein's bacilli, and consequently, modulate vaginal pH, such as the systemic or topic use of antibiotics, stress, immunity decrease, hormonal disorders, and modifications in estrogen levels during a woman's lifetime [28].

As a result of fetal exposure to maternal-placental estrogens in the first month of life, lactobacilli are abundant in the vagina, thus maintaining vaginal pH around 5. From the first month of life until puberty, the glycogen content of the vaginal epithelial cells decrease in response to decreased estrogen levels. Consequently, the production of lactic acid decreases while vaginal pH rises to about 7. This modification facilitates the growth of other bacteria, mainly *Staphylococcus epidermidis*, *Streptococcus*, and *E. coli* [28]. Estrogen levels increase again during reproductive years, due to the onset of ovarian activity, lowering vaginal pH to less than 5. This decrease in vaginal pH predisposes to the proliferation of lactobacilli, which accounts to 90% of all microorganisms present in the vagina at this time. Other bacteria such as *Corynebacterium*, *Staphylococcus*, *Streptococcus*, and *Bacterioides* correspond to 10% of this flora [29].

During the menstrual cycle, the vaginal pH becomes more acidic from the 2nd up to the 14th day of the cycle, ranging from 6.6 (± 0.3) to 4.2 (± 0.2) [29]. This acidic vaginal environment is toxic to sperm, for the optimal pH for sperm viability ranges between 7.0 and 8.5, and a reduction in sperm motility is seen at pH of less than 6.0 [2–5]. During sexual intercourse and as a result of sexual excitement, the vaginal epithelium produces a transudate that lubricates and also elevates the vaginal pH to 7.0 within seconds. This decrease in acidity can be maintained for up to 2 h after ejaculation [6]. This physiological modification, associated with the alkaline pH of semen, temporarily protects spermatozoa [30].

The vaginal pH also increases during menses, since blood is slightly alkaline, and also in patients with excessive cervical ectropion, that produces alkaline mucus [31]. Postmenopausal women have a lower amount of glycogen in the epithelial cells as a consequence of hypoestrogenism, and their vaginal pH is around 7 like in prepubescents. Increased vaginal pH in the aforesaid conditions predisposes to proliferation of pathogenic bacteria [32].

Variations in the vaginal pH diminish its defense and increase the susceptibility to infections that can indirectly affect fertility. An association of abnormal vaginal flora (bacterial vaginosis) with increased tumor necrosis factor alpha (TNF-α) and interferon-gamma (IFN-γ) levels in the cervical mucus has been described in patients with unexplained infertility [33]. In addition, concentrations of TNF-α and IFN-γ are significantly higher in the cervical mucus of infertile women with unexplained infertility compared with fertile controls [34]. These data suggest that an altered vaginal ecosystem can induce the production of proinflammatory cytokines which may play a role in the pathophysiology of unexplained infertility [33]. The mechanism by which these cytokines impair fertility is still unclear; however, it has been found that high levels of TNF-α and IFN-γ are associated with elevated levels of activated natural-killer (NK) cells [35].

Finally, semen deficiency to neutralize the acidic vaginal pH can also be an infertility factor since spermatozoa are vulnerable to vaginal acidity [6]. For instance, an abnormally low semen volume (hypospermia) negatively impacts fertility since the semen buffering capacity against vaginal acidity is decreased. The same is true when semen becomes acidic, which may occur as a result of obstruction in the ejaculatory ducts and due to hypoplastic seminal vesicles [36].

Sperm Transport at the Vaginal Level

Under normal conditions, only about 200 out of approximately 280 million spermatozoa deposited in the upper vagina upon ejaculation are capable of successfully transversing the cervical canal [37]. Almost immediately after ejaculation, the semen forms a coagulum that temporarily restricts the movement of sperm out of the seminal clot. Then, this coagulum is gradually liquefied by seminal-fluid proteolytic enzymes produced by the prostate gland during the next 20–30 min [2, 38, 39]. Deficiency in prostatic secretions, usually caused by infectious processes, is related with the absence of secondary liquefaction or partial liquefaction. As a consequence, clustered sperms are trapped within highly viscous semen, which can impair the sperm ability to transverse the cervix [9, 40].

Most spermatozoa are lost at the vaginal level with the expulsion of semen from the introitus. However, a variable number of spermatozoa are rapidly taken up by the cervical mucus in a process described as "rapid transport," leaving behind the seminal plasma [2, 7]. Rapid sperm transport may begin within seconds after ejaculation. In fact, spermatozoa are found in the mucus within 90 s postejaculation [38]. Despite helping sperm to reach the cervical mucus, sperm motility is not the main drive for sperm transit. Sperm movement is predominantly passive, resulting from coordinated vaginal, cervical, and uterine contractions that occur during coitus. Although these contractions are of short duration, they are believed to be the primary force responsible for the rapid progression of sperm to the upper female reproductive tract, like in other mammalian species [2, 41]. Although there are reports of motile sperm persisting within the vagina for up to 12 h after ejaculation, motility of most vaginal sperm is diminished within about 30 min, and after 2 h almost all sperm motility has been lost [39].

Other nonphysiological factors may play a role in sperm loss at the vaginal level. The use of vaginal lubricants during coitus, for instance, has been shown to be toxic to sperm [42–45]. Vaginal infectious processes increase the number of leukocytes in the vagina, thus enhancing sperm phagocytosis and reducing the number of spermatozoa that enter the tongues of cervical mucus extended over the ectocervix [7].

Cervix and Cervical Mucus

Cervix

The cervix, which is the lower narrow portion of the uterus where it joins with the top end of the vagina, generally functions as an effective barrier against sperm [7]. Several important functions have been attributed to the cervix and its secretion, including:

1. Protecting sperm from the hostile environment of the vagina [31, 46, 47]
2. Protecting sperm from phagocytosis by vaginal leukocytes [2, 7, 46, 47]
3. Preventing sperm, microorganisms and particulate matter to access the upper reproductive tract and thus, the peritoneal cavity [2]
4. Facilitating sperm transport during the periovulatory period and modulating at other cycle periods [2, 7, 46, 47]
5. Filtrating morphologically normal sperm [2, 7, 46, 47]
6. Preserving large numbers of sperm within the cervical crypts, providing a biochemical environment sufficient for sperm storage, capacitation, migration, and release of sperm into the upper genital tract [2, 7]

The anatomical and functional structure of the human cervix facilitates the performance of these aforesaid functions, but the production of mucus is probably the most important one. Throughout the menstrual cycle, the cervix changes in size and texture. Just prior to ovulation and as a result of estrogen levels rise, the cervix swells and softens and the external os dilates. Also, during this time, the cervix secretes more abundant, slippery, clear, and stretchy mucus, which exudes from cervix into the vagina, thus facilitating the entrance of sperm into the uterine cavity [2, 48]. In the periovulatory period, more than 96 % of cervical mucus is water, thus conferring the mucus high spinnbarkheit and pronounced ferning capacity; as such, sperm penetrability is highest at this time [46]. After ovulation, progesterone induces the cervix to harden, close and secrete thicker mucus, which acts as a plug, preventing bacteria and sperm from entering the uterus and making fertilization very unlikely [48].

The endocervical canal is lined by single layer of columnar epithelial cells, both ciliated and nonciliated. The cervix does not contain true glandular units; instead, the epithelium is thrown into longitudinal folds and invaginations with blind-ending tubules arising from the clefts forming crypts off the central canal. The nonciliated cells secrete mucin in granular form through exocytosis. There are several hundred mucus-secreting units in the cervical canal. The daily production varies in relation to the cyclical changes of the menstrual cycle, from 600 mg during midcycle to 20–60 mg during other periods of the cycle. A few ciliated cells among the secreting cells propel the cervical mucus from the crypt of origination toward the canal [2, 49, 12].

An uncommon cause of cervical infertility is a previous surgery on the cervix such as cryo- or electric cauterization, cone biopsy and loop electrosurgical excision procedure (LEEP). These interventions can alter the anatomy of the cervix canal and may lead to constriction or even stenosis. As a result, the production of mucus may be impaired due to the removal of secretory cells [8, 9]. Severe infections can also damage the mucus producing cells [12]. Interventions, such as curettage, can also block the canal or simply turn it into a pinpoint opening [9]. Birth defects can likewise affect the cervix. Most of such defects occur in women whose mothers had used diethylstilbestrol (DES), a synthetic nonsteroidal estrogen, which was banned from the marketplace in 1997 [11]. Anomalies in the müllerian ducts, which differentiate to form the fallopian tubes, uterus, the uterine cervix, and the superior aspect of the vagina, can also result in a defective cervix. Most müllerian duct anomalies are associated with functioning ovaries and age-appropriate external genitalia. These abnormalities are often recognized after the onset of puberty, but late presentations include infertility [10, 50]. All of these conditions may significantly impair the ability of sperm to trespass the cervix and enter the upper female reproductive tract [8–12, 50].

Cervical Mucus

The cervical mucus is a heterogeneous mixture of secretions whose rate of production depends on several factors. These factors include the number of mucus-secretory units in the cervical canal, the percentage of mucus-secreting cells per unit and the secretory activity of the cells in response to circulating hormones [12].

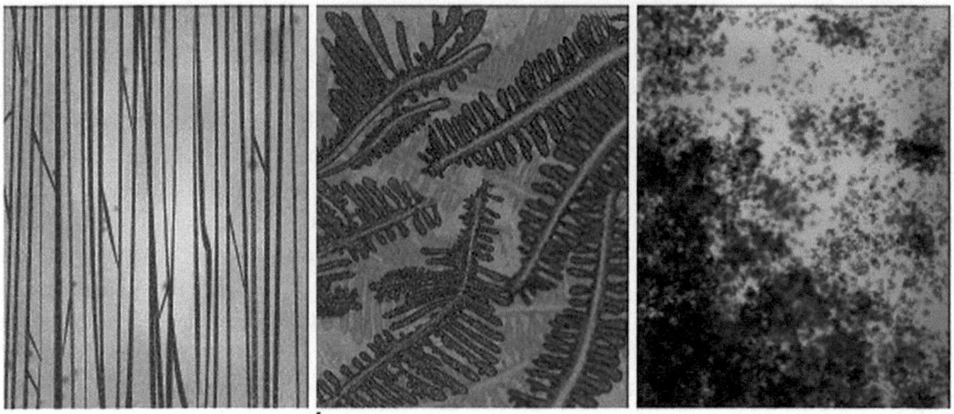

Fig. 16.1 Illustration depicting air-dried cervical mucus studied with *light* microscopy (× 40). **a** Es mucus: a parallel arrangement of crystals is close together but not joined, with or without short branches protruding from them. **b** El mucus: a typical ferning morphology. It has a structure composed of *straight or curved central axis* and with branches protruding from its *axis* at a 90° angle. These branches can also act as an *axis* for new branches, again at a 90° angle. **c** G mucus: a high free-crystal content with no predetermined form

There are several types of mucus, as characterized by Odeblad [51]. Type E is thin and watery (with approximately 98% of water), which is characteristic of estrogen dominance. Type G is thick and sticky, and reflects the stimulation of progestogenic hormones. Under the influence of progesterone, water content decreases to approximately 90% and the mucus becomes more viscous. Therefore, type E is predominant at the time of ovulation in a proportion of about 97% of type E and 3% of type G, while type G predominates during the normal luteal phase [12, 15, 51]. Both types are always present in different proportions during the menstrual cycle, varying according to the circulating progesterone and estrogen levels. Using nuclear magnetic resonance analysis, the aforementioned author established that the ovulatory mucus (E) is a mosaic composed of mucus "strings" (called Es) and "loaves" (labeled as El). The strings (Es) are fluid gels, and the loaves are more viscid gels (El). The Es–El system is very dynamic. Ovulatory mucus contains 20–25% type Es, 72–77% type El, and 3% type G. Since, Es and El differ in their molecular architecture and their protein content, not all areas of the cervical mucus are equally penetrable by the sperm. While the Es mucus conveys the spermatozoa from the vaginal pool, the El type has a very limited role in this respect [12, 52, 53]. The differences between each type of mucus can be observed in dried mucus sample studied in light microscopy. Cervical mucus forms fern-like patterns due to the crystallization of sodium chloride on its fibers, which vary according with the mucus type (Fig. 16.1) [54].

Ultrastructurally, the cervical mucus can be seen as a complex biphasic fluid with high-viscosity and low-viscosity components. It is a hydrogel composed of a low-molecular-weight component (cervical plasma) and a high-molecular-weight component (gel phase). The cervical plasma consists mainly of trace elements (zinc, copper, iron, manganese, selenium, sodium, and chloride ions), organic components of low molecular weight such as glucose and amino acids, and soluble proteins, such as albumin and globulins [12, 55, 56]. The gel phase consists of a glycoprotein network called mucin, presenting glycosylation variations according to the menstrual cycle, contributing to the changes in its physical properties. This extremely large macromolecule (about 10,000 KDa) is rich in carbohydrate content and is responsible for the high mucus viscosity [57]. The mucin macromolecules are thread-like and appear in long parallel bundles maintained by a peptide of 30 kDa. This peptide connects mucin molecules through disulphide bridges (S–S), thus forming mucin micelles of 100–1000 glycoprotein chains [55]. This system assembly, which varies both in diameter and arrangement, is called "micelle." Collectively, mucin molecules form a complex of interconnected micelles, which comprise a lattice whose interstices are capable of supporting the low viscosity phase, which is predominantly water. Protein content is low in the intermicellar spaces of Es mucus. The very low viscosity of Es intermicellar fluid allows very rapid sperm migration [12, 58]. In type G mucus, no micelle formation occurs, but the long macromolecules form a large, three-dimensional, irregular, dense network that does not allow spermatozoa to penetrate (Fig. 16.2) [59]. These channels or spaces vary in size according to the type of mucus: 2–5 μm wide (Es type mucus), 1–2 μm wide (El type mucus), and 0.3–1 μm wide (type G mucus). Therefore, intermicellar spaces play a key role in sperm migration [12].

Abnormalities of cervical mucus can result in infertility. For instance, chronic cervicitis is associated with alterations of cervical mucus. In this case, a different mucus pattern appears, defined as type Q by Odeblad, in which the mucus composition varies depending on the type, degree,

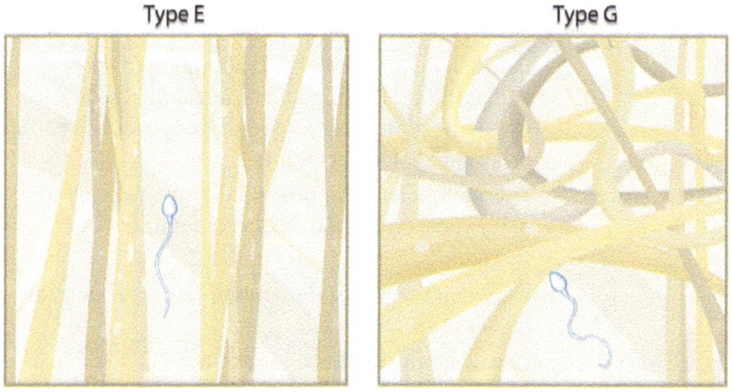

Fig. 16.2 Schematic representation of the gel structure of types E and G cervical mucus. In type E, mucin macromolecules lie together in long parallel bundles (micelles), which spaces in between are filled with cervical plasma. Spermatozoa can easily swim through these spaces. In type G, no micelle formation occurs, and long macromolecules form a large, three-dimensional, irregular, dense network. Spermatozoa are not allowed to penetrate

and duration of the inflammatory process. The crypts releasing this type of secretion have limited response to hormonal stimulation [51, 60]. In acute inflammatory conditions, the crypts can also produce a serous type of secretion of low viscosity but with high leukocyte content, classified as type V, which is unable to maintain sperm vitality. Therefore, common infections of the cervix such as those caused by sexually transmitted microorganisms (*Chlamydia trachomatis, Neisseria Gonorrhea, Trichomonas vaginalis, Mycoplasma hominis, and Ureaplasma urealyticum*) may result in cervical hostility [12].

Women with cystic fibrosis (CF) are also unable to produce the watery and stretchy mucus needed for optimal sperm penetrability. CF is caused by a mutation in the gene for the protein CF transmembrane conductance regulator (CFTR). This protein functions as a channel which transports negatively charged particles (chloride ions) inside and outside the cells. The transport of chloride ions helps to control the movement of water in tissues, which is necessary for the production of thin, freely flowing mucus. When the CFTR protein does not work properly, chloride (Cl^-) is trapped inside the cells. Because chloride is negatively charged, it creates a difference in the electrical potential inside and outside the cell causing sodium to cross into the cell. As a result, water movement from inside to outside cellular compartments is decreased, leading the mucus to be more viscous and less watery thus harming the sperm transport. Along with a loss of Cl^- conductance, mutations of CFTR protein also impede bicarbonate (HCO_3^-) transport. A HCO_3^- rich alkaline pH environment is crucial for optimal sperm motility and capacitation. During the process of releasing highly condensed mucins from intracellular granules, calcium (Ca^{2+}) and hydrogen (H^+) cations must be removed to enable the mucins to expand by as much as 1000 times, forming extracellular mucus–gel networks. It is suggested that HCO_3^- is essential to normal mucin expansion because it forms complexes with these cations. Due to defective HCO_3^- secretion in CF, mucins tend to remain aggregated, poorly solubilized, and less transportable. It is tempting to consider that some cases of reduced fertility in females might be associated with putative mild mutations in this gene with consequent abnormal cervix-uterine mucus release due to inadequate HCO_3^- secretion [14, 61, 62]. An example of this condition is the report of two infertile sisters with significantly abnormal cervical mucus who were found to be compound heterozygote carriers of the CF ΔF508 and R117H/7T mutations [13].

Many exogenous factors can render the cervical mucus hostile to sperm and, therefore, be implicated in the pathophysiology of unexplained infertility [12]. Clomiphene citrate (CC), frequently used to stimulate follicle growth and ovulation as a first line therapy in couples with unexplained infertility, can interfere with the cervical mucus. Clomiphene is structurally similar to estrogen, which allows CC to bind to estrogen receptors (ER) throughout the reproductive system. In contrast to estrogen, CC binds to nuclear ER for extended periods of time, that is, weeks rather than hours, which ultimately depletes ERs by interfering with the normal process of ER replenishment. Acting at the hypothalamic level, CC is effective in ovulation induction by inhibiting negative feedback of estrogen on gonadotropin release, leading to upregulation of the hypothalamic–pituitary–adrenal axis that, in turn, serve to drive ovarian follicular activity. At the same time, CC exerts undesirable and unavoidable adverse antiestrogenic effects in the periphery (endocervix and endometrium). Several studies have described that CC has adverse effects on the quality and quantity of cervical mucus based on cervical mucus score, the value of which is debatable. Despite that, available evidence and accumulated clinical experience support the notion that any adverse antiestrogenic effect presents a significant obstacle for the largest majority of women treated with ovulation induction drugs [16–18, 63, 64]. Another drug that deserves attention is propranolol, which accumulates extensively in the cervical mucus after oral administration; its concentration is fourfold higher in the mucus compared with in the blood. Despite not affecting mucus production, propranolol accumulation may impair sperm motility by its direct effect on sperm membrane ion transport and energy production [19, 65–67]. Nicotine and its metabolite cotinine are secreted into the cervical mucus, and can be found in the mucus even of passive smokers [68, 69]. A retrospective study evaluating smoking histories of 901 women with infertility due to different etiologies and 1264 pregnant women admitted for delivery suggested that smoking is a risk factor for cervical factor infertility (relative risk = 1.7; 95 % confidence interval of 1.0–2.7); however, its mechanism of action is unclear [70]. It has been suggested that nicotine could have toxic effects on spermatozoa, but *in vitro* studies have noted that the harmful effects of nicotine and cotinine to sperm occurs in extremely high concentrations, not seen in the seminal plasma or cervical mucus of smokers [20, 71].

Other Components of Cervical Mucus

The cervical mucus contains not only mucin but also other proteins such as albumin and globulin. The concentration of different proteins in the mucus varies during the menstrual cycle, being lowest at ovulation. Morales et al. (1993), studying the mucus' concentration of protein and its ability to sustain sperm migration, found that periovulatory mucus exhibited low protein concentrations as revealed by sodium dodecyl sulphate polyacrylamide gel electrophoresis (SDS-PAGE). Most of the soluble proteins found in the cervical mucus had their lowest concentration around the periovulatory period, when the mucus is most receptive to sperm penetration [72]. The authors of the aforementioned study concluded that there is a statistically significant inverse relationship between protein concentration in the mucus and its ability to sustain sperm migration.

The mucus also provides local immunity through a unique interaction of immunoglobulins (mainly IgA), cytokines, and reproductive hormones (estrogen and proegesterone). Also, the mucus is a rich source of antimicrobial proteins and peptides, including secretory leucocyte protease inhibitor (SLPI), lysozyme, calprotectin, lactoferrin, human neutophil peptides 1–3, and epithelial beta-defensin [12, 73]. Increased levels of cervical mucus IgA and IgG have been reported in 23 women with genital infections caused by *N. gonorrhea, T. vaginalis,* genital herpes, and nonspecific cervicitis in comparison with a control group of 23 uninfected women ($p<0.001$), thus indicating increased local immune response [74]. Furthermore, it has been suggested that leukocytes, mainly neutrophils, play a role in both the cervical cellular defense line and the "selective" mechanisms of sperm transport through the cervix (phagocytosis of abnormal spermatozoa) [75].

Prostagladins and trace elements also have hormone-dependent cyclical variation in the cervical mucus during the menstrual cycle. Prostaglandins found in the cervical mucus are PGE_1, PGE_2, PGD_2, $PGF_{1\alpha}$, and $PGF_{2\alpha}$, and their contents increase in the preovulatory period. However, their biological importance remains unclear [76]. Ryantová et al. (2008), evaluating PGE_2 levels in ovulatory cervical mucus of 120 women with unexplained miscarriages, found that PGE_2 levels were 6×, 13×, and 21× higher in patients with one, two, and three or more miscarriages compared with controls ($p<0.033$), respectively [77]. Iron and copper levels show marked fall from preovulatory to ovulatory phases. Interestingly, their levels in the cervical mucus were elevated both in patients with primary or secondary infertility couples compared with fertile counterparts. The real influence of these elements in fertility remains unclear, but a spermatotoxic effect of copper has been described [55, 78–80].

Table 16.1 Factors affecting fertility at the vaginal and cervical levels

Vagina	Increase in the vaginal pH: alteration in the vaginal flora, leading to an increased susceptibility to infectious processes (phagocytosis of sperm, proinflammatory cytokines)
	Sperm deficiency in neutralizing the vaginal pH: hypospermia and deficient-seminal vesicle secretion
	Deficiency in sperm liquefaction (e.g., abnormal prostatic secretions)
	Use of lubricants toxic to sperm
Cervix	Previous surgery (e.g., cauterization, cone biopsy, and curettage)
	Infections
	Müllerian abnormalities
	Exogenous: intrauterus diethylstilbestrol (DES)
Cervical mucus	Hormonal: abnormal estrogen levels and premature progesterone rise
	Inflammatory: chronic cervicitis/acute inflammatory conditions
	Genetics: cystic fibrosis
	Exogenous: clomiphene citrate, propranolol, nicotine
	Trace elements: excess levels of copper, iron, and selenium
	Male-related: asthenozoospermia and abnormal morphology
	Immunological: antisperm antibodies in the female serum and semen

Table 16.1 summarizes the conditions that may affect fertility at the vaginal and cervical levels.

Sperm Transport Through the Cervical Mucus

Sperm movement inside the cervical mucus occurs primarily through the interstitial spaces in the mucin micelles. Sperm progression depends mainly on the size of these spaces [81]. The spaces between these large glycoproteins reach their maximum at the midcycle estrogen peak, when there is an increase in mucus production and in its water content [53].

Besides hormonal factors, uterine contractions can also alter the spaces between these macromolecules by mechanical pressure. Furthermore, these mechanical forces contribute to the orientation of the mucin filaments. It is suggested that the outward flow of the cervical mucus establishes a linear alignment of parallel strands, creating aqueous channels between the filaments that direct sperm upward [2, 7, 58]. Given this longitudinal orientation, with mucus outflow originating in the crypts of the cervical epithelium, it has been postulated that spermatozoa are constrained to swim in the direction of least resistance, that is, along the tracts of mucus outflow in the direction of the cervical crypts

[82, 83]. This theory is in agreement with the notion that spermatozoa entering the cervix are directed toward the cervical crypts, which are the sites of mucus secretion that serve as possible sperm storage reservoir. The number of spermatozoa within the cervical mucus is relatively constant for the first 24 h after coitus. Spermatozoa may retain their fertilizing capacity in the human cervical mucus for up to 48 h and their motility for as long as 120 h after ejaculation. However, the number of motile sperm within the mucus is markedly decreased after 48 h [84–86]. From their temporary storage location within the cervical crypts, sperm can be released gradually over time, thus enhancing the probability of fertilization. As the size of the interstices is usually smaller than the size of sperm heads, spermatozoa must actively push their way through the mucus. Therefore, one cause of infertility, presumably, is the reduced sperm progressive motility that prevents sperm movement through the mucus [2, 7].

It is generally believed that another potentially important feature of human cervical mucus is its ability to restrict migration of abnormal spermatozoa, thus acting as a "filter" that eliminates deficient sperm [21, 87, 88]. It has been shown that abnormal sperm have poorer hydrodynamic profile compared with morphologically normal motile sperm [7, 21, 87, 88]. Moreover, sperm movement is probably influenced by the interaction between the mucus and the surface properties of the sperm head; for example, sperm antibodies on the sperm head inhibit sperm movement through the mucus [89].

Like the vagina, the cervix can assemble immune responses. Studies have shown that vaginal insemination stimulates the migration of leukocytes, particularly neutrophils and macrophages, into the cervix as well as into the vagina [90, 91]. This leukocytic invasion protects against microbes that are often seen in the semen, but it does not present a barrier to normal sperm under physiological conditions [88]. On the other hand, it has been demonstrated that neutrophils bind to and ingest human sperm if the female serum contain both serological complement and complement-fixing antisperm antibodies (ASA) [92]. This process occurs when the female becomes immunized against sperm antigens. As already mentioned, immunoglobulins, mainly IgG and IgA, have been detected in human cervical mucus. Secretory IgA is produced locally by plasma cells in subepithelial connective tissue. Although immunoglobulins provide protection from microorganisms, immunological infertility can occur when antibodies present in the cervical mucus recognize sperm-bound antigens [93]. Since complement proteins are present in the cervical mucus, antibody-mediated sperm destruction as well as leukocytic sperm capture may occur [94]. Despite the fact that not all ASA are complement-activated, they can still interfere with sperm progression by attaching the sperm head and avoiding spermatozoa to enter the microarchitecture of the cervical mucus network [93, 95]. Furthermore, the presence of ASA in the male can also result in infertility since such antibodies have been shown to affect sperm motility and function [22, 23, 36].

Conclusions

A substantial diminution in sperm number occurs as they transverse the cervix. From an average of 200 to 300 million sperm deposited in the vagina, only a few hundred achieve proximity to the oocyte. Given this expected high spermatozoa loss, slight modifications in the vaginal pH and cervical mucus may rapidly transform these compounds into a "hostile" environment that may prevent natural conception and be a cause of infertility. Among the several conditions that may be involved in the pathophysiology of unexplained infertility at the vaginal and cervical levels, physicians should pay particular attention to (1) inadequate buffering capacity of acid vaginal pH, (2) alterations in cervical anatomy caused by surgeries, birth defects, and infections, and (3) alterations in the cervical mucus caused by hormonal dysfunctions, inflammatory disorders, CF, exogenous and immunological factors.

Acknowledgment The authors are grateful to Mrs. Fabiola C. Bento for language revision.

References

1. Kelly KG. Tests on vaginal discharge. In: Walker HK, Hall WD, Hurst JW, editors. Clinical methods: the history, physical, and laboratory examinations. 3rd ed. Boston: Butterworths; 1990. p. 833–5.
2. Brannigan RE, Lipshultz LI. Sperm transport and capacitation. Global library of women's medicine. 2008. http://www.glowm.com/index.html?p=glowm.cml/section_view&articleid=315. Accessed 12 March 2013.
3. Makler A, David R, Blumenfeld Z, Better OS. Factors affecting sperm motility. VII. Sperm viability as affected by change of pH and osmolality of semen and urine specimens. Fertil Steril. 1981;36(4):507–11.
4. Peek JC, Matthews CD. The pH of cervical mucus, quality of semen, and outcome of the postcoital test. Clin Reprod Fertil. 1986;4(3):217–25.
5. Zavos PM, Cohen MR. The pH of cervical mucus and the postcoital test. Fertil Steril. 1980;34(3):234–8.
6. Fox CA, Meldrum SJ, Watson BW. Continuous measurement by radio-telemetry of vaginal pH during human coitus. J Reprod Fertil. 1973;33(1):69–75.
7. Speroff L, Fritz MA. Sperm and egg transport, fertilization, and implantation. In: Speroff L, Fritz MA, editors. Clinical gynecologic endocrinology and infertility. Philadelphia: Lippincott Williams & Wilkins; 2005. pp. 437–87.
8. Hammond RH, Edmonds DK. Does treatment for cervical intraepithelial neoplasia affect fertility and pregnancy? BMJ. 1990;301(6765):1344–5.
9. Jequier AM. Sperm transport in the human and mammalian cervix and genital tract: its relation to fertility. In: Jordan JA, Singer A, editors. The cervix. 2nd ed. Oxford: Blackwell; 2006. pp. 169–80.

10. Steinkeler JA, Woodfield CA, Lazarus E, Hillstrom MM. Female infertility: a systematic approach to radiologic imaging and diagnosis. Radiographics. 2009;29(5):1353–70.
11. Hoover RN, Hyer M, Pfeiffer RM, et al. Adverse health outcomes in women exposed in utero to diethylstilbestrol. N Engl J Med. 2011;365(14):1304–14.
12. Sharif K, Olufowobi O. The structure, chemistry and physics of human cervical mucus. In: Jordan JA, Singer A, editors. The cervix. 2nd ed. Oxford: Blackwell; 2006. p. 157–68.
13. Schoyer KD, Gilbert F, Rosenwaks Z. Infertility and abnormal cervical mucus in two sisters who are compound heterozygotes for the cystic fibrosis (CF) DeltaF508 and R117H/7T mutations. Fertil Steril. 2008;90(4):1201.e19–22.
14. Gervais R, Dumur V, Letombe B, et al. Hypofertility with thick cervical mucus: another mild form of cystic fibrosis? JAMA. 1996;276(20):1638.
15. Pommerenke WT. Cyclic changes in the physical and chemical properties of cervical mucus. Am J Obstet Gynecol. 1946;52(6):1023–31.
16. Roumen FJ. Decreased quality of cervix mucus under the influence of clomiphene: a meta-analysis. Ned Tijdschr Geneeskd. 1997;141(49):2401–5.
17. Annapurna V, Dhaliwal LK, Gopalan S. Effect of two antiestrogens, clomiphene citrate and tamoxifen, on cervical mucus and sperm-cervical mucus interaction. Int J Fertil Womens Med. 1997;42(3):215–8.
18. Massai MR, de Ziegler D, Lesobre V, Bergeron C, Frydman R, Bouchard P. Clomiphene citrate affects cervical mucus and endometrial morphology independently of the changes in plasma hormonal levels induced by multiple follicular recruitment. Fertil Steril. 1993;59(6):1179–86.
19. Turner P. Recent observations on drugs and human fertility. Postgrad Med J. 1988;64(754):578–80.
20. Augood C, Duckitt K, Templeton AA. Smoking and female infertility: a systematic review and meta-analysis. Hum Reprod. 1998;13(6):1532–9.
21. Katz D, Morales P, Samuels SJ, Overstreet JW. Mechanisms of filtration of morphologically abnormal human sperm by cervical mucus. Fertil Steril. 1990;54(3):513–6.
22. Shibahara H, Hirano Y, Takamizawa S, Sato I. Effect of sperm-immobilizing antibodies bound to the surface of ejaculated human spermatozoa on sperm motility in immunologically infertile men. Fertil Steril. 2003;79(3):641–2.
23. Shibahara H, Shiraishi Y, Hirano Y, Suzuki T, Takamizawa S, Suzuki M. Diversity of the inhibitory effects on fertilization by anti-sperm antibodies bound to the surface of ejaculated human sperm. Hum Reprod. 2003;18(7):1469–73.
24. Cohen L. Influence of pH on vaginal discharges. Brit J Vener Dis. 1969;45(3):241–7.
25. Redondo-Lopez V, Cook RL, Sobel JD. Emerging role of lactobacilli in the control and maintenance of the vaginal bacterial microflora. Rev Infect Dis. 1990;12(5):856–72.
26. Lepargneur JP, Rousseau V. Rôle protecteur de la flore de Doderleïn. J Gynecol Obstet Biol Reprod (Paris). 2002;31(5):485–94.
27. Eroschenko, VP. Female reproductive system. In: Eroschenko, VP, editor. Di Fiore's Atlas of histology with functional correlations. 11th ed. Philadelphia: Lippincott Williams & Wilkins; 2008. p. 439–88.
28. Sobel JD. Is there a protective role for vaginal flora? Curr Infect Dis Rep. 1999;1(4):379–83.
29. Wagner G, Ottesen B. Vaginal physiology during menstruation. Ann Intern Med. 1982; 96(6 Pt 2):921–3.
30. Masters WH, Johnson VE. The physiology of vaginal reproductive function. West J Surg Obstet Gynecol. 1961;69:105–20.
31. Almeida AB. Higiene Feminina. In: Halbe HW, editor. Tratado de Ginecologia. 3rd ed. Rio de Janeiro: Ed Roca; 2000. p. 107–12.
32. Roy S, Caillouete JC, Roy T, Faden JS. Vaginal pH is similar to follicle-stimulating hormone for menopause diagnosis. Am J Obstet Gynecol. 2004;190(5):1272–7.
33. Aboul Enien WM El Metwally HA. Association of abnormal vaginal flora with increased cervical tumour necrosis factor–alpha and interferon–gamma levels in idiopathic infertility. Egypt J Immunol. 2005;12(2):53–9.
34. Naz RK, Butler A, Witt BR, Barad D, Menge AC. Levels of interferon-gamma and tumor necrosis factor-alpha in sera and cervical mucus of fertile and infertile women: implication in infertility. J Reprod Immunol. 1995;29(2):105–17.
35. Thum MY, Abdalla HI, Bhaskaran S, et al. The relationship of systemic TNF-alpha and IFN-gamma with IVF treatment outcome and peripheral blood NK cells. Am J Reprod Immunol. 2007;57(3):210–7.
36. Esteves SC, Miyaoka R, Agarwal A. An update on the clinical assessment of the infertile male. [corrected]. Clinics (Sao Paulo). 2011;66(4):691–700. (2012;67(2):203. (Erratum in: Clinics, Sao Paulo))
37. Harper MJK. Sperm and egg transport. In: Austin CR, Short RV, editors. Reproduction in mammals: germ cells and fertilization. Cambridge: Cambridge University Press; 1982. p. 102–27.
38. Sobrero AJ, MacLeod J. The immediate postcoital test. Fertil Steril. 1962;13:184–9.
39. Moghissi KS. Cervical and uterine factors in infertility. Obstet Gynecol Clin North Am. 1987;14(4):887–904.
40. Du Plessis SS Gokul S Agarwal A. Semen hyperviscosity: causes, consequences, and cures. Front Biosci (Elite Ed). 2013;5:224–31.
41. Overstreet JW, Tom RA. Experimental studies of rapid sperm transport in rabbits. J Reprod Fertil. 1982;66(2):601–6.
42. Miller B, Klein TA, Opsahl MS. The effect of a surgical lubricant on in vivo sperm penetration of cervical mucus. Fertil Steril. 1994;61(6):1171–3.
43. Frishman GN, Luciano AA, Maier DB. Evaluation of astroglide, a new vaginal lubricant: effects of length of exposure and concentration on sperm motility. Fertil Steril. 1992;58(3):630–2.
44. Anderson L, Lewis SE, McClure N. The effects of coital lubricants on sperm motility in vitro. Hum Reprod. 1998;13(12):3351–6.
45. Kutteh WH, Chao CH, Ritter JO, Byrd W. Vaginal lubricants for the infertile couple: effect on sperm activity. Int J Fertil Menopausal Stud. 1996;41(4):400–4.
46. Tredway DR. The post coital test. Gynecology and obstetrics [CD-ROM]. Philadelphia: Lippincott Williams & Wilkins; 2004.
47. Lunenfeld B, Insler V, eds. Infertility. Berlin: Springer; 1978. p. 90–104.
48. Hatcher RA, Trussel J, Stewart F, Nelson A, Cates W, Guest F, Kowal D eds. Contraceptive technology, 18th ed. New York: Ardent Media Inc; 2004.
49. Hafez ESE. Functional anatomy of uterine cervix. In: Insler V, Lunenfeld B, editors. Infertility: male and female. Edinburgh: Churchill Livingstone; 1986. p. 3–25.
50. Golan A, Langer R, Bukovsky I, Caspi E. Congenital anomalies of the müllerian system. Fertil Steril. 1989;51(5):747–55.
51. Odeblad E. The functional structure of human cervical mucus. Acta Obstet Gynecol Scand. 1968;47:57–79.
52. Odeblad E. Physical properties of cervical mucus. Adv Exp Med Biol. 1977;89:217–25.
53. Overstreet JW, Katz DF, Yudin AI. Cervical mucus and sperm transport in reproduction. Semin Perinatol. 1991;15(2):149–55.
54. Menárguez M, Pastor LM, Odeblad E. Morphological characterization of different human cervical mucus types using light and scanning electron microscopy. Hum Reprod. 2003;18(9):1782–9.
55. Schumacher GF. Biochemistry of cervical mucus. Fertil Steril. 1970;21(10):697–705.
56. Gibbons RA, Selwood R. The macromolecular biochemistry of cervical secretions. In: Blandau RJ, Moghissi KS, editors. The biology of the cervix. Chicago: University of Chicago Press; 1973. p. 251–66.
57. Schumacher GF. The uterine cervix. In: Reproduction. Stuttgart: Georg Thieme; 1977. p. 101–7.
58. Katz DF, Drobnis EZ, Overstreet JW. Factors regulating mammalian sperm migration through the female reproductive tract and oocyte vestments. Gamete Res. 1989;22(4):443–69.

59. Odeblad E, Rudolfsson-Asberg C. Types of cervical secretions: biophysical characteristics. In: Blandau RA, Moghissi KS, editors. The biology of the cervix. Chicago: University of Chicago Press; 1973. p. 267–83.
60. Odeblad E. Micro-NMR in high permanent magnetic fields. Theoretical and experimental investigations with an application to the secretions from single glandular units in the human uterus cervix. Acta Obstet Gynecol Scand. 1966;45(Suppl 2):1–188.
61. Muchekehu RW, Quinton PM. A new role for bicarbonate secretion in cervico-uterine mucus release. J Physiol. 2010;588(Pt 13):2329–42.
62. Quinton PM. Cystic fibrosis: impaired bicarbonate secretion and mucoviscidosis. Lancet. 2008;372(9636):415–7.
63. Randall JM, Templeton A. Cervical mucus score and in vitro sperm mucus interaction in spontaneous and clomiphene citrate cycles. Fertil Steril. 1991;56(3):465–8.
64. Maxson WS, Pittaway DE, Herbert CM, Garner CH, Wentz AC. Antiestrogenic effect of clomiphene citrate: correlation with serum estradiol concentrations. Fertil Steril. 1984;42(3):356–9.
65. Peterson RN, Freund M. The inhibition of the motility of human spermatozoa by various pharmacologic agents. Biol Reprod. 1975;13(5):552–6.
66. Peterson RN, Freund M. Effects of (H+), (Na+), (K+) and certain membrane-active drugs on glycolysis, motility, and ATP synthesis by human spermatozoa. Biol Reprod. 1973;8(3):350–7.
67. Hong CY, Chaput de Saintonge DM, Turner P. The inhibitory action of procaine, (+)-propranolol and (+ /-)-propranolol on human sperm motility: antagonism by caffeine. Br J Clin Pharmacol. 1981;12(5):751–3.
68. Jones CJ, Schiffman MH, Kurman R, Jacob P 3rd, Benowitz N. Elevated nicotine levels in cervical lavages from passive smokers. Am J Public Health. 1991;81(3):378–9.
69. McCann MF, Irwin DE Walton LA, Hulka BS, Morton JL, Axelrad CM. Nicotine and cotinine in the cervical mucus of smokers, passive smokers, and nonsmokers. Cancer Epidemiol Biomarkers Prev. 1992;1(2):125–9.
70. Phipps WR, Cramer DW, Schiff I, Belisle S, Stillman R, Albrecht B, Gibson M, Berger MJ, Wilson E. The association between smoking and female infertility as influenced by cause of the infertility. Fertil Steril. 1987;48(3):377–82.
71. Gandini L, Lombardo F, Lenzi A, Culasso F, Pacifici R, Zuccaro P, Dondero F. The in-vitro effects of nicotine and cotinine on sperm motility. Hum Reprod. 1997;12(4):727–33.
72. Morales P, Roco M, Vigil P. Human cervical mucus: relationship between biochemical characteristics and ability to allow migration of spermatozoa. Hum Reprod. 1993;8(1):78–83.
73. Behrman SJ. Biosynthesis of immunoglobulins by the cervix. In: Blandau RJ, Moghissi KS, editors. The biology of the cervix. Chicago: University of Chicago Press; 1973. p. 237–49.
74. Chipperfield EJ, Evans BA. Effect of local infection and oral contraception on immunoglobulin levels in cervical mucus. Infect Immun. 1975;11(2):215–21.
75. Thompson LA, Tomlinson MJ, Barratt CL, Bolton AE, Cooke ID. Positive immunoselection—a method of isolating leucocytes from leukocytic reacted human cervical mucus samples. Am J Reprod Immunol. 1991;26(2):58–61.
76. Charbonnel B, Kremer M, Gerozissis K, Dray F. Human cervical mucus contains large amounts of prostaglandins. Fertil Steril. 1982;38(1):109–11.
77. Ryantová M, Ulcová-Gallová Z, Micanová Z, Bibková K, Sedivá B. Levels of prostaglandin E2 (PGE2) in cervical ovulatory mucus in women with spontaneous miscarriages. Ceska Gynekol. 2008;73(2):98–101.
78. Chowdhury AR, Singh S, Kutty D, Kamboj VP. Metallic ions in cervical mucus. Indian J Med Res. 1981;73:277–9.
79. Elstein M, Ferrer K. The effect of a copper-releasing intrauterine device on sperm penetration in human cervical mucus in vitro. J Reprod Fertil. 1973;32(1):109–11.
80. Randic L, Musacchio I, Epstein JA. Copper level in cervical mucus of women with copper-bearing and noncopper-bearing intrauterine devices. Biol Reprod. 1973;8(4):499–503.
81. Chretien FC. The saga of human spermatozoa throughout the jungle of the female genital tract. Prog Clin Biol Res. 1989;296:263–72.
82. Davajan V, Nakamura RM. The cervical factor. In: Behrman SJ, Kistner RW, editors. Progress in Infertility. 2nd ed. Boston: Little-Brown; 1975. p. 17–46.
83. Gibbons RA, Mattner P. Some aspects of the chemistry of cervical mucus. Int J Fertil. 1966;11(4):366–72.
84. Overstreet JW, Cooper GW. Sperm transport in the reproductive tract of the female rabbit: I. The rapid transit phase of transport. Biol Reprod. 1978;19(1):101–14.
85. Gould JE, Overstreet JW, Hanson FW. Assessment of human sperm function after recovery from the female reproductive tract. Biol Reprod. 1984;31(5):888–94.
86. Lambert H, Overstreet JW, Morales P, Hanson FW, Yanagimachi R. Sperm capacitation in the human female reproductive tract. Fertil Steril. 1985;43(5):325–7.
87. Morales P, Katz DF, Overstreet JW, Samuels SJ, Chang RJ. The relationship between the motility and morphology of spermatozoa in human semen. J Androl. 1988;9(4):241–7.
88. Suarez SS, Pacey AA. Sperm transport in the female reproductive tract. Hum Reprod Update. 2006;12(1):23–37.
89. Yudin AI, Hanson FW, Katz DF. Human cervical mucus and its interaction with sperm: a fine-structural view. Biol Reprod. 1989;40(3):661–71.
90. Tyler KR. Histological changes in the cervix of the rabbit after coitus. J Reprod Fertil. 1977;49(2):341–5.
91. Pandya IJ, Cohen J. The leukocytic reaction of the human uterine cervix to spermatozoa. Fertil Steril. 1985;43(3):417–21.
92. D'Cruz OJ, Wang BL, Haas GG Jr. Phagocytosis of immunoglobulin G and C3-bound human sperm by human polymorphonuclear leukocytes is not associated with the release of oxidative radicals. Biol Reprod. 1992;46(4):721–32.
93. Menge AC, Edwards RP. Mucosal immunity of the reproductive tract and infertility. In: Zaz RK, editor. Immunology of Reproduction. Boca Raton: CRC Press; 1993. p. 19–36.
94. Matthur S, Rosenlund C, Carlton M, et al. Studies on sperm survival and motility in the presence of cytotoxic sperm antibodies. Am J Reprod Immunol Microbiol. 1988;17(2):41–7.
95. Ulcova-Gallova Z. Ten-year experience with antispermatozoal activity in ovulatory cervical mucus and local hydrocortisone treatment. Am J Reprod Immunol. 1997;38(3):231–4.

Role of Endometrial Receptivity in Unexplained Infertility

17

Alfredo Guillén Antón and Juan Antonio García Velasco

Unexplained Infertility

Normal results encountered during a standard infertility investigation are the hallmark of unexplained infertility. Approximately 30–40 % of infertile couples will be included in this category [1]. While there is not a common definition in the literature of "unexplained infertility", the Practice Committee bulletin on effectiveness and treatment for unexplained infertility [2] refers that the basic evaluation "should provide evidence" of ovulation, adequate sperm production, and patency of the fallopian tubes.

Basically, a "lack of diagnosis" is what defines unexplained infertility after a normal semen analysis, tubal patency (hysterosalpingogram and/or laparoscopy), and normal ovulatory function are confirmed. Other causes for unexplained infertility may be explained on the basis of endocrinology, immunology, genetic, or reproductive physiology [3].

Obviously, with the crudeness of this evaluation described above coupled with the complexity of reproduction, this problem is ripe for further exploration to uncover a number of abnormalities that currently remain without diagnosis.

The current assessment of the reproductive system in humans is far from perfect and some authors claim that the term "unexplained infertility" should be abandoned as it depends on the quantity and quality of the diagnostic tests performed in the couple [4].

Some of these patients with the diagnosis of unexplained infertility may have an altered endometrial function resulting in an impaired dialogue between the embryo and the endometrium. We will try to look at this problem in more detail in this chapter.

J. A. García Velasco (✉) · A. G. Antón
Department of Reproductive Medicine IVI Madrid, Rey Juan Carlos University, Av del Talgo 68, 28023 Madrid, Spain
e-mail: juan.garcia.velasco@ivi.es

Embryo Implantation

Implantation is an extremely complex and yet elusive series of processes in which the blastocyst successfully communicates with the receptive endometrium. Synchrony between the development of the embryo and the changing endometrium is indispensable for a successful implantation (Fig. 17.1).

Three phases have been described in the human implantation process: apposition, adhesion (attachment), and invasion (penetration). The blastocyst communicates with the endometrium in the apposition phase. During the adhesion and invasion phases, the blastocyst attaches itself to the epithelium, orients itself 3-dimensionally and finally invades the underlying endometrial surface establishing a vascular relationship.

After 17β-estradiol priming for endometrial development and subsequent progesterone exposure, the endometrium becomes receptive for only a limited period of time. This window appears to be between days 19 and 21 of an idealized 28 day cycle (luteinizing hormone (LH) + 5 and 7). The dynamic changes in the endometrium described below enables embryo implantation.

Structural and molecular changes occur in the endometrium in the secretory phase during the WOI. Endocrine, paracrine, and autocrine factors are involved between the maternal tissue and the implanting blastocyst in a "cross-talk" that performs with limited efficiency in humans. Implantation requires the synchronous development of a competent blastocyst and an endometrium able to respond to the signals from the blastocyst [5]. The endometrium, with its orchestrated series of changes in preparation for implantation, will be destroyed leading to menstruation if the blastocyst fails to implant.

Endometrial receptivity is compounded of morphological features, molecular basis, and genetic evidence. Many approaches to assessing endometrial maturation and receptivity have been described and are outlined below along with their limitations [6, 7].

G. L. Schattman et al. (eds.), *Unexplained Infertility*, DOI 10.1007/978-1-4939-2140-9_17,

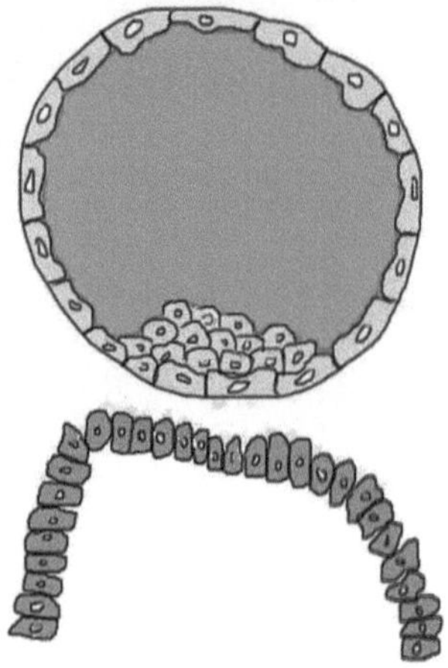

Fig. 17.1 Early stage of blastocyst implantation

Morphology

Ultrasound

In contrast with invasive techniques, transvaginal ultrasound examination is a simple method to measure the structure of the endometrium. Three key aspects can be assessed with ultrasound: structure, contractility, and uterine perfusion.

Structure

The endometrium starts to thicken from a single thin line after menstruation under an estrogenic influence. It will achieve a hypoechoic, trilaminar appearance at the end of the follicular phase. After ovulation the change to a secretory state starts by increasing its echogenicity beginning at the periphery and progressing toward the midline [8]. More structural changes during the luteal phase will continue to transform the endometrium to a homogenous and hyperechoic pattern relative to the myometrium. There is only a slight increase in endometrial thickness during the transition from the mid-follicular to the secretory phase. Data from stimulated and IVF cycles regarding the thickness of the endometrium are conflicting. There seems to be a minimal thickness of about 5 mm below which implantation rarely occurs. Although, data from another study [9] show relatively high success rates with very poor endometrial development, the number of patients was relatively low. Although, studies on endometrial volume measurements with three-dimensional ultrasound show contradictory results, most of them conclude that endometrial volume does not predict endometrial receptivity [10].

The endometrial pattern at the time of human chorionic gonadotropin triggering has shown better correlation to implantation than endometrial volume [11]. The highest pregnancy rates were achieved in patients who had a trilaminar appearing endometrium when compared with the homogenous pattern. Unfortunately, most of this data on endometrial appearance derives from ovulation induction with either oral agents or injectable gonadotropins, and extrapolating this data with multifollicular development and supraphysiologic hormone levels may not be valid compared to the natural cycle. The change to a secretory appearance may be a reflection of a rise in progesterone (perhaps premature) rather than an intrinsic defect of the endometrium.

Contractility

The study of uterine myometrial contractions has shown that there is a reduction in uterine contraction frequency in the mid-luteal phase. Increased wavelike activity may act against implantation in natural cycles [12]. Higher frequency and amplitude contractions lowered implantation rates of transferred day three embryos in an ART study. Nevertheless, it is difficult to extrapolate the results of this study to patients with unexplained infertility.

Uterine Perfusion

An adequate uterine and endometrial blood flow has long been considered a marker of endometrial receptivity. Few studies have been done with conflicting results. One study showed a reduction in endometrial vascular perfusion (vascularization index (VI)) that represents the relative proportion of power Doppler data within the defined volume and flow index (FI) that is the mean signal intensity of this power Doppler information) in patients with unexplained infertility irrespective of serum hormone concentrations [13].

Histology

The first criteria for endometrial "dating" were established more than 60 years ago by Noyes et al. and are still in use today [14]. There are, however, significant limitations of this test described below. Other endometrial tests to evaluate the chance for successful implantation are now available [15].

The morphological description of specific histologic features in the endometrium throughout the menstrual cycle and that change following progesterone exposure has been considered the gold standard test for diagnosis of luteal phase defect. These criteria are still in use for endometrial dating, nevertheless their accuracy as a predictor of endometrial receptivity has been questioned. Balasch et al. evaluated more than 1000 endometrial biopsies showing that luteal phase assessment by histological dating was not related to outcome (pregnancy) in infertile patients [16].

The interobserver variation and difficulties in interpretation of the described histologic changes, much like the description in the original paper, limit its use in the clinical setting [17, 18]. Murray included in their study normal cycling and proven fertile women in contrast to the population evaluated in the study by Noyes et al. Relevant findings in this study included: (a) abnormal and delayed endometrium is common even in fertile women; (b) between-cycle variations in the histology of the secretory endometrium are as common in fertile women as in infertile women; and (c) interobserver variability among different pathologists is common, which may change the diagnosis and subsequently treatment. Although the methodology employed in this study was more rigorous than what is used in clinical practice, they concluded that traditional histologic dating is not a valid tool to diagnose luteal phase defect or to guide treatment for patients with reproductive failure.

Similar conclusions were achieved by Coutifaris et al. [19] in 2004 after the evaluation of 619 biopsies in volunteers in a multicenter, randomized prospective study. Histologic dating was not able to discriminate between a fertile or infertile status, and therefore they postulate that timed endometrial biopsy followed by dating of the endometrium does not provide clinically useful information as a screening test.

Unfortunately, in the endometrial evaluation of unexplained infertility, endometrial histology is not a reliable diagnostic test and is therefore not included in most clinics first line investigations in couples with unexplained infertility.

Pinopodes

Pinopodes (pinopods or uterodomes) identified on scanning electron microscopy (SEM) have been suggested to be ultrastructural markers of endometrial receptivity. They were first described in the rat in 1973 [20], and soon proposed as reliable biomarkers of the human WOI.

Pinopodes are smooth or balloon-like structures that arise from the apical surface of the luminal epithelium of the endometrium in response to progesterone around the time that implantation would be occurring. There is no consensus in the literature as to the timing, function, and clinical value of pinopodes. The quantification of pinopodes is also subjective, and the absence may be interpreted differently as they may have disappeared or not even yet appeared. Due to the inconsistency of pinopode expression during the WOI as well as the requirement of SEM to evaluate for the presence or absence of pinopodes, this does not appear to be useful in the human as a reliable and consistent marker of endometrial receptivity [21].

Biomarkers

A number of factors produced by the endometrium during the so-called window of implantation (WOI) have been considered molecular biomarkers of endometrial receptivity.

Cytokines

Many cytokines participate in implantation [22]. Interleukin (IL)-1, IL-11, IL-6, IL-10, IL-15, IL-18, leukemia inhibitory factor (LIF), colony-stimulating factor (CSF), tumour necrosis factor (TNF), and transforming growth factor-beta (TGF-beta) have all been shown to play essential roles in human implantation.

Interleukin-1

IL-1 is a proinflamatory cytokine located in multiple tissues. It is present in the human endometrium and in the maternal-trophoblast interface during implantation. The importance of this molecule was shown by the use of IL-1 receptor antagonist significantly reducing the number of implanted embryos in mice [23].

Interleukin-6

IL-6 is expressed during the proliferative phase and reaches its peak during the mid-secretory phase. The activity of IL-6 is mediated by a high affinity receptor complex with two membrane proteins (IL-6R and gp130). The IL-6-R is predominantly localized in glandular epithelium, and to a lesser extent in the stroma, throughout the menstrual cycle [24]. IL-6 secretion has been measured in endometrial biopsies comparing fertile and infertile women in day LH+6 and LH+13 finding no difference. However, the level of secretion varied enormously from patient to patient. Nevertheless significantly lower levels of sgp130 were secreted by endometrial biopsies taken between days LH+6 and LH+13 in the infertile patient group compared with fertile controls [25].

Endometrial biopsies in the mid-secretory phase from women with proven fertility and women with recurrent miscarriage were compared in another study. It showed a reduced IL-6 mRNA and IL-1 mRNA expression in women with recurrent miscarriage [26].

Cytokine profiling of endometrial secretions may offer a novel approach in the study of the endometrial factor in human implantation [27]. This study showed that a profile of mediators (17 soluble cytokines, chemokines, and growth factors) involved in implantation and endometrial maturation could be quantified in endometrial secretions aspirated with the embryo transfer catheter prior to an embryo transfer. It was also confirmed that this technique was safe and can be used in the clinical setting (sufficient material for analysis in 99.5 % of cases).

Leukemia Inhibitory Factor

LIF is a multifunctional cytokine of the IL-6 family. LIF expression is low in the endometrium during the follicular phase. It rises after ovulation and reaches its maximal expression during the mid-late secretory phase. LIF mRNA is expressed on days 18–28 (LH+4 to LH+14) of the menstrual cycle in the endometrium of fertile women [28]. The blastocyst also expresses LIF receptor, which highlights the essential crosstalk between both agents in the implantation process. LIF acts through specific receptors on the cell surface sharing gp130 subunit as a common accessory signal transduction molecule [29]. Measurement of LIF secretion in uterine flushing samples is a noninvasive technique that has been used to determine LIF concentration during the late luteal phase in different studies. Mutations in the LIF gene have also been described in nulligravid infertile women, and may be related with transcription abnormalities and decreased LIF expression [28].

In women with unexplained infertility several studies have shown lower LIF concentrations compared to fertile women in uterine flushings, and also in endometrial explants, especially during the implantation window [30–32].

A recent study has been designed to investigate the expression of LIF and its receptor subunit gp130 in endometrium of infertile women in uterine flushing during the implantation window in patients with primary unexplained infertility [33]. LIF mRNA was expressed in the endometrium of all normal fertile women but was significantly decreased in infertile women. LIF was not detectable in 88 % of samples collected from infertile women. Gp130 mRNA was hardly detectable in both fertile and infertile women with no difference between them. Infertile women secreted significantly less LIF and gp130 molecules in the uterine flushing compared with normal fertile women. They concluded that the measurement of secreted LIF and gp130 molecules in uterine flushing could be another useful technique for predicting successful implantation.

Unfortunately, what appears to be a breakthrough in the laboratory does not always translate into clinical benefit. In a randomized controlled trial, the use of this molecular biomarker and supplementing women with rLIF in patients with unexplained implantation failure did not improve implantation or pregnancy rates compared with placebo [34]. Measurement of LIF concentrations in endometrial secretions and addition of LIF to culture media or into the endometrium at the time of embryo transfer are still in need of further investigation.

Cellular Adhesion Molecules Family

Integrins

Integrins are one of the families of the cell adhesion molecules (CAM). Integrin β-3 expression is up-regulated during the WOI, while α-4 integrin is down-regulated in the same period of time. Integrin αvβ3 and its ligand osteopontin (OPN) have been extensively studied. Apart from immunohistochemical methods, Horcajadas et al. showed that OPN is up-regulated during the WOI when compared with both the late proliferative phase and the early secretory phase with microarray technology [35]. Abnormal integrin expression was found in women with unexplained infertility [36, 37]. It has also been described an aberrant expression of αvβ3 integrin in patients with endometriosis and absence of expression in patients with IVF failure but adequate embryo quality and/or endometriosis. The hypothesis that this marker would return after a 3-month course of GnRH agonist, and that this would predict which patients with endometriosis would benefit from the treatment before an IVF cycle could not be proven [38].

Selectins

Selectins are a group of CAM's that includes P-selectin, L-selectin, and E-selectin. Selectins seem to take part in the very early stages of blastocyst interaction with the maternal endometrial epithelium. L-selectine consists of a large, highly glycosylated extracellular domain, a single spanning trans-membrane domain, and a small cytoplasmic tail. It is expressed on vessel walls capturing leukocytes and binding them after activation at the site where they are needed [39]. A similar hypothesis can be made between leukocyte's "rolling" phenomenon and the blastocyst apposition to the endometrial epithelium [40]. Selecting oligosaccharide-based ligand expression is also up-regulated during the WOI [41]. Immunohistochemical techniques of uterine epithelium for the expression of selectin ligands (MECA-79 and HECA-452) were compared in fertile women and in patients with unexplained infertility [42]. During the secretory phase in natural cycles, MECA-79 was more strongly expressed in fertile women compared to infertile patients. It was also shown that the expression of GlcNAc6ST-2 is decreased in infertile patients when compared with fertile women, which correlates with the decrease in MECA-79 expression.

The expression of L-Selectin was also compared in a pilot study in 20 patients with recurrent implantation failure and 20 fertile women [43]. In the RIF patients, those with negative result for the MECA-79 tests did not become pregnant, postulating that screening for the absence of this ligand may identify a poor prognosis group of patients.

Growth Factors

In the vast families of growth factors, the members of the epidermal growth factor (EGF) family, and the insulin-like growth factors (IGF) play decisive roles in the implantation process. Heparin-binding epidermal growth factor (HB-EGF) plays a role in implantation and embryonic development reaching its maximal expression during the period of endometrial receptivity [44, 45]. Following the hypothesis that women with unexplained infertility may show deficiencies in a series of biochemical markers reflecting impaired endometrial development, Aghajova studied HB-EGF endometrial expression. They compared the endometrium from women with unexplained infertility with endometrium from women with male factor infertility or healthy fertile controls. HB-EGF expression was lower in women with unexplained infertility and the authors postulated that abnormal expression of this member of the EGF family may contribute to infertility in some patients with unexplained infertility [46].

Proprotein Convertase 5/6 (PC6)

PC6 is a serine protease, which has an essential role as a regulator for implantation [47]. PC6 achieves its maximum expression during the WOI.

Uterine lavages were obtained in patients ($n=103$) diagnosed with unexplained infertility and compared to fertile controls in a recent study. In a subgroup of unexplained infertility patients, the PC6 activity was significantly lower than the activity in another group of unexplained infertility patients and highly significantly lower than fertile women. Unfortunately, there is not a description of the two subgroups of patients with unexplained infertility with such a different PC6 activity. The assessment of PC6 with in uterine fluid may lead to the establishment a less invasive marker for the evaluation of endometrial receptivity [48], although no treatment exists for those with reduced levels.

Molecular Approaches

New molecular technologies are being used to identify biomarkers of the WOI and thus to assess endometrial receptivity. During the last decade global gene expression analysis has tried to identify genes associated with human endometrial receptivity [49–59]. Many different genes have been evaluated and only a small fraction of them have been selected for their potential role in the endometrial receptivity. Selecting specific sets of genes important during the WOI is made more difficult due to discrepancies among studies in design, data analysis, and microarray platforms. Altmäe et al. published their experience in 2010 comparing endometrial biopsy samples from healthy women with proven fertility and patients with unexplained infertility demonstrating that the endometrial gene expression pattern at the time of implantation is different between these two populations of patients [60]. The endometrial samples were obtained on cycle day LH+7. Microarray analysis was performed using the Whole Human Genome Oligo Microarray (Agilent Technologies) and gene expression profiles were compared. A total of 260 differentially expressed genes were identified, 145 were significantly up-regulated and 115 down-regulated in the endometria of infertile patients compared with fertile controls. Among other findings, there was a significant dysregulation in the leukocyte extravasation-signaling pathway in infertile women, in concordance with previous studies [40].

The experience of our group in this field led to the development of a customized gene expression microarray—endometrial receptivity array (ERA), a bioinformatic predictor for endometrial dating and in addition to define a transcriptomic signature for human endometrial receptivity [61].

Previous work from our group analyzed the different gene expression profile between prereceptive and receptive endometrium [62] in healthy fertile donors and IVF patients. The raw expression data from this study were used to select the candidate genes using endometrial samples from a prereceptive group LH+1, LH+3, and LH+5 and a receptive group LH+7. A total of 238 genes were found to be differentially expressed in the receptive phase, and therefore included in the ERA design.

Once the ERA was designed, another set of endometrial biopsies (training set) was used to train the predictor [61] to date the endometrium and to define the receptivity expression signature. This new set of sample came from fertile women in different moments during the cycle (receptive LH+7, prereceptive LH+1 to LH+5, and proliferative day 8–12 of the cycle) and also from patients with pathology in LH+7 (implantation failure and hydrosalpinx).

A clustering of the ERA genes in the different scenarios in the cycle was performed to detect similar expressions from the proliferative to the secretory phase. In order to define the transcriptomic signature for endometrial receptivity, different gene expressions in ERA were compared: receptive vs. prereceptive and receptive vs. proliferative. A total of 134 genes with statistically significance resulted from these comparisons isolating 74 up-regulated and 60 down-regulated genes. In our study, the endometrial dating classify an LH+7 endometrium (R) in transcriptomic terms with a specificity and sensitivity of 0.8857 and 0.99758, respectively; and a specificity of 0.1571 and a sensitivity of 0.995 for the pathological classification.

The limitations of the histological dating are confirmed once again in the comparison with the ERA [63], changing the point of view and initiating a transformation from the anatomic to molecular medicine. Our group compared the endometrial dating according to the histologic features (Noyes criteria) between two pathologists and the ERA predictor in samples from oocyte donors. Also, a reproducibility study was performed in a small group with samples obtained in the same day of the cycle 29–40 months later. The results of this study showed that the ERA was more accurate than histologic dating and that the reproducibility of the ERA test was 100% consistent.

Table 17.1 Usefulness of specific diagnostic tools for endometrial receptivity

		Usefulness
Morphological studies	US	+
	Histology	−
	Pinopodes	−
Biomarkers	Cytokines	+
	CAM	+
	Growth factors	+
Molecular tests	ERA	++

CAM cell adhesion molecules, *ERA* endometrial receptivity array

The ERA test is included in the clinical protocol of implantation failure in our group as it has been proven an accurate method to discriminate among patients with receptive and nonreceptive endometrium on day LH + 7, or after 5 days of progesterone in a programmed cycle [63]. Nevertheless in terms of implantation, the clinical relevance of this molecular tool for endometrial receptivity has not been yet elucidated in randomized controlled trials.

Conclusions

Human embryo implantation is not completely understood. A number of defects in the endometrium have been identified and may play a decisive role in identifying a cause of unexplained infertility. Histologic tests are not reliable, and endometrial biopsies or aspirates to identify a single biomarker have limited usefulness in the clinical setting. The use of the ultrasound examination provides limited information about endometrial appearance and some correlation to implantation potential but the picture is incomplete. Molecular gene expression tools are being investigated for the possible diagnosis of endometrial abnormalities as a cause for previously unexplained infertility (Table 17.1).

References

1. Smith S, Pfiefer SM, Collins J. Diagnosis and management of female infertility. JAMA. 2003;290(13):1767–70.
2. ASRM. Diagnostic evaluation of the infertile female: a committee opinion. Fertil Steril. 2012;98:302–7.
3. Pellicer A, Albert C, Mercader A, Bonilla-Musoles F, Remohi J, Simon C. The follicular and endocrine environment in women with endometriosis: local and systematic cytokine production. Fertil Steril. 1998;70:425–31.
4. Gleicher N, Barad D. Unexplained infertility: does it really exist? Hum Reprod. 2006;21(8):1951–5.
5. Nardo LG, Li TC, Edwards RG. Introduction: human embryo implantation failure and recurrent miscarriage: basic science and clinical practice. Reprod Biomed Online. 2006;13:11–2.
6. Achache H, Revel A. Endometrial receptivity markers, the journey to successful embryo implantation. Hum Reprod Update. 2006;12:731–46.
7. Diedrich K, Fauser BCJM, Devroey P, et al. On behalf of the Evian Annual Reproduction (EVAR) workshop group: the role of the endometrium and embryo in human implantation. Hum Reprod Update. 2007;13:365–77.
8. Killick SR. Ultrasound and the receptivity of the endometrium. Reprod Biomed Online. 2007;15(1):63–7.
9. Richter KS, Bugge KR, Bromer JG, Levy MJ. Relationship between endometrial thickness and embryo implantation, based on 1294 cycles of in vitro fertilization with transfer of two blastocyst-stage embryos. Fertil Steril. 2007;87(1):53–9.
10. Alcázar JL. Three-dimensional ultrasound assessment of endometrial receptivity: a review. Reprod Biol Endocrinol. 2006;4:56.
11. Kupesic S, Bekavac I, Bjelos D, Kurjak A. Assessment of endometrial receptivity by transvaginal color doppler and three- dimensional power doppler ultrasonography in patients undergoing in vitro fertilization procedures. J Ultrasound Med. 2001;20:125–34.
12. Ijland MM, Evers JL, Hoogland HJ. Velocity of endometrial wavelike activity in spontaneous cycle. Fertil Steril. 1997;68:72–5.
13. Raine-Fenning NJ, Campbell BK, Kendall NR, et al. Endometrial and subendometrial perfusion are impaired in women with unexplained subfertility. Hum Reprod. 2004;19:2605–14.
14. Noyes RW, Hertig AT, Rock J. Dating the endometrial biopsy. Fertil Steril. 1950;1:3–17.
15. Ray A, Shah A, Gudi A, Homburg R. Unexplained infertility: an update and review of practice. Reprod Biomed Online. 2012;24(6):591–602.
16. Noyes RW, Hertig AT, Rock J. Dating the endometrial biopsy. Fertil Steril. 1950;1:3–17.
17. Balasch J, Fábregues F, Creus M, Vanrell JA. The usefulness of endometrial biopsy for luteal phase evaluation in infertility. Hum Reprod. 1992;7(7):973–7.
18. Murray MJ, Meyer WR, Zaino RJ, Lessey BA, Novotny DB, Ireland K, et al. A critical analysis of the accuracy, reproducibility, and clinical utility of histologic endometrial dating in fertile women. Fertil Steril. 2004;81:1333–43.
19. Coutifaris C, Myers ER, Guzick DS, Diamond MP, Carson SA, Legro RS, et al. Histological dating of timed endometrial biopsy tissue is not related to fertility status. Fertil Steril. 2004;82:1264–72.
20. Enders AC, Nelson DM. Pinocytotic activity of the uterus of the rat. Am J Anat. 1973;138:277–99.
21. Quinn CE, Casper RF. Pinopodes: a questionable role in endometrial receptivity. Hum Reprod Update. 2009;15:229–36.
22. Dimitriadis E, White CA, Jones RL, Salamonsen LA. Cytokines, chemokines and growth factors in endometrium related to implantation. Hum Reprod Update. 2005;11:613–30.
23. Simon C, Caballero-Campo P, Garcia-Velasco JA, Pellicer A. Potential implications of chemokines in reproductive function: an attractive idea. J Reprod Immunol. 1998;38:169–93.
24. Tabibzadeh S, Babaknia A. The signals and molecular pathways involved in implantation, a symbiotic interaction between blastocyst and endometrium involving adhesion and tissue invasion. Hum Reprod. 1995;10:1579–602.
25. Sherwin JR, Smith SK, Wilson A, Sharkey AM. Soluble gp130 is up-regulated in the implantation window and shows altered secretion in patients with primary unexplained infertility. J Clin Endocrinol Metab. 2002;87:3953–60.
26. Jasper MJ, Tremellen KP, Robertson SA. Reduced expression of IL-6 and IL-1alpha mRNAs in secretory phase endometrium of women with recurrent miscarriage. J Reprod Immunol. 2007;73:74–84.
27. Boomsma CM, Kavelaars A, Eijkemans MJ, Amarouchi K, Teklenburg G, Gutknecht D, Fauser BJ, Heijnen CJ, Macklon NS. Cytokine profiling in endometrial secretions: a non-invasive window on endometrial receptivity. Reprod Biomed Online. 2009;18(1):85–94.
28. Arici A, Engin O, Attar E, Olive DL. Modulation of leukemia inhibitory factor gene expression and protein biosynthesis in human endometrium. J Clin Endocrinol Metab. 1995;80(6):1908–15.
29. Steck T, Giess R, Suetterlin MW, Bolland M, Wiest S, Poehls UG, Dietl J. Leukemia inhibitory factor (LIF) gene mutations in women with unexplained infertility and recurrent failure of implantation after IVF and embryo transfer. Eur J Obstet Gynecol Reprod Biol. 2004;112:69–73.

30. Laird SM, Tuckerman EM, Dalton CF, Dunphy BC, Li TC, Zhang X. The production of leukemia inhibitory factor by human endometrium: presence in uterine flushing and production by cells in culture. Hum Reprod. 1997;12:569–74.
31. Dimitriadis E, Stoikos C, Stafford-Bell M, Clark I, Paiva P, Kovacs G, Salamonsen LA. Interleukin-11, IL-11 receptor α and leukemia inhibitory factor are dysregulated in endometrium of infertile women with endometriosis during implantation window. J Reprod Immunol. 2006;69:53–64.
32. Hambartsoumain E. Endometrial leukemia inhibitory factor as a possible cause of unexplained infertility and multiple failures of implantation. Am J Reprod Immunol. 1998;39:137–43.
33. Tawfeek MA, Eid MA, Hasan AM, Mostafa M, El-Serogy HA. Assessment of leukemia inhibitory factor and glycoprotein 130 expression in endometrium and uterine flushing: a possible diagnostic tool for impaired fertility. BMC Womens Health. 2012;12:10.
34. Brinsden PR, Alam V, de Moustier B, Engrand P. Recombinant human leukemia inhibitory factor does not improve implantation and pregnancy outcomes after assisted reproductive techniques in women with recurrent unexplained implantation failure. Fertil Steril. 2009;91:1445–7.
35. Horcajadas JA, Riesewijk A, Dominguez F, Cervero A, Pellicer A, Simon C. Determinants of endometrial receptivity. Ann N Y Acad Sci. 2004;1034:166–75.
36. Lessey BA, Castelbaum AJ, Sawin SW, Sun J. Integrins as markers of uterine receptivity in women with primary unexplained infertility. Fertil Steril. 1995;63(3):535–42.
37. Klentzeris LD, Bulmer JN, Trejdosiewicz LK, Morrison L, Cooke ID. Beta-1 integrin cell adhesion molecules in the endometrium of fertile and infertile women. Hum Reprod. 1993;8:1223–30.
38. Surrey E, Lietz A, Gustofson R, Minjarez D, Schoolcraft W. Does endometrial integrin expression in endometriosis patients predict enhanced in vitro fertilization cycle outcomes after prolonged GnRH agonist therapy? Fertil Steril. 2010;93(2):646–51.
39. Alon R, Feigelson S. From rolling to arrest on blood vessels: leukocyte tap dancing on endothelial integrin ligands and chemokines at sub-second contacts. Semin Immunol. 2002;14:93–104.
40. Dominguez F, Yanez-Mo M, Sanchez-Madrid F, Simon C. Embryonic implantation and leukocyte transendothelial migration: different processes with similar players? FASEB J. 2005;19:1056–60.
41. Genbacev OD, Prakobphol A, Foulk RA, Krtolica AR, Ilic D, Singer MS, Yang ZQ, Kiessling LL, Rosen SD, Fisher SJ. Trophoblast L-selectin- mediated adhesion at the maternal–fetal interface. Science. 2003;299:405–8.
42. Margarit L, Gonzalez D, Lewis PD, Hopkins L, Davies C, Conlan RS, et al. L-selectin ligands in human endometrium: comparison of fertile and infertile subjects. Hum Reprod. 2009;24:2767–77.
43. Foulk RA, Zdravkovic T, Genbacev O, Prakobphol A. Expression of L-selectin ligand MECA-79 as a predictive marker of human uterine receptivity. J Assist Reprod Genet. 2007;24:316–21.
44. Leach RE, Khalifa R, Ramirez ND, et al. Multiple roles for heparin-binding epidermal growth factor-like growth factor are suggested by its cell-specific expression during the human endometrial cycle and early placentation. J Clin Endocrinol Metab. 1999;84:3355–63.
45. Yoo HJ, Barlow DH, Mardon HJ. Temporal and spatial regulation of expression of heparin-binding epidermal growth factor-like growth factor in the human endometrium: a possible role in blastocyst implantation. Dev Genet. 1997;21:102–8.
46. Aghajanova L, Bjuresten K, Altmäe S, Landgren BM, Stavreus-Evers A. HB-EGF but not amphiregulin or their receptors HER1 and HER4 is altered in endometrium of women with unexplained infertility. Reprod Sci. 2008;15(5):484–92.
47. Nie G, Li Y, Wang M, Liu YX, Findlay JK, Salamonsen LA. Inhibiting uterine pc6 blocks embryo implantation: an obligatory role for a proprotein convertase in fertility. Biol Reprod. 2005;72:1029–36.
48. Heng S, Hannan NJ, Rombauts LJ, Salamonsen LA, Nie G. PC6 levels in uterine lavage are closely associated with uterine receptivity and significantly lower in a subgroup of women with unexplained infertility. Hum Reprod. 2011;26(4):840–6.
49. Carson DD, Lagow E, Thathiah A, Al-Shami R, Farach-Carson MC, Vernon M, Yuan L, Fritz MA, Lessey B. Changes in gene expression during the early to mid-luteal (receptive phase) transition in human endometrium detected by high-density microarray screening. Mol Hum Reprod. 2002;8:871–9.
50. Kao LC, Tulac S, Lobo S, Imani B, Yang JP, Germeyer A, Osteen K, Taylor RN, Lessey BA, Giudice LC. Global gene profiling in human endometrium during the window of implantation. Endocrinology. 2002;143:2119–38.
51. Borthwick JM, Charnock-Jones DS, Tom BD, Hull ML, Teirney R, Phillips SC, Smith SK. Determination of the transcript profile of human endometrium. Mol Hum Reprod. 2003;9:19–33.
52. Riesewijk A, Martin J, van Os R, Horcajadas JA, Polman J, Pellicer A, Mosselman S, Simon C. Gene expression profiling of human endometrial receptivity on days LH þ 2 versus LH þ 7 by microarray technology. Mol Hum Reprod. 2003;9:253–64.
53. Horcajadas JA, Riesewijk A, Martin J, Cervero A, Mosselman S, Pellicer A, Simon C. Global gene expression profiling of human endometrial receptivity. J Reprod Immunol. 2004;63:41–9.
54. Mirkin S, Arslan M, Churikov D, Corica A, Diaz JI, Williams S, Bocca S, Oehninger S. In search of candidate genes critically expressed in the human endometrium during the window of implantation. Hum Reprod. 2005;20:2104–17.
55. Simon C, Oberye J, Bellver J, Vidal C, Bosch E, Horcajadas JA, Murphy C, Adams S, Riesewijk A, Mannaerts B, et al. Similar endometrial development in oocyte donors treated with either high- or standard-dose GnRH antagonist compared to treatment with a GnRH agonist or in natural cycles. Hum Reprod. 2005;20:3318–27.
56. Talbi S, Hamilton AE, Vo KC, Tulac S, Overgaard MT, Dosiou C, Le Shay N, Nezhat CN, Kempson R, Lessey BA, et al. Molecular phenotyping of human endometrium distinguishes menstrual cycle phases and underlying biological processes in normo-ovulatory women. Endocrinology. 2006;147:1097–121.
57. Feroze-Zaidi F, Fusi L, Takano M, Higham J, Salker MS, Goto T, Edassery S, Klingel K, Boini KM, Palmada M, et al. Role and regulation of the serum- and glucocorticoid-regulated kinase 1 in fertile and infertile human endometrium. Endocrinology. 2007;148:5020–9.
58. Haouzi D, Assou S, Mahmoud K, Tondeur S, Reme T, Hedon B, De Vos J, Hamamah S. Gene expression profile of human endometrial receptivity: comparison between natural and stimulated cycles for the same patients. Hum Reprod. 2009;24:1436–45.
59. Haouzi D, Mahmoud K, Fourar M, Bendhaou K, Dechaud H, De Vos J, Reme T, Dewailly D, Hamamah S. Identification of new biomarkers of human endometrial receptivity in the natural cycle. Hum Reprod. 2009;24:198–205.
60. Altmäe S, Martínez-Conejero JA, Salumets A, Simón C, Horcajadas JA, Stavreus-Evers A. Endometrial gene expression analysis at the time of embryo implantation in women with unexplained infertility. Mol Hum Reprod. 2010;16(3):178–87.
61. Díaz-Gimeno P, Horcajadas JA, Martínez-Conejero JA, Esteban FJ, Alama P, Pellicer A, et al. A genomic diagnostic tool for human endometrial receptivity based on the transcriptomic signature. Fertil Steril. 2011;95:50–60.
62. Horcajadas JA, Riesewijk A, Mínguez P, Dopazo J, Esteban FJ, Domínguez F, et al. Controlled ovarian stimulation induces a functional genomic delay of the endometrium with potential clinical implications. J Clin Endocrinol Metab. 2008;93:4500–10.
63. Díaz-Gimeno P, Ruiz-Alonso M, Blesa D, Bosch N, Martínez-Conejero JA, Alamá P, Garrido N, Pellicer A, Simón C. The accuracy and reproducibility of the endometrial receptivity array is superior to histology as a diagnostic method for endometrial receptivity. Fertil Steril. 2013;99(2):508–17.

Fallopian Tube Dysfunction in Unexplained Infertility

18

Thalia R. Segal and Avner Hershlag

Normal Tubal Physiology

The human oviduct is a tubular, seromuscular structure that attaches distally to the ovary and proximally to the uterine fundus. The length of the human oviduct averages around 12 cm and can be divided into four parts: the infundibulum, the ampullary region, the isthmic portion, and the intramural portion. The infundibulum is the trumpet-shaped distal portion of the tube that communicates with the peritoneal cavity and ovary. It contains an outer longitudinal and inner circular muscle layers and a lumen lined with cilia concentrated at the fimbria. The muscular layers of the myosalpinx provide peristalsis to facilitate gamete union and transport back to the uterus [1].

The fallopian tube is lined by epithelium composed of 70% ciliated cells in the infundibulum and the remaining nonciliated secretory cells in the ampulla [2] (Fig. 18.1). Secretory cells release important cytoplasmic factors for egg passage and implantation [3]. During the estrous cycle, epithelial height and secretory activity increase, reaching a plateau before ovulation. After ovulation, cell height decreases as the material is evacuated into the tubal lumen.

Ciliated epithelium has adhesive features that assist in ovum transport. Cilia beat in the direction of the uterus. This is the site of ovum capture and accounts for distal tubal dysfunction. The ampulla is 5–8 cm long and is the site of fertilization and early cleavage of the human embryo. This is also the most common site of tubal ectopic pregnancies.

The isthmus extends from the ampulla to the uterus and is the site of proximal tubal obstructions, which may inhibit spermatozoa from reaching the egg. The length of the isthmus is 2–3 cm and is the most muscular portion of the fallopian tube with the narrowest lumen. The mucosa is arranged in folds and is less ciliated compared with the distal tube. The intramural segment is the portion of tube that extends into the uterine cavity. It has three layers of muscle and has been described as the sphincter between the uterus and tube.

Tubal Fluid

Tubal fluid plays a critical role in providing the right environment for gametes traveling through the tube and optimizing circumstances for sperm capacitation and fertilization of the egg. In addition, in the past decade, evidence from in vitro fertilization (IVF) data has shed light over the role of tubal fluid in implantation. Specifically, IVF in patients with hydrosalpinx results in a ~50% reduction in pregnancy rates compared with patients without tubal disease [4]. In patients in whom the diseased tubes have been surgically removed, pregnancy rates have improved back to control values [5, 6]. Follicular fluid (FF) has been shown to be toxic to embryos in vitro [7]. Tubal fluid is composed of electrolytes, specifically high levels of potassium and bicarbonate compared with plasma. In addition, glycoproteins, glucose, pyruvate, lactate, and 17 different amino acids have been identified in tubal secretions [8]. The concentration of glucose fluctuates with the menstrual cycle. Following ovulation, the concentration of glucose decreases tenfold [9]. Tubal lumen glucose concentration drops from 3.1 mM in the follicular phase to 0.5 mM midcycle [10]. Human and animal studies have shown that estrogen and progesterone modulate oviductal fluid secretion by the epithelium [11, 12]. Estrogen causes hypertrophy, maturation, and the differentiation of the ciliated phenotype in fallopian tube epithelial cells in vitro [13]. Conversely, progesterone causes atrophy and decreases secretory production during the luteal phase.

Tubal fluid also contains glycoproteins, which may have a role in early development of the oocyte and embryos, enhance adherence of spermatozoa to the isthmus of the fallopian tube, and improve fertilization. Prior to ovulation, an oviduct-specific glycoprotein (OSGP) has been identified to enhance sperm capacitation, bind to the zona pellucida,

A. Hershlag (✉) · T. R. Segal
Department of Obstetrics, Gynecology and Reproductive Medicine, North Shore-Long Island Jewish Hospital of Hofstra University School of Medicine, 300 Community Drive, Manhasset, NY 11030, USA
e-mail: hershlag@nshs.edu

T. R. Segal
e-mail: thalia.segal@gmail.com

G. L. Schattman et al. (eds.), *Unexplained Infertility,* DOI 10.1007/978-1-4939-2140-9_18,

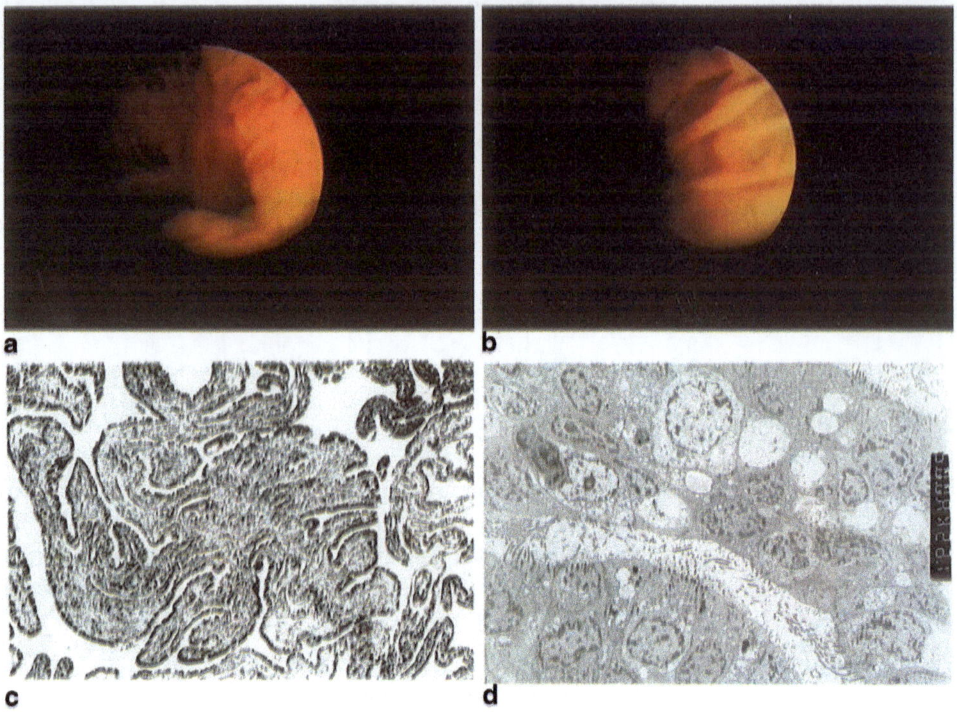

Fig. 18.1 Normal fallopian tube. Salpingoscopy reveals normal-looking mucosa in the ampullary (**a**) and infundibular (**b**) regions. A thin section of the ampulla (**c**) shows normal ciliated endosalpinx. Electron microscopy (**d**) shows evidence of normal homogenous cytoplasm, abundant mitochondria, columnar-shaped cells, normal nuclei, and a normal complement of cilia. (Reprinted from Hershlag et al. 1991, with permission from Wolters Kluwer Health)

and facilitate sperm penetration [14]. Others have postulated that OSGP and other glycoproteins increase the viscosity of the oviductal fluid, which serves as a buffer for the embryo against osmotic changes in the luminal fluid and also as protection against immunologic factors [15].

Spermatozoa undergo capacitation and antigenic changes through exposure to the uterus and tubal fluid, containing copious amounts of β-amylase [16]. This step is followed by the acrosome reaction, hyperactivation, and successful penetration of the zona pellucida of the oocyte.

In conclusion, the delicate composition of tubal fluid plays a critical role in fertilization of the egg, as well as embryo development and transport to the uterus. Any disturbance in the production of tubal fluid due to an erratic hormone milieu, destruction of secretory cells by fibrosis, or infection could potentially lead to altered sperm and egg transport and fertilization.

Tubal Inflammation

It is unclear what proportion of acute episodes of salpingitis is subclinical. Many young women may experience no symptoms or a low-grade fever or nonspecific abdominal pain. Oftentimes, these women do not seek medical care or get misdiagnosed. Physicians should therefore have a low threshold for diagnosis and treatment of subclinical or "silent" salpingitis to prevent future ectopic pregnancies and infertility.

Subclinical Infection

In the 9 months following HSG and/or laparoscopy in ovulatory women with patent tubes, patients with *Chlamydia trachomatis* IgG seropositivity have a 33% lower conception rate compared with seronegative patients [17]. The changes caused by *C. trachomatis* are intraluminal, and histological changes have been observed by salpingoscopy and biopsies of luminal epithelium (Figs. 18.2 and 18.3). Normal architecture of the fallopian tube is lost as neutrophils invade the tubal plicae and cause edema and congestion acutely. Long-term sequelae include scarring, fibrosis, and loss of luminal folds, normal epithelium, and cilia [18]. In addition, antibodies from a chronic inflammatory reaction elicits an autoimmune response to release human heat shock proteins (HSPs) [19]. These human HSPs can have a negative influence on the developing embryo during tubal transport as well as during implantation.

Acute Salpingitis

Acute salpingitis is usually secondary to sexually transmitted infection by *Neisseria gonorrhoeae*, *C. Trachomatis*, *Mycoplasma*, streptococci, staphylococci, coliform bacilli, and anaerobes, which reach the tube usually directly from the uterus attached to sperm or by blood vessels or lymphatic drainage. Clinically, young women may experience fever, leukocytosis, and adnexal tenderness [20]. The tube is

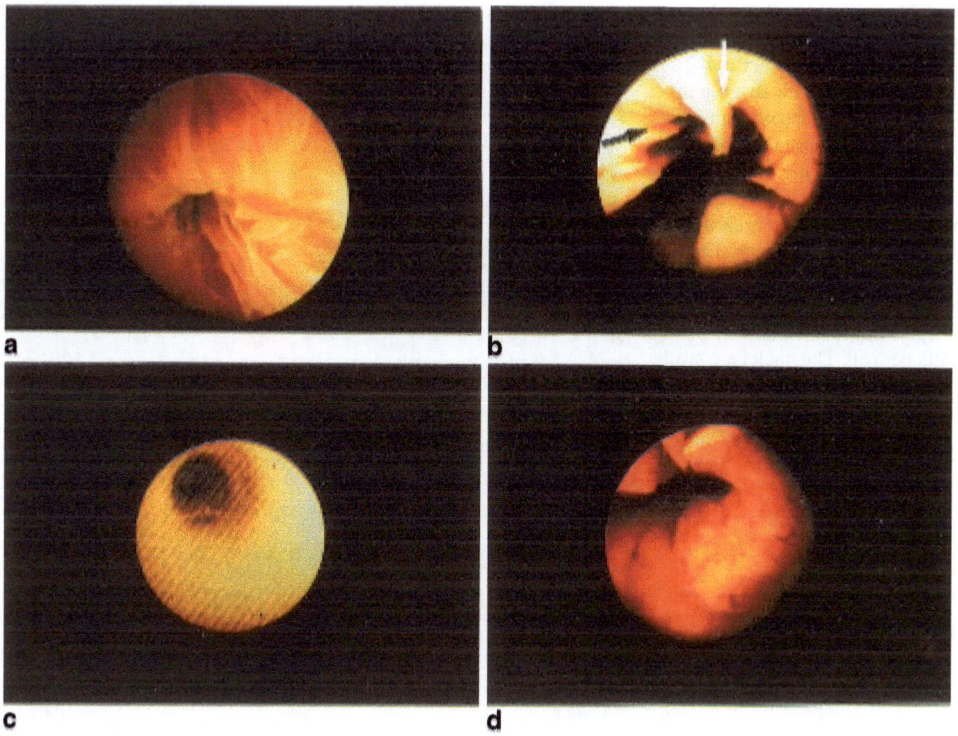

Fig. 18.2 Salpingoscopic view of a normal ampulla (**a**, **b**). *Black* and *white arrows* denote primary and secondary folds, respectively (**b**). An intraluminal adhesion is shown in the isthmus (**c**) via flexible salpingoscope. The ampullary lumen in a patient with severe hydrosalpinx (**d**) is devoid of primary and secondary folds, with abnormal vessel formation. (Reprinted from Hershlag et al. 1991, with permission from Wolters Kluwer Health)

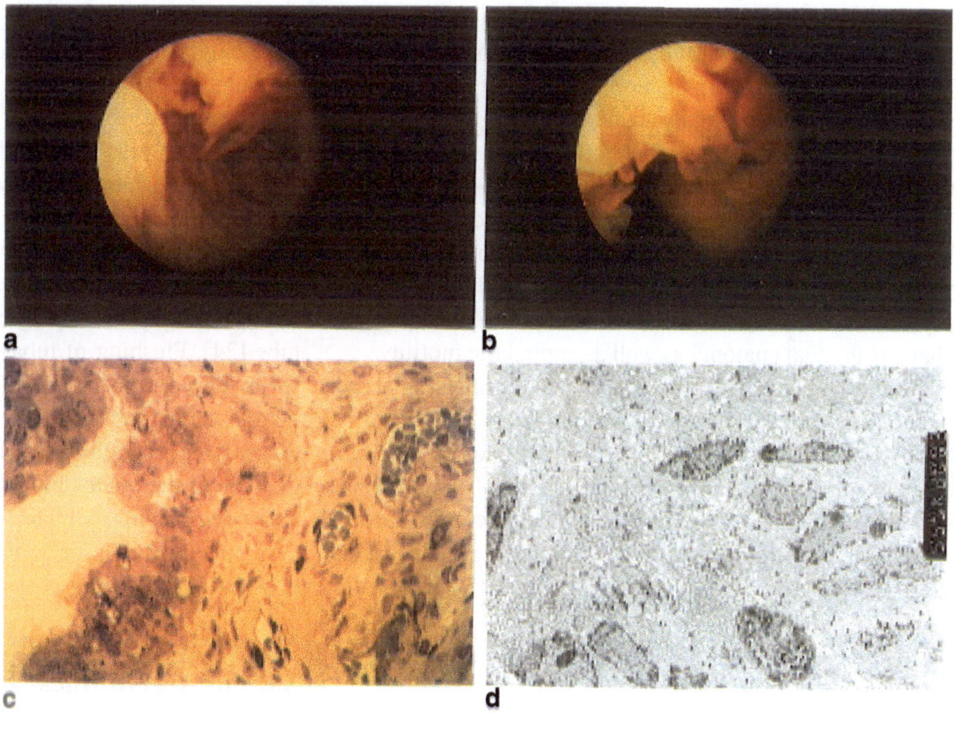

Fig. 18.3 Moderate tubal disease. Rigid salpingoscopy shows moderate attenuation of the epithelial folds (**a**) and increased vascularity (**b**). Histology (**c**) of the ampulla shows evidence of epithelial proliferation, thickening of the lamina propria, and increased vascularity. Electron microscopy (**d**) shows broken plasmalemma, swollen mitochondria, and vacuolated cytoplasm. (Reprinted from Hershlag et al. 1991, with permission from Wolters Kluwer Health)

usually enlarged, erythematous, and edematous. There can be exudates and an associated tubo-ovarian abscess. Microscopically, there are numerous neutrophils, congestion, and edema.

Chronic Salpingitis

Chronic salpingitis frequently goes unrecognized. In patients with no known antecedent history of sexually transmitted diseases (STDs), 35.9 % of them tested positive for

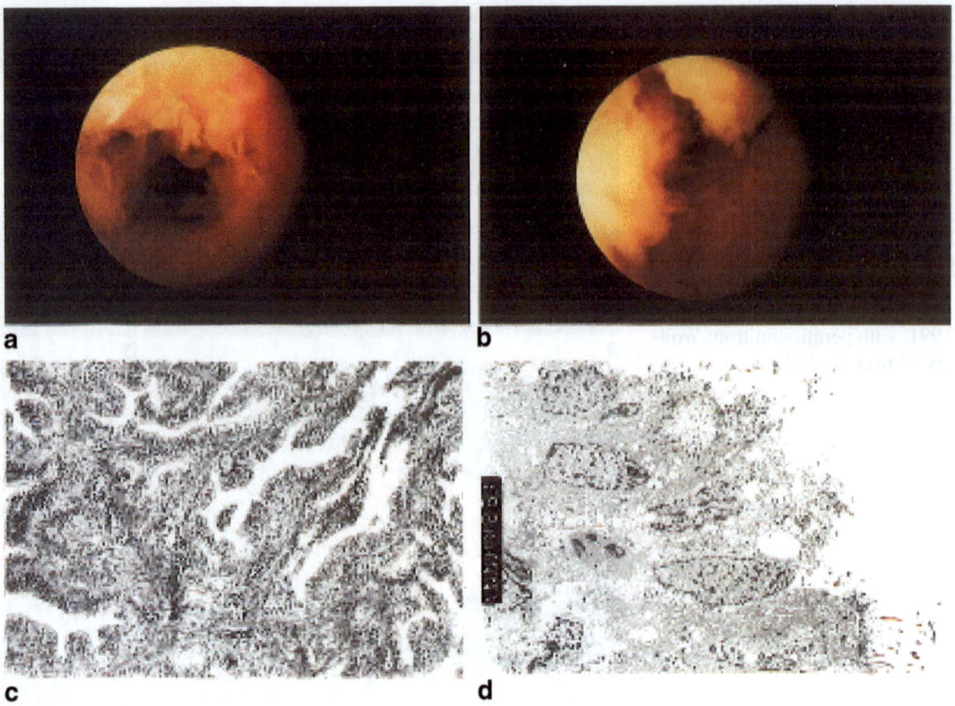

Fig. 18.4 Moderate tubal disease. Rigid salpingoscopy shows attenuation of ampullary epithelial folds (**a**) with absence of secondary folds and widening of spaces between primary folds (**b**). Histology (**c**) of the infundibulum of the same tube shows evidence of conglutination and muscular hypertrophy of the fimbrial stalk. On electron microscopy (**d**), the epithelial cells are cuboidal in shape, with sparse numbers of cilia per cell. The nuclei are swollen and large vacuoles are present. (Reprinted from Hershlag et al. 1991, with permission from Wolters Kluwer Health)

C. trachomatis antibody titer and had tuboperitoneal abnormalities found during an infertility workup [21]. What is better to have: a *diagnosed* or an *undiagnosed* salpingitis? This is yet another question that has not been fully studied. While the acute salpingitis may be more severe, because of symptoms, it is usually promptly treated with aggressive antibiotics, thus allowing some tubes to heal without significant scarring, while others may not escape long-term damage. The undiagnosed and therefore untreated kind, on the other hand, may represent a lower level of inflammation, but it is yet to be determined whether it could more likely to cause permanent tubal dysfunction secondary to subtle chronic changes in tubal anatomy as well as contractile motility.

The chronically inflamed tube can become enlarged, distorted, or adherent to other pelvic organs. There can be hydro- or pyosalpinx in which the tube is full of fluid or exudates, respectively. Microscopically, the tubal folds may be shortened, blunted, or fibrotic (Fig. 18.3). There is a chronic inflammatory infiltrate and flattening of the epithelial lining (Fig. 18.4).

Isthmic Plugs

Since the isthmus is less than 1 mm in diameter compared with the ampullary portion, which is 1 cm wide, mucus plugs may represent a relatively common and frequently unrecognized underlying cause of unexplained infertility.

Histologically, endotubal isthmic plugs consist of casts of histiocytes mixed with endometrial stroma or mesothelial cells [22]. Several studies have observed isthmic secretions increase with estrogen exposure and decrease after ovulation as the corpora lutea forms. Hypotheses on the origin of these isthmic plugs include retrograde menstrual flow, a sign of early pelvic infection, or secondary to cyclical estrogen prior to ovulation.

There are several lines of evidence that mucus plugs may play a major role in unexplained infertility. In a study by Sulak et al. [23], the majority of fallopian tubes diagnosed as obstructed by HSG were found to have only a mucus plug. Successful tubal cannulation either through hysteroscopy or novy cornual cannulation may also be partially attributable to dislodging a mucus plug rather than dilating an obstructed tube [24]. Flushing of tubal plugs could be the reason why for many years it has been known that performing an HSG demonstrating tubal patency is associated with a relative increase in fecundability of up to 20 % [25]. In many patients, dislodging the mucus plug may be all it takes to reopen the sperm–egg highway. Unfortunately, identifying the presence of a mucous plug prior to dislodging it during an HSG is not possible.

Salpingitis Isthmica Nodosa

Salpingitis isthmica nodosa, or SIN, is an old HSG diagnosis for a nodular proximal tubal occlusion. The fallopian tube has nodular thickening of the tunica muscularis in the proximal isthmus enclosing dilated glands, which causes complete obliteration of the lumen [26]. The incidence of SIN in healthy fertile women ranges from 0.6 to 11 %, with a mean age of 26 years, and predisposes patients to infertility and ectopic pregnancies [27, 28]. It is bilateral in 85% of cases [29]. The etiology is unknown, but some hypothesize a postinflammatory effect [30]. On salpingoscopy, this entity may present with no apparent lesion or gray–white nodules up to 2 cm in size in the isthmic portion of the fallopian tube. Microscopically, one can see nodules, cystic and dilated tubal epithelium with hypertrophic muscularis, and normal tubes distally. SIN is considered a risk factor for ectopic pregnancy [31].

How relevant is the diagnosis of SIN in the IVF era? The incidence of SIN in women with an ectopic pregnancy is 10% compared with 0.2% in the control group [32]. Patients with bilateral SIN should not attempt repair since the success rate is extremely poor with a high risk of ectopic pregnancy, and these patients should be immediately referred to IVF.

Granulomatous Salpingitis

Tuberculosis was probably at one point the most common reason of irreversible infertility in endemic areas, giving the typical lead pipe appearance on HSG. Genital tuberculosis involves the fallopian tubes bilaterally in 90% of women [33]. The most common cause of granulomatous salpingitis is *Mycobacterium tuberculosis* or *Mycobacterium bovis*. Grossly, there is thickening and nodularity in the wall, serosal tubercles, or caseous luminal exudate. In severe forms, there may be adhesions between the ovaries and other organs in the pelvis. Interestingly, the ostium usually remains open in contrast to many other forms of chronic salpingitis. Histologically, the mucosa has caseating granulomas, inflammatory changes, and fibrosis. There are epithelial hyperplasia and Schaumann bodies. Other less common causes of granulomatous salpingitis include leprosy [34], Crohn's disease [35], sarcoidosis [36], chronic pelvic inflammatory disease [37], endometriosis [38], pelvic radiation [39], and giant cell arteritis [40].

Patients who had an intrauterine device (IUD) are most at risk for actinomycosis of the fallopian tubes, a disease caused by the *Actinomyces* species such as *Actinomyces israelii*. It affects both tubes in 50% of cases, which may spread to the ovaries [41]. It is estimated that 7% of women using an IUD have colonization with an *Actinomyces* species on a cervical smear [42]. If a patient is asymptomatic, there is no need for antimicrobial treatment or IUD removal. However, if a woman with an IUD has pelvic symptoms and a positive cervical smear for *A. israelii*, they are four times more likely to develop pelvic inflammatory disease [43]. Diagnosis can be made with Pap smear, computed tomography-guided tissue biopsy [44], or laparoscopically with a culture from the fimbrial lumen or posterior cul-de-sac [45]. On gross inspection, there can be small yellow flecks composed of sulfur granules within the tubal lumen. Sequelae of this infection include fistula communication between bowel, bladder, or skin. Histological examination shows granules of gram-positive filamentous bacteria surrounded by purulent exudates [46].

Although rare, there have been case reports of granulomatous salpingitis caused by blastomycosis [47] and coccidioidomycosis [48]. These fungal infections usually present as a tubo-ovarian abscess with peritoneal nodules, and the organisms are identified microscopically.

Parasitic Salpingitis

Parasites such as *Schistosoma haemotobium* have been found to cause nodularity and scarring with the histological finding of characteristic ova surrounded by fibrosis. Pinworms caused by *Enterobius vermicularis* have been identified as nodular thickening in the tubal wall. They spread from anal infections to the genital tract. The characteristics include eosinophilic infiltrates, giant cells, granulation tissue, and fibrous tissue. Cysticercosis has also been reported in the tube, with its characteristic calcified larvae surrounded by granulomatous salpingitis [49].

Physiological Salpingitis

Physiological salpingitis is a nonbacterial inflammatory reaction that can be found in women at the time of menstruation or the peripartum period [50]. Clinically, patients are usually asymptomatic. The diagnosis was made from routine analysis of tubes removed at the time of hysterectomy or sterilization. Histologically, there is edema, lymphatic dilation, and infiltration with polymorphonuclear lymphocytes in the tubal plicae [51]. However, unlike infectious salpingitis, there is no necrosis, ulceration, or bacterial infection. Menstrual debris causes an inflammatory reaction in the tubal epithelium and stroma, but rarely involve the muscular walls. There are no known long-term sequelae from physiologic salpingitis. However, women are more susceptible to pelvic infections during menses due to low estrogen, less cervical mucous to block ascension of bacteria, and the presence of this physiologic salpingitis could facilitate infectious spread [52].

Endometriosis

Similar to endometriotic lesions of other pelvic organs, it is unclear how the involvement of the fallopian tube in endometriosis affects fertility in most cases. Only a full obstruction of both tubes or unilateral obstruction where the other tube is absent represents a clear association. However, such instances are uncommon. The most common site of endometrial foci in the fallopian tube is the serosa, but the myosalpinx and mucosa can also be involved [53]. Endometrial tissue may spread from the uterus to the isthmic portion of the tube along with mucosal changes such as obstructing endometrial polyps [54]. These intratubal polyps are associated with ectopic pregnancy and infertility, especially if they are bilateral [55]. In one review, the prevalence of intramural tubal polyps was 3.8% in a group of infertile women, where 50% had unexplained infertility [56]. The diagnosis can be made by HSG. The lesions are typically broad based, 0.1–1.3cm, pink to red, smooth protrusions from the mucosa. Microscopically, one can see non-functioning endometrium covering the polyp.

In addition to obstructing lesions, endometriosis causes elevated oxidative stress, increased immunologic factors, and changes in the hormonal levels in peritoneal and FF. Reactive oxidative species (ROS) produced by erythrocytes, macrophages, and apoptotic endometriotic cells induce oocyte degeneration, DNA damage, increased cell membrane permeability [57], and cell death [58]. ROS negatively impacts fertilization through increased DNA fragmentation in spermatozoa [59] and inhibition of the acrosome reaction [60]. Nitrous oxide (NO) is higher in patients with endometriosis from the presence of macrophages. NO is toxic to embryos and decreases sperm motility [61].

Endometriosis has also been shown to affect the sperm interaction with the tubal epithelium. The tubal ampulla binds significantly more spermatozoa in women with endometriosis leaving less freely motile spermatozoa for fertilization [62]. Another study found cilia to beat at a lower frequency when exposed to peritoneal fluid from women with endometriosis [63].

Endometriosis may impair fertilization and implantation through decreasing oocyte quality, decreasing sperm motility, and/or exposure of the gametes/embryo to toxic peritoneal and FF. The FF of women with endometriosis decreases sperm binding to the zona pellucida [64]. Women with endometriosis have decreased levels of vascular endothelial growth factor (VEGF), which has been associated with reduced embryo quality and implantation defects [65]. Increased levels of circulating immunoglobulins and complement deposits have been detected in the peritoneal fluid of patients with endometriosis. This local inflammatory cascade has been proposed to increase ectopic endometrial implants, promote its growth, and release free radicals.

There are increased E2 levels in peritoneal fluid that stimulates cycle-oxygenase-2 (COX-2) enzyme, which then upregulates prostaglandin E2 (PGE2) production. PGE2 stimulates aromatase expression in endometrial tissue, which then produces more E2 and continues a vicious cycle of proliferation and cytokine induction [66]. Specifically, interleukin (IL)-6, and IL-1a cytokine produced by endometrial and epithelial cells in response to E2, has been shown to decrease sperm motility within the uterus [67].

The impact of endometriosis on fertility is widespread and still has many unanswered questions. Even with fertility treatments such as IVF, pregnancy rates are lower in women with endometriosis compared with controls (tubal factor) [68]. Should these patients be treated like unexplained infertility, especially if the diagnosis was found incidentally? There is still no clear answer for targeted treatment. Differentiating mild from severe endometriosis may help stratify who should be offered laparoscopic treatment, expectant management, or immediate assisted reproduction techniques (ART). The current recommendations are to treat patients with mild endometriosis similarly to patients with unexplained infertility, especially when invasive surgeries have not been shown to have a better clinical outcome [69].

Late Sequelae of Chronic Salpingitis

Fimbrial Agglutination

Fimbrial agglutination can cause distal tubal obstruction and can range from mild adhesions to phimosis, or narrowing of the tube to severe occlusion (Fig. 18.3). Complete occlusion can prevent ovum capture, while phimosis may decrease ovum pick-up. Microsurgery such as fimbrioplasty and neosalpingostomy can open the tubes to restore fimbria and patency.

Intraluminal Fibrosis

Intraluminal fibrosis is a late sequelae of chronic salpingitis and is irreversible. The fallopian tubes appear anatomically patent and normal. The definitive diagnosis of intraluminal fibrosis can only be made with salpingoscopy; however, most people rely on HSG or laparoscopic tubal lavage to diagnose tubal obstruction, techniques that are incapable of making such a specific diagnosis. A definitive diagnosis can be made by pathologists on analysis of surgically -removed fallopian tubes. According to a study of histological features of surgically removed tubes, 35.5% of specimens showed plical fibrosis [70]. Mild to moderate fibrosis was found in patients at an average age of 28 years and severe fibrosis at an average age of 42 years. Several studies have shown that there is a steady increase in plical fibrosis and the relative amount of plicae occupying the lumen in the fallopian tube from birth to menopause [71]. These age-groups represent the majority of patients who present for infertility evaluation.

Ciliary Dysfunction

The tubal cilia provide a delicate mechanism of propagating gametes toward the uterus in a unidirectional beat. In a study in rabbits, a segment of the ampulla was reversed so that the cilia beat toward the ovary. The experiment did not affect fertilization, but it did arrest the egg from moving to the uterus, and no pregnancy occurred [72]. Kartagener's syndrome serves as an interesting model of what happens when the ultramicroscopic structure of the cilia is abnormal (congenital absence of dynein arms) [73]. This rare syndrome may, at times, be associated with female subfertility, ectopic pregnancy, and male infertility with impaired sperm motility [74]. While patients with Kartagener's syndrome are natural candidates for ciliary dysfunction and therefore male and female infertility, they do not have an increased rate of ectopic pregnancies documented in the literature. Pregnancies in women with this syndrome have been reported, which highlights the importance of the tubal musculature and peristalsis to facilitate oocyte transport to the uterus.

Ciliary function changes during the menstrual cycle, depending on the relative concentrations of estrogen and progesterone, with variations in the respective receptors. In vivo studies show that progesterone decreases ciliary beat frequency (CBF) by 40–50%, which correlates to the proliferative phase allowing maximal fertilization time of the ovum. Estradiol inhibits the antagonistic effect of progesterone on CBF. From these studies, it can be hypothesized that ovulatory dysfunction could lead to defective CBF and therefore inhibit transport of the ovum along the fallopian tube. At this point, the question of whether ovulation induction agents such as clomiphene citrate and/or gonadotropins could fail because of their adverse affect on ciliary function remains unanswered.

Tubal Motility

It is unclear whether cilia or tubal muscular contractions provide the propulsive force to transport sperm and the oocyte as the data are conflicting. In one study, interference with muscular contractility in the rabbit did not block egg transport [75]. In another study on rabbits, blocking smooth muscle with nicardipine caused oviduct stasis and inhibited egg movement even with unaffected ciliary beating [76]. In addition, reversal of a segment of the ampulla so that cilia beat in the other direction did not block fertilization but did arrest egg transport [77]. Therefore, both the myosalpinx and cilia beating are critical for egg transport. At ovulation, waves of intermittent smooth muscle contraction in the myosalpinx move the egg from the infundibular ostium to the ampullary-isthmic junction, in a prouterine direction [78]. Cilia in the isthmus beat toward the ampullary-isthmic junction at the time of ovulation [79].

After fertilization, the musculature of the distal isthmus relaxes and the egg passes into the uterus. The isthmic musculature (adrenergic innervation) is upregulated by estrogen prior to ovulation, allowing for constriction and therefore retention of the egg for adequate fertilization time in the ampulla [80]. Progesterone binds to β-adrenergic receptors and causes isthmic smooth muscle relaxation [81]. In theory, cases of tubal spasm can be attributed to dysregulation of the myosalpinx by erratic steroid hormone production in women with irregular ovulatory cycles. In a study of human fallopian tubes, muscular contractions were significantly increased by PGE2 and F2α and downregulated by progesterone, levonorgestrel, mifepristone, oxytocin, and human chorionic gonadotropin [82].

How does the fallopian tube pace itself? The action of the myosalpinx is controlled by the pacemaker activity in the interstitial cells of Cajal of the oviduct [83]. Interstitial cells of Cajal line the oviducts and provide pacemaker activity to regulate the peristalsis of the oviduct essential for the transport of the oocyte and sperm. Damage to these cells could lead to intrinsic pacemaker dysfunction and pseudo-obstruction of the tube [84]. Infections such as with *Chlamydia* cause dilated oviducts and pyosalpinx due to the loss of normal muscle contraction and retention of fluid within the tube. Electrophysiological analysis showed loss of pacemaker activity without loss of muscle potential.

The question whether emotional stress can cause infertility has not been properly studied. That stress plays a part in many couples with otherwise unexplained infertility may be evident from treatment-independent pregnancies in couples with multiple IVF failures subsequent to removal of stressors (vacation, adoption, etc). According to Foldes et al., tubal occlusion may be caused by spasms operating under stress. The intricate biochemical influences on the musculature surrounding the tiny (less than 1 mm) lumen of the isthmus effectively protect women under stress from conception. Other studies, including a large meta-analysis, found that emotional stress has no effect on IVF outcomes [85].

Tubal Surgery

Much of the aforementioned tubal pathology can be directly visualized by the salpingoscope, a tiny endoscopic device aimed at scoping the entire length of the tube. Earlier work by Confino et al. [86] and Hershlag et al. [87] found reasonable correlation between salpingoscopic findings and histology. Since this technique was developed right when IVF became more successful, interest in the interior of the fallopian tube as well as diagnosing and treating tubal epithelial abnormalities ceased to gain momentum.

By definition, unexplained infertility must have patent tubes as demonstrated by HSG or laparoscopic chromopertubation. Using aqua dissection and tubal cannulation, the salpingoscope can be used to treat proximal tubal occlusion by removal of plugs of amorphous cellular debris, lysis of adhesions, and endotuboplasty [88]. It can also identify nonobstructive tubal disease such as fibrosis, stenosis,

Table 18.1 Various etiologies of fallopian tube dysfunction identified by salpingoscopy and histological examination

Study (*n*=patients)	Obstructive debris (%)	Stenosis (%)	Obliterative fibrosis (%)	Salpingitis isthmica nodosa (%)	Intratubal polyps (%)	Hydrosalpinx (%)	Chronic inflammation (%)	Tubal tuberculosis (%)	Intramucosal endometriosis (%)	References
Kerin et al. (n=75)	6	18	7	5	6	6	–	–	–	[89]
Fortier et al. (*n*=42)	–	–	38.1	23.8	–	–	21.4	–	14.3	[91]
Punnonen et al. (*n*=25)	–	–	12	60	–	–	8	4	12	[92]
Zhang et al. (*n*=33)	–	–	7.84	5.88	–	–	70.59	3.92	9.80	[93]
Wiedemann et al. (*n*=53)	–	–	61	42	–	–	57	–	–	[94]

nonobstructive adhesions, debris, polyps, or loss of normal epithelium and abnormal vasculature [89]. Nakagawa et al. [90] used the salpingoscope to assess adhesions, loss of mucosal folds, rounded edges of mucosal folds, debris, foreign bodies, and abnormal vessels (Figs. 18.1–18.4). The various causes of tubal obstruction identified by salpingoscopy and pathological examination are summarized in Table 18.1 [89, 91–94]. Indeed, had the initial interest in evaluating pathologic abnormalities of the fallopian tube endothelium continued, many patients currently diagnosed as "unexplained" may have been identified with salpingoscopy. While this may have given patients a sense of relief to be labeled with a cause for their infertility, the treatment would still be IVF to bypass the defective fallopian tube. Once patients have a diagnosis, they can be treated as tubal factor with relief of the obstruction or IVF if the occlusion is bilateral or cannot be cannulated, flushed, or catheterized.

Conclusion

So, does the tube matter? In a way, IVF has done to the study of fallopian tube pathologies what intracytoplasmic sperm injection (ICSI) has done to male factor infertility. With ICSI, the sperm–egg barrier has been circumvented, thus making the understanding of sperm–egg interaction, and a multitude of efforts at improving normal fertilization in vivo or in vitro, obsolete. Similarly, IVF serves as a "bypass" procedure. With the accelerating success of IVF, the fallopian tube has lost its prime time as the site for sperm–egg interaction, fertilization, and preliminary embryo development. The study of tubal physiology was all but halted, and microsurgery of the fallopian tube with its limited success is now a historical chapter taught to medical students. In patients unwilling to utilize modern approaches such as ART for suspected/diagnosed tubal pathology, proximal tubal obstruction may be treated by tubal cannulation in young women with no other significant infertility factors [95]. Laparoscopic fimbrioplasty or neosalpingostomy is also an option for women with mild hydrosalpinges [96]. In cases of severe or irreparable hydrosalpinges, laparoscopic salpingectomy improves IVF pregnancy rates compared with controls. Tubal reversal in appropriate candidates (less than 40 years old with residual healthy fallopian tubes equal to or greater than 4 cm in length) is still a valid alternative to IVF [97]. However, these approaches are not equivalent to the success with ART and not without risk of surgical complications, failure, or ectopic pregnancy. Additionally, fewer and fewer surgeons are being trained to successfully perform laparoscopic or conventional microsurgery of the fallopian tube.

So what relevance remains for the fallopian tube today?

Clearly, identifying and treating disorders of the fallopian tube that have a reasonable chance of success are warranted. Tubal pathology cannot be suspected based on history, and even women without risk factors or utilizing ART might benefit from a preliminary evaluation of their tubes. The fact that some patients who did not conceive through IVF have conceived naturally is evidence that the moratorium on the fallopian tubes has been premature and hasty.

References

1. Eddy CA, Pauerstein CJ. Anatomy and physiology of the fallopian tube. Clin Obstet Gynecol. 1980;23(4):1177–93.
2. Brosens IA, Vasquez G. Fimbrial microbiopsy. J Reprod Med. 1976;16:171.
3. Speroff L, Fritz MA. Female infertility. In: Speroff L, Fritz MA, editors. Clinical gynaecologic endocrinology and infertility. 7th ed. Philadelphia: Lippincott Williams & Wilkins; 2005. pp. 1046–55.
4. Camus E, Poncelet C, Goffinet F, Wainer B, Meriet F, Nisand I, et al. Pregnancy rates after in-vitro fertilization in cases of tubal infertility with and without hydrosalpinx: a meta-analysis of published comparative studies. Hum Reprod. 1999;14:1243–9.
5. Practice Committee of the American Society for Reproductive Medicine. Salpingectomy for hydrosalpinx prior to in vitro fertilization. Fertil Steril. 2008;90:S66–8.
6. Johnson N, et al. Surgical treatment for tubal disease in women due to undergo in vitro fertilisation. Cochrane Database Syst Rev. 2010;(1):CD002125.
7. Copperman A, Wells V, Luna M, Kalir T, Sandler B, Mukherjee T. Presence of hydrosalpinx correlated to endometrial inflammatory response in vivo. Fertil Steril. 2006;86(4):972–6.
8. Tay JJ, Rutherford AJ, Killick SR, Maguiness SD, Patridge RJ, Leese HJ. Human tubal fluid: production, nutrient composition, and response to adrenergic agents. Hum Reprod. 1997;12(11):2451–6.

9. Nichol R, Hunter RHF, Garner DK, Leese HJ, Cooke GM. Concentrations of energy substrates in oviductal fluid and blood plasma during the peri-ovulatory period. J Reprod Fertil. 1992;96:699–707.
10. Tay JJ, Rutherford AJ, Killick SR, maguiness SD, Patridge RJ, Leese HJ. Human tubal fluid: production, nutrient composition, and response to adrenergic agents. Hum Reprod. 1997;12(11):2451–6.
11. Mcdonald MF, Bellve AR. Influence of oestrogen and progesterone on flow of fluid from the fallopian tube in the ovariectomized ewe. J Reprod Fertil. 1969;20:51–61.
12. Mastroianna L, Beer F, Shah V, Clewe TH. Endocrine regulation of oviduct secretions in the rabbit. Endocrinology. 1961;68:92–100.
13. Comer MT, Leese HJ, Southgate J. Induction of a differentiated ciliated cell phenotype in primary cultures of fallopian tube epithelium. Hum Reprod. 1998;13:3114–20.
14. Verhage HG, Fazleabas AT, Mavrogiannis PA, O'Day-Bowman MB, Donelly KM, Arias EB, Jaffe RC. The baboon oviduct: characteristics of an oestradiol-dependent oviduct-specific glycoprotein. Hum Reprod. 1997;3:541–52.
15. Hunter RHF. Modulation of gamete and embryonic microenvironment by oviduct of glycoproteins. Mol Reprod Dev. 1994;39:176–81.
16. Johnson WL, Hunter AG. Seminal antigens: their alteration in the genital tract of female rabbits and during partial in vitro capacitation with beta amylase and beta glucuronidase. Biol Reprod. 1972;7(3):332–40.
17. Coppus SFPJ, Land JA, Opmeer BC, Teures P, Eijkemans MJC, Hompes PGA, Bossuyt PMM, van der Veen F, Mol BWJ, van der Steeg JW. Chlamydia trachomatis IgG seropositivity is associated with lower natural conception rates in ovulatory subfertile women without visible pathology. Human Reprod. 2011;26(11):3061–7.
18. Young RH, Clement PB. The fallopian tube and broad Ligament. In: Mills SE, editor. Sternberg's diagnostic surgical pathology. 5th ed. Philadelphia: Lippincott Williams & Wilkins; 2010. pp. 2372–3004.
19. Neuer A, Lam KN, Tiller FW, Kiesel L, Witkin SS. Humoral immune response to membrane components of *Chlamydia trachomatis* and expression of human 60 kDa heat shock protein in follicular fluid of in-vitro fertilization patients. Hum Reprod. 1997;12:925–9.
20. Sweet RL. Diagnosis and treatment of acute salpingitis. J Reprod Med. 1997;19(1):21–30.
21. Veenemans LMW, van der Linden PJQ. The value of *Chlamydia trachomatis* antibody testing in predicting tubal factor infertility. Hum Reprod. 2002;17(3):695–8.
22. Kerin JF, Surrey ES, Williams DB, Daykhovsky L, Grundfest WS. Falloposcopic observations of endotubal isthmic plugs as a cause of reversible obstruction and their histological characterization. J Laparoendosc Surg. 1991;1:103–10.
23. Sulak PJ, Letterie GS, Hayslip CC, Coddington CC, Klein TA. Hysteroscopic cannulation and lavage in the treatment of proximal tubal occlusion. Fertil Steril. 1987;48(3):493–4.
24. Confino E, Tur-Kaspa I, DeCherney A, Corfoman R, Coulam C, Robinson E, Haas G, Katz E, Vermesh M, Gleicher N. Transcervical balloon tuboplasty. A multicenter study. JAMA. 1990;264(16):2078–82.
25. Vandekerckhove P, Watson A, Likford R, et al. Therapeutic effect of oil-soluble and water-soluble media used for tubal patency testing (hysterosalpingography or laparoscopy) on pregnancy rates in infertility patients (Cochrane Review). In the Cochrane Library 1999, Issue 4. Update Software, Oxford, UK.
26. Karasick S, Karasick D, Schilling J. Salpingitis isthmica nodosa in female infertility. J Can Assoc Radiol. 1985;36(2):118–21.
27. Young RH, Clement PB. The fallopian tube and broad Ligament. In: Mills SE, editor. Sternberg's diagnostic surgical pathology, 5th ed. Philadelphia: Lippincott Williams & Wilkins; 2010. pp. 2372–3004.
28. Jenkins CS, Williams SR, Schmidt GE. Salpingitis isthmica nodosa: a review of the literature, discussion of clinical significance, and consideration of patient management. Fertil Steril. 1993;60(4):599–607.
29. Wrork OH, Broders AC. Adenomyosis of the fallopian tubes. Am J Obstet Gynecol. 1942;44:412–32.
30. Azad S, Chawla N, Kudesia S, Rai S, Singhal M. Salpingitis isthmica nodosa. Indian J Pathol Microbiol. 2009;52(3):434.
31. Majmudar B, Henderson PH, 3rd, Semple E. Salpingitis isthmica nodosa: a high-risk factor for tubal pregnancy. Obstet Gynecol. 1983;62(1):73–8.
32. Saracoglu FO, Mungan T, Tanzer F. Salpingitis isthmica nodosa in infertility and ectopic pregnancy. Gynecol Obstet Invest. 1992;34(4):202–5.
33. Nogales-Ortiz F, Tarancon I, Nogales FF. The pathology of female genital tuberculosis. Obstet Gynecol. 1979;53:422–8.
34. Bonar BE, Rabson AS. Gynecologic aspects of leprosy. Obstet Gynecol. 1957;9:33–43.
35. Brooks JJ, Wheeler JA. Granulomatous salpingitis secondary to Crohn's disease. Obstet Gynecol. 1977;49:S31–3.
36. Kay S. Sarcoidosis of the fallopian tubes. Report of a case. Br J Obstet Gynaecol. 1956;63:871–4.
37. McEntee GP, Coughlan M, Corrigan T, Dervan P. Pelvic Inflammatory pseudotumor: problems in clinical and histolgical diagnosis. Case report. Br J Obstet Gynaecol. 1985;92:1067–9.
38. Clement PB, Young RH, Scully RE. Necrotic pseudoxanthomatous nodules of ovary and peritoneum in endometriosis. Am J Surg Pathol. 1988;12:390–7.
39. Herrera GA, Riemann BE, Greenberg HL. Pimentosus tubae, a new entity: light and electron microscopic study. Obstet Gynecol. 1983;61:S80–3.
40. Bell DA, Mondschein M, Scully RE. Giant cell arteritis of the female genital tract. A report of three cases. Am J Surg Pathol. 1986;10:696–701.
41. Paalman RJ, Dockerty MB, Mussey RD. Actinomycosis of ovaries and fallopian tubes. Am J Obstet Gynecol. 1949;58:419–31.
42. Westhoff C. IUDs and colonization or infection with actinomyces. Contraception. 2007;75(6):S48–50.
43. Kelly J, Aaron J. Pelvic actinomycosis and usage of intrauterine contraceptive devices. Yale J Bio Med. 1982;55:453–61.
44. Lee YC, Min D, Holcomb K, Buhl A, DiMaio T, Abulafia O. Computed tomography guided core needle biopsy diagnosis of pelvic actinomycosis. Gynecol Oncol. 2000;2:318–23.
45. Brihmer C, Kallings I, Nord CE, Brundin J. Salpingitis; aspects of diagnosis and etiology; a 4 year study from a Swedish capital hospital. Eur J Obstet Gynecol Reprod Biol. 1987;24:211–20.
46. Braby HH, Dougherty CM, Mickal A. Actinomycosis of the female genital tract. Obstet Gynecol. 1964;23:580–3.
47. Murray JJ, Clark CA, Lands RH, Heim CR, Burnett LS. Reactivation blastomycosis presenting as a tuboovarian abscess. Obstet Gynecol. 1984;64:828–30.
48. Bylund DJ, Nanfro JJ, Marsh WL. Coccidiodomycosis of the female genital tract. Arch Pathol Lab Med. 1986;110:232–5.
49. Abraham JL, Spore WW, Benirschke K. Cysticercosis of the fallopian tube: histology and microanalysis. Hum Pathol. 1982;13(7):665–70.
50. Nassberg S, McKay DG, Hertig AT. Physiological salpingitis. Am J Obstet Gynecol. 1954;67(1):130–7.
51. Smith HA, Greene RR. Physiologic endosalpingitis. Am J Obstet Gynecol. 1956;72(1):174–9.
52. Ringrose CAD. Clinical, etiological, and economic aspects of salpingitis. Can Med Assoc J. 1960;83(2):53–58.
53. Sheldon RS, Wilson RB, Dockerty MB. Serosal endometriosis of the fallopian tubes. Am J Obstet Gynecol. 1967;99:882–4.
54. Lisa JR, Gioia JD, Rubin IC. Observations on the interstitial portion of the fallopian tube. Surg Gynecol Obstet. 1954;99:159–69.
55. David MP, Ben-Zwi D, Kanger L. Tubal intramural polyps and their relationship to infertility. Fertil Steril. 1981;35:526–31.
56. Wansaicheong GK, Ong CL. Intramural tubal polyps—a villain in the shadows? Singap Med J. 1998;39(3):97–100.
57. Agarwal A, Gupta S, Sikka S. The role of free radicals and antioxidants in reproduction. Curr Opin Obstet Gynecol. 2006;18:325–32.
58. Bedaiwy MA, Falcone T, Sharma RK, Goldberg JM, Attaran M, Nelson DR, et al. Prediction of endometriosis with serum and peritoneal fluid markers: a prospective controlled trial. Hum Reprod. 2002;17:426–31.

59. Mansour G, Goldberg J, Agarwal A, Sharma R, Mahfouz R, Falcone T. Correlation between sperm DNA damage, stage of endometriosis and the duration of infertility. ASRM 63rd annual meeting; 15–17 Oct. 2007; Washington, DC.
60. Baker MA, Aitken RJ. The importance of redox regulated pathways in sperm cell biology. Mol Cell Endocrinol. 2004;216:47–54.
61. Osborn BH, Haney AF, Misukonis MA, Weinberg JB. Inducible nitric oxide synthase and alpha(v)beta(3) integrin in women with endometriosis. Fertil Steril. 2002;78:860–4.
62. Reeve L, Lashen H, Pacey AA. Endometriosis affects sperm-endosalpingeal interactions. Hum Reprod. 2005;20:448–51.
63. Lyons RA, Djahanbakhch O, Saridogan E, Naftalin AA, Mahmood T, Weekes A, Chenoy R. Peritoneal fluid, endometriosis, and ciliary beat frequency in the human fallopian tube. Lancet. 2002;360(9341):1221–2.
64. Qiao J, Yeung WS, Yao YQ, Ho PC. The effects of follicular fluid from patients with different indications for IVF treatment on the binding of human spermatozoa to the zona pellucida. Hum Reprod. 1998;13:128–31.
65. Pellicer A, Albert C, Garrido N, Navarro J, Remohi J, Simon C. The pathophysiology of endometriosis-associated infertility: follicular environment and embryo quality. J Reprod Fertil Suppl. 2000;55:109–19.
66. Noble LS, Takayama K, Zeitoun KM, Putnam JM, Johns DA, Hinshelwood MM, et al. Prostaglandin E2 stimulates aromatase expression in endometriosis-derived stromal cells. J Clin Endocrinol Metab. 1997;82:600–6.
67. Pellicer A, Albert C, Mercader A, Bonilla-Musoles F, Remohi J, Simon C. The follicular and endomcrine environment in women with endometriosis: local and systemic cytokine production. Fertil Steril. 1998;70:425–31.
68. Barnhart K, Dunsmoor R, Coutifaris C. Effect of endometriosis on in vitro fertilization. Fertil Steril. 2002;77:1148–55.
69. Siristatidis C, Bhattacharya S. Unexplained infertility: does it really exist? Does it matter? Hum Reprod. 2007;22(8):2084–7.
70. Hunt JL, Lynn AA. Histologic features of surgically removed fallopian tubes. Arch Pathol Lab Med. 2002;126:951–5.
71. Pinero DA, Foraker AG. Aging in the fallopian tube. Am J Obstet Gynecol. 1963;86:397–400.
72. Eddy CA, Flores JJ, Archer DR, Pauerstein CJ. The role of cilia in infertility: an evaluation by selective microsurgical modification of the rabbit oviduct. Am J Obstet Gynecol. 1978;132(7):814–21.
73. Talbot P, Geiske C, Knoll M. Oocyte pickup by the mammalian oviduct. Mol Biol Cell. 1999;10:5–8.
74. Afzelius BA, Eliasson R. Male and female infertility problems in the immotile-cilia syndrome. Eur J Respir Dis Suppl. 1983;127:144–7.
75. Halbert SA, Tam BY, Blandau RJ. Egg transport in the rabbit oviduct: the roles of cilia and muscle. Science. 1976;191:1052–3.
76. Dixon RE, Hwang SJ, Hennig GW, Ramsey KH, Justin H, et al. *Chlamydia* infection causes loss of pacemaker cells and inhibits oocyte transport in the mouse oviduct. Biol Reprod. 2009;80(4):665–73.
77. McComb PF, Halbert SA, Gomel V. Pregnancy, ciliary transport and the reversed ampullary segment of the rabbit fallopian tube. Fertil Steril. 1980;34:386–90.
78. Harper MJK. The mechanisms involved in the movement of newly ovulated eggs through the ampulla of the rabbit fallopian tube. J Reprod Fertil. 1961;2:522–4.
79. Blandau RJ, Gaddum-Rosse P. Mechanism of sperm transport in pig oviducts. Fertil Steril. 1974;25:61–7.
80. Howe GR, Black DL. Autonomic nervous system and oviduct function in the rabbit. J Reprod Fertil. 1973;13:425–30.
81. Boling JL, Blandau RJ. Egg transport through the ampulla of the oviducts of rabbits under various experimental conditions. Biol Reprod. 1971;4:174–84.
82. Wanggren K, Stavreus-Evers A, Olsson C, Andersson E, Gemzell-Danielsson K. Regulation of muscular contractions in the human fallopian tube through prostaglandis and progestagens. Hum Reprod. 2008;23:2359–68.
83. Dixon RE, Hwang SJ, Hennig GW, Ramsey KH, Schripsema JH, Sanders KM, Ward SM. *Chlamydia* infection causes loss of pacemaker cells and inhibits oocyte transport in the mouse oviduct. Biol Reprod. 2008;80:665–73.
84. Popescu LM, Ciontea SM, Cretoiu D. Interstitial Cajal-like cell in human uterus and fallopian tube. Ann N Y Acad Sci. 2007;1101:139–65.
85. Boivin J, Griffiths E, Venetis CA. Emotional distress in infertile women and failure of assisted reproductive technologies: meta-analysis of prospective psychosocial studies. Br Med J. 2011;342:223–31.
86. Confino E, Friberg J, Gleicher N. Transcervical balloon tuboplasty. Fertil Steril. 1986;46:963–6.
87. Hershlag A, Seifer DB, Carcangiu ML, Patton DL, Diamond MP, DeCherney AH. Salpingoscopy: light microscopic and electron microscopic correlations. Obstet Gynecol. 1991;77(3):399–405.
88. Kerin JF, Surrey ES, Williams DB, Daykhovsky L, Grundfest WS. Falloposcopic observations of endotubal isthmic plugs as a cause of reversible obstruction and their histiological characterization. J Laparoendosc Surg. 1991;1(2):103–10.
89. Kerin JF, Williams DB, San Roman GA, Pearlstone AC, Grundfest WS, Surrey ES. Falloposcopic classification and treatment of fallopian tube lumen disease. Fertil Steril. 1992;57(4):731–41.
90. Nakawaga K, Inoue M, Nishi Y, Sugiyama R, Motoyama K, Kuribayashi Y, Akira S, Sugiyama R. A new evaluation score that uses salpingoscopy to reflect fallopian tube function in infertile women. Fertil Steril. 2010;94(7):2753–7.
91. Fortier KJ, Haney AF. The pathologic spectrum of uterotubal junction obstruction. Obstet Gynecol. 1985;65(1):93–8.
92. Punnonen R, Söderström KO, Alanen A. Isthmic tubal occlusion: etiology and histology. Acta Eur Fertil. 1984;15(1):39–42.
93. Zhang D, Zeng Y, Chen X. Pathological findings of proximal tubal occlusive infertility. Zhonghua Fu Chan Ke Za Zhi. 1995;30(6):352–5.
94. Wiedemann R, Sterzik K, Gombisch V, Stuckensen J, Montag M. Beyond recanalizing proximal tube occlusion: the argument for further diagnosis and classification. Hum Reprod. 1996;11(5):986–91.
95. Honore GM, Holden AE, Schenken RS. Pathophysiology and management of proximal tubal blockage. Fertil Steril. 1999;5:785–95.
96. American Fertility Society. The American Fertility Society classifications of adnexal adhesions, distal tubal occlusion, tubal occlusion secondary to tubal ligation, tubal pregnancies, Mullerian anomalies and intrauterine adhesions. Fertil Steril. 1988;49:944–55.
97. Boeckxstaens A, Devroey P, Collins J, Tournaye H. Getting pregnant after tubal sterilization: surgical reversal or IVF? Hum Reprod. 2007;22:2660–4.

Subtle Endometriosis and Unexplained Infertility

19

Paula Andrea de Albuquerque de Salles Navarro, Anderson Sanches de Melo and Rui Alberto Ferriani

Unexplained infertility (UI) is a diagnosis of exclusion for infertile couples whose examinations for semen analysis, assessment of tubal permeability, and confirmation of ovulation do not reveal abnormalities [1]. The incidence of UI varies according to age, geographic area, and the selection criteria used in the different studies, affecting 15–37 % of all infertile couples [2, 3]. The spontaneous pregnancy rate of couples with UI has been reported to be 2–4 % per menstrual cycle [4], 15 % at the end of 1 year, and 35 % after 2 years [3]. The prognosis for natural conception with expectant management in couples with UI depends on factors such as age of the female partner, length of infertility, primary or secondary infertility, and semen parameters. For this reason, if the pregnancy prognosis is good, expectant management can be suggested [1, 5]. Other factors are important in making this recommendation, like the anxiety of the couple.

In infertile patients with no other associated symptoms, with a normal clinical examination and with an ultrasound evaluation revealing no pelvic pathology, undiagnosed pelvic disease may still be present. The only way to make this diagnosis would be a diagnostic laparoscopy. Although controversial and based on cost/benefit analyses, the guidelines of professional organizations such as the American Society of Reproductive Medicine [6] and the National Institute for Health and Clinical Excellence in the UK (NICE [1]) do not include routine laparoscopy in the routine investigation of infertile couples. On this basis, we may speculate whether UI is really unexplained or just "undiagnosed" as there may be subtle pathological pelvic conditions that might contribute to the infertility.

Endometriosis may inhibit conception at all stages of the process from oocyte development to ovulation, fertilization, and embryo implantation and therefore there is speculation about its role in cases of UI. Laparoscopy has demonstrated that approximately 75 % of patients with UI have a diagnosis of endometriosis, with most patients having stage I (minimal) or stage II (mild) disease (70 % of cases) [7], suggesting that endometriosis may be underdiagnosed in couples classified as having UI.

The laparoscopic diagnosis of endometriosis is difficult even for experienced surgeons because the disease shows macroscopic diversity of atypical lesions [8], especially in patients classified as having minimal and mild disease. Although the guidelines of the European Society of Human Reproduction and Embryology (ESHRE) recommend histological confirmation of suspected lesions visualized by laparoscopy, negative histology does not exclude a diagnosis of endometriosis [9]. For this reason, endometriosis may not be detected in women with UI and, according to some researchers, UI may even represent a preclinical microscopic stage of endometriosis [10], especially in asymptomatic women (2–22 % of all cases of endometriosis) [11]. The ASRM recommends a biopsy only when the diagnosis cannot be made by macroscopic visualization of lesions suspected to represent endometriosis [6].

Pathophysiology of Infertility Associated with Endometriosis

Endometriosis is frequently associated with infertility, being present in more than 30 % of infertile women [12], with 30–50 % of women with known endometriosis experiencing difficulties in having children. The actual incidence of endometriosis in UI is unknown since not all patients undergo laparoscopy. We also do not know the actual incidence of endometriosis in the all reproductive aged women, although it is estimated to be present in 2–8 % of the general population [13]. Despite a lack of solid epidemiologic evidence to support an association between endometriosis and infertility, several lines of investigation support its association with infertility, even in its mildest forms. However, the mechanisms

R. A. Ferriani (✉) · P. A. de A. de S. Navarro · A. S. de Melo
Department of Obstetrics and Gynecology, University of São Paulo, Av Bandeirantes 3900, Ribeirão Preto, São Paulo, 14049900, Brazil
e-mail: ruiferriani@gmail.com

G. L. Schattman et al. (eds.), *Unexplained Infertility*, DOI 10.1007/978-1-4939-2140-9_19,

involved in the pathogenesis of endometriosis-associated infertility, especially in women with early stage pelvic disease (i.e., minimal and mild endometriosis, defined as stages I and II, respectively), who show no anatomical changes in the reproductive tract, have not been fully elucidated [13]. Several mechanisms relating endometriosis and infertility are possible (Fig. 19.1), but most of the studies were more focused on severe cases of the disease, and not on subtle endometriosis.

Pathogenesis of Endometriosis

Several theories and hypotheses have attempted to explain the origin of endometriosis and how the different stages of the disease can affect fertility. The various mechanisms possibly involved in the pathogenesis of the disease may also be related to the pathophysiology of infertility associated with endometriosis. In general, there are theories proposing that the implants originate from the uterine endometrium and other suggesting that they originate from extrauterine tissues [14]. Within these theories, triggering factors for disease development and potential genetic susceptibility have been studied and their roles are beginning to be delineated. Unfortunately, these theories are not sufficiently established to confirm a cause-effect relationship in the development of the disease or in the disease's role in perturbations of normal physiologic mechanisms. Studies correlating endocrine disruptors with endometriosis [15] have suggested that these factors, together with endogenous/exogenous estrogens, may be potential candidates favoring the implantation of endometriotic implants. The action of these agents and their influence on other systems that predispose to endometriosis, such as endocrine factors, progenitor stem cells, immune system, and epigenetic modifications should be considered [16].

Among the theories proposing a nonuterine origin of endometriosis, the coelomic metaplasia theory suggests the occurrence of transformation of normal peritoneal tissue

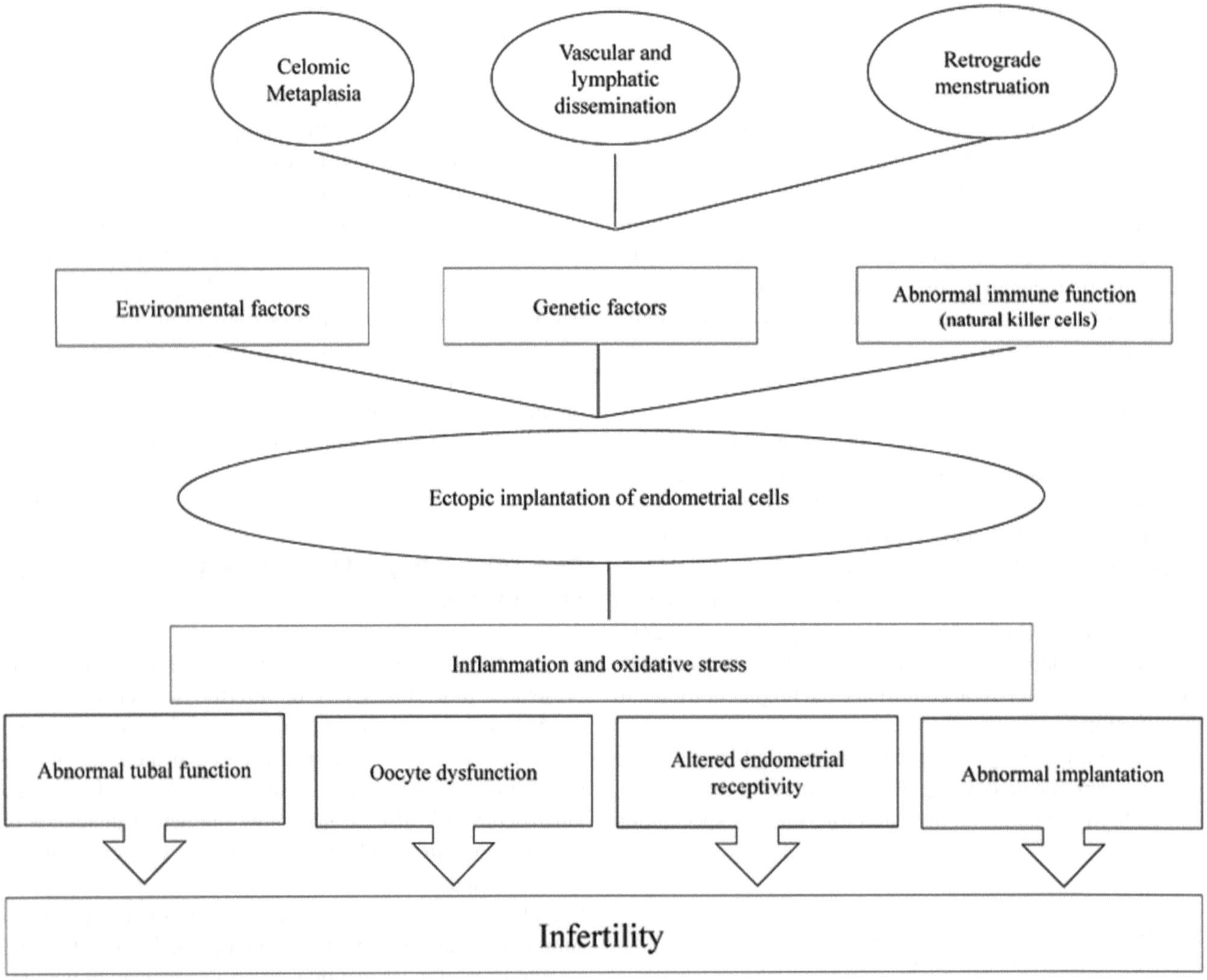

Fig. 19.1 Physiopathology of infertility associated with endometriosis

to ectopic endometrial tissue [17]. The agents responsible for this transformation are poorly known, even though endocrine disruptors are potential candidates [15]. Among the theories that propose a uterine origin of the disease is the theory of benign metastasis which is the most commonly accepted theory of origin for most endometriotic implants. This theory proposes that ectopic endometrial implants are the result of lymphatic or hematogenic dissemination of endometrial cells [18]. The theory of retrograde menstruation, which is supported by several lines of scientific evidence is the most accepted explanation of most lesions of endometriosis [18]. Although retrograde menstruation explains the physical displacement of endometrial fragments towards the peritoneal cavity, this occurs in most menstruating women and additional steps are needed for the development of endometriotic implants, such as escape from the immunological defense system, fixation in the peritoneal epithelium, invasion of the epithelium, the establishment of local neovascularization, and continued growth and survival. Investigations of the physiopathology of endometriosis have revealed several molecular markers of the disease, such as genetic predisposition, estrogen dependence, resistance to progesterone, and inflammation, factors that may be related to the lower fecundability of patients with the disease.

As can be seen, the pathogenesis of endometriosis has not been well defined, and it is possible that infertility may be the result of ectopic endometrial foci with or without anatomical changes. However, since the condition involves multiple factors, these factors may, in and of themselves predispose to infertility regardless of the presence of the disease. In fact, the disease may be a marker for infertility!

Subtle Endometriosis and Infertility—Possible Mechanisms

New approaches to the treatment of endometriosis-related infertility include the use of assisted reproduction techniques (ART). Contradictory results of in vitro fertilization (IVF) have been reported for patients with endometriosis [19, 20]. Several studies have found that the rates of fertilization, implantation, and pregnancy are lower in women with endometriosis than in women without the condition who undergo IVF [21]. These poorer outcomes may be due to impaired oocyte quality and, consequently, to impaired embryo quality, endometrial defects, and/or impaired interactions between the endometrium and the embryo [22, 23]. However, since the presence of endometriosis in donor oocyte recipients does not decrease implantation or pregnancy rates, it is possible that impaired implantation in women with endometriosis is mainly related to oocyte abnormalities [20, 24], although this subject remains controversial. In a recent meta-analysis, we observed that women with endometriosis undergoing ART have the same chance of achieving a clinical pregnancy and live birth as women with other causes of infertility. No relevant difference was observed in the chance of achieving clinical pregnancy and live birth following ART when comparing women with stage III/IV endometriosis with women who have stage I/II endometriosis [25].

Oocyte Quality and Endometriosis

Oocyte quality depends on the appropriate acquisition of cytoplasmic and nuclear maturation, with the latter depending on the presence of a normal cell spindle [26, 27]. The meiotic spindle of human oocytes in metaphase II (MII) is a temporary dynamic structure consisting of microtubules associated with the oocyte cortex and their network of subcortical microfilaments [28, 29]. This microtubular structure functions primarily by assisting chromatid segregation, concomitant with the extrusion of the second polar body, ensuring the end of the meiotic process. The meiotic spindle of the oocyte is extremely sensitive to factors such as oxidative stress (OS), which promotes meiotic anomalies and chromosome instability and is associated with increased apoptosis and impairment of preimplantation embryo development [29–31].

Noninvasive spindle analysis of in vivo matured oocytes from infertile patients with mild (stages I and II) and advanced (stages III and IV) endometriosis, and patients without endometriosis undergoing stimulated cycles for intracytoplasmic sperm injection (ICSI) did not demonstrate significant differences between groups in terms of the nuclear maturation stage, the percentage of oocytes in metaphase II with visible spindles, and the spindle localization [32]. However, it is important to state that there are no studies evaluating the accuracy of PolScope microscopy for the detection of meiotic anomalies in human oocytes (by comparing noninvasive analyses with invasive analyses after immunostaining for morphological visualization of both microtubules and chromatin by high-performance confocal microscopy). Thus, although no differences were observed in the percentage of oocytes in metaphase II with visible spindles between infertile women with and without endometriosis, we cannot conclude that the percentage of meiotic anomalies in oocytes matured in vivo would be similar for the two groups.

Endometriosis may be associated with OS [33, 34]. The disease is associated with chronic inflammation, and reactive oxygen species (ROS) are inflammatory mediators that modulate cell proliferation [34]. Endometriotic cells may suffer endogenous OS due to increased ROS production, changes in the pathways of ROS detoxification, and a fall in catalase levels, as observed in tumor cells [35]. In the presence of pelvic endometriosis, there may be macrophage activation in the peritoneal cavity, which in turn may promote an increased production of ROS, nitrogen, cytokines, prostaglandins, and growth factors. As a consequence, OS occurs, generating lipid peroxidation as well as peroxidation of their degradation products and of the products formed by its interaction with low-density lipoproteins and other proteins. OS may also damage endometrial mesothelial cells and induce the onset of adhesion sites for endometrial cells, favoring the development and progression of endometriotic foci [36]. The activity of superoxide dismutase (SOD), one of the enzymes responsible for ROS neutralization, appears to be significantly higher in the ectopic endometrium of endometriomas than in eutopic endometrium [36, 37].

The data suggest a tendency to a higher production of free radicals in women with endometriosis, associated with a potential change in antioxidant capacity, which may supposedly contribute to the occurrence of OS. This, in turn, may be related to the pathogenesis of the disease, its progression and its possible consequences regarding fertility. However, this increase in the levels of antioxidant enzymes in the eutopic and ectopic endometrium of women with endometriosis may be both a primary event and an event secondary to the increased production of ROS in an attempt to prevent oxidative damage.

There is a positive association between infertility related to endometriosis, advanced disease stage and increased serum hydroxyperoxide levels, suggesting an increased production of systemic reactive species in women with endometriosis [38]. These data, taken together with the reduction of serum vitamin E and glutathione levels observed by our group, suggest the occurrence of systemic OS in women with infertility associated with endometriosis.

The peritoneal fluid (PF) of women with endometriosis promoted meiotic oocyte anomalies and embryo apoptosis in an experimental murine model, with OS being the potential mediator [39]. However, these authors used mice as the experimental model, limiting the extrapolation to humans of the data obtained. Preliminary results from our laboratory regarding the cell spindle and chromosome distribution of in vitro matured oocytes obtained from stimulated cycles of infertile women with endometriosis have suggested a potential delay or impairment of meiosis I, supporting the correlation between endometriosis and meiotic oocyte anomalies [40].

Since the follicular environment is extremely important for the process of oocyte maturation, changes in the composition of the follicular fluid (FF) may influence the maturation and quality of oocytes, affecting fertilization, early embryo development and subsequent pregnancy [41]. Differences in the constituents of FF have been reported between women with and without endometriosis [20, 34, 42, 43], suggesting that FF may influence the acquisition of oocyte competence in women with this condition. We investigated also if OS in the follicular microenvironment may be involved in female infertility by comparing FF from infertile women undergoing controlled ovarian hyperstimulation (COH) for ICSI between women who achieved pregnancy and those who did not. We compared the levels of five OS markers in the FF and found higher total antioxidant capacity (TAC) in the FF of infertile women who did not achieve clinical pregnancy compared to those who did, suggesting that the occurrence of OS in this microenvironment may be related to compromised ICSI outcome, a fact that needs further confirmation [44].

Due to inconsistent results about the association between minimal and mild endometriosis and infertility [13, 45], and in order to examine the mechanisms of infertility related to mild endometriosis, we evaluated the effect of FF from infertile women with mild endometriosis on nuclear maturation and the genesis of meiotic oocyte anomalies during in vitro maturation (IVM) of bovine oocytes. We found that FF from infertile women with mild endometriosis may compromise nuclear maturation and the meiotic spindles of in vitro matured bovine oocytes [46]. In fact, markers of OS have been observed in the FF of infertile women with endometriosis who underwent ovarian stimulation for assisted reproduction procedures [47]. As previously mentioned, OS may promote meiotic oocyte anomalies and chromosome instability, and is associated with increased apoptosis and impairment of preimplantation embryo development [29–31]. These findings led us to hypothesize that OS in the follicular microenvironment may impair nuclear maturation and may promote the genesis of meiotic oocyte anomalies in infertile women with endometriosis. Our results open new insights into the pathogenic mechanisms of infertility related to mild endometriosis, suggesting that FF from infertile women with mild endometriosis may be involved in the worsening of oocyte quality of these women, a hypothesis that should be evaluated in future studies, including patients with UI.

Some authors have also associated minimal endometriosis with a defect of steroidogenesis in granulosa cells, represented not only by reduced basal aromatase activity, but also by lower progesterone production in nonstimulated and stimulated cycles [48, 49]. A functional oocyte defect due to abnormal follicular function may be caused by endometriosis [50]. Several other factors were related to abnormal folliculogenesis in endometriosis patients, like a longer follicular phase in IVF cycles, slower follicular growth rate, and reduced dominant follicle size [34]. Thus, anomalies of folliculogenesis associated with endometriosis, if confirmed, may be a potential cause of impaired oocyte quality.

Another way to assess oocyte quality indirectly is the analysis of different markers in cumulus cells (CC). During follicular development, the granulosa cells differentiate into two distinct phenotypes, i.e., the mural population lining the follicular antrum and the population of CC surrounding the oocyte. The former is essential for the production of estrogen and for follicular rupture, while the latter is closely associated with oocyte development. CC function is regulated in part by factors derived from oocytes and the CC, in turn, contribute to oocyte maturation and the oocytes potential for development [51, 52]. In addition, it should be emphasized that CC protect the oocytes from entering apoptosis induced by OS. Some studies have suggested that analysis of gene expression of CC may be used as an indirect predictor of oocyte quality and of the results of ART, with several possible clinical applications [53–55]. Thus, we started studies focusing on gene expression in the CC population. There is a lower expression of the *CYP19A1 (aromatase)* gene in the CC of infertile women with minimal and mild endometriosis compared to controls [56]. This study opens a new perspective for understanding the pathogenesis of endometriosis-related infertility, suggesting that reduced expression of the *CYP19A1* gene in CC might be involved in the impairment of oocyte quality associated with endometriosis. This hypothesis should be confirmed in future studies.

Other Possible Alterations in Endometriosis Related to Infertility

Alterations in immune function are also possible in patients with endometriosis [34]. An increased percentage of B lymphocytes, natural killer cells, and monocyte macrophages in the FF have been noted in a case-control study of patients with endometriosis compared to those with other causes of infertility. This suggests the possibility of an altered immunologic function in the FF of patients with endometriosis [57].

Alterations in both humoral and cell-mediated immunity have been found in the peritoneal environment of endometriosis patients [58], although it is not possible to say at the present time if these alterations are a cause or an effect of ectopic endometrium implantation. In addition, immunoglobulins and complement deposits were observed in the eutopic endometrium of patients with endometriosis [59]. The various components of cell-mediated immunity such as activated pelvic macrophages are increased in the PF of infertile patients with endometriosis resulting in a local peritoneal inflammatory cascade [60]. It was proposed that this inflammatory response can lead to increased ectopic implantation of endometrial tissue, as well as its growth and proliferation [34], although a similar picture may be seen in response to the ectopic implantation of endometrial tissue.

Although there is no consensus, women with endometriosis may have a decreased implantation capacity resulting in lower pregnancy rates, even with IVF. Reduced endometrial receptivity may be secondary to delayed histologic maturation, biochemical disturbances [61] or disturbance in cellular adhesion molecules such as avb3 integrin [61, 62]. It was also found that dysregulation of other select genes in the endometrium of patients with endometriosis may lead to impaired embryonic attachment, embryotoxicity, immune dysfunction, and apoptosis during the window of implantation (WOI) [63].

Related to answer to infertility treatment in women with endometriosis, it was described that they had a worse prognosis than couples with male factor infertility undergoing COH and intrauterine insemination (IUI) [64]. In IVF, there are mixed reports with some studies observing a detrimental effect of endometriosis on success rates and others not finding an adverse effect on success rates [13]. In general, IVF has a proven benefit over all other treatments, although sporadic reports suggested that endometriosis reduced the success rates with IVF. However, we observed that women with endometriosis undergoing ART have the same chance of clinical pregnancy and live birth, as women with other causes of infertility [25]. Other modalities of adjuvant treatment before IVF were proposed for women with endometriosis and infertility, i.e., medical suppression of their disease with GnRH analogs or surgery with subsequent ovulation induction or IVF. Outcomes may differ when surgery is followed by ovulation induction, compared with surgery followed by expectant management. During IVF cycles, outcome might be affected by prolonged use of GnRH agonists or oral contraceptives before the start of the cycle. Suppression of disease before IVF using GnRH analogs might interfere with the negative effect of endometriosis on cycle outcome since long luteal suppression with GnRH analogs was shown to improve outcomes compared with shorter courses of luteal suppression [65]. Medical treatment of endometriosis alone with oral contraceptives or GnRH analogs has not been shown to increase cycle fecundity rates once the treatment is stopped and only serves to delay attempts at conception [65]. Cumulative pregnancy rates in women with mild endometriosis had a 45 % chance for conception after expectant management, whereas only 20 % conceived with stage III and none with stage IV endometriosis [66]. Laparoscopy excision of mild endometriosis had only a modest benefit on fertility [67].

Since the pathophysiology of endometriosis involves an inflammatory response, cell survival, proliferation, migration, adhesion, invasion, and neoangiogenesis, a high number of medications were tested in preclinical models of endometriosis. This was done due to their theoretic capacity of disrupting important pathophysiologic pathways of the disease, such as inflammatory response, angiogenesis and cell survival, proliferation, migration, adhesion, and invasion [68]. Most of these agents have not been tried in the clinical setting, but further study may help to elucidate the physiopathology pertubations of endometriosis -associated infertility.

Conclusions

There is no consensus about whether milder stages of endometriosis are a cause of infertility or merely an incidental finding in some patients with UI. Studies by our group and others have shown that even cases of milder disease may inhibit the mechanisms involved in fertility, such as follicular steroidogenesis and oocyte competence. There seems to be an increase in OS in both the follicular and peritoneal compartments of patients with endometriosis, as well as a possible increase in enzyme expression in CC which may alter oocyte development. The discordant results in the literature are due in part to limitations of study design including a heterogeneous patient population, differences in disease severity, lack of fertile patients with endometriosis as controls, different medical and surgical therapeutic modalities used for treating endometriosis, varying IVF outcomes studied, lack of stringent inclusion criteria, and other compounding factors that influence IVF outcomes in endometriosis and UI patients [34].

Cases of UI, especially those with a long duration of infertility, may have subtle endometriosis and possible changes in the intimate mechanisms of fertilization involving oocyte maturation and response, as well as later embryonic implantation. Without laparoscopic verification of the presence or absence of disease, endometriosis may not be able to be ruled out as a contributing factor in couples with UI. Even the absence of visible disease does not exclude subtle, atypical endometriosis as an etiology since these types of lesions can be difficult to assess. While the necessity of laparoscopy is being debated purely on a cost/benefit assessment, the decreasing role of laparoscopy in the basic evaluation will continue to contribute a larger population of patients with UI that might otherwise have a diagnosis. Additionally, the lack of this diagnosis prevents further research into the role of subtle endometriosis as a factor in infertility. Fortunately, these patients can achieve a pregnancy as the assisted reproductive technologies are a good therapy that can overcome the possible intrinsic disturbances of fertilization in patients with UI and undiagnosed endometriosis.

References

1. National Institute of Clinical Excellence. Clinical guideline. Fertility: assessment and treatment for people with fertility problems (update); May 2012. http://www.nice.org.uk/nicemedia/live/12157/59278/59278.pdf. Accessed 21 June 2014.
2. Aboulghar MA, Mansour RT, Serour GI, Al-Inany HG. Diagnosis and management of unexplained infertility: an update. Arch Gynecol Obstet. 2003;267(4):177–88.
3. Isaksson R, Tiitinen A. Present concept of unexplained infertility. Gynecol Endocrinol. 2004;18(5):278–90.
4. Polyzos NP, Tzioras S, Mauri D, Tsappi M, Cortinovis I, Tsali L, Casazza G. Treatment of unexplained infertility with aromatase inhibitors or clomiphene citrate: a systematic review and meta-analysis. Obstet Gynecol Surv. 2008;63(7):472–9.
5. Brandes M, Hamilton CJ, van der Steen JO, de Bruin JP, Bots RS, Nelen WL, Kremer JA. Unexplained infertility: overall ongoing pregnancy rate and mode of conception. Hum Reprod. 2011;26(2):360–8.
6. American Society for Reproductive Medicine (ASRM). Endometriosis and infertility: a committee opinion. Fertil Steril. 2012;98(3):591–5.
7. Bonneau C, Chanelles O, Sifer C, Poncelet C. Use of laparoscopy in unexplained infertility. Eur J Obstet Gynecol Reprod Biol. 2012;163(1):57–61.
8. Cook AS, Rock JÁ. The role of laparoscopy in the treatment of endometriosis. Fertil Steril. 1995;55:663–80.
9. Johnson NP, Hummelshoj L, World Endometriosis Society Montpellier Consortium. Consensus on current management of endometriosis. Hum Reprod. 2013;28(6):1552–68.
10. Guidice LC, Kao LC. Endometriosis. Lancet. 2004;364:1789–1799.
11. Cramer DW, Missmer SA. The epidemiology of endometriosis. Ann N Y Acad Sci. 2002;955:11–22. (discussion 34–6, 396–406).
12. Augoulea A, Alexandrou A, Creatsa M, Vrachnis N, Lambrinoudaki I. Pathogenesis of endometriosis: the role of genetics, inflammation and oxidative stress. Arch Gynecol Obstet. 2012;286(1):99–103.
13. Holoch KJ, Lessey BA. Endometriosis and infertility. Clin Obstet Gynecol. 2010;53(2):429–38.
14. Burney RO, Giudice LC. Pathogenesis and pathophysiology of endometriosis. Fertil Steril. 2012;98(3):511–9.
15. Crain DA, Janssen SJ, Edwards TM, Heindel J, Ho SM, Hunt P, Iguchi T, Juul A, McLachlan JA, Schwartz J, Skakkebaek N, Soto AM, Swan S, Walker C, Woodruff TK, Woodruff TJ, Giudice LC, Guillette LJ Jr. Female reproductive disorders: the roles of endocrine-disrupting compounds and developmental timing. Fertil Steril. 2008;90(4):911–40.
16. Bulun SE. Endometriosis. N Engl J Med. 2009;360(3):268–79.
17. Iwanoff N. Dusiges cystenhaltiges uterusfibromyom compliciert durch sarcom und carcinom. (Adenofibromyoma cysticum sarcomatodes carcinomatosum). Monatsch Geburtshilfe Gynakol. 1898;7:295–300.
18. Sampson A. Peritoneal endometriosis due to menstrual dissemination of endometrial tissue into the peritoneal cavity. Am J Obstet Gynecol. 1927;14:442–69.
19. Garcia-Velasco JA, Arici A. Is the endometrium or oocyte/embryo affected in endometriosis? Hum Reprod. 1999;14(Suppl 2):77–89.
20. Garrido N, Navarro J, Remohí J, Simón C, Pellicer A. Follicular hormonal environment and embryo quality in women with endometriosis. Hum Reprod Update. 2000;6(1):67–74.
21. Barnhart K, Dungsmoor-Su R, Coutifaris C. Effect of endometriosis on in vitro fertilization. Fertil Steril. 2002;77(6):148–55.
22. Brizek CL, Schlaff S, Pellegrini VA, Frank JB, Worrilow KC. Increased incidence of aberrant morphological phenotypes in human embryogenesis-an association with endometriosis. J Assist Reprod Genet. 1995;12(2):106–12.
23. Pellicer A, Oliveira N, Ruiz A, Remohí J, Simón C. Exploring the mechanism(s) of endometriosis-related infertility: an analysis of embryo development and implantation in assisted reproduction. Hum Reprod. 1995;10(Suppl 2):91–7.
24. Pellicer A, Navarro J, Bosch E, Garrido N, Garcia-Velasco JA, Remohí J, Simón C. Endometrial quality in infertile women with endometriosis. Ann N Y Acad Sci. 2001;943:122–30.
25. Barbosa MAP, Teixeira DM, Navarro PAAS, Ferriani RA, Nastri CO, Martins WP. The impact of endometriosis and its staging on assisted reproduction outcomes: a systematic review and meta-analysis. Ultrasound Obstet Gynecol. 2014;44(3):261–78.
26. Albertini DF. Cytoplasmic microtubular dynamics and chromatin organization during mammalian oogenesis and oocyte maturation. Mutat Res. 1992;296(1/2):57–68.
27. Ferreira EM, Vireque AA, Adona PR, Meirelles FV, Ferriani RA, Navarro PA. Cytoplasmic maturation of bovine oocytes: structural and biochemical modifications and acquisition of developmental competence. Theriogenology. 2009;71(5):836–48.
28. Wang WH, Keefe DL. Prediction of chromosome misalignment among *in vitro* matured human oocytes by spindle imaging with the Polscope. Fertil Steril. 2002;78(5):1077–81.
29. Navarro PA, Liu L, Keefe DL. In vivo effects of arsenite on meiosis, preimplantation development and apoptosis in the mouse. Biol Reprod. 2004;70(4):980–5.
30. Navarro PA, Liu L, Ferriani, RA, Keefe DL. Arsenite induces aberrations in meiosis that can be rescued by co-administration of N-acetylcysteine in mice. Fertil Steril. 2006;85(Suppl 1):1187–94.
31. Liu L, Trimarchi JR, Navarro P, Blasco MA, Keefe DL. Oxidative stress contributes to arsenic-induced telomere attrition, chromosome instability, and apoptosis. J Biol Chem. 2003;278(34):31998–2004.

32. Dib LA, Araújo MCPM, Giorgenon RC, Romão GS, Ferriani RA, Navarro PAAS. Noninvasive imaging of the meiotic spindle of in vivo matured oocytes from infertile women with endometriosis. Reprod Sci. 2013;20(4):456–62.
33. Agarwal A, Aponte-Mellado A, Premkumar BJ, Shaman A, Gupta S. The effects of oxidative stress on female reproduction: a review. Reprod Biol Endocrinol. 2012;10(1):49.
34. Gupta S, Goldberg JM, Aziz N, Goldberg E, Krajcir N, Agarwal A. Pathogenic mechanisms in endometriosis-associated infertility. Fertil Steril. 2008;90(2): 247–57.
35. Ngô C, Chéreau C, Nicco C, Weill B, Chapron C, Batteux F. Reactive oxygen species controls endometriosis progression. Am J Pathol. 2009;175(1):225–34.
36. Alpay Z, Saed GM, Diamond MP. Female infertility and free radicals: potential role in adhesions and endometriosis. J Soc Gynecol Investig. 2006;13(6):390–8.
37. Oner-Iyidoğan Y, Koçak H, Gürdöl F, Korkmaz D, Buyru F. Indices of oxidative stress in eutopic and ectopic endometria of women with endometriosis. Gynecol Obstet Invest. 2004;57(4):214–7.
38. Andrade AZ, Rodrigues JK, Dib LA, Romão GS, Ferriani RA, Jordão Junior AA, Navarro PA. Serum markers of oxidative stress in infertile women with endometriosis. Rev Bras Ginecol Obstet. 2010;32(6):279–85.
39. Mansour G, Abdelrazik H, Sharma RK, Radwan E, Falcone T, Agarwal A. L-carnitine supplementation reduces oocyte cytoskeleton damage and embryo apoptosis induced by incubation in peritoneal fluid from patients with endometriosis. Fertil Steril. 2009;91:2079–86.
40. Barcelos ID, Vieira RC, Ferreira EM, Martins WP, Ferriani RA, Navarro PA. Comparative analysis of the spindle and chromosome configurations of in vitro-matured oocytes from patients with endometriosis and from control subjects: a pilot study. Fertil Steril. 2009;92(5):1749–52.
41. Ma CH, Yan LY, Qiao J, Sha W, Li L, Chen Y, Sun QY. Effects of tumor necrosis factor-alpha on porcine oocyte meiosis progression, spindle organization, and chromosome alignment. Fertil Steril. 2010;93:920–6.
42. Jackson LW, Schisterman EF, Dey-Rao R, Browne R, Armstrong D. Oxidative stress and endometriosis. Hum Reprod. 2005;20:2014–20.
43. Campos Petean C Ferriani RA Reis RM de Moura MD Jordao AA Jr Navarro PA. Lipid peroxidation and vitamin E in serum and follicular fluid of infertile women with peritoneal endometriosis submitted to controlled ovarian hyperstimulation: a pilot study. Fertil Steril. 2008;90:2080–5.
44. Da Broi MG Andrade AZ Rodrigues JK Paz CCP. Total antioxidant capacity (TAC) levels in follicular fluid of infertile patients undergoing ICSI: a possible predictor of clinical pregnancy. Fertil Steril. 2013;100(3):S425.
45. Matorras R, Corcostegui B, Esteban J, Ramon O, Prieto B, Exposito A, Pijoan JI. Fertility in women with minimal endometriosis compared with normal women was assessed by means of a donor insemination program in unstimulated cycles. Am J Obstet Gynecol. 2010;203:341–5.
46. Da Broi MG Malvezzi H Paz CC Ferriani RA Navarro PA. Follicular fluid from infertile women with mild endometriosis may compromise the meiotic spindles of bovine metaphase II oocytes. Hum Reprod. 2014;29(2):315–23.
47. Prieto L, Quesada JF, Cambero O, Pacheco A, Pellicer A, Codoceo R, Garcia-Velasco JA. Analysis of follicular fluid and serum markers of oxidative stress in women with infertility related to endometriosis. Fertil Steril. 2012;98:126–30.
48. Harlow CR, Cahill DJ, Maile LA, Talbot WM, Mears J, Wardle PG, Hull MG. Reduced preovulatory granulosa cell steroidogenesis in women with endometriosis. J Clin Endocrinol Metab. 1996;81(1):426–9.
49. Gomes FM, Navarro PA, de Abreu LG, Ferriani RA, dos Reis RM, de Moura MD. Effect of peritoneal fluid from patients with minimal/mild endometriosis on progesterone release by human granulosa-lutein cells obtained from infertile patients without endometriosis: a pilot study. Eur J Obstet Gynecol Reprod Biol. 2008;138(1):60–5.
50. Wardle PG, Mitchell JD, McLaughlin EA, Ray BD, McDermott A, Hull MG. Endometriosis and ovulatory disorder: reduced fertilisation in vitro compared with tubal and unexplained infertility. Lancet. 1985;2(8449):236–9.
51. Eppig JJ, Wigglesworth K, Pendola FL. The mammalian oocyte orchestrates the rate of ovarian follicular development. Proc Natl Acad Sci U S A. 2002;99(5):2890–4.
52. Tanghe S, Van Soom A, Nauwynck H, Coryn M, de Kruif A. Minireview: functions of the cumulus oophorus during oocyte maturation, ovulation, and fertilization. Mol Reprod Dev. 2002;61(3):414–24.
53. Hamel M, Dufort I, Robert C, Gravel C, Leveille MC, Leader A, et al. Identification of differentially expressed markers in human follicular cells associated with competent oocytes. Hum Reprod. 2008;23(5):1118–27.
54. Haouzi D, Hamamah S. Pertinence of apoptosis markers for the improvement of in vitro fertilization (IVF). Curr Med Chem. 2009;16(15):1905–16.
55. Tesfaye D, Ghanem N, Carter F, Fair T, Sirard MA, Hoelker M, et al. Gene expression profile of cumulus cells derived from cumulus-oocyte complexes matured either in vivo or in vitro. Reprod Fertil Dev. 2009;21(3):451–61.
56. Barcelos ID, Donabella FC, Ribas CP, Meola J, Ferriani RA, Navarro PAAS. Gene expression of aromatase (CYP19A1) and 3β-hydroxysteroid dehydrogenase in cumulus oophorus cells of endometriosis and control infertile patients submitted to ICSI. Fertil Steril. 2011;96(3):S75.
57. Lachapelle MH, Hemmings R, Roy DC, Falcone T, Miron P. Flow cytometric evaluation of leukocyte subpopulations in the follicular fluids of infertile patients. Fertil Steril. 1996;65:1135–40.
58. Oosterlynck DJ, Meuleman C, Waer M, Koninckx PR, Vandeputte M. Immunosuppressive activity of peritoneal fluid in women with endometriosis. Obstet Gynecol. 1993;82:206–12.
59. Weed JC, Arquembourg PC. Endometriosis: can it produce an autoimmune response resulting in infertility? Clin Obstet Gynecol. 1980;23:885–93.
60. Lebovic DI, Mueller MD, Taylor RN. Immunobiology of endometriosis. Fertil Steril. 2001;75:1–10.
61. Lessey BA, Castelbaum AJ, Buck CA, Lei Y, Yowell CW, Sun J. Further characterization of endometrial integrins during the menstrual cycle and in pregnancy. Fertil Steril. 1994;62:497–506.
62. Lessey BA, Castelbaum AJ, Sawin SW, Buck CA, Schinnar R, Bilker W, et al. Aberrant integrin expression in the endometrium of women with endometriosis. J Clin Endocrinol Metab. 1994;79:643–9.
63. Kao LC, Germeyer A, Tulac S, Lobo S, Yang JP, Taylor RN, et al. Expression profiling of endometrium from women with endometriosis reveals candidate genes for disease-based implantation failure and infertility. Endocrinology. 2003;144:2870–81.
64. Hughes EG. The effectiveness of ovulation induction and intrauterine insemination in the treatment of persistent infertility: a meta-analysis. Hum Reprod. 1997;12:1865–72.
65. Lessey BA. Medical management of endometriosis and infertility. Fertil Steril. 2000;73:1089–96.
66. Olive DL, Stohs GF, Metzger DA, et al. Expectant management and hydrotubations in the treatment of endometriosis associated infertility. Fertil Steril. 1985;44:35–41.
67. Marcoux S, Maheux R, Berube S. Laparoscopic surgery in infertile women with minimal or mild endometriosis. Canadian collaborative group on endometriosis. N Engl J Med. 1997;337:217–22.
68. Soares SR, Martinez-Varea A, Hidalgo-Mora JJ, Pellicer A. Pharmacologic therapies in endometriosis: a systematic review. Fertil Steril. 2012;98:529–55.

Part IV
Evaluation

Evaluation of Women with Unexplained Infertility

20

Richard P. Dickey

Introduction

The causes of infertility in 14,141 couples compiled from 21 reports in 1995 were: ovulatory disorder 27 %, abnormal semen 25 %, tubal occlusion 22 %, endometriosis 5 %, and unexplained 17 %. [1]. The proportion with unexplained infertility ranged from 0 to 26 % in these reports with the differences due largely to whether or not a post coital test (PCT) was performed, and the age of the female partner. The causes of infertility in over 12,000 pregnancies conceived following infertility treatment 1976–2010 at the Fertility Institute of New Orleans are shown in Table 20.1. Causes of infertility in couples referred for additional treatment after three or more cycles of clomiphene citrate (CC) are shown in Table 20.2. Cervical factor and thin endometrial lining were the primary cause of infertility in 20 % of couples who became pregnant and in 49 % of couples referred for failure to conceive after three or more cycles of CC. Two medical conditions, insulin resistance and hypothyroidism were contributing factors in 17 % of CC failures [2].

The goal of evaluation of the infertile couple is to identify the cause of their infertility or subfertility, which may be due to a medical or surgically correctable disorder in either partner. Modern infertility treatment with ovulation induction (OI) and in vitro fertilization (IVF) make it possible to circumvent most causes of unexplained infertility. However, proceeding directly to OI and IVF without diagnosing and treating the underlying cause may adversely affect the pregnancy and the fetus.

Conception requires ovulation of a mature oocyte, normal fallopian tubes, the presence of progressively motile sperm in the female reproductive tract, and an endometrium favorable for implantation. Evaluation of unexplained infertility assumes that a semen analysis, and diagnostic tests for ovulation and tubal patency are normal, and that sufficient time has elapsed for conception to occur naturally.

R. P. Dickey (✉)
The Fertility Institute, 800 N Causeway Blvd., Ste. 2C, Mandeville, LA 70448, USA

Table 20.1 Causes of infertility at the fertility institute of New Orleans: 1976–2010. (Adapted from [2]. With permission from Cambridge University Press)

Factor	Incidence (%)
Male	40
Ovulatory dysfunction	35
Uterine-tubal	25
Peritoneal/endometriosis	15
Cervical mucus	10
Under developed endometrium	10

Table 20.2 Infertility factors in 100 couples referred to the fertility institute of New Orleans due to failure to conceive after three or more cycles of clomiphene citrate (CC). (Adapted from [2]. With permission from Cambridge University Press)

Factor	Incidence (%)
Cervical	39
Peritoneal (endometriosis)	31
Male (undiagnosed)	25
Tubal	24
Insulin Resistance	12
Endometrial (thin endometrium)	10
Hypothyroidism	5

Evaluation proceeds in a step wise manner from the least to the most complex and invasive tests.

The first step in evaluation of unexplained infertility is to rule out medical conditions as a cause. At a minimum, TSH and fasting insulin and glucose should be measured. Dehydroepiandrosterone sulfate (DHEAS) alone or with testosterone and 17-Hydroxyprogesterone (17-OHP) should be measured if there is clinical evidence of excessive androgen. Immunological testing other than for antisperm antibodies is not indicated. Antiphospholipid syndrome and anti-thyroid antibodies have been associated with recurrent pregnancy loss, not with infertility.

The second step is to re-examine whether the results of initial tests of semen quality and quantity, ovulation, and tubal patency were truly normal.

G. L. Schattman et al. (eds.), *Unexplained Infertility,* DOI 10.1007/978-1-4939-2140-9_20,

The third step is to determine whether endometrial development at the time of ovulation is normal and progressively motile sperm are present within the cervical canal 6–12 h after coitus which evaluates both coital and cervical mucus, significant infertility factors that are not evaluated by the traditional triad of tests.

The fourth step, when there are findings of either suboptimal ovulation or less than optimal progressively motile sperm in the cervical mucus is a three month trial of intrauterine insemination (IUI), CC induction of ovulation, or both.

The fifth and final step is IVF with split insemination, a portion of oocytes exposed to sperm in vitro and a portion of oocytes subjected to intracytoplasmic sperm injection (ICSI). If embryos develop to blastocyst stage but fail to implant PGS may be considered.

Step One: Tests for Medical Conditions

Overweight, Underweight

Ovulation disorders due to stress, exercise, and eating or weight disorders are caused by abnormalities in the pulsatile secretion of hypothalamic gonadotropin releasing hormone (GnRH). Obesity (BMI≥25) is a common cause of anovulation. It has been estimated that 50 % of women who are more than 20 % over their ideal weight will be anovulatory or have luteal insufficiency. Often a 9 kg (20 lb) or 5 % reduction in body weight is all that is required to restore ovulation and potentially fertility. Underweight (BMI<18.5) due to voluntary caloric restriction and hypoglycemia are dietary disorders associated with suboptimal ovulation. Both disorders may be diagnosed by a 4 h glucose tolerance test. A return to fasting serum glucose level 1 h after ingestion of a glucose load indicates inadequate carbohydrate in the diet. It can be corrected by consuming a diet containing 200 plus grams of carbohydrates, the "carb up" diet employed by Marathon runners. A serum glucose level of 60 mg/dL or less 3–4 h after a 75 g glucose load indicates hypoglycemia, correctable by replacing sugar and fructose in the diet with complex carbohydrates contained in wheat, rice, and other grains.

Insulin Resistance

Obesity is associated with insulin resistance, but many patients with incipient insulin resistance may have normal weight. Insulin resistance was the primary cause in 12 % of patients who failed to conceive after three or more cycles of CC-IUI Table 20.2. Evidence of excessive androgen (excessive body and facial hair, oily scalp, and in young women acne) are commonly present in insulin resistant women due to elevated IGF1 levels and acanthosis nigricans, a thickening and darkening of the skin on the back of the neck and inner thighs is pathognomonic for insulin resistance. Hyperinsulinemia, if left untreated can lead to hypertension and an increased risk of cardiovascular disease as well as gestational diabetes. Insulin resistance is considered to be one component of a condition formerly called syndrome X and now labeled metabolic syndrome. In addition to insulin resistance and obesity, the metabolic syndrome requires there to be three or more of the following: [3]

- Hypertension 130/85 mm Hg or higher
- Triglyceride levels 150 mg/dL or higher
- HDL-cholesterol levels less than 50 mg/dL
- Abdominal obesity waist circumference greater than 35 in.
- Fasting glucose 110 mg/dL or higher

Laboratory findings in IR are: fasting insulin levels greater than 20 μU/mL, and a fasting glucose to fasting insulin ratio less than 4.5 [4]. The first line of treatment for women with borderline and mild IR should be weight loss. Metformin 500–1000 mg twice a day with meals is indicated for women with sub-optimal ovulation who continue to have elevated insulin levels after weight loss. Addition of CC is often necessary as these women often remain anovuatory [5].

Adrenal Hyperplasia

Congenital adrenal hyperplasia is an autosomal-recessive inherited enzyme defect that results in metabolic disorders and in the classical form (complete enzyme block) masculinization of newborn females, salt wasting, and potentially death if not diagnosed in a timely fashion. It is fortunately rare. A mild form of adrenal hyperplasia with onset at or following menarche, is variously labeled, late-onset, adult onset, acquired, partial, attenuated, or nonclassical adrenal hyperplasia. Clinical signs include: hirsutism, mild acne; increased scalp sebum, and possibly mild hypertension. The diagnosis is confirmed by 17-hydroxy P levels ≥200 ng/dL or DHEAS sulfate levels ≥180 ug/dL. ACTH stimulated levels of 17-OHP can also be used to differentiate mild forms with borderline baseline levels. Elevated DHEAS is more common in mild cases and can be measured first. Treatment for either defect is low dose corticosteroid (0.5 mg dexamethasone or 5 mg prednisone) daily at bedtime. The addition of CC is often necessary for ovulation.

Thyroid

Hypothyroidism was identified in 5 % of patients who failed to conceive after three or more cycles of CC-IUI (Table 20.2). Hypothyroidism and hyperthyroidism are associated with menstrual dysfunction, with hypothyroidism being more common. Thyroid stimulating hormone (TSH) levels less than 0.4 μU/mL are abnormal and indicate the need for additional studies to diagnose hyperthyroidism. Although TSH levels ≥4.5 µU/mL are generally accepted as diagnostic of subclinical hypothyroidism, many medical and reproductive endocrinologists consider TSH levels ≥2.5 µU/mL as abnormal and may contribute to ovulatory dysfunction. Hypothyroidism during pregnancy is linked to miscarriage and mental retardation in children. Patients with TSH levels ≥4.5 should be treated with levothyroxine (LTX) 50–75 mcg per day before attempting pregnancy. Treatment with LTX 25–50 mcg per day may be considered for anovulatory patients when TSH levels are between 2.5 and 4.5 µU/mL. While pregnant, patients with TSH levels ≥2.0 µU/mL should be retested monthly during the first trimester and again post partum. Newly pregnant patients already using LTX should have the dose increased by 20–50 % (at least 25 mcg) as soon as pregnancy is confirmed. TSH levels are approximately 30 % lower when measured while patients are fasting.

Hyperprolactinemia

Mildly elevated prolactin levels < 35 ng/mL are not associated with unexplained infertility but may be secondary to hypothyroidism. Moderate elevation of prolactin above 35–100 ng/ml can be associated with abnormal folliculogenesis and luteal phase dysfunction. The incidence of hyperprolactinemia in an infertile population has been reported to be as high as 20 % [6]. Causes of mild to moderate increases in prolactin include antidepressant and antipsychotic medications, physical activity, stress, nipple stimulation, high carbohydrate meal, etc.; mildly elevated levels should be repeated early am and fasting.

Step Two: Reexamination of Initial Tests of Semen, Ovulation, and Tubal Patency

Semen Analysis

A comprehensive semen analysis requires strict morphology by Kruger [7] criteria and is difficult to obtain from commercial and hospital or non specialty clinical laboratories. Until 1980, the standards for normal semen were those established by MacLeod and Gold in 1951, who analyzed the sperm counts of 1000 fertile and 1000 infertile men. They observed that 19 % of infertile men had counts of less than 20 million/ml compared to 8 % of fertile men [8]. On this basis they stated that men with sperm counts above 20 million/ml were fertile, and men with counts below that concentration were subfertile, even though they had not further stratified counts of less than 20 million. They proposed that a minimum of 50 million total sperm, 30 % "active" sperm and 55 % normal morphology were necessary for normal male fertility [9]. Although reports with lower thresholds were subsequently published by others and had been published previously, MacLeod and Gold's values were used to define male infertility for the next 30 years.

In 1980, the WHO published new standards for normal semen parameters. These were 20 million per ml, 40 million total count, 50 % forward progression, and 30 % normal forms [10]. In the fourth edition of The WHO Laboratory manual for the "Examination of Human Semen and Sperm-Cervical Mucus Interaction" published in 1999, there were two important changes [11] (Table 20.3). The first was that the new reference value for normal motility could be either 50 % overall motility or 25 % rapid progressive motility (PM) within 60 min of ejaculation. The second was a new reference value for normal morphology of 15 % by strict Kruger criteria based on results of IVF studies [12]. When evaluated by strict criteria, sperm with 15 % or greater normal forms were observed to have normal fertilization capability in vitro. Sperm with 5–14 % normal forms had intermediate, and sperm with < 5 % normal forms had poor fertilization capability in vitro [12]. Significantly, Kruger arrived at his definition of normal from the shape and measurements of progressively motile sperm found in cervical mucus 9–12 h after coitus [7]. When evaluating semen analysis reports from commercial centers, hospitals, and non-specialty laboratories, it is necessary to know which WHO criteria is being used and to realize that these criteria are very likely to change again.

Initial fresh semen quality necessary for normal pregnancy rates in IUI cycles differs from the WHO standard for semen analysis with respect to concentration (count per ml),

Table 20.3 World Health Organization reference values for normal sperm. (Adapted from [11]. Reprinted with the permission of Cambridge University Press)

Parameter	Reference value
Volume	≥2.0 ml
Sperm concentration	≥20 × 10^6/ml
Total sperm count	≥40 × 10 million per ejaculate
Motility	≥50 % motile or 25 % with PM
Morphology	≥30 % normal forms or ≥15 % using strict criteria
TMS	≥25 × 10 million per ejaculate
Grade of progression	3–4
Agglutination	0–1
Liquefaction	complete in 20–30 min.
Viscosity	0–1
pH	7.2–7.8
Viability	≥75 % or > 12–15 % difference from % motility
PMNS (WBC)	< 1 million/ml

Total motile normal sperm (TMNS) derived from above, ≥3 × 10 million per ejaculate
TMS: Total motile spermatozoa
PMNS: Polymorphonuclear granulocytes

and total sperm count because the entire volume is used to prepare the insemination specimen, the sperm are placed directly into the uterine cavity and fallopian tubes bypassing the cervix. Based on semen analysis performed before preparation for timed IUI in 4056 spontaneous, clomiphene, or gonadotropin cycles, sperm criteria for pregnancy rates of ≥ 8 % per IUI cycle (threshold levels) were: 5 million sperm per ml, 10 million total count, 30 % progression motility, 5 million total motile sperm (TMS) and 5 % normal forms. (Table 20.4) [13]. Pregnancy rates per cycle were 2.5 % when values were lower than these threshold levels. Pregnancy rates were 50 % higher when the total count was more than 80 million, forward motility was greater than 50 %, or TMS were more than 40 million. Pregnancy rates did not increase when there were more than 5 % normal forms.

Table 20.4 Relation of initial sperm quality to per-cycle pregnancy rate. (Adapted from [13]. With permission from Elsevier)

Sperm variable	No. of cycles	No. of pregnancies	Pregnancy rate per cycle (%)
Concentration: (× 10^6/mL)			
<5	121	3	2.5
5–10[a]	221	19	8.6
10–20	434	38	8.8
20–40	794	306	10.4
≥40	2486	306	12.3
Total sperm count (× 10^6 per ejaculate)			
<10	102	1	1.0
10–20[a]	183	15	8.2
20–40	352	29	8.2
40–80	647	55	8.5
≥80	2772	349	12.6
Sperm motility (%)			
<20	80	1	1.2
20–30	194	7	3.6
30–40[a]	555	54	9.7
40–50	955	123	12.9
≥50	2272	264	
Percent normal forms (%)			
<5	11	0	0
5–10[a]	34	3	10.7
10–20	127	16	12.7
20–30	248	29	11.7
30–60	1804	209	11.6
≥60	1719	175	10.2
Total motile sperm (× 10^6 per ejaculate)			
<5	175	4	2.3
5–10[a]	193	16	8.3
10–20	402	33	8.2
20–40	658	59	9.0
≥40	2626	337	12.8
[a]*Threshold level*			

[a] Less than threshold value vs. threshold value; Fisher's exact test

Ovulation

Ovulation may have been confirmed during an initial evaluation of the infertile female by physiological, histological, or hormonal test but could still be an incomplete or suboptimal ovulation. Lutenized unruptured follicle (LUF) syndrome is an old term used to describe a condition in which ovulation appears to have occurred on the basis of hormonal or histological tests but the oocyte did not appear to be released by ultrasound (US) or other criteria. In most cases it is due to inaccuracy of the tests used to "confirm" ovulation or to an inadequate LH surge. Suboptimal ovulation is a more correct term for a common condition usually called luteal insufficiency (LI) where the oocyte is released but P levels or endometrial biopsy results are suboptimal. The underlying defect may be either inadequate follicular development or a weak LH surge. Tests used to evaluate ovulation and their interpretations are shown in Fig. 20.1. In patients with unexplained infertility, either US or laparoscopy, before and after presumptive ovulation, is necessary to confirm lack of ovulation. In the controversial LUF syndrome, ovulation is suspected not to have occurred despite an LH surge, or physiological changes normally associated with ovulation (shift in basal body temperature, mid cycle pain, cervical mucus thickening). However, no change in size of the dominant follicle on US and no operculum (stigma of ovulation) found at laparoscopy post LH surge would be presumptive evidence of this. Unfortunately, because of these requirements, definitive evidence for this disorder is lacking.

Luteal insufficiency (LI) is a subtle abnormality of ovulation characterized by abnormally low levels of P production by the corpus luteum or a short luteal phase [14, 15]. Patients with LI ovulate but it has been hypothesized that pregnancy fails to occur or ends in early miscarriage. It is one of the most common ovulatory disorders in patients over the age of 28. Estimates of the prevalence of LI in fertility and women with recurrent early pregnancy loss range from 3.5 to 60 %

Ovulation Function Evaluation

- Physiological
  - Normal; Basal Temperature >98.0 degrees Fahrenheit (37 degrees Celcius) x 14 days.
  - Abnormal: Increase in premenstrual cramping, clotting
- Histological:
  - Normal; In Phase Endometrial biopsy,
  - Abnormal: > 2 day lag in development
- Hormonal Progesterone
  - Normal; ≥18 ng/mL 4-7 days after ovulation
  - Abnormal: <18 ng/mL = Luteal Insufficiency
  - Abnormal: < 7 ng/ml = anovulation
- Other: Pre & Post-ovulation US, Laparoscopy
  - Only absolute confirmation of ovulation.

Fig. 20.1 Ovulation function evaluation

[15]. Luteal phase P is principally produced by theca-luteal cells derived from granulosa cells in the preovulatory follicle. Low levels of luteal phase P may be due to inadequate FSH stimulation in the proliferative phase or inadequate LH stimulation in the luteal phase. P is released in pulsatile fashion in time with LH pulses and has considerable diurnal variation [14]. Low levels of both estradiol and P indicate deficient granulosa cell numbers or activity. If only P is low and estradiol is ≥180 pg/ml, the problem may be deficient LH stimulation, defective theca-luteal cells secondary to a hemorrhagic CL cyst, or the level being tested during the nadir of pulsatile P secretion.

At one time the diagnosis of LI was made by endometrial biopsy, a procedure that was uncomfortable and risked injury to an implanted embryo. Today, the diagnosis is more often based on serum P levels and the appearance of the endometrium on US. Although some textbooks and laboratory manuals report serum P concentrations of 500–1000 ng/dL (0.5–1.0 pg/mL) as evidence of normal ovulation, many infertility experts and the current author included, believe that levels lower than 1600–1800 ng/dl (1.6–1.8 pg/ml) are associated with failure to implant or early miscarriage [16]. Others believe that P levels must be below 1000 ng/dl (10 pg/ml) on repeated sampling in order to diagnose LI [14]. On US, the midluteal phase endometrium should have a thickness≥9 mm and the endometrial pattern should be homogeneous and hyperechogenic [17].

Tubal Patency

Tubal obstruction and tubal adhesions are responsible for 25% of identified cases of infertility. Causes of tubal disease include: infection (primarily *Chlamydia trachomatis*, but also tuberculosis in some countries), endometriosis, pelvic surgery and rarely uterine fibroids. Hysterosalpingogram and sonohysterogram alone are inadequate for comprehensive evaluation. A hysterosalpingogram (HSG), can provide detailed information about the uterine cavity that laparoscopy, without the addition of hysteroscopy, cannot. Laparoscopy is necessary to provide information about tubal adhesions to the ovaries and other pelvic structures and to diagnose endometriosis. Endometriosis and adenomyosis, as a cause of tubal occlusion were identified in 15% of infertility patients who eventually conceived (Table 20.1), and were a factor in 31% of patients who failed to conceive after three or more cycles of CC-IUI (Table 20.2).

An infertility evaluation is incomplete until a diagnostic laparoscopy has been performed, but the question is when in the course of the infertility work up it should be done. In the absence of clinical findings or symptoms of pelvic pathology, tubal evaluation may be reasonably postponed until after three or four cycles of IUI alone or CC-IUI. Tubal evaluation should be performed before beginning gonadotropins, a more costly and intrusive procedure. The decision about whether to perform HSG or laparoscopy before starting any form of infertility treatment is aided by testing for serum chlamydia IGG and CA-125 early in the diagnostic workup.

Step Three: Evaluation of Endometrium Development and Cervical Mucus

Endometrium Thickness and Pattern

Insulin resistance was the primary cause in 10% of patients who conceived following infertility treatment (Table 20.1) and also 10% of patients referred because of failure to conceive after three or more cycles of CC-IUI (Table 20.2). Endometrial thickness and pattern on the day of the spontaneous LH surge or hCG administration are intimately associated with implantation success or failure in IUI and IVF cycles [17–19]. Conception rarely occurs in OI-IUI cycles when endometrial thickness is<6 mm on the day of spontaneous LH surge or hCG; conception and delivery rates are highest when endometrial thickness was ≥9 mm (Chap. 27, Table 27.4) [17, 19]. Endometrial thickness was less than 9 mm in 65% and less than 6 mm in 8.7% of spontaneous ovulatory cycles during initial evaluation of infertile couples. (Table 20.5) [17]. Six to seven days after a spontaneous LH surge or hCG injection, the endometrium should show a completely homogeneous hyperechogenic pattern. A mixed or triple line pattern at the time of implantation have been associated with inadequate 17OH-P (luteal insufficiency) and a lower pregnancy rate [17, 19, 20]. Other endometrial and uterine abnormalities that affect endometrial thickness or may have an adverse effect on implantation include intrauterine synechiae (Asherman's syndrome), endometrial polyps, endometrial hyperplasia, endometrial fluid, and submucosal fibroids [21].

Cervical Mucus

Cervical factor was the presumed etiology of infertility in 10% of patients who conceived following infertility

Table 20.5 Endometrial thickness according to OI regimen: percent cycles. (Reprinted by permission from the American Society for Reproductive Medicine [19])

Regimen	No. cycles	<6 mm	6–8 mm	≥9 mm
None	23	8.7%	56.5%	34.8%
CC	197	9.1%	43.6%	47.2%
hMG	49	2.0%	38.8%	59.2%
hMG+CC	205	11.2%	55.6%	33.2%

CC Clomiphene, *hMG* human menopausal gonadotropin, *OI* = ovulation induction treatment (Table 20.1) and in 39% of patients referred because of failure to conceive after three or more cycles of CC-IUI (Chap. 27, Table 27.2) [21]. The appropriately timed Sims-Huhner post coital test (PCT) evaluates coital technique, mucus quality and quantity, and the ability of sperm to enter and survive in the cervical canal. A simple practice such as use of a petroleum based lubricant or other spermicidal lubricants may be all that is preventing conception in some couples. In addition, infections that may cause hostile cervical mucus (Ureaplasma, Coagulase positive Staphylococcus, Enterococcus) or other bacteria associated with adverse delivery outcome (Streptococcus) may be detected and treated. A good to excellent semen analysis does not eliminate the possible need for IUI, where as a good to excellent PCT may delay the need for a more formal semen analysis (without strict morphology recommended before IVF). The presence of any sperm with rapid PM argues against significant male or cervical factor as a cause of infertility, and the presence of large numbers of PM sperm is presumptive evidence that IUI is unnecessary and will not increase the possibility of pregnancy [22]. The presence of progressively motile sperm without evidence of clumping is also presumptive evidence for the lack of significant anti sperm antibodies. However, sperm penetration into cervical mucus and fertilization in IVF fertilization are not significantly impaired unless 50% or more of motile sperm exhibit head-head clumping, indicating potentially the presence of anti-sperm antibodies. [23].

The PCT using ≥5 PM sperm per high-power field as a cutoff point has been a standard part of infertility evaluation in the USA for many years. However, the presence of a single motile sperm is evidence that pregnancy is possible and the presence of ≥20 progressively motile sperm indicates both that neither sperm or cervical mucus is responsible for the unexplained infertility and that IUI will most likely not substantially improve the chance of conception [24, 25]. The sensitivity and specificity of a 6–10 h PCT with mucus collected from within the cervical canal depend on whether the criteria for a positive test was set at ≥1, ≥5, or ≥20 PM sperm per hpf [25]. (Table 20.6) The predictive power of a PCT overrides that of semen analysis except when sperm numbers are severely depleted. [26].

Table 20.6 Sensitivity and specificity of post coital test (PCT) according to sperm criteria[a]. (Adapted from [25]. With permission from Oxford University Press)

Motile sperm per field (×400)	Sensitivity[b]	Specificity[c]
≥1	0.62	0.80
≥5	0.84	0.44
≥20	0.90	0.30

[a] Studies with 200+couples, weighted averages
[b] Sensitivity=ability to identify infertile couples
[c] Specificity=ability to identify fertile couples

Table 20.7 Infertility work practices of 397 reproductive endocrinologists. (Adapted from [28]. With permission from Elsevier)

Semen analysis	100%
Hysterosalpingogram	96%
Laparoscopy	89%
PCT	79%[a]
Prolactin	66%
TSH	59%
US	54%

[a] 92% private practice, 73% academic practice
PCT post coital test
TSH thyroid stimulating hormone
US ultrasound

The value of the PCT has been questioned because of its inability to predict fertility (specificity) or non-fertility (sensitivity) in 100% of couples, because of the lack of standardization as to number of sperm that constitute a positive test and because it is possible to recover peritoneal sperm despite a poor PCT [27]. With few exceptions, peritoneal sperm recovery studies have involved intra-cervical insemination of sperm and small numbers of patients. Recently, there has been a trend in the USA and Europe, to bypass the PCT and treatment of mucus disorders and proceed directly to IUI in couples with unexplained infertility and patients treated with OI drugs. However, a 1998 report of a survey of Board Certified Reproductive Endocrinology Infertility (REI) specialists in the USA found that 92% in private practice and 73% in academic practice employed the PCT in their initial evaluation of infertile couples (Table 20.7) [28].

The PCT should be performed 9–12 h after intercourse, the length of time presumed to be required for capacitation in order to evaluate sperm survival and behavior. It should be performed 1–3 days before ovulation occurs, in order to evaluate mucus quality when it is at its peak [29]. When the PCT is abnormal and the semen analysis is normal, empiric treatment of the cervical mucus with antibiotics like a cephalosporin for Staphylococcus) or doxycycline for other bacteria, quanefesin for viscous mucus or precoital alkaline douche may be tried before moving to IUI.

Step Four: Clomiphene, IUI

The rational for using CC alone and with IUI for unexplained infertility is that it may increase the number of ovulated eggs and/or correct subclinical ovulatory dysfunction and a "luteal phase defect" [30]. The advantages of CCs over gonadotrophin for OI include: a low incidence of multiple pregnancies and ovarian hyperstimulation syndrome (OHSS), low cost, oral administration and less need for cycle monitoring. For patients under age 40, administration of CC or IUI alone for three cycles, followed by CC plus IUI for three cycles, followed by low doses of gonadotropin plus IUI for three to six cycles is the traditional protocol for the treatment of unexplained infertility [31]. During the 1980s the traditional protocol was modified to include IVF after three unsuccessful cycles of COH-IUI. An important reason for use of CC or CC-IUI before COH is that it reduces the risk of twins and triplets and higher order multiple pregnancy (HOMP) [32, 33]. A recent alternative to the traditional protocol is to eliminate COH-IUI and proceed directly to IVF when pregnancy does not occur after three cycles of CC-IUI [34].

The rational for IUI is that by concentrating motile sperm in the upper genital tract, it increases the probability of fertilization when 5 million or more total motile sperm with 30% or greater PM are available in the pre wash semen specimen and that it by passes deficient or hostile cervical mucus. The anti-estrogen affects of CC on the endometrium and cervical mucus are significant in a least 20% of treatment cycles so that effective use of CC requires monitoring with US and PCT (in cycles where intercourse and not IUI is planned), even though sperm were plentiful in the mucus and endometrial thickness was ≥9 mm in a non treatment cycle. US monitoring initially and before ovulation also reduces the risk of multiple pregnancy. Polycystic ovaries are not always apparent on screening US during the initial evaluation of infertility and may appear only during OI. The pregnancy rate per cycle is dependent on the number of preovulatory follicles that develop in response to stimulation and patient's age. Traditionally CC use in unexplained infertility is usually limited to three cycles, however CC and CC-IUI may be continued for up to six cycles with a reasonable chance of success if fewer than three follicles develop or patients are older, there is a satisfactory endometrial lining and cervical mucus and no evidence of tubal adhesions or untreated endometriosis on laparoscopy [35]. If the anti-estrogen effects of CC are predominant (thin endometrium, thick or hostile mucus, more than one or two preovulatory follicles), tamoxifen may be substituted for CC rather than switching to gonadotropins for ovulation induction with their greater risk of multiple pregnancy.

Step Five: IVF

In 2010, 12,420 IVF cycles representing 13% of all IVF cycles in the USA, were performed for unexplained infertility. IVF allows assessment of oocyte quality, sperm-oocyte interaction, embryo development as far as the blastocyst stage, and implantation of morphologically normal embryos. If PGS is performed with analysis of all 23 chromosome pairs, the ratio of abnormal (aneuploid) to normal (euploid) to embryos and type of aneuploidy can be determined [36]. On average, greater than 50% of embryos are aneuploid and the percent of aneuploid embryos increases with advancing female age [37]. During IVF cycles, the ovaries are subject to gonadotropin stimulation. If the number of preovulatory

Table 20.8 Relationship age, FSH and antral follicles to eggs, embryos, and pregnancy. (Adapted from [2]. With permission from Cambridge University Press)

Age (years)	25–29	30–34	35–39	40–44
Antral follicles	13.5	10.9	9.6	7.6
Preovulation follicles	21.6	20.6	15.8	9.2
% Antral follicles	160	189	165	121
Oocytes	11.2	9.5	6.8	
% Antral follicles	86	103	99	76
% Preovulation follicles	54	54	60	63
Good quality embryos	6.1	5.8	4.2	2.0
% Antral follicles	45	53	44	27
% Preovulation follicle	28	28	27	22
% Oocytes inseminated	52	52	44	35
% Sacs/Embryos trans	50	48	38	27
Pregnancy/Cycle %	60	56	48	43
Cont. pregnancy/cycle %	52	38	23	19

Relationship good embryos to: number preovulation follicles ≥10 mm r=0.50, antral follicle count r=0.39, patient age r=−0.31, FSH r=−0.23

follicles that develop in response to stimulation, the number of oocytes retrieved or the number of good quality embryos per oocyte are less than average for other patients of the same age, this may provide an explanation for unexplained infertility.

The probability of pregnancy in IVF cycles is most closely related to age. Between the ages of 25 and 40, the average number of antral follicles and oocytes decrease by approximately 3% per year, while the number of preovulatory follicles ≥12 mm, good quality embryos and implantations per transferred embryo decrease by approximately 4.0 to 4.5% per year Table 20.8 [2]. The percent of oocytes retrieved per preovulatory follicles does not decrease with age. The percents of preovulatory follicle per antral follicle and good quality embryos per preovulatory follicle do not decrease until after age 40. Therefore the probability of pregnancy and live birth can be predicted by age and antral follicle count (r=0.39) and even more reliably by age and number of preovulatory follicles (r=0.50) although the implantation rate per embryo transferred does not vary dramatically between "good" responders and "low" responders. The improvement in pregnancy rates, therefore appears to be more closely linked to a difference in number of embryos transferred and embryo selection.

Other methods to predict fecundity include the anti-Müllerian hormone (AMH), inhibin B concentration (IHB), day 3 follicular stimulating hormone (FSH) levels, clomiphene challenge test (CCT) and ovarian volume on the third to fifth cycle day. The sensitivity, specificity, and predictive value of these tests have been reviewed recently [38]. In a single cycle, the predictive ability was: inhibin B 71%, FSH 77%, AFC 80%, CCT 81%, and AMH 92%. Results of any tests must be interpreted to the patient with caution, because patients with abnormal levels in one cycle may become pregnant in a later cycle.

Summary

Fertility requires motile sperm in adequate numbers, a favorable cervical mucus, unobstructed fallopian tubes with fimbria capable of touching the surface of the ovary, a mature oocyte that is released from the ovary, endometrium adequate for implantation and ovarian or exogenous P levels to support the endometrium until the placenta assumes that role. Thorough evaluation of all factors is necessary before declaring infertility as "unexplained." The success of IUI alone, CC-IUI and COH IUI in treatment of unexplained infertility is evidence that cervical mucus plays a role and should be evaluated or bypassed and that oocyte maturation represented by preovulatory follicle size and estrogen level per follicle, and in the luteal phase by estradiol and P levels, are intimately associated with fecundity. Capability of the fimbria to reach the site of ovulation cannot be verified without laparoscopy. Lastly, oocyte maturity and capability of fertilization and development of an embryo with normal chromosome component would require IVF with embryo trophectoderm biopsy and genetic testing for aneuploidy. Unfortunately, resorting to IVF may or may not identify the problem and even if identified, may require IVF for future pregnancies, since these steps are not yet correctable.

References

1. Collins HA. Unexplained infertility. In: Keye WR, Chang RJ, Rebar RW, Soules MR, editors. Infertility: evaluation and treatment. Philadelphia: WB Saunders; 1995. p. 249–62.
2. Dickey RP, Brinsden PR. Female causes of infertility: evaluation and treatment chapter 3. In: Dickey RP, Brinsden PR, Pyrzak P, editors. Manual of intrauterine insemination and ovulation induction. Cambridge: Cambridge University Press; 2010. p. 19–30.
3. Expert Panel on Detection Evaluation and Treatment of High Blood Cholesterol in Adults. Executive summary of the third report of the National Cholesterol Education Program (NCEP) expert panel on detection, evaluation, and treatment of high blood pressure in adults (Adult Treatment Panel III). JAMA. 2001;285:2486–97.
4. Legro RS, Finegood D, Dunaif A. A fasting glucose to insulin ratio is a useful measure of insulin sensitivity in women with polycystic ovary syndrome. J Clin Endocrinol Metab. 1998;83:2694–8.
5. Legro RS, Barnhart HX, Schlaff WD, Carr BR, Diamond MP, Carson SA, et al. Clomiphene, metformin, or both for infertility in the polycystic ovary syndrome. N Engl J Med. 2007;356:551–66.
6. Liu JH. Hypothalamic-pituitary disorders. In: Key WR, Chang RJ, Rebar RW, Soules MR, editors. Infertility: evaluation and treatment. Philadelphia: WB Saunders; 1995. p. 154–67.
7. Kruger TF, Menkveld R, Stander FSH, Lombard CJ, Van der Merwe JP, Van Zyl JA, et al. Sperm morphologic features as a prognostic factor in vitro fertilization. Fertil Steril. 1986;46:1118–23.
8. MacLeod J, Gold RZ. The male factor in fertility and infertility. II Spermatozoon counts in 1000 men of known fertility and in 1000 cases of infertile marriage. J Urol. 1951;66:436–49.
9. MacLeod J. Semen quality in one thousand men of known fertility and in eight hundred cases of infertile marriage. Fertil Steril. 1951;2:115–39.
10. World Health Organization. WHO laboratory manual for the examination of human semen and sperm-cervical mucus interaction. 1st ed. Singapore: Press Concern. 1980.
11. World Health Organization. WHO laboratory manual for the examination of human semen and sperm-cervical mucus interaction. 4th ed. Cambridge: Cambridge University Press; 1999. p. 60–1.
12. Kruger TF, Acosta AA, Simmons KF, Swanson RJ, Matta JF, Oehninger S. Predictive value of abnormal sperm morphology in in vitro fertilization. Fertil Steril. 1988;49:112–17.
13. Dickey RP, Taylor SN, Rye PH, Lu PY, Pyrzak R. Comparison of the sperm quality necessary for successful intrauterine insemination with World Health Organization threshold values for normal sperm. Fertil Steril. 1999;71:684–89.
14. Soules MR. Luteal phase deficiency a subtle abnormality of ovulation. In: Keye WR, Chang RJ, Rebar RW, Soules MR, editors. Infertility: evaluation and treatment. Philadelphia: WB Saunders; 1995. p. 178–94.
15. Speroff L, Fritz MA. Clinical gynecologic endocrinology and infertility. 7th ed. Philadelphia: Lippincott Williams & Wilkins; 2005. p. 1030–7.
16. Dickey RP. Evaluation and management of threatened and habitual first trimester abortion. In: Osofsky H, editor. Advances in clinical obstetricts and gynecology (vol. 2, chap. 2). Chicago: Yearbook Medical Publishers; 1984. p. 329–88.
17. Dickey RP, Olar TT, Taylor SN, Curole DN, Harrigill K. Relationship of biochemical pregnancy to preovulatory endometrial thickness and pattern in patients undergoing ovulation induction. Hum Reprod. 1993;8:327–30.
18. Strowitzki T, Germeyer A, Popovici R, von Wolff M. The human endometrium as a fertility-determining factor. Hum Reprod Update. 2006;12:617–30.
19. Dickey RP, Olar TT, Taylor SN, Curole DN, Matulich EM. Relationship of endometrial thickness and pattern to fecundity in ovulation induction cycles: effect of clomiphene citrate alone and with human menopausal gonadotropin. Fertil Steril. 1993;59:756–60.
20. Smith B, Porter R, Ahuja K, Craft I. Ultrasonic assessment of endometrial changes in stimulated cycles in an in vitro fertilization and embryo transfer program. J IVF-ET. 1984;1:233–8.
21. Dickey RP. Ultrasonography in OI and IUI. in evaluation and treatment chapter 9. In: Dickey RP, Brinsden PR, Pyrzak P, editors. Manual of intrauterine insemination and ovulation induction. Cambridge: Cambridge University Press; 2010. p. 93–107.
22. QuagliarelloJ, Arny M. Intracervical versus intrauterine insemination: correlation of outcome with antecedent postcoital testing. Fertil Steril. 1986;46:870–5.
23. Ayvaliotis B, Bronson R, Rosenfeld D, Cooper G. Conception rates in couples where autoimmunity to sperm is detected. Fertil Steril. 1985;43:739–42.
24. Eimers JM, te Velde ER, Gerritse R, van Kooy RJ, Kremer J, Habbema JD. The validity of the postcoital test estimating the probability of conceiving. Am J Obstet Gynecol. 1994;171:65–70.
25. Oei SG, Helmerhost EM, Kerise MJN. When is the postcoital test normal? A critical appraisal. Hum Reprod. 1995;10:1711–4.
26. Hull MGR, Evers JLH. Postcoital testing. BMJ 1999;318:1007 (Letter).
27. Griffith CS, Grimes DA. The validity if the postcoital test. Am J Obstet Gynecol. 1990;162:615–20.
28. Glatstein IZ, Harlow BL, Hornstein MD. Practice patterns among reproductive endocrinologists: further aspects of the infertility evaluation. Fertil Steril. 1998;70:263–9.
29. World Health Organization. WHO laboratory manual for the examination of human semen and sperm-cervical mucus interaction. 4th ed. Cambridge: Cambridge University Press; 1999. p. 56–8.
30. Dickey RP, Holtkamp D. Development, pharmacology, and clinical experience with clomiphene citrate. Hum Reprod Rev. 1996;2:485–506.

31. Practice Committee of the American Society for Reproductive Medicine. Effectiveness and treatment for unexplained infertility. Fertil Steril. 2006;86:(Suppl 4):S111–4.
32. Dickey RP, Taylor NN, Lu PY, Sartor MM, Pyrzak, R. Clomiphene citrate intrauterine insemination (IUI) before gonadotropin IUI affects the pregnancy rate and high order multiple pregnancy. Fertil Steril. 2004;81:545–50.
33. Dickey RP. Strategies to reduce multiple pregnancies due to ovulation stimulation. Mod Trends Fertil Steril. 2009;91:1–17.
34. Reindollar RH, Regan MM, Neumann PJ, Levine BS, Thornton KL, Alper MM, et al. A randomized clinical trial to evaluate optimal treatment for unexplained infertility: the fast tract and standard treatment (FASTT) trial. Fertil Steril. 2010;94:888–9.
35. Dickey RP, Taylor NN, Lu PY, Sartor MM, Rye PH, Pyrzak R. Effect of diagnosis, age, sperm quality, and number of preovulatory follicles on the outcome of multiple cycles of clomiphene citrate-intrauterine insemination. Fertil Steril. 2002;78;1088–95.
36. Brezina PR, Brezina DS, Kearns WG. Preimplantation genetic testing. BMJ. 2012;345:e5908.
37. Kearns WG. Personal communication, Oct 25, 2012.
38. Sun W, Stegmann BJ, Henne M, Catherino WH, Segars JH. A new approach to ovarian reserve testing. Fertil Steril. 2008;90;2196–202.

Evaluation of Men with Unexplained Infertility

21

Marcello Cocuzza and Bruno Camargo Tiseo

Introduction

Infertility affects the male, the couple, and also the society. Approximately 10 % of all couples seek fertility assessment. Although assisted reproductive techniques (ART) remain an effective option for infertile couples, the cost is considerable, and there is a small but definite risk of ovarian hyperstimulation as well as fetal and maternal consequences associated mainly with multiple gestations.

In half of infertility cases, a male factor is involved. When possible, identifying the pathology and treating the male may allow couples to regain fertility and conceive through natural intercourse. The goal of specific treatments of infertility is to overcome identifiable disorders by increasing the fertility status, thus allowing pregnancy achievement.

Any process that influences sperm production and/or sperm function is potentially harmful to male fertility. There are many causes of male infertility including cryptorchidism, varicocele, primary testicular failure, genetic conditions, gonadotoxin exposure, hormonal dysfunction, immunological conditions, ejaculatory dysfunction, systemic diseases, and genital tract obstruction or infection. However, in spite of advancements in the diagnostic work-up of infertile men, about 22–28 % men exhibit normal semen analyses and still are unable to conceive spontaneously [1]. This condition is referred to as unexplained male infertility, and nonspecific treatments, based on theoretical concepts, are usually applied. Empiric therapies may be used and a variety of empiric medical therapies have been recommended to treat these patients [2]. However, with few exceptions, most of the recommendations are not based on controlled studies, and large placebo controlled trials are still lacking in this area.

Unexplained infertility might result from numerous discrete defects in sperm production and maturation that are yet unidentified. A better understanding of these defects will yield more effective treatment options and appropriate triage of patients to specific therapeutic regimens, avoiding unnecessary use of ART. The application of these methods in the majority of infertile couples would definitely represent overtreatment.

The goal of this chapter is to provide the reader with a foundation for a comprehensive evaluation of the male partner presenting with normal seminal parameters, providing to the urologist the essential elements necessary to understand the ideal evaluation of unexplained male infertility.

Clinical Evaluation

Initial assessment of infertile male patients should be meticulous and detailed in order to rule out any obscure cause of infertility before delving deeper into evaluating the potential etiologies of unexplained male infertility. In these couples, particular attention should be given to identifying occult female factor fertility issues, as well as assessing coital frequency to optimize reproductive timing for conception. Almost two thirds of infertility can be attributed to the female side, either wholly or in combination with male factors. Failure to include these considerations into the evaluation and management can result in unsuccessful and unnecessarily costly treatment courses.

A thorough history is important including information about not only medical and surgical problems, but also developmental issues, occupational and social habits and exposures [3]. Sperm production is a very sensitive production cycle to overall body health and problems that make the body ill will often influence spermatogenesis.

Simple problems of coital timing and frequency can be corrected by a review of the couple's sexual habits. An appropriate frequency of intercourse is every 2 days, performed within the periovulatory period, the window of time surrounding ovulation when egg fertilization is possible. Couples should be counseled to avoid lubricants if at all possible. It is also wise to discontinue any superfluous medications

M. Cocuzza (✉) · B. C. Tiseo
Department of Urology, University of Sao Paulo (USP),
Rua Adma Jafet, 50 151/152, Sao Paulo, SP 01308-050, Brazil
e-mail: mcocuzza@uol.com.br

G. L. Schattman et al. (eds.), *Unexplained Infertility*, DOI 10.1007/978-1-4939-2140-9_21,

Table 21.1 Medications and substances that impair male fertility

Substance	Effect	Reference
Alcohol	Inhibit testosterone synthesis	[5]
Anticonvulsants	Sperm abnormalities	[6]
Arsenic	Decrease sperm concentration and motility	[7]
Cadmium	Decreased acrosome reaction	[8]
Caffeine	Lower sperm concentration	[9]
Calcium channel blockers	Impairs sperm biding function	[10]
Cimetidine	Androgen antagonist/lower sperm count	[11]
Ketoconazole	Inhibit testosterone synthesis	[12]
Lead	Lower sperm count and motility	[13]
Marijuana	Reduces sperm motility	[14, 15]
Medroxyprogesterone	Azoospermia	[16]
Mercury	Lower sperm count and motility	[17]
Nitrofurantoin	Sperm immobilization	[18]
Pesticides	Reduction in sperm concentration	[19]
Solvents	Lower sperm count and motility	[20]
Sulfasalazine	Decreased semen quality	[21]
Tobacco	Higher incidence of oligozoospermia	[22]
Tricyclic antidepressants	Induces DNA fragmentation Spermicidal activity	[23, 24]

during attempts to conceive [4]. Other coital toxins comprise heat exposure from regular saunas, hot saunas, hot tubs, or Jacuzzis and the use of cigarettes, cocaine, marijuana, and excessive alcohol [3]. Table 21.1 summarizes substances and medications related to infertility and its possible effects on sperm.

It is also important to keep in mind that any generalized condition such as a fever, viraemia, or other acute infection can decrease testis function and semen quality for a variable period of time. The effects of such insults are not noted in the semen immediately after the event, because spermatogenesis requires approximately 60 days to be completed.

Aging

Infertility services are increasingly being utilized due to the later age of first pregnancy and associated reduction in female fertility. The considerable decline in fertility associated with advancing maternal age prompt the question whether advanced paternal age is also associated with compromised fertility. Changes in human reproductive behavior including prolonged life expectancy and improvements in assisted reproductive techniques have led to an increase in average paternal age [25]. Moreover, delayed childbearing is a common phenomenon in industrialized countries and age-related changes in the male reproductive system are becoming commonly recognized. Although men at any age can establish pregnancy in a woman, we still do not know how safe and wise it is to attain pregnancy through assisted reproductive techniques at an advanced age. Although the effect of male age is less prominent than of the female, this becomes especially significant when the female partner is also of advanced age [26].

Probably, men start contributing to a decline in the couple's fertility in their late thirties and to a decrease in fecundity in early forties [27]. Changes in male reproductive and sexual physiology clearly occur with aging, but the real impact of these changes on male fertility is not completely established. Currently, there is evidence that birth defects, especially those arising from new autosomal mutations, increase with paternal age [28]. Also, advanced paternal age is associated with new mutations in paternal genome and increased risk of aneuploidy in the fetus. These findings suggest that genetic risks associated to increased paternal age should be of high interest to andrologists counseling older men who wish to father a child or those for whom ageing could be an associated cause of infertility.

Spermatozoa are susceptible to the damage induced by excessive reactive oxygen species (ROS) because their cytoplasm contains low concentrations of antioxidant scavenging enzymes [29]. It is already known that with advancing age an organism is under a greater oxidative stress (OS) as the result of impairment of the function of the mitochondrial respiratory chain [30].

Recent data showed that seminal ROS levels are significantly higher in healthy fertile men older than 40 years [31]. Also, these high levels of ROS are significantly correlated with age among fertile men. As high ROS levels have been associated with the pathogenesis of male infertility, these findings suggested that delayed fatherhood may reduce the chances of pregnancy.

Seminal OS causes impairment of semen quality by multiple mechanisms including damage of sperm DNA integrity.

Recently, a significant age related increase of DNA fragmentation has been reported [32]. The risk of miscarriage in couples with paternal age over 40 years may be attributed to the greater DNA fragmentation found in older men, possibly as a result of a less efficient apoptotic mechanism [26, 32].

There are many other factors that could be involved in sperm dysfunction, independent of age. These factors include environmental pollution, lifestyle (smoking, caffeine intake, or alcohol), occupational exposure to industrial agents and heavy metals [33]. However, the andrologists should be aware that our population is aging and the age of prospective patients has increased. Therefore, there is an increasing concern about the notion that aging may affect spermatogenesis and fertility potential.

Behavior and Lifestyle

A detailed history should include a comprehensive assessment of environmental and occupational exposures that can impact fertility. Unfortunately, the impacts of environmental and occupational exposures on spermatogenesis are extremely difficult to prove and quantify.

Evidence indicative of harmful effects of occupational exposure on the reproductive system and related outcomes has gradually accumulated in recent decades, and is further compounded by persistent environmental endocrine disrupting chemicals [33]. Effects of chemicals on reproduction may be induced directly by a chemical itself on reproductive organs or indirectly through the influence in altering hormonal regulation, which is responsible for growth, sexual development, and many other essential physiological functions. A number of occupations are being reported to be associated with reproductive dysfunction in males as well as in females.

The overall functioning of the reproductive system is controlled by the nervous system and the hormones produced by the endocrine glands. The reproductive neuroendocrine axis of males involves principally the anterior pituitary gland and the testes. Toxicants that damage the Leydig cells can lead to reduced secretion of testosterone, which in turn affects the Sertoli cell function and spermatogenesis. Most reproductive toxicants are thought to act directly on the testes. There are some indications that substances interacting with the pituitary secretion of gonadotropin (FSH, LH) and hypothalamic neuroendocrine releasing factors may also play an important role in sperm quality [34].

Various behaviors and lifestyles have been associated with increased ROS production. An association between cigarette smoking and reduced seminal quality has been identified [35]. Harmful substances including alkaloids, nitrosamines, nicotine, cotinine, and hydroxycotinine are present in cigarettes and produce free radicals [36]. In a prospective study, Saleh et al. compared infertile men who smoked cigarettes with nonsmoker infertile men [37]. Smoking was associated with a significant increase (approximately 50%) in seminal leukocyte concentrations, a 107% ROS level increase, and a 10 point decrease in reactive oxygen species and total antioxidant capacity (ROS-TAC score). Also, infertile men who smoke cigarettes present higher seminal ROS levels than infertile nonsmokers, possibly due to the significant increase in leukocyte concentration in their semen. An earlier study also reported an association between cigarette smoking in infertile men and increased leukocyte infiltration in the semen [38]. Significantly higher levels of DNA strand breaks have also been identified in men who smoke. DNA strand breaks may be resulting from the presence of carcinogens and mutagens in cigarette smoke [39].

In recent decades, evidence suggestive of the harmful effects of occupational exposure to endocrine disruptive chemicals on the reproductive system has gradually accumulated [34]. Environmental pollution is a major source of ROS production and has been implicated in the pathogenesis of poor sperm quality [40]. OS is hypothesized to play an important role in the development and progression of adverse health effects due to such environmental exposure [41].

Sperm quality can be influenced for all potential causative factors mentioned above and another that has not received much attention to date. It is well known that weight gain in men, particularly the deposition of adipose tissue around the waist, can depress serum total testosterone levels and increase serum estradiol levels [42]. The interaction between obesity and fertility has received increased attention owing to the rapid increase in the prevalence of obesity in the developed world [43]. Increase in mean male weight coupled with type 2 diabetes and metabolic syndrome could explain some of the observed declines of sperm quality in specific populations of men studied. The relationship between high levels of body mass index and changes in altered standard semen analysis parameters are already described in the literature [44, 45]. Furthermore, more recent studies revealed that increased body mass index values are associated with decreased mitochondrial activity and progressive motility and increased DNA fragmentation [46].

Usually, behavior and lifestyle modification should be the first steps in reducing ROS. Unfortunately, only some data link changes in these exposures to decrease in OS and subsequent increases in human fertility. Although it is likely good medical practice to recommend modifications of unhealthy lifestyles or exposures, definitive evidence awaits additional studies.

Immunologic Infertility

The testis is an interesting organ in which it is an immunologically privileged site, probably owing to the blood–testis barrier. The tight Sertoli–cell junctions provide the testis with a barrier that prevents the immune system from coming in contact with the post-meiotic germ cells. Autoimmune infertility may be a result of certain conditions such as previous genital tract infection, testicular biopsy, testicular trauma, testicular torsion, and vasectomy [47–49]. After the blood–testis barrier is broken, the body is exposed to sperm antigens resulting in an immune response presented as antisperm antibodies (ASA). An immunologic basis for some cases of infertility has been identified in a significant number of infertile men, suggesting that ASA may have a harmful effect on fertilization [50, 51].

Immunologic infertility is characterized by the presence of antibodies against spermatozoa in three locations; serum, seminal plasma, and sperm surface. Among these, sperm surface antibodies are the most clinically relevant and the antibody classes that appear to be clinically relevant include immunoglobulin G (IgG) and IgA, as IgM has high molecular weight and cannot penetrate the blood–testis barrier. The IgG antibody is derived from local production and from transudation from the bloodstream, whereas IgA is thought to be purely locally derived. It is thought that antibodies bound to the sperm head might interfere with sperm–egg interaction and fertilization capacity, whereas tail bound antibodies may be more likely to influence sperm transport through the female reproductive tract [52].

Testing for antisperm antibodies is classically indicated when: (1) the semen analysis reveals aggregates of sperm; (2) there are isolated asthenospermia; or (3) there is a risk of autoimmune infertility (i.e. prior testicular trauma or torsion). Indications of ASA tests are listed in Table 21.2. Moreover, in men with unexplained infertility, it has been suggested that ASA should be routinely tested due to the high frequency of normal routine seminal parameters in men with elevated ASA [53]. Although, approximately 10 % of infertile men will present with ASA as compared with 2 % of fertile men [54], ASA formation has been reported in up to 42 % of men with unexplained infertility [55, 56].

Typically performed with antibody coated, polyacrylamide spheres, an ASA test with at least 50 % of sperm bound with antibodies is considered clinically significant. The presence of multiple ASA can lead to impaired sperm transport through the reproductive tract, immobilization, and/or agglutination of spermatozoa, which blocks sperm–egg interaction. They can also prevent implantation, and/or arrest embryo development [49, 57].

Table 21.2 Indications for antisperm antibody test

Indications for antisperm antibodies test
History of testicular torsion
Sperm aggregates in sperm analysis
Isolated asthenospermia
Postcoital test with poor sperm motility or shaking motility
All other causes excluded in men with normal sperm analysis

The real significance of ASA in infertile men is controversial and currently, there are no standardized treatment regimens [58]. Oral corticoids are commonly used to suppress antibody production, but to date; no double-blind, randomized trial has confirmed their efficacy. Intracytoplasmic sperm injection (ICSI) is considered to be the treatment of choice for patients with severe sperm autoimmunity [59].

Low Leukocytes Levels in Semen

The prevalence of leukocytospermia (> 10^6 WBC/mL semen) among male infertility patients is approximately 10–20 % [60]. Under a wet mount microscopy, both leukocytes and immature germ cells have a similar appearance and are properly termed "round cells." Although many laboratories improperly report all round cells as white blood cells, the clinician must make sure that the two types of cells are differentiated. Leukocytes are difficult to differentiate from immature germ cells without the use of traditional cytology staining and immunohisthochemical techniques [61]. The World Health Organization (WHO) considers leukocytospermia to be a condition in which leukocyte levels are equal to or exceed 1×10^6/mL [62]. As a consequence, all seminal analysis containing leukocyte levels below this limit are considered "normal". In spite of that, recent studies reported that leukocyte counts below 1×10^6/mL were significantly correlated with the production of seminal ROS as well as decreased sperm DNA integrity, despite the seminal parameters between the reference ranges [63–66]. All men with elevated seminal white blood cell levels (> 1×10^6/mL) should be evaluated for a genital tract infection or inflammation, and a semen culture should be performed. Unexpectedly, approximately 80 % of leukocytospermic samples are microbiologically negative [60, 67].

The significance of white blood cells in semen is controversial. Most studies found that leukocytospermia is associated with decreased sperm motility and fertilization capacity [68–72]. However, El-Demiry et al. reported no association between standard seminal parameters and the leukocyte concentration in human semen [73]. This discrepancy may be due to the fact that different techniques were used to determine the leukocyte concentration in semen. In addition, the studies differed in regard to the lower leukocyte concentration responsible for sperm damage [63, 65, 74]. Infections located in the testis and epididymis produce ROS that are particularly harmful to sperm due to their lack of a pro-oxidant defense system.

The most commonly found Gram-positive and Gram-negative bacteria are *Streptococcus fecalis* and *Escherichia coli*, respectively [75]. Also, *Chlamydia trachomatis* and *Ureaplasma urealyticum* are often involved. Once the responsible microorganism has been identified, antibiotic therapy is initiated. However, culture-negative patients should be treated with anti-inflammatory therapy and frequent ejaculation because empiric antibiotic therapy generally provides no benefit and may be harmful [76, 77]. In cases of refractory leukocytospermia, sperm washing can be performed before intrauterine insemination to remove the white cells. Although antibacterial therapy can reduce inflammatory influences when administered in patients with genital tract infection, there are no available studies on this subject that show improved pregnancy rates [78].

Seminal Parameters Limitations

A carefully performed semen analysis is the primary source of information on sperm production and reproductive tract patency. However, it is not a measure of fertility. An abnormal semen analysis simply suggests the likelihood of decreased fertility and normal seminal parameters are not assuredness of fertility.

Routine semen parameters such as sperm count, percentage motility, and morphology have a limited value mainly because there is not any consistent data that could distinguish between fertile and infertile samples in both in vitro and in vivo [79]. There are just reference values determined by the WHO over the last decades [62, 80, 81].

Approximately half of men presenting for an infertility evaluation will have seminal parameters between the "normal" reference values, representing a particularly difficult task to assign an etiology for subfertility and reinforcing the inherent inability of standard seminal parameters to assess sperm function.

We must keep in mind that the interpretation of the new reference ranges for seminal parameters proposed by the WHO, in 2010, requires an understanding that seminal parameters within the 95 % reference interval do not guarantee fertility nor do the values outside those limits necessarily indicate male infertility [80]. However, as the new lower reference limits are even lower than the previous "reference" values, clinicians will more frequently face men with semen parameters within the "normal" reference limits. Due to these seminal parameters markedly lower, a higher percentage of men will not be even referenced for an andrologic evaluation [82]. They will be inaccurately diagnosed as potential unexplained male infertility and sent to an in vitro fertilization (IVF) clinic for treatment. This may illustrate an urgent need for new diagnostic tools in the evaluation of these men.

Studies on sperm donors with known fertility status reveal a significant overlap in the sperm characteristics between fertile and subfertile men [54, 83]. The current normal values fail to satisfy clinical and statistical standards and pose the risk of misclassifying a subject's true fertility status [83]. Moreover, introduction in clinical practice of new values likely result in a reclassification of many infertile couples [82]. Specifically, those couples previously classified as having male factor infertility with sperm parameters greater than the new reference limits but less than the previous values will now be diagnosed as having unexplained or female factor infertility. In fact, using the WHO actual cutoff values most likely some patients previously categorized as having an abnormal semen analysis will now be considered "normal," with referral for evaluation postponed or not undertaken [82, 84].

Postcoital Test

To reach the site of fertilization, the spermatozoa must be able to successfully cross the cervix and the cervical mucus. The cervical mucus demonstrates cyclical changes in consistency being highly receptive around the time of ovulation. Increase in penetrability is often observed one day before the LH surge. Also, cervical mucus has been shown to protect the spermatozoa from the hostile environment of the vagina. The postcoital test (PCT) is a conventional test to evaluate the cervical environment as a cause of infertility. The PCT is the microscopic examination of the cervical mucus, performed shortly before expected ovulation and within hours after intercourse, to identify the presence of motile sperm in the mucus. So, accurate timing is crucial because it must be conducted when the cervical mucus is thin and clear just before ovulation.

In this test, cervical mucus is examined 2–8 h after normal intercourse. Progressively motile sperm superior than 10–20 per HPF is classified as normal. Practical guidelines of the American Society of Reproductive Medicine recommend PCT in a few situations including hyperviscous semen, unexplained infertility, or low-volume semen with normal sperm count [85]. The medical history and semen analysis can predict the result of the PCT in approximately 50 % of the subfertile couples with a regular cycle, without compromising its potential to predict pregnancy [85]. Impaired seminal parameters most likely will result in poor PCT. Despite that, couples with an abnormal PCT may benefit from intrauterine insemination which bypasses the hostile cervical factors [54]. There are other causes of irregular PCT including anatomic abnormalities, improperly performed intercourse, inappropriate timing of the test, abnormal seminal parameters, and cervical or seminal mucus antisperm antibodies. Of note, persistently abnormal PCT in the presence of adequate seminal parameters should indicate poor cervical mucus quality. The finding of good quality mucus with non-motile spermatozoa demonstrating shaking motion should call attention to evaluate both partners for the presence of antisperm antibodies. Occasionally, antisperm antibodies in the cervical mucus may inhibit sperm motility in vivo and prevent fertilization.

This situation can be quantified with indirect antisperm antibody testing of the cervical mucus, although an in vivo assessment of the compatibility of sperm with the cervical mucus can be provided with the PCT.

Although the PCT utility and predictive value have been seriously questioned, some practitioners still consider it a useful diagnostic test since it may help to identify ineffective coital technique or a cervical factor not otherwise suspected on the basis of history and physical examination [86, 87]. Also, a more recent study showed that the PCT has prognostic value but does not add substantially as a prognostic tool for spontaneous pregnancy [88].

Contemporary treatments for otherwise unexplained infertility, such as intrauterine insemination or in vitro fertilization, successfully reverse any unrecognized cervical factors. Currently, PCT is not recommended routinely, especially for men who have abnormal semen analyses. In addition, the test may be reserved for patients in whom results will influence treatment strategy.

Sperm Penetration Assay and Sperm Zona Binding Tests

The removal of the zona pellucida from hamster oocytes allows human spermatozoa to fuse with hamster ova. This procedure is termed as sperm penetration assay (SPA). The SPA determines the functional capacity of the spermatozoa necessary to fertilize an oocyte, which determines the ability of sperm to successfully undergo capacitation, acrosome reaction, membrane fusion with oocytes, and chromatin decondensation. The zona pellucida is stripped, allowing cross-species fertilization. Normally, 10–30 % of ova are penetrated [62].

Infertile sperm would be expected to penetrate as well as fertilize a lower fraction of eggs than normal sperm. The indications for the diagnostic SPA are limited but could be used to further evaluate couples with unexplained infertility and to help couples decide whether to undergo with intrauterine insemination, when presenting good SPA result, or to proceed to IVF. Although SPA has low predictive power, but is positively correlated with spontaneous pregnancy outcomes [89]. The monthly fecundity rate at any time during a 30-month interval of follow-up is twice as great for men with normal SPA values as for those with abnormal values [89]. However, this test should be reserved for patients in whom results may influence treatment strategy. Many versions of the SPA have been used clinically, and the value of the test results depends, in part, on the experience of the laboratory performing the assay [90].

Compared with SPA, the zona binding test uses oocytes that failed to fertilize in IVF clinics. A meta-analysis of sperm function assays by Oehninger and colleagues showed a high predictive power of sperm zona pellucida binding assays over SPA for fertilization and IVF outcome [91]. Also, the findings indicated a poor clinical value of the SPA as predictor of fertilization. On the other hand, the need for human oocyte supply remains an important limitation to the use of zona binding test in the clinical settings.

Acrosome Reaction

The acrosome is a membrane-bound organelle that covers the anterior two thirds of the sperm head. After capacitation, the sperm fuses with the ovum plasma membrane and releases acrosomal enzymes that will allow sperm penetration and fertilization. Acrosome reaction is an essential precondition for successful fertilization. Although transmission electron microscopy is the procedure of choice to detect acrosome reaction defects is a labor-intensive and also an expensive test.

The acrosome reaction test may be recommended in cases of profound abnormalities of head morphology or in the setting of unexplained fertility in patients with poor IVF cycles results [92]. Samples presenting normal seminal parameters demonstrate spontaneous acrosome reaction rates of less than 5 % and induced acrosome reaction rates of 15–40 %. On the other hand, infertile populations have shown high spontaneous rates of acrosome-reacted sperm and low rates of induced-acrosome reactions. Despite of that, acrosome reaction testing is not widely practiced in laboratories and only remains a research interest.

Oxidative Stress

Free radicals are a group of highly reactive chemical molecules that have one or more unpaired electrons and can oxidatively modify biomolecules that they encounter. This causes them to react almost instantly with any substance in their vicinity [93]. Generally, free radicals attack the nearest stable molecule, "stealing" its electron, beginning a chain reaction. Once the process is started, it can cascade and ultimately lead to the disrupting of living cells.

Human semen consists of different types of cells such as mature and immature spermatozoa, round cells from different stages of the spermatogenic process, leukocytes, and epithelial cells. Of these, leukocytes (neutrophils and macrophages) and immature spermatozoa are the two main sources of ROS [94, 95]. Leukocytes can be activated by infection and/or inflammation, in which situation they are capable of producing 100 times superior amounts of ROS than inactivated leukocytes [74].

Spermatozoa produce small amounts of ROS that are essential to many of the physiological processes such as capacitation, hyperactivation, and sperm–oocyte fusion [29, 96].

In the context of human reproduction, an equilibrium usually exists between ROS production and antioxidant scavenging activities in the male reproductive system. Minimal amounts of ROS remain in the system since they are needed for the regulation of normal sperm functions such as sperm capacitation, the acrosome reaction, and sperm–oocyte fusion [97].

In most cases, free radical-induced damage can be repaired. Unfortunately, spermatozoa are unable to repair the damage induced by ROS because they lack the cytoplasmic enzyme systems required to accomplish this [98, 99]. The pathological levels of ROS detected in the semen of infertile men are more likely caused by increased ROS production than by the reduced antioxidant capacity of the seminal plasma [29].

The production of excessive amounts of ROS in semen can overwhelm the antioxidant defense mechanisms of spermatozoa and seminal plasma causing oxidative stress. OS is a common condition caused by biological systems in aerobic conditions that results in an extreme generation of ROS, which damages cells, tissues, and organs [100, 101]. Numerous assays for ROS measurement have been introduced in the last decade [97]. The chemiluminescence method is the most commonly used technique for measuring ROS produced by spermatozoa [102]. This assay quantifies both intracellular and extracellular ROS. Depending on the probe used, this method can differentiate between the production of superoxide and hydrogen peroxide by spermatozoa.

Measurement of ROS is a helpful tool in the initial evaluation and follow-up of infertile male patients because high levels of OS seem to be strongly correlated with reduced fertility [103]. Recent studies have reported high levels of ROS in the semen in up to 40% of infertile men [104]. In addition, elevated ROS levels can be found in up to 11% of infertile patients with normal semen parameters [105].

High levels of ROS are negatively correlated with sperm concentration and sperm motility [106]. Additionally, Aitken et al. reported that men with elevated ROS levels in semen have a sevenfold reduction in conception rates when compared with men having low ROS [107]. Table 21.3 summarizes the data of ROS action in sperm.

Although, seminal parameters still constitutes the initial evaluation of male fertility in an infertile couple, basic semen analysis does not satisfactorily reflect all the parameters of semen quality and function that are mandatory for an optimum fertility evaluation even more in cases of unexplained male infertility [113]. Men classified as having unexplained infertility usually present with higher seminal ROS levels and lower antioxidant properties than healthy controls [101]. Also, some studies have shown that seminal parameters do not always correlate with ROS levels in semen [114, 115]. As reported by Aitken et al., low hydrogen peroxide concentrations do not influence sperm motility, but do suppress human sperm competence during oocyte fusion [116]. In specific situations, ROS levels are not high enough to impair standard seminal parameters but can cause defects in other processes that are required for fertilization, such as sperm–oocyte interaction. These findings suggest a satisfactory explanation why patients with normal routine semen parameters can experience infertility.

Table 21.3 Summary of evidence of ROS effect in sperm

Effect	Reference
Reduce sperm motility	[108]
Increase DNA fragmentation	[63]
Increase DNA fragmentation and apoptosis	[109]
Reduce sperm quality	[110]
DNA damage and abnormal morphology	[111]
DNA fragmentation and reduces sperm concentration	[112]

Conflicting studies make it difficult to establish the clinical value of ROS measurement in medical practice. There is no clear evidence whether high ROS levels are a cause or an effect of abnormal semen parameters [117]. However, a more recent study reported high levels of ROS as an independent marker of male factor infertility, irrespective of whether these patients have normal or abnormal semen parameters [118]. These findings suggest that ROS measurement should be used as a diagnostic tool in infertile men especially in cases of unexplained infertility.

Presently there is no consensus regarding the inclusion of ROS measurements in the routine evaluation of fertility potential in men with varicocele, and the more recent WHO manual still describes the measurement of ROS as a research procedure [80]. This may be due to a lack of standardization of the normal values of ROS in the fertile and infertile populations [65, 119]. Perhaps in the near future, measurement of seminal ROS levels could help to better evaluate men with no evident cause of infertility with normal semen parameters.

Role of Sperm Chromatin Structure Damage in Male Infertility

The sperm genetic material is structured in a particular manner that keeps the nuclear chromatin extremely compact as well as stable. Also, the regular DNA structure is capable of decondensation at the appropriate time transferring the packaged genetic information to the egg without defects in the fertilization process. The cause of DNA damage in sperm can be attributed to various pathological conditions including the presence of varicose, fever, drugs, aging, or leukocytospermia [119–124]. Environmental conditions can also be responsible as radiation, air pollution, smoking, pesticides, chemicals, heat, and ART prep protocols [39, 111, 125, 126]. The majority of these agents may not only disrupt hormone levels but also induce oxidative stress, which could damage sperm DNA [127].

Table 21.4 Commonly used DNA damage tests

Test	Aspect evaluated	Reference
Sperm chromatin structure assay	Susceptibility of sperm DNA to denaturation	[133]
Nuclear protein composition (by protein separation)	Sperm histone and protamine levels	[134]
Sperm nuclear maturity test (by nuclear staining)	Chromatin compaction, protamine content	[135]
Comet assay (by single-cell gel electrophoresis)	Double-stranded DNA breaks (neutral assay)	[136, 137]
TUNEL assay	Double-stranded DNA breaks	[138]
DNA oxidation	8-hydroxy-2-deoxyguanosine	[139]

Excessive generation of ROS in the reproductive tract not only attacks the fluidity of the sperm plasma membrane, but also the integrity of DNA in the sperm nucleus. DNA bases are susceptible to oxidative damage resulting in base modification, strand breaks, and chromatin cross-linking. DNA damage in the male germ line has been associated with poor semen quality, low fertilization rates, impaired preimplantation development and increased abortion [128, 129]. The causes of this DNA damage are still uncertain but the major candidates are OS and aberrant apoptosis.

Fertile healthy men with normal seminal parameters almost consistently have low levels of DNA breakage, whereas infertile men, in particular those with abnormal seminal parameters, have a higher fraction of sperm DNA damage [130]. However, infertile men even presenting normal routine seminal parameters may have abnormal DNA integrity [130–132].

The structure of sperm chromatin can be measured by several techniques and the ability of these techniques to accurately estimate sperm DNA damage depends on many technical and biological aspects, see Table 21.4. On the other hand, to establish a threshold level between the fertile population and the lowest sperm DNA integrity required for achieving pregnancy remains extremely challenging.

Currently, both direct (fragmentation, oxidation) and indirect (sperm chromatin compaction), methods are available to evaluate the integrity of sperm DNA. Direct methods for detecting DNA breaks include the single-gel electrophoresis assay ("Comet assay") and terminal deoxynucleotidyl transferase-mediated 2′-deoxyuridine 5′-triphosphate (dUTP)-nick end-labelling (TUNEL) [112, 130]. Indirect methods for assessing DNA damage include the sperm chromatin structure assays (SCSA) which use chromatin and/or DNA intercalating dyes such as acridine orange to differentiate single-strand and double-stranded DNA [130, 140, 141].

All methods nowadays lack a threshold, except for the sperm chromatin structure assay, which assesses the ability of the DNA to resist denaturation by acid or heat, using flow cytometry, and the damage is expressed as the DNA fragmentation index (DFI) [142]. In clinical applications, the DFI not only distinguishes fertile men from those who were infertile, but also identified samples that were compatible with in vivo and in vitro pregnancy [143].

Abnormally fragmented sperm DNA rarely occurs in fertile men, but can be found in 5% of infertile men with normal semen analyses and 25% of infertile men with abnormal semen analyses [107]. This test can detect infertility that is missed on a conventional semen analysis.

The decision to incorporate a new test into clinical practice depends on the volume and quality of currently existing literature. Current data on the relationship between abnormal DNA integrity and reproductive outcomes are limited and not analyzed systematically [144]. The Practice Committee of the American Society for Reproductive Medicine summarizes the current understanding of the impact of abnormal sperm DNA integrity on reproductive outcomes [132]. This Committee concluded that there are not enough data to make DNA testing routine in infertility testing and that treatments have yet to prove their clinical value. Prior to sperm DNA damage analysis is introduced routinely in clinical practice, studies with adequate sample size must be conducted evaluating outcomes and tests' role in the management of male infertility [144].

Sperm chromatin structure damage tests applications to research can provide greater insights to infertility and andrology. If tests on this become standardized, inexpensive, accessible, and reliable in their application, testing for DNA fragmentation defects can help couples decide on what fertility modality and possible lifestyle modifications they can employ that may increase their chances of conception.

Genetics

Male fertility largely depends on the quality of sperm production, which may be affected by genetic factors. Genetic alterations have a profound impact on the formation and function of the genitourinary system. Thus, some of these genetic alterations have obvious effects early in life including chromosomal alterations such as Kleinfelter's syndrome or trisomy 21. On the other hand, some affect patients later in life including some of the single gene defects, such as autosomal dominant polycystic kidney disease or the androgen insensitivity syndrome. Some may have an isolated effect on fertility including a Y microdeletion. However, others may be multifactorial and involve an interaction between genetic and environmental resulting in prostate cancer or vesicoureteral reflux.

Several reports have shown the occurrence of disomy for autosomes and sex chromosomes is 0.11 and 0.44% for normozoospermic infertile men, and the rate of diploidy is 0.3–1% [145, 146]. The occurrence of sex chromosomal abnormalities is 15 times greater in infertile men than in the general population, while autosomal abnormalities occur with six times greater frequency [105]. Gene mutations and polymorphism have been also recognized in infertile men with normal spermiograms. The polymerase gamma (POLG) gene polymorphism should be considered as a possible contributing factor in patients with unexplained infertility [147].

The tremendous advances in the area of genetics have allowed us to understand more about the contribution that genetic alterations make to urologic diseases. As urologists, we are increasingly expected to be experts on the genetic basis of the diseases we treat and be knowledgeable about genetic counseling. Knowing the genetic cause is the first step in finding ways to cure and prevent abnormalities, especially during the management of infertility.

Genetic mechanisms, especially autosomal disorders, may account for many cases heretofore labelled unexplained. Overall, approximately 30% of male infertility is currently unexplained and it is likely that much of this has a genetic basis. Ideally, cause-specific therapy of male factor infertility would minimize the use of ART, avoiding the costs, complications, and treatment of the unaffected female partner.

There is no doubt that ICSI overcome natural barriers resulting in transmission of possible genetic abnormalities to offspring. Infertility could be, in some way, a natural mechanism to block the transmission of these undesirable genetic traits to any offspring. Although researchers believe that approximately 75% or more cases of all infertility have a contributing genetic basis, presently our real ability to diagnose these defects remains limited [148]. There is no better example of this phenomenon than performing ICSI as a treatment for azoospermic men. Before the development of ART, these men basically could not have reproduced by any means at all.

Interest has been renewed in genetic studies to determine underlying causes of unexplained male infertility, but the overwhelming trend has been to sidestep improvements in diagnostic evaluation in favor of a more expensive, albeit efficacious option, ART [149].

Future of Semen Analyses

The prevalence of male infertility and the availability of new highly successful therapeutic options make the testing of sperm functional competence mandatory. It may help in diagnosing the exact condition that impairs patient's sperm function.

Advances in biomolecular techniques are transforming the scientific landscape of sperm cell biology. Novel tests are emerging from andrology research laboratories that may soon become clinically available. The omics revolution, as it is termed, refers to the study of genes (genomics), transcripts (transcriptomics), proteins (proteomics), and the various metabolites (metabolomics) [92]. With these technologies, inventories of lipids, proteins, metabolites, and RNA species may be determined. The application of omics technologies to spermatozoa, in concert with detailed assessments of their functional competence, may provide insights into the biochemical basis of defective semen quality.

Microarray technology emerges as a promising diagnostic tool. Garrido et al. conducted microarray analysis of sperm mRNAs of men with normal semen parameters [150]. The authors compared infertile men versus fertile controls and showed a profound differential expression of hundreds of genes between the two study groups. Although, the authors presented only preliminary results, these findings could represent a potential diagnostic tool.

Blumer et al. also investigated DNA fragmentation in patients with varicocele with normal seminal parameters compared with normal subjects and found a lower percentage of sperm with intact DNA in varicocele group [151]. OS is suspected to be involved in DNA fragmentation and probably due to decrease in amount of antioxidant leading to changes in spermatogenesis [95]. This technique may be applied in patients with normal sperm analysis and may help to understand subfertile man's etiology and aid clinical decision.

Others tests are available and might assist diagnose in patients already extensively investigated that still were unable to conceive, even with IVF. Acrosomal impaired function may affect fertility by not allowing sperm–oolemma fusion leading to IVF failure [152]. It can be assessed with another challenge that induces the enzymatic release. Semen samples with 5–30% of reacted spermatozoa have higher fertility potential and reproductive outcome [153].

The decision between IVF and ICSI can be facilitated with hemizona assays that evaluate binding between sperm and the oocytes. Sperm zona binding is assessed comparing with fertile sperm donors by a ratio, as described before. Poor zona binding have been correlated with poor fertilization rates using IVF and those patients should be counseled to ICSI [92].

Spermatozoa ability to undergo capacitation, acrosome reaction, fusion, and penetration through the oolemma is assessed by sperm penetration assay that is conducted using a hamster oocyte with zona pellucida removed and incubated with the patient's spermatozoa. This test is one of the most sensitive measures of sperm function available [92]. It is associated with good IVF outcome and the achievement of pregnancy by infertile males with unexplained infertility [107].

Impaired sperm function can be associated with oxidative stress created by excess reactive oxygen species and can be evaluated by chemiluminescent assay [119]. A signal is generated by stressed spermatozoa in the presence of redox-sensitive probes and the intensity of this signal have been negatively associated with sperm function reflecting the fertilizing potential of spermatozoa in vivo and in vitro [154]. Men with high levels of reactive oxygen species should be considered for antioxidant therapy to allow improvement of semen quality affecting pregnancy rates and IVF outcome [155].

Clearly, the future of infertile man's evaluation is to find the exact cause of impaired sperm function. All new assays are being studied to bring new light to a problem not fully comprehended and also become promising evaluation tools in unexplained infertility management. These tests may help investigation but still lack of clinical significance and require more information to determine its potential for predicting fertility and defining management.

It is crucial to point out that the targets to which male infertility therapy is aimed today have been lightened by the huge advances of ART. The modern view of male infertility approach gives a new meaning to the term "male infertility therapy," which goes away beyond the identification and elimination of the cause. These facts have by some means changed the andrologist's therapeutic strategies, which in a recent past was only attempting to achieve a simple increase in the sperm concentration. However, we are moving forward and now our main target is to improve the "quality" of spermatozoa, that means, improve the real "fertility potential." This approach is thus especially recommended in patients with unexplained infertility, usually undergoing ART, which are currently feasible with a single spermatozoa.

It also is imperative that urologists work intimately with reproductive specialists, because timing and coordination of care may help achieve the ultimate goals in addition to the better management of unexplained infertility to maximize the conceiving potential of these patients. In an ideal world, cause-specific therapy of male factor infertility would decrease the use of ART, avoiding the costs, risks, complications, and treatment of the unaffected female partner.

Take Home Message

Despite the diagnostic advances in the field of male infertility, many patients will still have no discernible cause for infertility. Better understanding of the factors that control spermatogenesis possibly will reveal the underlying pathology of many of these disorders and will permit better management.

Although it is anticipated that future developments will allow identification of the etiology for subfertility in these patients, at present they are considered unexplained disorders that defy specific treatment recommendations. In the absence of obvious causality, empiric medical therapy or ART remain the only options for these infertile patients. Despite the tremendous success of ICSI, most couples would prefer to conceive offspring naturally.

Normal routine seminal parameters do not guarantee fecundity. This premise is important for anyone involved in infertility management. At present, one of the main objectives of the male infertility research is to develop a "magic" diagnostic test that competently correlates with sperm fertilizing capacity. Unexplained infertility may result from multiple discrete defects in sperm generation and/or maturation that are still object of investigation. A better understanding of these defects using all available tools for evaluation of men presenting with an initial diagnosis of unexplained infertility will yield an appropriate triage of patients to specific therapeutic regimens.

References

1. Kamath MS, Bhattacharya S. Demographics of infertility and management of unexplained infertility. Best Prac Res Clin Obstet Gynaecol. 2012;26(6):729–38. PubMed PMID: 22951769.
2. Kamischke A, Nieschlag E. Analysis of medical treatment of male infertility. Human reproduction (Oxford, England). 1999;14(Suppl 1):1–23. PubMed PMID: 10573021. eng.
3. Shefi S, Turek PJ. Definition and current evaluation of subfertile men. Int Braz J Urol. 2006;32(4):385–97. PubMed PMID: 16953904. eng.
4. Agarwal A, Deepinder F, Cocuzza M, Short RA, Evenson DP. Effect of vaginal lubricants on sperm motility and chromatin integrity: a prospective comparative study. Fertil Steril. 2007;89(2): 375–9. PubMed PMID: 17509584. Eng.
5. La Vignera S, Condorelli RA, Balercia G, Vicari E, Calogero AE. Does alcohol have any effect on male reproductive function? A review of literature. Asian J Androl. 2013;15(2):221–5. PubMed PMID: 23274392. Epub 2013/01/01. eng.
6. Isojarvi JI, Lofgren E, Juntunen KS, Pakarinen AJ, Paivansalo M, Rautakorpi I, et al. Effect of epilepsy and antiepileptic drugs on male reproductive health. Neurology. 2004;62(2):247–53. PubMed PMID: 14745062. Epub 2004/01/28. eng.
7. Xu W, Bao H, Liu F, Liu L, Zhu YG, She J, et al. Environmental exposure to arsenic may reduce human semen quality: associations derived from a Chinese cross-sectional study. Environ Health. 2012;11:46. PubMed PMID: 22776062. Pubmed Central PMCID: 3419631. Epub 2012/07/11. eng.
8. Benoff S, Jacob A, Hurley IR. Male infertility and environmental exposure to lead and cadmium. Hum Reprod Update. 2000;6(2):107–21. PubMed PMID: 10782569. eng.
9. Jensen TK, Swan SH, Skakkebaek NE, Rasmussen S, Jorgensen N. Caffeine intake and semen quality in a population of 2,554 young Danish men. Am J Epidemiol. 2010;171(8):883–91. PubMed PMID: 20338976. Epub 2010/03/27. eng.

10. Benoff S, Cooper GW, Hurley I, Mandel FS, Rosenfeld DL, Scholl GM, et al. The effect of calcium ion channel blockers on sperm fertilization potential. Fertil Steril. 1994;62(3):606–17. PubMed PMID: 8062958. Epub 1994/09/01. eng.
11. Wang C, Lai CL, Lam KC, Yeung KK. Effect of cimetidine on gonadal function in man. Br J Clin Pharmacol. 1982;13(6):791–4. PubMed PMID: 6807332. Pubmed Central PMCID: 1402017. Epub 1982/06/01. eng.
12. Roth MY, Nya-Ngatchou JJ, Lin K, Page ST, Anawalt BD, Matsumoto AM, et al. Androgen synthesis in the gonadotropin-suppressed human testes can be markedly suppressed by ketoconazole. J Clin Endocrinol Metab. 2013;98(3):1198–206. PubMed PMID: 23348398. Pubmed Central PMCID: 3590466. Epub 2013/01/26. eng.
13. Naha N, Chowdhury AR. Inorganic lead exposure in battery and paint factory: effect on human sperm structure and functional activity. J UOEH. 2006;28(2):157–71. PubMed PMID: 16780224. Epub 2006/06/20. eng.
14. Rossato M, Ion Popa F, Ferigo M, Clari G, Foresta C. Human sperm express cannabinoid receptor Cb1, the activation of which inhibits motility, acrosome reaction, and mitochondrial function. J Clin Endocrinol Metab. 2005;90(2):984–91. PubMed PMID: 15562018. Epub 2004/11/25. eng.
15. Whan LB, West MC, McClure N, Lewis SE. Effects of delta-9-tetrahydrocannabinol, the primary psychoactive cannabinoid in marijuana, on human sperm function in vitro. Fertil Steril. 2006;85(3):653–60. PubMed PMID: 16500334. Epub 2006/02/28. eng.
16. Gu YQ, Tong JS, Ma DZ, Wang XH, Yuan D, Tang WH, et al. Male hormonal contraception: effects of injections of testosterone undecanoate and depot medroxyprogesterone acetate at eight-week intervals in chinese men. J Clin Endocrinol Metab. 2004;89(5):2254–62. PubMed PMID: 15126550. Epub 2004/05/06. eng.
17. Mocevic E, Specht IO, Marott JL, Giwercman A, Jonsson BA, Toft G, et al. Environmental mercury exposure, semen quality and reproductive hormones in Greenlandic Inuit and European men: a cross-sectional study. Asian J Androl. 2013;15(1):97–104. PubMed PMID: 23223027. Epub 2012/12/12. eng.
18. Albert PS, Mininberg DT, Davis JE. The nitrofurans as sperm immobilising agents: their tissue toxicity and their clinical application. Br J Urol. 1975;47(4):459–62. PubMed PMID: 171024. Epub 1975/08/01. eng.
19. Abell A, Ernst E, Bonde JP. Semen quality and sexual hormones in greenhouse workers. Scand J Work Environ Health. 2000;26(6):492–500. PubMed PMID: 11201396. Epub 2001/02/24. eng.
20. Cherry N, Moore H, McNamee R, Pacey A, Burgess G, Clyma JA, et al. Occupation and male infertility: glycol ethers and other exposures. Occup Environ Med. 2008;65(10):708–14. PubMed PMID: 18417551. Epub 2008/04/18. eng.
21. Delaere KP, Strijbos WE, Meuleman EJ. Sulphasalazine-induced reversible male infertility. Acta Urol Belg. 1989;57(1):29–33. PubMed PMID: 2566274. Epub 1989/01/01. eng.
22. Coelho C, Julio C, Silva G, Neves A. Tobacco and male infertility: a retrospective study in infertile couples. Acta Med Port. 2009;22(6):753–8. PubMed PMID: 20350458. Epub 2010/03/31. Tabaco e infertilidade masculina: estudo retrospectivo em casais inferteis. por.
23. Tanrikut C, Feldman AS, Altemus M, Paduch DA, Schlegel PN. Adverse effect of paroxetine on sperm. Fertil Steril. 2010;94(3):1021–6. PubMed PMID: 19515367. Epub 2009/06/12. eng.
24. Kumar VS, Sharma VL, Tiwari P, Singh D, Maikhuri JP, Gupta G, et al. The spermicidal and antitrichomonas activities of SSRI antidepressants. Bioorg Med Chem Lett. 2006;16(9):2509–12. PubMed PMID: 16464584. Epub 2006/02/09. eng.
25. Heck KE, Schoendorf KC, Ventura SJ, Kiely JL. Delayed childbearing by education level in the United States, 1969–1994. Matern Child Health J. 1997;1(2):81–8. PubMed PMID: 10728230. eng.
26. de la RE, Thonneau P. Paternal age and maternal age are risk factors for miscarriage; results of a multicentre European study. Hum Reprod (Oxford, England). 2002;17(6):1649–56. PubMed PMID: 12042293.
27. Kuhnert B, Nieschlag E. Reproductive functions of the ageing male. Hum Reprod Update. 2004;10(4):327–39. PubMed PMID: 15192059.
28. Rolf C, Nieschlag E. Reproductive functions, fertility and genetic risks of ageing men. Exp Clin Endocrinol Diabetes. 2001;109(2):68–74. PubMed PMID: 11341301. eng.
29. Lewis SE, Boyle PM, McKinney KA, Young IS, Thompson W. Total antioxidant capacity of seminal plasma is different in fertile and infertile men. Fertil Steril. 1995;64(4):868–70. PubMed PMID: 7672165.
30. Wei YH, Lu CY, Wei CY, Ma YS, Lee HC. Oxidative stress in human aging and mitochondrial disease-consequences of defective mitochondrial respiration and impaired antioxidant enzyme system. Chin J Physiol. 2001;44(1):1–11. PubMed PMID: 11403514.
31. Cocuzza M, Athayde KS, Agarwal A, Sharma R, Pagani R, Lucon AM, et al. Age-related increase of reactive oxygen species in neat semen in healthy fertile men. Urology. 2008;71(3):490–4. PubMed PMID: 18342194.
32. Moskovtsev SI, Willis J, Mullen JB. Age-related decline in sperm deoxyribonucleic acid integrity in patients evaluated for male infertility. Fertil Steril. 2006;85(2):496–9. PubMed PMID: 16595239. eng.
33. Aitken RJ, Koopman P, Lewis SE. Seeds of concern. Nature. 2004;432(7013):48–52. PubMed PMID: 15525979. eng.
34. Kumar S. Occupational exposure associated with reproductive dysfunction. J Occup Health. 2004;46(1):1–19. PubMed PMID: 14960825.
35. Kunzle R, Mueller MD, Hanggi W, Birkhauser MH, Drescher H, Bersinger NA. Semen quality of male smokers and nonsmokers in infertile couples. Fertil Steril. 2003;79(2):287–91. PubMed PMID: 12568836. eng.
36. Traber MG, van der Vliet A, Reznick AZ, Cross CE. Tobacco-related diseases. Is there a role for antioxidant micronutrient supplementation? Clin Chest Med. 2000;21(1):173–87, x. PubMed PMID: 10763098. eng.
37. Saleh RA, Agarwal A, Sharma RK, Nelson DR, Thomas AJ, Jr. Effect of cigarette smoking on levels of seminal oxidative stress in infertile men: a prospective study. Fertil Steril. 2002;78(3):491–9. PubMed PMID: 12215323.
38. Close CE, Roberts PL, Berger RE. Cigarettes, alcohol and marijuana are related to pyospermia in infertile men. J Urol. 1990;144(4):900–3. PubMed PMID: 2398564. eng.
39. Potts RJ, Newbury CJ, Smith G, Notarianni LJ, Jefferies TM. Sperm chromatin damage associated with male smoking. Mutat Res. 1999;423(1–2):103–11. PubMed PMID: 10029686. eng.
40. Gate L, Paul J, Ba GN, Tew KD, Tapiero H. Oxidative stress induced in pathologies: the role of antioxidants. Biomed Pharmacother. 1999;53(4):169–80. PubMed PMID: 10392289.
41. Fowler BA, Whittaker MH, Lipsky M, Wang G, Chen XQ. Oxidative stress induced by lead, cadmium and arsenic mixtures: 30-day, 90-day, and 180-day drinking water studies in rats: an overview. Biometals. 2004;17(5):567–8. PubMed PMID: 15688865.
42. Kaukua J, Pekkarinen T, Sane T, Mustajoki P. Sex hormones and sexual function in obese men losing weight. Obes Res. 2003;11(6):689–94. PubMed PMID: 12805389. eng.
43. Pasquali R, Patton L, Gambineri A. Obesity and infertility. Curr Opin Endocrinol Diabetes Obes. 2007;14(6):482–7. PubMed PMID: 17982356. eng.

44. Hammoud AO, Wilde N, Gibson M, Parks A, Carrell DT, Meikle AW. Male obesity and alteration in sperm parameters. Fertil Steril. 2008;90(6):2222–5. PubMed PMID: 18178190. eng.
45. Hammoud AO, Gibson M, Peterson CM, Meikle AW, Carrell DT. Impact of male obesity on infertility: a critical review of the current literature. Fertil Steril. 2008;90(4):897–904. PubMed PMID: 18929048. eng.
46. Fariello RM, Pariz JR, Spaine DM, Cedenho AP, Bertolla RP, Fraietta R. Association between obesity and alteration of sperm DNA integrity and mitochondrial activity. BJU Int. 2012;110(6):863–7. PubMed PMID: 22300410. eng.
47. Arap MA, Vicentini FC, Cocuzza M, Hallak J, Athayde K, Lucon AM, et al. Late hrmonal levels, semen parameters and presence of antisperm antibodies in patients treated for testicular torsion. J Androl. 2007;28(4):528–32. PubMed PMID: 17287456. Eng.
48. Broderick GA, Tom R, McClure RD. Immunological status of patients before and after vasovasostomy as determined by the immunobead antisperm antibody test. J Urol. 1989;142(3):752–5. PubMed PMID: 2671415. eng.
49. Koide SS, Wang L, Kamada M. Antisperm antibodies associated with infertility: properties and encoding genes of target antigens. Proc Soc Exp Biol Med Society. 2000;224(3):123–32. PubMed PMID: 10865226. eng.
50. Rumke P, Hellinga G. Autoantibodies against spermatozoa in sterile men. Am J Clin Pathol. 1959;32:357–63. PubMed PMID: 14440176. eng.
51. Esteves SC, Schneider DT, Verza S, Jr. Influence of antisperm antibodies in the semen on intracytoplasmic sperm injection outcome. Int Braz J Urol. 2007;33(6):795–802. PubMed PMID: 18199347. eng.
52. Turek PJ, Lipshultz LI. Immunologic infertility. Urol Clin North Am. 1994;21(3):447–68. PubMed PMID: 8059500. eng.
53. Munuce MJ, Berta CL, Pauluzzi F, Caille AM. Relationship between antisperm antibodies, sperm movement, and semen quality. Urol Int. 2000;65(4):200–3. PubMed PMID: 11112869. eng.
54. Guzick DS, Overstreet JW, Factor-Litvak P, Brazil CK, Nakajima ST, Coutifaris C, et al. Sperm morphology, motility, and concentration in fertile and infertile men. N Engl J Med. 2001;345(19):1388–93. PubMed PMID: 11794171.
55. Haas GG Jr, Cines DB, Schreiber AD. Immunologic infertility: identification of patients with antisperm antibody. N Engl J Med. 1980;303(13):722–7. PubMed PMID: 7402269. eng.
56. Pattinson HA, Mortimer D. Prevalence of sperm surface antibodies in the male partners of infertile couples as determined by immunobead screening. Fertil Steril. 1987;48(3):466–9. PubMed PMID: 3305089. eng.
57. Haas GG Jr. The inhibitory effect of sperm-associated immunoglobulins on cervical mucus penetration. Fertil Steril. 1986;46(2):334–7. PubMed PMID: 3732542. eng.
58. Marshburn PB, Kutteh WH. The role of antisperm antibodies in infertility. Fertil Steril. 1994;61(5):799–811. PubMed PMID: 8174713. eng.
59. Check ML, Check JH, Katsoff D, Summers-Chase D. ICSI as an effective therapy for male factor with antisperm antibodies. Arch Androl. 2000;45(3):125–30. PubMed PMID: 11111859. eng.
60. Wolff H. The biologic significance of white blood cells in semen. Fertil Steril. 1995;63(6):1143–57. PubMed PMID: 7750580. eng.
61. Wolff H, Anderson DJ. Immunohistologic characterization and quantitation of leukocyte subpopulations in human semen. Fertil Steril. 1988;49(3):497–504. PubMed PMID: 3342902. eng.
62. WHO. World Health Organization: WHO Laboratory manual for the examination of human semen and sperm-cervical mucus interaction. New York: Cambridge University Press; 1999.
63. Henkel R, Kierspel E, Stalf T, Mehnert C, Menkveld R, Tinneberg HR, et al. Effect of reactive oxygen species produced by spermatozoa and leukocytes on sperm functions in non-leukocytospermic patients. Fertil Steril. 2005;83(3):635–42. PubMed PMID: 15749492. eng.
64. Henkel R, Maass G, Hajimohammad M, Menkveld R, Stalf T, Villegas J, et al. Urogenital inflammation: changes of leucocytes and ROS. Andrologia. 2003;35(5):309–13. PubMed PMID: 14535861.
65. Athayde KS, Cocuzza M, Agarwal A, Krajcir N, Lucon AM, Srougi M, et al. Development of normal reference values for seminal reactive oxygen species and their correlation with leukocytes and semen parameters in a fertile population. J Androl. 2007;28(4):613–20. PubMed PMID: 17409462. Eng.
66. Sharma RK, Pasqualotto AE, Nelson DR, Thomas AJ Jr, Agarwal A. Relationship between seminal white blood cell counts and oxidative stress in men treated at an infertility clinic. J Androl. 2001;22(4):575–83. PubMed PMID: 11451354.
67. Jennings MG, McGowan MP, Baker HW. Is conventional bacteriology useful in the management of male infertility? Clin Reprodand Fertil. 1986;4(6):359–66. PubMed PMID: 3594346. eng.
68. Aitken RJ, Buckingham D, West K, Wu FC, Zikopoulos K, Richardson DW. Differential contribution of leucocytes and spermatozoa to the generation of reactive oxygen species in the ejaculates of oligozoospermic patients and fertile donors. J Reprod Fertil. 1992;94(2):451–62. PubMed PMID: 1317451.
69. Aitken RJ, West K, Buckingham D. Leukocytic infiltration into the human ejaculate and its association with semen quality, oxidative stress, and sperm function. J Androl. 1994;15(4):343–52. PubMed PMID: 7982803.
70. Wolff H, Politch JA, Martinez A, Haimovici F, Hill JA, Anderson DJ. Leukocytospermia is associated with poor semen quality. Fertil Steril. 1990;53(3):528–36. PubMed PMID: 2407566. eng.
71. Berger RE, Karp LE, Williamson RA, Koehler J, Moore DE, Holmes KK. The relationship of pyospermia and seminal fluid bacteriology to sperm function as reflected in the sperm penetration assay. Fertil Steril. 1982;37(4):557–64. PubMed PMID: 6896033. eng.
72. Maruyama DK Jr, Hale RW, Rogers BJ. Effects of white blood cells on the in vitro penetration of zona-free hamster eggs by human spermatozoa. J Androl. 1985;6(2):127–35. PubMed PMID: 3838741. eng.
73. el-Demiry MI, Young H, Elton RA, Hargreave TB, James K, Chisholm GD. Leucocytes in the ejaculate from fertile and infertile men. Br J Urol. 1986;58(6):715–20. PubMed PMID: 3801833. eng.
74. Shekarriz M, Sharma RK, Thomas AJ Jr, Agarwal A. Positive myeloperoxidase staining (Endtz test) as an indicator of excessive reactive oxygen species formation in semen. J Assist Reprod Genet. 1995;12(2):70–4. PubMed PMID: 7545483.
75. March MR, Isidori A. New frontiers in the treatment of male sterility. Contraception. 2002;65(4):279–81. PubMed PMID: 12020778. eng.
76. Comhaire FH, Rowe PJ, Farley TM. The effect of doxycycline in infertile couples with male accessory gland infection: a double blind prospective study. Int J Androl. 1986;9(2):91–8. PubMed PMID: 3539821. eng.
77. Yanushpolsky EH, Politch JA, Hill JA, Anderson DJ. Antibiotic therapy and leukocytospermia: a prospective, randomized, controlled study. Fertil Steril. 1995;63(1):142–7. PubMed PMID: 7805903. eng.
78. Weidner W. Which efforts towards conservative treatment of male infertility will be successful? Antibiotic therapy. Andrologia. 1999;31(5):297. PubMed PMID: 10526640. eng.
79. Aziz N, Fear S, Taylor C, Kingsland CR, Lewis-Jones DI. Human sperm head morphometric distribution and its influence on human fertility. Fertil Steril. 1998;70(5):883–91. PubMed PMID: 9806571.
80. WHO. World Health Organization: WHO Laboratory manual for the examination and processing of human semen—5th ed. Geneva: WHO Press; 2010.

81. WHO. World Health Organization: WHO Laboratory manual for the examination of human semen and sperm-cervical mucus interaction. Cambridge: Cambridge University Press; 1992.
82. Esteves SC, Zini A, Aziz N, Alvarez JG, Sabanegh ES Jr, Agarwal A. Critical appraisal of World Health Organization's new reference values for human semen characteristics and effect on diagnosis and treatment of subfertile men. Urology. 2012;79(1):16–22. PubMed PMID: 22070891. eng.
83. Nallella KP, Sharma RK, Aziz N, Agarwal A. Significance of sperm characteristics in the evaluation of male infertility. Fertil Steril. 2006;85(3):629–34. PubMed PMID: 16500330.
84. Andersen AG, Jensen TK, Carlsen E, Jorgensen N, Andersson AM, Krarup T, et al. High frequency of sub-optimal semen quality in an unselected population of young men. Hum Reprod (Oxford, England). 2000;15(2):366–72. PubMed PMID: 10655308. eng.
85. van der Steeg JW, Steures P, Eijkemans MJ, Habbema JD, van der Veen F, Bossuyt PM, et al. Should the post-coital test (PCT) be part of the routine fertility work-up? Hum Reprod (Oxford, England). 2004;19(6):1373–9. PubMed PMID: 15070874. eng.
86. Oei SG, Helmerhorst FM, Bloemenkamp KW, Hollants FA, Meerpoel DE, Keirse MJ. Effectiveness of the postcoital test: randomised controlled trial. BMJ (Clinical research ed). 1998;317(7157): 502–5. PubMed PMID: 9712594. eng.
87. Glatstein IZ, Harlow BL, Hornstein MD. Practice patterns among reproductive endocrinologists: further aspects of the infertility evaluation. Fertil Steril. 1998;70(2):263–9. PubMed PMID: 9696218. eng.
88. Leushuis E, van der Steeg JW, Steures P, Koks C, Oosterhuis J, Bourdrez P, et al. Prognostic value of the postcoital test for spontaneous pregnancy. Fertil Steril. 2011;95(6):2050–5. PubMed PMID: 21444078. eng.
89. Corson SL, Batzer FR, Marmar J, Maislin G. The human sperm-hamster egg penetration assay: prognostic value. Fertil Steril. 1988;49(2):328–34. PubMed PMID: 3338589. eng.
90. Smith RG, Johnson A, Lamb D, Lipshultz LI. Functional tests of spermatozoa. Sperm penetration assay. Urol Clin North Am. 1987;14(3):451–8. PubMed PMID: 3617267. eng.
91. Oehninger S, Franken DR, Sayed E, Barroso G, Kolm P. Sperm function assays and their predictive value for fertilization outcome in IVF therapy: a meta-analysis. Hum Reprod Update. 2000;6(2):160–8. PubMed PMID: 10782574. eng.
92. Agarwal A, Bragais FM, Sabanegh E. Assessing sperm function. Urol Clin North Am. 2008;35(2):157–71, vii. PubMed PMID: 18423237. eng.
93. Warren JS, Johnson KJ, Ward PA. Oxygen radicals in cell injury and cell death. Pathol Immunopathol Res. 1987;6(5–6):301–15. PubMed PMID: 3333183.
94. Aitken RJ, West KM. Analysis of the relationship between reactive oxygen species production and leucocyte infiltration in fractions of human semen separated on Percoll gradients. Int J Androl. 1990;13(6):433–51. PubMed PMID: 1965724.
95. Hendin BN, Kolettis PN, Sharma RK, Thomas AJ Jr, Agarwal A. Varicocele is associated with elevated spermatozoal reactive oxygen species production and diminished seminal plasma antioxidant capacity. J Urol. 1999;161(6):1831–4. PubMed PMID: 10332447.
96. Sies H. Strategies of antioxidant defense. Eur J Biochem. 1993;215(2):213–9. PubMed PMID: 7688300.
97. Sharma RK, Agarwal A. Role of reactive oxygen species in male infertility. Urology. 1996;48(6):835–50. PubMed PMID: 8973665. eng.
98. Irshad M, Chaudhuri PS. Oxidant-antioxidant system: role and significance in human body. Indian J Exp Biol. 2002;40(11):1233–9. PubMed PMID: 13677624.
99. Ochsendorf FR. Infections in the male genital tract and reactive oxygen species. Hum Reprod Update. 1999;5(5):399–420. PubMed PMID: 10582780.
100. Aitken RJ, Baker HW. Seminal leukocytes: passengers, terrorists or good samaritans? Hum Reprod (Oxford, England). 1995;10(7):1736–9. PubMed PMID: 8582971.
101. Pasqualotto FF, Sharma RK, Kobayashi H, Nelson DR, Thomas AJ Jr, Agarwal A. Oxidative stress in normospermic men undergoing infertility evaluation. J Androl. 2001;22(2):316–22. PubMed PMID: 11229806.
102. Agarwal A, Allamaneni SS, Said TM. Chemiluminescence technique for measuring reactive oxygen species. Reprod Biomed Online. 2004;9(4):466–8. PubMed PMID: 15511350.
103. Sharma RK, Pasqualotto FF, Nelson DR, Thomas AJ Jr, Agarwal A. The reactive oxygen species-total antioxidant capacity score is a new measure of oxidative stress to predict male infertility. Hum Reprod (Oxford, England). 1999;14(11):2801–7. PubMed PMID: 10548626.
104. Padron OF, Brackett NL, Sharma RK, Lynne CM, Thomas AJ Jr, Agarwal A. Seminal reactive oxygen species and sperm motility and morphology in men with spinal cord injury. Fertil Steril. 1997;67(6):1115–20. PubMed PMID: 9176453.
105. Hamada A, Esteves SC, Nizza M, Agarwal A. Unexplained male infertility: diagnosis and management. Int Braz J Urol. 2012;38(5):576–94. PubMed PMID: 23131516. eng.
106. Agarwal A, Said TM. Oxidative stress, DNA damage and apoptosis in male infertility: a clinical approach. BJU Int. 2005;95(4): 503–7. PubMed PMID: 15705068.
107. Aitken RJ, Irvine DS, Wu FC. Prospective analysis of sperm-oocyte fusion and reactive oxygen species generation as criteria for the diagnosis of infertility. Am J Obstet Gynecol. 1991;164(2):542–51. PubMed PMID: 1992700.
108. Kao SH, Chao HT, Chen HW, Hwang TI, Liao TL, Wei YH. Increase of oxidative stress in human sperm with lower motility. Fertil Steril. 2008;89(5):1183–90. PubMed PMID: 17669405. eng.
109. Moustafa MH, Sharma RK, Thornton J, Mascha E, Abdel-Hafez MA, Thomas AJ Jr, et al. Relationship between ROS production, apoptosis and DNA denaturation in spermatozoa from patients examined for infertility. Hum Reprod (Oxford, England). 2004;19(1):129–38. PubMed PMID: 14688171.
110. Wang X, Sharma RK, Sikka SC, Thomas AJ Jr, Falcone T, Agarwal A. Oxidative stress is associated with increased apoptosis leading to spermatozoa DNA damage in patients with male factor infertility. Fertil Steril. 2003;80(3):531–5. PubMed PMID: 12969693. eng.
111. Said TM, Agarwal A, Sharma RK, Thomas AJ Jr, Sikka SC. Impact of sperm morphology on DNA damage caused by oxidative stress induced by beta-nicotinamide adenine dinucleotide phosphate. Fertil Steril. 2005;83(1):95–103. PubMed PMID: 15652893.
112. Oger I, Da Cruz C, Panteix G, Menezo Y. Evaluating human sperm DNA integrity: relationship between 8-hydroxydeoxyguanosine quantification and the sperm chromatin structure assay. Zygote. 2003;11(4):367–71. PubMed PMID: 15085738.
113. Nallella KP, Sharma RK, Allamaneni SS, Agarwal A. Identification of male factor infertility using a novel semen quality score and reactive oxygen species levels. Clinics. 2005;60(4):317–24. PubMed PMID: 16138239.
114. Whittington K, Harrison SC, Williams KM, Day JL, McLaughlin EA, Hull MG, et al. Reactive oxygen species (ROS) production and the outcome of diagnostic tests of sperm function. Int J Androl. 1999;22(4):236–42. PubMed PMID: 10442296.
115. Pasqualotto FF, Sharma RK, Nelson DR, Thomas AJ, Agarwal A. Relationship between oxidative stress, semen characteristics, and clinical diagnosis in men undergoing infertility investigation. Fertil Steril. 2000;73(3):459–64. PubMed PMID: 10688996.
116. Aitken RJ, Buckingham D, Harkiss D. Use of a xanthine oxidase free radical generating system to investigate the cytotoxic effects

of reactive oxygen species on human spermatozoa. J Reprod Fertil. 1993;97(2):441–50. PubMed PMID: 8388958.
117. Agarwal A, Prabakaran S, Allamaneni S. What an andrologist/urologist should know about free radicals and why. Urology. 2006;67(1):2–8. PubMed PMID: 16413322.
118. Agarwal A, Sharma RK, Nallella KP, Thomas AJ Jr, Alvarez JG, Sikka SC. Reactive oxygen species as an independent marker of male factor infertility. Fertil Steril. 2006;86(4):878–85. PubMed PMID: 17027357. eng.
119. Cocuzza M, Sikka SC, Athayde KS, Agarwal A. Clinical relevance of oxidative stress and sperm chromatin damage in male infertility: an evidence based analysis. Int Braz J Urol. 2007;33(5):603–21. PubMed PMID: 17980058.
120. Saleh RA, Agarwal A, Sharma RK, Said TM, Sikka SC, Thomas AJ Jr. Evaluation of nuclear DNA damage in spermatozoa from infertile men with varicocele. Fertil Steril. 2003;80(6):1431–6. PubMed PMID: 14667879.
121. Evenson DP, Jost LK, Corzett M, Balhorn R. Characteristics of human sperm chromatin structure following an episode of influenza and high fever: a case study. J Androl. 2000;21(5):739–46. PubMed PMID: 10975421.
122. Chatterjee R, Haines GA, Perera DM, Goldstone A, Morris ID. Testicular and sperm DNA damage after treatment with fludarabine for chronic lymphocytic leukaemia. Hum Reprod (Oxford, England). 2000;15(4):762–6. PubMed PMID: 10739816. eng.
123. Singh NP, Muller CH, Berger RE. Effects of age on DNA double-strand breaks and apoptosis in human sperm. Fertil Steril. 2003;80(6):1420–30. PubMed PMID: 14667878.
124. Erenpreiss J, Hlevicka S, Zalkalns J, Erenpreisa J. Effect of leukocytospermia on sperm DNA integrity: a negative effect in abnormal semen samples. J Androl. 2002;23(5):717–23. PubMed PMID: 12185107.
125. Aitken RJ, Bennetts LE, Sawyer D, Wiklendt AM, King BV. Impact of radio frequency electromagnetic radiation on DNA integrity in the male germline. Int J Androl. 2005;28(3):171–9. PubMed PMID: 15910543.
126. Bennetts LE, Aitken RJ. A comparative study of oxidative DNA damage in mammalian spermatozoa. Mol Reprod Dev. 2005;71(1):77–87. PubMed PMID: 15736137.
127. Sharma RK, Said T, Agarwal A. Sperm DNA damage and its clinical relevance in assessing reproductive outcome. Asian J Androl. 2004;6(2):139–48. PubMed PMID: 15154089.
128. Henkel R, Hajimohammad M, Stalf T, Hoogendijk C, Mehnert C, Menkveld R, et al. Influence of deoxyribonucleic acid damage on fertilization and pregnancy. Fertil Steril. 2004;81(4):965–72. PubMed PMID: 15066449.
129. Tomsu M, Sharma V, Miller D. Embryo quality and IVF treatment outcomes may correlate with different sperm comet assay parameters. Hum Reprod (Oxford, England). 2002;17(7):1856–62. PubMed PMID: 12093852.
130. Zini A, Bielecki R, Phang D, Zenzes MT. Correlations between two markers of sperm DNA integrity, DNA denaturation and DNA fragmentation, in fertile and infertile men. Fertil Steril. 2001;75(4):674–7. PubMed PMID: 11287017.
131. Kodama H, Yamaguchi R, Fukuda J, Kasai H, Tanaka T. Increased oxidative deoxyribonucleic acid damage in the spermatozoa of infertile male patients. Fertil Steril. 1997;68(3):519–24. PubMed PMID: 9314926.
132. Practice Committee of the American Society for Reproductive Medicine. The clinical utility of sperm DNA integrity testing. Fertil Steril. 2006;86(Suppl 1): S35–7.
133. Evenson DP. Sperm chromatin structure assay (SCSA(R)). Methods Mol Biol (Clifton, NJ). 2013;927:147–64. PubMed PMID: 22992911. eng.
134. Miller D, Paradowska A. Evaluating the localization and DNA binding complexity of histones in mature sperm. Methods Mol Biol (Clifton, NJ). 2013;927:459–75. PubMed PMID: 22992937. eng.
135. Kazerooni T, Asadi N, Jadid L, Kazerooni M, Ghanadi A, Ghaffarpasand F, et al. Evaluation of sperm's chromatin quality with acridine orange test, chromomycin A3 and aniline blue staining in couples with unexplained recurrent abortion. J Assist Reprod Genet. 2009;26(11–12):591–6. PubMed PMID: 19894107. eng.
136. Chi HJ, Chung DY, Choi SY, Kim JH, Kim GY, Lee JS, et al. Integrity of human sperm DNA assessed by the neutral comet assay and its relationship to semen parameters and clinical outcomes for the IVF-ET program. Clini Exp Reprod Med. 2011;38(1):10–7. PubMed PMID: 22384412. eng.
137. Simon L, Carrell DT. Sperm DNA damage measured by comet assay. Methods Mol Biol (Clifton, NJ). 2013;927:137–46. PubMed PMID: 22992910. eng.
138. Henkel R, Hoogendijk CF, Bouic PJ, Kruger TF. TUNEL assay and SCSA determine different aspects of sperm DNA damage. Andrologia. 2010;42(5):305–13. PubMed PMID: 20860629. eng.
139. Meseguer M, Martinez-Conejero JA, O'Connor JE, Pellicer A, Remohi J, Garrido N. The significance of sperm DNA oxidation in embryo development and reproductive outcome in an oocyte donation program: a new model to study a male infertility prognostic factor. Fertil Steril. 2008;89(5):1191–9. PubMed PMID: 17681311. eng.
140. Spano M, Bonde JP, Hjollund HI, Kolstad HA, Cordelli E, Leter G. Sperm chromatin damage impairs human fertility. The Danish first pregnancy planner study team. Fertil Steril. 2000;73(1):43–50. PubMed PMID: 10632410.
141. Evenson DP, Jost LK, Marshall D, Zinaman MJ, Clegg E, Purvis K, et al. Utility of the sperm chromatin structure assay as a diagnostic and prognostic tool in the human fertility clinic. Hum Reprod (Oxford, England). 1999;14(4):1039–49. PubMed PMID: 10221239.
142. Evenson DP, Larson KL, Jost LK. Sperm chromatin structure assay: its clinical use for detecting sperm DNA fragmentation in male infertility and comparisons with other techniques. J Androl. 2002;23(1):25–43. PubMed PMID: 11780920.
143. Agarwal A, Said TM. Role of sperm chromatin abnormalities and DNA damage in male infertility. Hum Reprod Update. 2003;9(4):331–45. PubMed PMID: 12926527.
144. Agarwal A, Allamaneni SS. Sperm DNA damage assessment: a test whose time has come. Fertil Steril. 2005;84(4):850–3. PubMed PMID: 16213833.
145. Egozcue S, Blanco J, Vendrell JM, Garcia F, Veiga A, Aran B, et al. Human male infertility: chromosome anomalies, meiotic disorders, abnormal spermatozoa and recurrent abortion. Hum Reprod Update. 2000;6(1):93–105. PubMed PMID: 10711834. eng.
146. Rives N, Saint Clair A, Mazurier S, Sibert L, Simeon N, Joly G, et al. Relationship between clinical phenotype, semen parameters and aneuploidy frequency in sperm nuclei of 50 infertile males. Hum Genet. 1999;105(3):266–72. PubMed PMID: 10987656. eng.
147. Jensen M, Leffers H, Petersen JH, Nyboe Andersen A, Jorgensen N, Carlsen E, et al. Frequent polymorphism of the mitochondrial DNA polymerase gamma gene (POLG) in patients with normal spermiograms and unexplained subfertility. Hum Reprod (Oxford, England). 2004;19(1):65–70. PubMed PMID: 14688158. eng.
148. Alukal JP, Lamb DJ. Intracytoplasmic sperm injection (ICSI)-what are the risks? Urol Clin North Am. 2008;35(2):277–88, ix-x. PubMed PMID: 18423248. eng.

149. Kim HH, Schlegel PN. Endocrine manipulation in male infertility. Urol Clin North Am. 2008;35(2):303–18, x. PubMed PMID: 18423250. eng.
150. Garrido N, Martinez-Conejero JA, Jauregui J, Horcajadas JA, Simon C, Remohi J, et al. Microarray analysis in sperm from fertile and infertile men without basic sperm analysis abnormalities reveals a significantly different transcriptome. Fertil Steril. 2009;91(Suppl 4):1307–10. PubMed PMID: 18367176. eng.
151. Blumer CG, Fariello RM, Restelli AE, Spaine DM, Bertolla RP, Cedenho AP. Sperm nuclear DNA fragmentation and mitochondrial activity in men with varicocele. Fertil Steril. 2008;90(5):1716–22. PubMed PMID: 18155699. eng.
152. von Bernhardi R, de Ioannes AE, Blanco LP, Herrera E, Bustos-Obregon E, Vigil P. Round-headed spermatozoa: a model to study the role of the acrosome in early events of gamete interaction. Andrologia. 1990;22(1):12–20. PubMed PMID: 2281873. eng.
153. Sigman M, Baazeem A, Zini A. Semen analysis and sperm function assays: what do they mean? Semin Reprod Med. 2009;27(2): 115–23. PubMed PMID: 19247913. eng.
154. Said TM, Agarwal A, Sharma RK, Mascha E, Sikka SC, Thomas AJ Jr. Human sperm superoxide anion generation and correlation with semen quality in patients with male infertility. Fertil Steril. 2004;82(4):871–7. PubMed PMID: 15482762.
155. Greco E, Scarselli F, Iacobelli M, Rienzi L, Ubaldi F, Ferrero S, et al. Efficient treatment of infertility due to sperm DNA damage by ICSI with testicular spermatozoa. Hum Reprod (Oxford, England). 2005;20(1):226–30. PubMed PMID: 15539441.

Part V

Expectant, Medical and Surgical Treatment

The Role of Expectant Management for Couples with Unexplained Infertility

22

N. M. van den Boogaard, Fulco van der Veen and Ben Willem Mol

Infertility is defined as a failure to conceive after at least 1 year of regular unprotected intercourse [1]. It affects approximately 10% of couples in their reproductive lives [2, 3]. Unexplained infertility is defined as infertility without any demonstrable cause after the basic fertility workup, including assessment of ovulation, semen analysis and evaluation of tubal patency. The incidence of infertility is increasing in the developed world mainly due to postponement of maternity. After a basic fertility workup, about 25% of couples will be diagnosed with unexplained infertility [4, 5].

As in unexplained infertility, a causal explanation for the failure of conception is by definition lacking; natural conception should never be excluded in couples diagnosed as such. Consequently, expectant management (EM) may be a good option, especially when the prognosis for natural conception is reasonable.

The Evidence

A recent update of a Cochrane review on intra uterine insemination (IUI) for couples with unexplained infertility was published in 2012 [6]. One trial was included that compared IUI in a natural cycle with EM and showed no evidence of increased live births (334 women: OR 1.6, 95% CI: 0.92–2.8). Two trials compared EM with IUI with ovarian stimulation (OS) and both concluded there was no evidence of a difference in pregnancy rate (in total 304 women: data could not be pooled) [6]. In the last comparison (IUI-OS versus EM) one large multicentre randomised controlled trial (RCT) from the Netherlands was included. This RCT randomised 253 couples with unexplained infertility and intermediate prognosis of natural conception between either 6 months of EM or immediate start with OS and IUI. Within 6 months, the ongoing pregnancy rate in the EM group was 27% and in the OS group with IUI 24% (RR 0.85 CI: 0.63–1.1) [7]. The couples were then treated according to the centre's standard protocol, usually OS with IUI, followed by IVF. Three years after randomisation, the cumulative ongoing pregnancy rates were 72 and 73% for EM and OS with IUI, respectively (RR 0.99 (95% CI: 0.85–1.1). The time of ongoing pregnancy also did not differ between groups (log-rank test, $p=0.98$) [8]. An RCT from the UK included 334 couples with unexplained infertility that were randomised to EM, oral clomiphene citrate or unstimulated IUI. After 6 months, a live birth rate of 23% was obtained in the IUI group versus 16% in the EM group, which was not significantly different (OR 1.60, 95% CI 0.92) [9].

A systematic Cochrane review on in vitro fertilisation (IVF) for couples with unexplained infertility concluded that the added value of IVF in relation to EM or IUI with or without OS in couples with unexplained infertility has not been conclusively proven due to a paucity of data: only one trial with 51 women compared IVF with EM and the live birth rate per woman was significantly higher with IVF (45.8%) compared to EM (3.7%; OR 22, 95% CI 2.5–189) [10].

Thus, RCTs in couples with unexplained infertility comparing EM with IUI with or without OS, OS alone with timed intercourse (TI) or IVF so far do not provide irrefutable evidence of a beneficial effect of treatment over EM.

High rates of natural conception have also been observed in several cohort studies. In one cohort study that included 652 couples with unexplained infertility, the cumulative live birth rate after 36 months was 33% [11]. In another study, 218 couples with unexplained infertility were included and the cumulative live birth rate within 36 months was 60% [12]. And in a third cohort study of 443 couples with unexplained infertility, EM was advised in couples with good prospects of natural conception. The chance of natural conception within 12 months was determined according the prognostic model of Hunault; and if less than 30%, couples

N. M. van den Boogaard (✉)
Gynaecology and Obstetrics and Reproductive medicine, VU medical centre Amsterdam, Pieter Lodewijk Takstraat 31, 1073 KJ Amsterdam, The Netherlands
e-mail: n.m.vandenboogaard@amc.nl

F. van der Veen
Department of Gynecology, Academic Medical Center, Amsterdam, The Netherlands

B. W. Mol
Department Gynecology/Obstetrics, Academic Medical Center at the University of Amsterdam, Amsterdam, The Netherlands

G. L. Schattman et al. (eds.), *Unexplained Infertility,* DOI 10.1007/978-1-4939-2140-9_22,

were counselled to continue to try on their own for up to 2 years, and if still not pregnant, they would undergo up to six cycles of IUI with controlled ovarian stimulation (COS-IUI) [13]. If no pregnancy was achieved, up to three cycles of IVF were recommended. If the chance of natural conception was greater than 30% and the female's age was greater than 38 years, 3–6 cycles of IUI-COS cycles were offered before IVF was started. If female age was ≥38 years, IVF was offered directly. Patients were followed until their first ongoing pregnancy, which caused variation in the follow-up period per couple from 2 to 8 years. After the fertility work-up, 93% (408/437) couples were eligible for EM. In total, 37% (163/437) couples started with IUI and 15% (64/437) couples started with IVF. Of all couples, 81.5% (356/437) achieved an ongoing pregnancy and 73.9% (263/356) of the pregnancies were conceived naturally. IUI and IVF were responsible for 12.6% (45/356) and 13.5% (48/356) of all pregnancies, respectively. Of all the pregnancies, 98.6% were conceived within 3 years after first visit to the hospital. Predictors for overall pregnancy chance and mode of conception were duration of infertility, female age and obstetrical history [14].

When to Use Expectant Management

The most difficult problem to overcome with recommending EM is how to identify couples that would benefit from EM over treatment; and how to convince the patient frustrated with her monthly failures of conception to continue to "do nothing" but keep on trying. Gynaecologists differ widely in estimating fertility prognoses in subfertile couples. Prognostic models may be of help here [11]. For several treatment policies, prognostic models have been developed. For eight models, the validity has been assessed in populations other than the one in which the model was developed (external validation), and only three of these showed good performance. One model predicting the chance of natural conception has reached the phase of impact analysis [11, 15]. This prognostic model is based on three prognostic models: data of these three models [12, 16, 17] were pooled and integrated in a synthesis model. This synthesis model predicts the chance of live birth, and contains the variables: female age, duration of subfertility/infertility, infertility being primary or secondary, semen motility and referral status and is available in a version with and without the post-coital test (PCT) as a predictor. The Dutch guideline for unexplained infertility recommends the use of this prognostic model and EM for 6–12 months in couples with a good prognosis (>30%) [18]. In agreement with this, both the European Society of Human Reproduction and Embryology (ESHRE) guidelines and the guidelines of the National Institute of Clinical Excellence (NICE) emphasize that couples should not be exposed to unnecessary risks or ineffective treatments, and encourage that each couple should receive information about the estimate of their chances of natural conception [19, 20]. Guidelines from the Royal College of Obstetricians and Gynaecologists (RCOG, 1998) have recommended that couples should have tried EM before assisted reproductive treatment.

Implementation of Expectant Management

It is unclear how EM for subfertile couples with good chances of natural conception is being implemented; but, two large prospective cohort studies suggest that it is not being implemented optimally [11, 21, 22]. Optimal implementation of EM for 6–12 months for subfertile couples with good chances of natural conception (>30% in 12 months) can cause a reduction in healthcare costs without compromising on overall live birth rates. Besides cost reduction, optimal implementation of EM is likely to lead to a decrease in the number of multiple pregnancies. Even though multiple pregnancy rates per treatment cycle are decreasing, the risks are still substantially higher than those in natural conceptions and almost all multiples occurring in natural conceptions are twins, not higher order multiples. Multiple pregnancies, even twins, are associated with a higher morbidity and mortality in both mothers and neonates [23]. Finally, fertility treatments carry a significant physical and psychological burden [24, 25]

To improve the implementation of EM, it must be tailored to the individual couple (TEM) and a systematic approach is needed including: acquiring data of current practice; identification of potential determinants; analysis of barriers and facilitators for implementation, development of an implementation strategy and finally an evaluation of the effectiveness of the implementation strategy. The first steps of this systematic approach have been taken. A qualitative study was performed to identify the barriers and facilitators of EM. Subfertile patients who were counselled to try EM and professionals within the field of reproductive medicine were interviewed. Among infertile couples, the main barriers to utilizing EM were a lack of confidence that it would result in natural conception, a perception that EM is a waste of time, inappropriate expectations prior to the first consultation, misunderstanding the reason for EM and overestimation of the success rates of treatment. Both couples and professionals saw the lack of patient information materials as a barrier. Among the professionals, limited knowledge about prognostic models leading to a decision in favour of EM or treatment was recognized as the main barrier. A main facilitator mentioned by the professionals was better management of patients' expectations [26, 27]. An implementation strategy focussing on these barriers and facilitators has been developed and this implementation strategy is being tested in a multicentre cluster randomised trial in the Netherlands (The Improvement study).

Conclusion

EM in couples with unexplained infertility and good prospects of natural conception is an effective strategy. Estimating a couples chances of natural conception can be done, however, convincing patients that this is the right approach can prove challenging. Optimal implementation of EM in couples with good prospects of natural conception can prevent unnecessary treatments, complications and costs. Barriers that patients and health care professionals have identified leading to limited implementation of this strategy are being addressed and studied in a multicentre cluster RCT [28].

References

1. Zegers-Hochschild F, Adamson GD, de MJ, Ishihara O, Mansour R, Nygren K, et al. The International Committee for Monitoring Assisted Reproductive Technology (ICMART) and the World Health Organization (WHO) revised glossary on ART terminology, 2009. Hum Reprod. 2009;24(11):2683–7.
2. Boivin J, Bunting L, Collins JA, Nygren KG. International estimates of infertility prevalence and treatment-seeking: potential need and demand for infertility medical care. Hum Reprod. 2007;22(6):1506–12.
3. Gnoth C, Godehardt D, Godehardt E, Frank-Herrmann P, Freundl G. Time to pregnancy: results of the German prospective study and impact on the management of infertility. Hum Reprod. 2003;18(9):1959–66.
4. Brandes M, Hamilton CJ, de Bruin JP, Nelen WL, Kremer JA. The relative contribution of IVF to the total ongoing pregnancy rate in a subfertile cohort. Hum Reprod. 2010;25(1):118–26.
5 Collins JA, Van SA. Overall prognosis with current treatment of infertility. Hum Reprod Update. 2004;10(4):309–16.
6. Veltman-Verhulst SM, Cohlen BJ, Hughes E, Heineman MJ. Cochrane review: intra-uterine insemination for unexplained subfertility. Cochrane Database Syst Rev. 2012;9:CD001838.
7. Steures P, van der Steeg JW, Hompes PG, Habbema JD, Eijkemans MJ, Broekmans FJ, et al. Intrauterine insemination with controlled ovarian hyperstimulation versus expectant management for couples with unexplained subfertility and an intermediate prognosis: a randomised clinical trial. Lancet. 2006;368(9531):216–21.
8. Custers IM, van Rumste MM, van der Steeg JW, van WM, Hompes PG, Bossuyt P, et al. Long-term outcome in couples with unexplained subfertility and an intermediate prognosis initially randomized between expectant management and immediate treatment. Hum Reprod. 2012;27(2):444–50.
9. Bhattacharya S, Harrild K, Mollison J, Wordsworth S, Tay C, Harrold A, McQueen D, Lyall H, Johnston L, Burrage J, et al. Clomifene citrate or unstimulated intrauterine insemination compared with expectant management for unexplained infertility: pragmatic randomised controlled trial. BMJ. 2008; 337:a716.
10. Pandian Z, Gibreel A, Bhattacharya S. In vitro fertilisation for unexplained subfertility. Cochrane Database Syst Rev. 2012;4:CD003357.
11. van der Steeg JW, Steures P, Eijkemans MJ, Habbema JD, Hompes PG, Broekmans FJ, van Dessel HJ, Bossuyt PM, van der Veen F, Mol BW. Pregnancy is predictable: a large-scale prospective external validation of the prediction of spontaneous pregnancy in subfertile couples. Hum Reprod. 2007;22: 536–42.
12. Collins JA, Burrows EA, Wilan AR. The prognosis for live birth among untreated infertile couples. Fertil Steril. 1995;64(1):22–8.
13. Hunault CC, Habbema JD, Eijkemans MJ, Collins JA, Evers JL, te Velde ER. Two new prediction rules for spontaneous pregnancy leading to live birth among subfertile couples, based on the synthesis of three previous models. Hum Reprod. 2004;19(9):2019–26.
14. Brandes M, Hamilton CJ, van der Steen JO, de Bruin JP, Bots RS, Nelen WL, et al. Unexplained infertility: overall ongoing pregnancy rate and mode of conception. Hum Reprod. 2011;26(2):360–8.
15. Leushuis E, van der Steeg JW, Steures P, Bossuyt PM, Eijkemans MJ, van der Veen F, Mol BW, Hompes PG. Prediction models in reproductive medicine: a critical appraisal. Hum Reprod Update. 2009;15(5):537–52.
16. Eimers JM, te Velde ER, Gerritse R, Vogelzang ET, Looman CW, Habbema JD. The prediction of the chance to conceive in subfertile couples. Fertil Steril. 1994;61(1):44–52.
17. Snick HK, Snick TS, Evers JL, Collins JA. The spontaneous pregnancy prognosis in untreated subfertile couples: the Walcheren primary care study. Hum Reprod. 1997;12(7):1582–8.
18. NVOG: Dutch national guideline subfertility. http://nvog-documenten.nl/uploaded/docs/Landelijke%20netwerkrichtlijn%20Subfertiliteit%20def.pdf (2011). Accessed 10 Feb 2014.
19. ESHRE. Guidelines for counseling infertility. http://www.eshre.com/binarydata.aspx?type=doc/psyguidelines.pdf (1999). Accessed 10 Feb 2014.
20. NICE. Guideline fertility: assessment and treatment for people with fertility problems. http://www.nice.org.uk/nicemedia/pdf/CG011publicinfoenglish.pdf (2004). Accessed Feb 2014.
21. Kremer JA, Bots RS, Cohlen B, Crooij M, van Dop PA, Jansen CA, L and JA, Laven JS, Kastrop PM, Naaktgeboren N, et al. Ten years of results of in-vitro fertilisation in the Netherlands 1996–2005. Ned Tijdschr Geneeskd. 2008;152:146–52.
22. Mourad SM, Hermens RP, Cox-Witbraad T, Grol RP, Nelen WL, Kremer JA. Information provision in fertility care: a call for improvement. Hum Reprod. 2009;24:1420–6.
23. Helmerhorst FM, Perquin DA, Donker D, Keirse MJ. Perinatal outcome of singletons and twins after assisted conception: a systematic review of controlled studies. BMJ. 2004;328(7434):261.
24. Verberg MF, Eijkemans MJ, Heijnen EM, Broekmans FJ, de Klerk C, Fauser BC, Macklon NS. Why do couples drop-out from IVF treatment? A prospective cohort study. Hum Reprod. 2008;23:2050–5.
25. Verhaak CM, Smeenk JM, Nahuis MJ, Kremer JA, Braat DD. Long-term psychological adjustment to IVF/ICSI treatment in women. Hum Reprod. 2007;22:305–8.
26. van den Boogaard NM, van den Boogaard E, Bokslag A, van Zwieten MC, Hompes PG, Bhattacharya S, et al. Patients' and professionals' barriers and facilitators of tailored expectant management in subfertile couples with a good prognosis of a natural conception. Hum Reprod. 2011;26(8):2122–8.
27. van den Boogaard, N. M., Ouderengering, K., Steures, P., Bossuyt, P. M., Hompes, P. G., van der Veen, F., Mol, B. W., van der Steeg, J. W. Tailored expectant management: risk factors for non-adherence. Hum Reprod. 2011:26(7):1784–1789.
28. van den Boogaard, N.M., Kersten, F., Goddijn, M., Bossuyt, P., van der Veen, F., Hompes, P., Hermens, R., Braat, D., Mol, B.W., Nelen, W. Improving the implementation of tailored expectant management. Implement Sci. 2013;8:53.

Treatment and Prognosis of Immunological Factors in Unexplained Male Infertility

23

Darius Paduch and Ali A. Dabaja

Introduction

It is widely accepted that immunological infertility is one of the major causes of infertility in humans. On average, infertility occurs in one in ten couples of reproductive age and in about 10–20 % of them, the reason for infertility is unexplained. A subset of infertile patients has been found to possess antisperm antibodies (ASA) in semen, blood, cervical mucus, or follicular fluid. Clinically, these patients are classified as being immunologically infertile. Investigations on the potential role of ASA in infertile couples have been performed extensively during the past three decades. Until now, there have been no randomized double-blinded clinical trials to support a uniform treatment protocol of ASA-mediated infertility. Published literature on the treatment of infertile men with ASA is often contradictory. Beside the utilization of assisted reproductive technologies (ART), there have been very few meaningful advances in the treatment of immunological infertility in the last 10 years.

To understand the treatment strategies of immunological factors in male infertility, it is essential to understand the mechanisms of how ASA can lead to infertility. The presence of ASA may not effect spermatogenesis, but will limit sperm survival, limit sperm transport and motility and therefore the passage through the female reproductive tract specifically the cervix, inhibits sperm oocyte binding, prevent capacitation and acrosome reaction, effect embryo development and implantation, and might lead to spontaneous miscarriage [1–3].

ASA can be detected on spermatozoa, in seminal plasma and semen, and in female serum and cervical mucus. The clinical importance of circulating ASA is limited, but there is a clear association between sperm surface antibodies and male fertility potential. When diagnosing ASA, indirect antibody agglutination assays are used to detect ASA in serum (usually immunoglobulin G (IgG)) or seminal plasma, and direct immunobead test, using mixed agglutination reaction (MAR) or immunobead tests, to detect IgG and IgA bound to the sperm head or tail [4]. There is no consensus on what titer levels are considered positive for ASA in serum. On the other hand, a direct test is considered weakly negative or weakly positive when ≤50 % of the motile spermatozoa are carrying immunoglobulins.

ASA-associated sperms have a limited ability to penetrate into the cervical mucus [5, 6]. Sperm coated with ASA can stimulate the complement cascade and cause a significant reduction (87–43 %) in mobility and morphology with subsequent sperm lysis in vitro [7]. Components of the complement cascades are present in low concentration in the cervical mucus as well as other part of the female reproductive tract and are capable of inducing time-sensitive immobilization or lysis in up to 70 % of ASA-coated sperm [8]. Therefore, minimizing exposure time might be important to prevent immobilization and sperm lysis. Sperm-bound immunoglobulins are associated with sperm autoagglutination in 80 % of the ejaculates and they decreased sperm penetration into cervical mucus in 97.6 % of the cases; furthermore, the proportion of ASA-bound sperm correlates with sperm penetration into cervical mucus [9–11]. It has been suggested that the cervical mucus aids in the selection of the most fertile sperm of an ejaculate by acting as an immunological filter, preventing the passage of sperm coated with ASA [12]. The binding of immunoglobulin A (IgA) ASA that is usually directed against the sperm head and IgG against the sperm principal piece can severely impair the ability of sperm to penetrate cervical mucus [13, 14]. To the contrary, the binding of ASA to the tail did not appear to affect the ability of sperm to penetrate the cervical mucus [15]. Therefore, artificially bypassing the cervical mucus (as with artificial insemination) and preventing the ASA from binding to the head of the sperm as in fertilization antigen-1 (FA-1) are important techniques to overcome infertility in this subgroup of patients. FA-1 is a sperm-specific glycoprotein found in both human and mouse

D. Paduch (✉) · A. A. Dabaja
Department of Urology, Weill Cornell Medical College, New York-Presbyterian Hospital, 525 East 68th Street Starr Pavilion, 9th floor, Room 900, NY 10065, USA
e-mail: dap2013@med.cornell.edu

G. L. Schattman et al. (eds.), *Unexplained Infertility*, DOI 10.1007/978-1-4939-2140-9_23,

germ cells. Functional studies demonstrated that antibody against FA-1 inhibits sperm penetration of zona pellucida (ZP)-free hamster eggs [16].

The interaction between the sperm and oocyte is highly regulated by specific receptor–ligand binding. The binding of head-directed ASA to sperm reduces sperm binding to human ZP without affecting motility [17–19]. ASA modulate ZP binding, which lowers the ability of the sperm to penetrate the oocyte and fuse with the oolemna. Numerous investigators have shown that human ASA against specific-sperm proteins are capable of inhibiting sperm–hamster oocyte penetration [20–22]. In this group of patients, intracytoplasmic sperm injection (ICSI) may be the best treatment option.

Negative effects of sperm-bound ASA on embryonic development and implantation have also been suggested. ASA can significantly inhibit early embryonic cleavage, thereby reducing the number of high-quality embryos. Oocytes from women with serum ASA had a lower embryo cleavage rate than oocytes from women without ASA [23]. Evidence that ASA influence the rate of miscarriage is seen in in vitro fertilization (IVF) settings where couples with ASA + sperm undergoing ICSI were found to have higher rate of spontaneous miscarriages compared to couples with normal sperm [24]. In this chapter, we will review the different treatment strategies for the male partners of infertile couples that are diagnosed with immunological infertility.

Treatment of Immunologic Infertility

Several strategies are used to overcome potentially deleterious effects of ASA-mediated infertility. The basic approaches for the treatment of men with ASA are: minimizing exposure to sperm antigen, decrease ASA production by immunosuppression, removal of sperm-bound ASA by a combination of laboratory techniques and sperm washing, and ART. Each of these strategies theoretically minimizes proportion of ASA-bound gametes, resulting in improved gamete function.

Minimizing Exposure to Sperm Antigen

Prevention

In couples practicing anal intercourse, an increase in the prevalence of ASA has been observed but not all authors agree that types of sexual practices correlates with prevalence of ASA in females [25]. To lower the risk of ASA formation, it is recommended that couples should try to avoid such exposure, but limited data exist to support such recommendations. Inflammation or infection of the genitourinary tract such as orchitis, prostatitis, or urethritis may lead to exposure of the immune system to highly antigenic sperm. Prompt and successful treatment of such infections may theoretically decrease the period of exposure. Furthermore, sexually transmitted diseases are associated with the development of ASA formation and early antibiotic treatment can prevent the formation of ASA [26].

Condom

Theoretically, repeated or multiple sperm exposure to the female reproductive tract results in ASA formation. Therefore, condom use would decrease sperm exposure, resulting in a concomitant decline in ASA production. In fact, in their original report, Franklin suggested that the condom therapy was an effective therapy for some patients. It was believed that if a systematic approach is used to gradually decrease coitus with condoms after a period of normal sexual intercourse it has theoretic immunologic merit in bringing about pregnancies [27]. However, studies that looked at couples with IgG and IgA ASA on the spermatozoa or in the cervical mucus and the use of condoms for 6 months did not yield any favorable results [28]. The evidence for the temporary use of condoms for ASA-related infertility is questionable; it might be that condoms might help a certain subset of couples with ASA as it is known from animal models and clinical observation that HLA composition modulates immunological response.

Immunosuppressive Therapies

Suppression of immunological response is believed to lower the burden of ASA in males and potentially benefit the couple. The method of immunosuppression that is most commonly used is glucocorticosteroids (GCSs) therapy. Corticosteroids prevent the chemotaxis of inflammatory cells, impede cytokine release, decrease antibody production, and weaken antigen–antibody association [29]. The exact mechanism of how GCSs help with immunological infertility is not well known and is believed to result in global decrease in immunological response during treatment. It is assumed that GCSs suppress ASA production and as ASA are being cleared, the levels of ASA decrease. The measure of effectiveness of immunosuppression treatment on immunological infertility is very difficult because the studies reported in the literature employed different laboratory techniques in detecting and measuring ASA, and lacked appropriate placebo controls. Moreover, multiple protocols with different dose regiments of various immunosuppressive drugs have been reported, which makes comparing the outcomes difficult (Table 23.1).

Improvement in the pregnancy rates has been reported after GCSs therapy [30, 31]. Studies have reported between 0 and 40% pregnancy rates after treatment. In a prospec-

Table 23.1 Summary of protocols used for immunosuppression in ASA patients

Reference	Protocol	Success of pregnancy
Shulman et al. [50]	Male patients receive 96 mg/day methylprednisolone from days 21 to 28 of the female menstrual cycle	44 % pregnancy rate in first 12 months
Hendry et al. [31]	Male patients receive 40 mg/day methylprednisolone on day 1 of the female menstrual cycle followed by 5 mg/day from days 11 to 12	33 % pregnancy rate/treatment cycle
De Almeida et al. [33]	Male patients receive 2 mg/day of dexamethasone for a total of 13 weeks	Success measured by reduction of ASA titers (rate of reduction is between 0 and 50 %)
Haas et al. [32]	96 mg/day methylprednisolone in three divided doses for 7 days followed by a 2-day tapering of the drug, repeated for three cycles	Decrease of sperm-associated IgG
Hendry et al. [34]	Male patients receive 20 mg twice daily on days 1–10 of the female partner's menstrual cycle, followed by 5 mg on days 11 and 12	31 % pregnancy rate in 9 months treatment cycle

tive, double-blind, placebo-controlled study of 43 men given three repeated monthly regiments of 96 mg methylprednisolone in three divided doses for 7 days followed by a 2-day tapering of the drug, corticosteroids did not have any effect on semen parameters, sperm-associated IgA, and plasma IgG ASA, or pregnancy rate. However, corticosteroids significantly reduced sperm-associated IgG, with no translation into any clinical benefit [32]. Similarly, other studies that looked at the effect of prednisone showed no significant effect on fertility, serum antibody levels, semen parameters, and sperm characteristics, but a slight decrease in the titer of seminal antibodies was observed [33]. Other protocols showed slightly favorable outcomes. In a cohort of subfertile men that were enrolled in a double-blinded crossover trial with circulating antibodies to spermatozoa who received prednisolone (20 mg twice daily on days 1–10 of the female partner's menstrual cycle, followed by 5 mg on days 11 and 12) for 9 months resulted in a pregnancy rate of 31 % in the treatment group compared with a 9 % in the untreated group. However, there were no changes in the semen parameters in this cohort of patients [34]. The response to GCSs treatment is more likely in men with persistent level of ASA than in men with an acute autoimmunological response. Infertile men with ASA detectable for more than 1 year and treated with steroid responded effectively in suppressing all isotypes of ASA, and improved sperm motility. Further, the presence of high titers of isotype IgG against the tails of spermatozoa, and sperms with type I motility were predictors of pregnancy [35]. Comparing GCSs to other treatment modalities in a crossover randomized study, the effectiveness of intrauterine insemination (IUI) was significantly better than timed intercourse with cyclic low dose (20 mg) prednisolone therapy. The pregnancy rate before crossover for the IUI group was 16.7 %, whereas no pregnancies occurred in the steroid-treated group.

The benefit of steroid treatment, if any, must be judged against the potential adverse effects. Steroid therapy may cause several side effects, such as acne, dyspepsia, skin rashes, fluid retention, and mood changes [36]. The potential adverse effects and the lack of effectiveness in many cases have decreased the enthusiasm for steroid use. Interest in the use of other immunosuppressing agents such cyclosporine in autoimmune orchitis showed some promising results [37]. In men with ASA treated with cyclosporin A (5–10 mg/kg/day) for 6 months the serum ASA fell in 33 % of the subjects on treatment, and sperm count and motility increased substantially in some [38]. However, this was a very small study with no placebo controls and conclusions cannot be drawn.

Laboratory Techniques and Sperm Washing

Sperm preparation, in subjects with ASA, as a preparation for artificial insemination, was first tried by Halim [39]. Since then, multiple techniques for sperm preparation and washing have evolved. The concept of removing ASA from semen or ASA bound to sperm can be classified into three categories: (1) preventing the binding of ASA to sperms, (2) removing bound ASA from sperm surface by immunobead exchange or by using proteases that will cleave the immunoglobulin, and (3) separating ASA-coated sperms from non-coated sperms. Even though some of these techniques are promising, conflicting outcomes, and the technical challenges needed to master some of these techniques have prevented them from wide utilization in clinical practice.

Preventing ASA Sperm Binding

In the effort to prevent the binding of ASA to the sperm, multiple techniques have been employed. In the past, it was thought antibodies are secreted from the prostate and seminal vesicle, and that ASA bind to sperm during or after ejaculation [40]. To stop the ASA binding to sperm, semen is collected into a medium containing 50 % heterologous serum or albumin, followed by rapid dilution or washing to increase the proportion of antibody-free spermatozoa in the specimen. Studies have suggested that combining this technique with IVF increased the rate of fertilization, but it is not clear if the success is due to the decrease in the ASA binding to sperm or to selecting good sperm in the washing process [41]. However, subsequent analysis have proven that rapid dilution or washing to be ineffective in collecting sperm that is free of bound ASA [42]. The efficacy of rapid dilution of semen on sperm-bound spermatozoa followed by swim up in HAM F-10 and 10% human serum was evaluated, and it was found that the diluting semen after ejaculation did not significantly change sperm-bound antibodies detected [43]. To the contrary, antibody secretion and biodistribution studies in the male reproductive tract using 125I-labeled anti-FA-1 IgG in mice revealed that the antibodies are preferentially secreted in epididymis and vas deferens to bind to sperm cells. These findings indicate that antibodies bind to sperm before ejaculation not after ejaculation as it was initially thought [44]. Hence, rapid washing and dilution of the ejaculate will not affect the binding of the antibodies to the sperm.

Eliminating Bound ASA from Sperm Surface

The use of immunobead incubation to treat ASA-positive sperm has been described. Assessment of sperm incubation with immunobeads showed that both serum and semen immunoglobulin binding to sperm decrease over time. It was thought that sperm-covered ASA and immunobead coincubation results in a decrease in the number of sperm bound to ASA, improving outcome [45, 46]. The use of immunobead adsorption itself seems striking for the removal of ASA off the spermatozoa, but the efficacy is not completely clear. Studies that used lyophilized immunobead adsorption concluded that this technique can be applied in the selection of antibody-free spermatozoa, and the rate of recovery of spermatozoa decreases as the number of antibodies bound to sperm increases [47]. The success of immunobead incubation in the treatment of immunologic infertility seems to be limited with no consistent benefits observed. According to the published literature, there are still plenty of questions that need to be addressed regarding the effect of this technique on the sperm membrane. Despite the limitation of the immunobead test in treating men with ASA, the information provided by the test results when it is performed is a very important prognostic tool. The immunobead test can help to identify the immunoglobulin subtype and the location of the antibody on the sperm [48]. The test is widely available, simple to run, and provides titers that are useful in monitoring patients who are being treated for ASA (i.e., corticosteroid treatment).

Simple centrifugation and washing of the sperm was first reported by Hanson et al. [49]. It is a very simple technique that is utilized in sperm preparation for IUI. Fresh seminal fluid from men with ASA is centrifuged and suspended in an albumin solution or nutrient medium before using it for insemination [50]. The effectiveness of sperm washing is dependent on the time of ejaculation to washing, limited to the IgG subtype, and it is less likely to yield motile sperms when compared to the swim-up method of preparation [51]. The use of centrifugation and simple wash procedure in men with immunological infertility has multiple drawbacks. Cell debris, white blood cells, bacteria, and sometime free ASA are part of the pellet and they are capable of causing irreversible damage to the viable sperms [52]. One way to filter the sperm from other elements is to use the ability of the sperm to swim. Both the swim-up and swim-down methods can be used to separate motile sperms up or down, respectively, in a nutrient rich medium. The efficiency of these techniques depends on the quality of the original specimen, and the quantity of sperm and ASA. Antibodies on the sperm surface cause agglutinated and poorly progressive spermatozoa, and therefore this results in limited recovery of sperm using the swim-up or swim-down methods [53]. This limitation makes these methods of sperm preparation poor treatment options for patient with ASA.

Enzymatic cleavage of immunoglobulin has also been proposed as a treatment option for men with ASA. IgA proteases derived from *Neisseria gonorrhoeae*, whose substrate specificity is limited to Fc region of human IgA type 1, have the ability to cleave IgA and reduce the total number bound to sperms with improvement in sperm cervical mucus penetration ability [54, 55]. However, IgA proteases are very specific and it is not clear how effective they are in clearing other antibody isotopes. In addition, since the site of the cleavage is in the Fc region, part of the immunoglobulin remains attached to the sperm. Since IgM, IgG, and IgA2 are not cleaved with IgA proteases, other proteases have been used with some success. It have been previously demonstrated that the three enzymes, trypsin (500 U/ml), chymotrypsin (500 U/ml), and papain (50 U/ml), are capable of decreasing immunologically agglutinated spermatozoa with no detrimental effect on sperm motility or vitality [56]. The efficacy of these enzymes and possible negative effect on sperm are not completely understood. Post-treatment testing showed some mixed results, the incubation of normal spermatozoa with either chymotrypsin or papain resulted in impairment of oocyte penetration in the zona-free hamster egg penetration test. The use of trypsin, while significantly improving oocyte penetration of spermatozoa had no effect on the sperm mucus interaction [57].

Magnetic isolation of antibody-coated sperm from antibody-free sperm to avoid potential damage to fragile sperm through centrifugation has been tried. Superparamagnetic polymer microspheres coated with monoclonal antibodies are used to isolate antibody labeled from antibody-free spermatozoa (see Fig. 23.1). Using magnetic isolation, viable spermatozoa are isolated, but the motility of the isolated

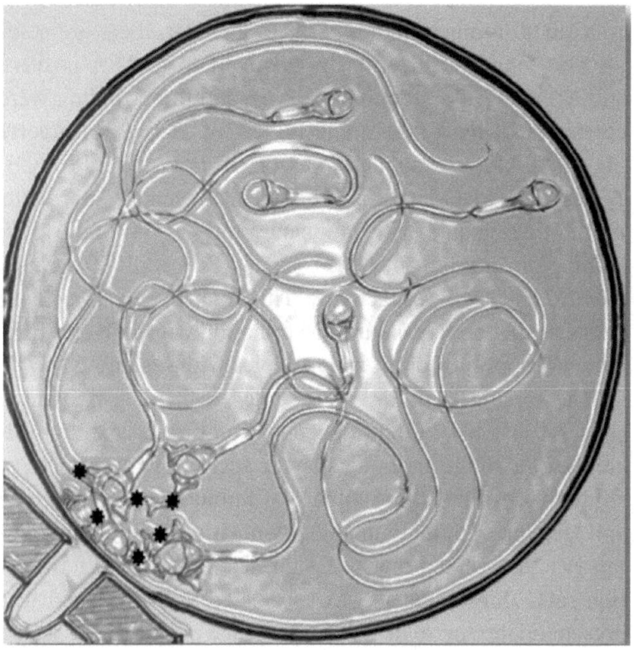

Fig. 23.1 Magnetic separation of antibody-labeled from antibody-free spermatozoa, a magnet separates ASA-bound spermatozoa by attraction of magnetic beads; only ASA-free sperm last in the supernatant

spermatozoa deteriorated rapidly [58]. ICSI would, therefore, be necessary for fertilization with the antibody-free sorted sample.

The different techniques that attempted to select sperm with no ASA showed some success, but most of the published studies are small series with no randomized control trials [47]. Although sperm preparation techniques are capable of separating ASA-free sperm, they still require the utilization of intrauterine IUI, or ART-like ICSI to achieve pregnancy. Furthermore, the consequence of these techniques on sperm is not completely understood.

Assisted Reproductive Technologies

There is a growing body of knowledge about interrelationship between ASA and ART. Although ART may be used to overcome ASA-related infertility, ASA may have a detrimental effect on ART outcome. Several studies have examined the use of IUI, gamete intrafallopian transfer (GIFT), IVF, and ICSI procedures for the treatment of immune infertility.

The results of the technique for ASA detection must be taken into account with regard to the selection of the best assisted reproductive technique. If sperm was found on a postcoital cervical mucus test, then IUI, to bypass the mucus, might be a good and inexpensive option. In the patient that has antibodies to the head of sperm, ICSI should be considered. Two factors need to be taken into account in presence of ASA when considering ART. First, ASA interfere with sperm passage through the female genital tract or with egg fertilization. ART itself may lead to ASA production in the female partner after sperm introduction (i.e., IUI). When offering couples ART, it is important to be aware of the female ASA titers. The presence of ASA in the female partner has multiple implications; IUI in the presence of ASA has the potential to be secreted in the female genital tract and impedes the sperm progressive motility. In such circumstance, it is reasonable to skip artificial insemination and to proceed directly to IVF [59]. Oocytes from females with positive ASA titers should be washed very carefully from follicular fluid since they will also be positive for ASA. Therefore, the evaluation of the presence of ASA in the serum of women involved in IVF treatment should be performed to avoid unexplained failure and unnecessary treatments.

Intrauterine Insemination

The use of various techniques as were discussed earlier to obtain ASA-free sperms has been very unpromising. Therefore, the recovery of motile antibody-free sperm makes the use of IUI limited to certain subsets of patients. One of the causes of immune-mediated infertility is the inability of sperm to penetrate the cervical mucus. Therefore, the rationale for IUI in this situation is to place the sperm beyond the cervix [60]. (See Fig. 23.2) There is a lack of controlled, prospective studies evaluating the outcomes in the patient with immune infertility being treated with IUI. When women who are positive for ASA in the cervical mucus are partnered with

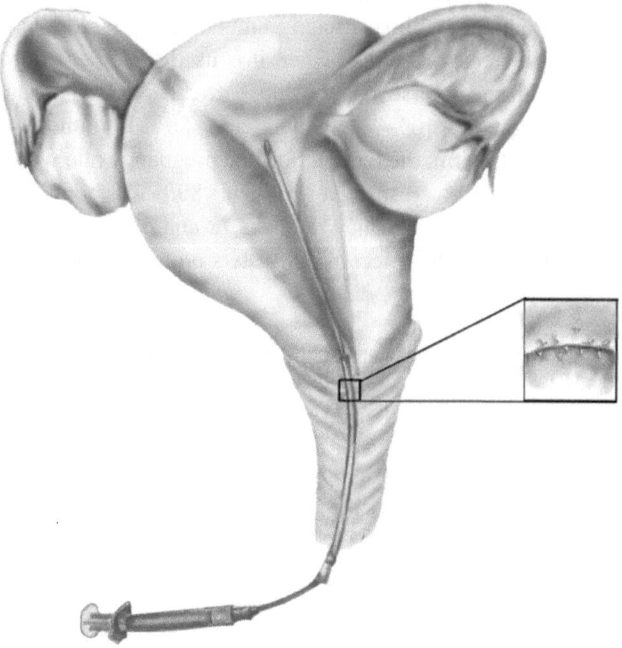

Fig. 23.2 IUI to bypass cervical mucus ASA

a male partner who is ASA negative, the pregnancy rate after IUI was identical to women who did not have ASA [61]. These findings were not consistently seen in other studies. Nevertheless, in the setting of controlled ovarian stimulation, IUI significantly improved pregnancy rates [62, 63]. In the setting of men with documented ASA, investigators have shown sperm washing before IUI might have little or no effect on improving the probability of pregnancy with some investigators reporting a 0% success rate [64–66]. There is no good evidence that IUI alone or in combination with specific-sperm preparation techniques might help ASA-positive infertile men. However, some studies have reported a good pregnancy rate after IUI in ASA-positive infertile men with a poor postcoital test compared to IUI in ASA-negative infertile men [67] with ASA-positive men achieving near 33% pregnancy rate with IUI compared to 19% in IUI couples for other reasons [68].

In Vitro Fertilization

IVF requires low number of sperms (100,000) to fertilize retrieved oocytes, and only enough viable sperms are needed as mature oocytes, making it useful to treat couples with male factor infertility. Studies on fertilization rates following IVF have reported contradictory results in couples identified as having ASA. Some studies demonstrated a detrimental effect of ASA on fertilization and pregnancy rates and others did not. However, comparing such studies is a challenge because of the heterogeneity in study design, ASA test type, and the wide range of ASA cutoff levels that are used (Table 23.2). Several studies have shown that IVF used to treat patients with suspected immunological factors have lower pregnancy rate than when it is used for other etiologies, with an inverse relationship between ASA titers and fertilization rates [69–73]. In men with > 80% immunoglobulin-bound sperm, the fertilization and pregnancy rate was as low as 27 and 0%, respectively. When < 80% was bound, the fertilization and pregnancy rate was 72 and 67% [74]. This correlation and the effect of ASA titers on fertilization were confirmed in other studies [75]. In contrast, there are studies that found fertilization to be identical in ASA-positive and ASA-negative populations [76], and these finding were corroborated by a systematic review of 16 studies involving 4209 ART treatment cycles (1508 IVF and 2701 ICSI cycles). The meta-analysis concluded that semen ASA status was not associated with pregnancy rates in IVF and ICSI, and the mean pregnancy rates for the IVF and ICSI groups were 23 and 36%, respectively. This extensive meta-analysis suggests that both standard insemination with IVF and ICSI are viable options for infertile couples with semen ASA [77].

The prognosis of IVF in couples with male ASA as a cause of infertility might dependent on the class and physical location of the antibodies on the sperm. In a retrospective study that evaluated the impact of immunoglobulin isotype and location of binding in 48 ASA-positive couples undergoing IVF, they noted that IgA significantly reduced fertilization rates only when it was associated with IgM and was present on the sperm head. The presence of IgM either on the sperm head or end of the tail also adversely affected fertilization rates [78]. Despite the reported success of IVF in these populations, it is important to note that the quality of embryos obtained after IVF using sperm from ASA-positive men is generally poorer when compared to embryos from ASA-negative men [24]. Unexpected fertilization failure happens rarely when the male has normal semen parameters. This can be due to an oocyte defect or a sperm defect and certainly ASA have been implicated in complete failure of fertilization despite normal semen parameters. The discussion with the couple undergoing treatment about this possibility should be part of every IVF consent consultation.

Intracytoplasmic Sperm Injection

IVF and ICSI have become a routine and widely acceptable procedure to treat infertility. In the ICSI procedure, a single sperm is injected into the cytoplasm of the oocyte. When immune infertility is not overcome by standard IVF despite normal fertilization rates, ICSI should also be considered

Table 23.2 ART and pregnancy rates in men with antisperm antibodies (ASA), immunobead binding test (IBT), and mixed antiglobulin reaction (MAR)

Study	Total ART cycles	Total cycles with ASA	ART procedure	Assay used for detection	Percent pregnancy
Lahteenmaki [75]	156	47	IVF	IBT and MAR	24
Acosta et al. [71]	67	38	IVF	IBT	39
Vujisic et al. [72]	52	14	IVF	IBT	29
Clarke [73]	89	38	IVF	IBT	8
Nagy et al. [83]	1822	54	ICSI	MAR	28
Clarke et al. [80]	179	39	ICSI	IBT	13
Check et al. [81]	93	26	ICSI	Not reported	42
Esteves et al. [82]	351	49	ICSI	IBT	53

[79–82]. ICSI has the potential to overcome antibody-mediated infertility that interferes with the interaction between the sperm and the oocyte's ZP and oolemna. In a study looking at 29 infertile ASA-positive couples treated with ICSI after failing fertilization with IVF, the fertilization and cleavage rates were not significantly different between ASA-positive and ASA-negative groups: 79 vs. 89 % [24]. A retrospective analysis of 55 ICSI cycles for 32 different couples with greater than 80 % of ASA-bound sperm demonstrated no difference in pregnancy rate (30 %) between the ASA-positive and ASA-negative groups undergoing ICSI [83]. Generally, there are no relationships between ASA levels and pregnancy rates or fertilization rate, and the use of ICSI leads to a better prognosis in couples where the man is ASA positive [77]. Despite the relatively good prognosis, care should be taken when counseling patients with ASA infertility since there is some evidence that ASA can have postfertilization effects on the preimplantation and developing embryo [84].

Antibodies to Specific Antigen

As we discussed earlier, the interaction between the sperm and oocyte is highly regulated by specific receptor–ligand binding. Antibodies to FA-1 antigen inhibit human sperm–zona interaction and block human sperm capacitation and acrosome reaction [84]. FA-1 antigen is involved in human immunological infertility in both men and women. The presence of these antibodies may interfere with fertilization in the IVF procedure and leads to fertilization failure. Antigen-specific immune absorption that is aimed at a specific antibodies, rather than all immunoglobulins, has been previously shown to be effective in removing and neutralizing anti-FA-1 antibodies in infertile men [85]. Adsorption with FA-1 antigen helps to remove autoantibodies from the cell surface of sperm cells and increases the acrosome reaction rate by 10 %. If this technique is successful, then IUI of FA-1-treated antibody-free sperm may lead to normal pregnancies and healthy babies, providing that this antigen treatment does not have a deleterious effect on implantation, embryonic, or fetal development [86].

Predicting Success

Decision making and counseling with male infertility factor for IUI, IVF, or ICSI is often difficult. Semen parameters are poor predictors of ART outcomes. However, the challenge is to identify the couple who will benefit from ART and the couple who will not. While the routine semen analysis is useful in identifying subfertile men, it has poor capacity to predict IUI outcome in couples. Models that evaluated IUI outcome in couples with male subfertility found that female age, duration of subfertility, secondary subfertility, the presence of anovulation and cervical hostility, cycle number and the absence of ovarian hyperstimulation are independent factors in determining success [87]. Furthermore, the presence of ASA in male patients increased the predictive capacity of these independent factors [88]. As such, ASA testing may be a useful adjunct to proper and thorough patient counseling. Couples that require IVF or ICSI have excellent outcomes despite having ASA. Studies that examine the relationship between ASA and reproductive outcomes after IVF or IVF with ICSI found no relationship between semen parameters (sperm concentration, motility, and strict morphology), ASA levels and fertilization or clinical pregnancy rate after IVF and IVF/ICSI. Having the capability of predicting success of the different procedures can help eliminate the cost and emotional stress of the couples that are undergoing treatment.

References

1. Mathur S, Rosenlund C, Carlton M, et al. Studies on sperm survival and motility in the presence of cytotoxic sperm antibodies. Am J Reprod Immunol Microbiol. 1988;17:41–7.
2. Check JH, Adelson HG, Bollendorf A. Effect of antisperm antibodies on computerized semen analysis. Arch Androl. 1991;27:61–3.
3. Upadhyaya M, Hibbard BM, Walker SM. Antisperm antibodies and male infertility. Br J Urol. 1984;56:531–6.
4. Practice Committee of American Society for Reproductive M. Diagnostic evaluation of the infertile male: a committee opinion. Fertil Steril. 2012;98:294–301.
5. Jager S, Kremer J, van Slochteren-Draaisma T. A simple method of screening for antisperm antibodies in the human male. Detection of spermatozoal surface IgG with the direct mixed antiglobulin reaction carried out on untreated fresh human semen. Int J Fertil. 1978;23:12–21.
6. Haas GG, Jr., Schreiber AD, Blasco L. The incidence of sperm-associated immunoglobulin and C3, the third component of complement, in infertile men. Fertil Steril. 1983;39:542–7.
7. D'Cruz OJ, Haas GG, Jr., Wang BL, DeBault LE. Activation of human complement by IgG antisperm antibody and the demonstration of C3 and C5b-9-mediated immune injury to human sperm. J Immunol. 1991;146:611–20.
8. Price RJ, Boettcher B. The presence of complement in human cervical mucus and its possible relevance to infertility in women with complement-dependent sperm-immobilizing antibodies. Fertil Steril. 1979;32:61–6.
9. De Almeida M, Soumah A, Jouannet P. Incidence of sperm-associated immunoglobulins in infertile men with suspected autoimmunity to sperm. Int J Androl. 1986;9:321–30.
10. Busacca M, Fusi F, Brigante C, Doldi N, Smid M, Vigano P. Evaluation of antisperm antibodies in infertile couples with immunobead test: prevalence and prognostic value. Acta Eur Fertil. 1989;20:77–82.
11. Menge AC, Beitner O. Interrelationships among semen characteristics, antisperm antibodies, and cervical mucus penetration assays in infertile human couples. Fertil Steril. 1989;51:486–92.
12. Mortimer D, Pandya IJ, Sawers RS. Relationship between human sperm motility characteristics and sperm penetration into human cervical mucus in vitro. J Reprod Fertil. 1986;78:93–102.
13. Kremer J, Jager S. Characteristics of anti-spermatozoal antibodies responsible for the shaking phenomenon with special regard

to immunoglobulin class and antigen-reactive sites. Int J Androl. 1980;3:143–52.
14. Witkin SS, Viti D, David SS, Stangel J, Rosenwaks Z. Relation between antisperm antibodies and the rate of fertilization of human oocytes in vitro. J Assist Reprod Genet. 1992;9:9–13.
15. Wang C, Baker HW, Jennings MG, Burger HG, Lutjen P. Interaction between human cervical mucus and sperm surface antibodies. Fertil Steril. 1985;44:484–8.
16. Hall JL, Engel D, Naz RK. Significance of antibodies against human sperm FA-1 antigen in immunoinfertility. Arch Androl. 1994;32:25–30.
17. Bronson RA, Cooper GW, Rosenfeld DL. Sperm-specific isoantibodies and autoantibodies inhibit the binding of human sperm to the human zona pellucida. Fertil Steril. 1982;38:724–9.
18. Mahony MC, Blackmore PF, Bronson RA, Alexander NJ. Inhibition of human sperm-zona pellucida tight binding in the presence of antisperm antibody positive polyclonal patient sera. J Reprod Immunol. 1991;19:287–301.
19. Naz RK, Brazil C, Overstreet JW. Effects of antibodies to sperm surface fertilization antigen-1 on human sperm-zona pellucida interaction. Fertil Steril. 1992;57:1304–10.
20. Abdel-Latif A, Mathur S, Rust PF, Fredericks CM, Abdel-Aal H, Williamson HO. Cytotoxic sperm antibodies inhibit sperm penetration of zona-free hamster eggs. Fertil Steril. 1986;45:542–9.
21. Shibahara H, Shigeta M, Inoue M, et al. Diversity of the blocking effects of antisperm antibodies on fertilization in human and mouse. Hum Reprod. 1996;11:2595–9.
22. Francavilla F, Romano R, Santucci R, Marrone V, Properzi G, Ruvolo G. Occurrence of the interference of sperm-associated antibodies on sperm fertilizing ability as evaluated by the sperm-zona pellucida binding test and by the TEST-yolk buffer enhanced sperm penetration assay. Am J Reprod Immunol. 1997;37:267–74.
23. Tian X, Zhang L, Wu Y, Yang C, Liu P. Relationship between serum antisperm antibodies and anticardiolipin antibodies and clinical pregnancy outcome in an in vitro fertilization and embryo transfer program. Chin Med J (Engl). 1999;112:34–6.
24. Lahteenmaki A, Reima I, Hovatta O. Treatment of severe male immunological infertility by intracytoplasmic sperm injection. Hum Reprod. 1995;10:2824–8.
25. Wolff H, Schill WB. Antisperm antibodies in infertile and homosexual men: relationship to serologic and clinical findings. Fertil Steril. 1985;44:673–7.
26. Greskovich F, Mathur S, Nyberg LM, Jr., Collins BS. Effect of early antibiotic treatment on the formation of sperm antibodies in experimentally induced epididymitis. Arch Androl. 1993;30:183–91.
27. Greentree LB. Antisperm antibodies in infertility: the role of condom therapy. Fertil Steril. 1982;37:451–2.
28. Kremer J, Jager S, Kuiken J. Treatment of infertility caused by antisperm antibodies. Int J Fertil. 1978;23:270–6.
29. Rosse WF. Quantitative immunology of immune hemolytic anemia: II. The relationship of cell-bound antibody to hemolysis and the effect of treatment. J Clin Invest. 1971;50:734–43.
30. Turek PJ, Lipshultz LI. Immunologic infertility. Urol Clin North Am. 1994;21:447–68.
31. Hendry WF, Treehuba K, Hughes L, Stedronska J, Parslow JM, Wass JA, Besser GM. Cyclic prednisolone therapy for male infertility associated with autoantibodies to spermatozoa. Fertil Steril. 1986;45(2):249–54.
32. Haas GG, Jr., Manganiello P. A double-blind, placebo-controlled study of the use of methylprednisolone in infertile men with sperm-associated immunoglobulins. Fertil Steril. 1987;47:295–301.
33. De Almeida M, Feneux D, Rigaud C, Jouannet P. Steroid therapy for male infertility associated with antisperm antibodies: results of a small randomized clinical trial. Int J Androl. 1985;8:111–7.
34. Hendry WF, Hughes L, Scammell G, Pryor JP, Hargreave TB. Comparison of prednisolone and placebo in subfertile men with antibodies to spermatozoa. Lancet. 1990;335:85–8.
35. Sharma KK, Barratt CL, Pearson MJ, Cooke ID. Oral steroid therapy for subfertile males with antisperm antibodies in the semen: prediction of the responders. Hum Reprod. 1995;10:103–9.
36. Hoes JN, Jacobs JW, Verstappen SM, Bijlsma JW, Van der Heijden GJ. Adverse events of low- to medium-dose oral glucocorticoids in inflammatory diseases: a meta-analysis. Ann Rheum Dis. 2009;68:1833–8.
37. Sakamoto Y, Matsumoto T, Kumazawa J. Cell-mediated autoimmune response to testis induced by bilateral testicular injury can be suppressed by cyclosporin A. J Urol. 1998;159:1735–40.
38. Bouloux PM, Wass JA, Parslow JM, Hendry WF, Besser GM. Effect of cyclosporin A in male autoimmune infertility. Fertil Steril. 1986;46:81–5.
39. Halim A, Antoniou D, Leedham PW, Blandy JP, Tresidder GC. Investigation and treatment of the infertile male. Proc R Soc Med. 1973;66:373–8.
40. Bronson R. Immunity in sperm and in vitro fertilization. J In Vitro Fert Embryo Transf. 1987;4:195–7.
41. Elder KT, Wick KL, Edwards RG. Seminal plasma anti-sperm antibodies and IVF: the effect of semen sample collection into 50% serum. Hum Reprod. 1990;5:179–84.
42. Lenzi A, Gandini L, Claroni F, Lombardo F, Morrone S, Dondero F. Immunological usefulness of semen manipulation for artificial insemination homologous (AIH) in subjects with antisperm antibodies bound to sperm surface. Andrologia. 1988;20:314–21.
43. Windt ML, Menkveld R, Kruger TF, van der Merwe JP, Lombard CJ. Effect of rapid dilution of semen on sperm-bound autoantibodies. Arch Androl. 1989;22:227–31.
44. Naz RK, Bhargava KK. Antibodies to sperm surface fertilization antigen (FA-1): their specificities and site of interaction with sperm in male genital tract. Mol Reprod Dev 1990;26:175–83.
45. Gould JE, Brazil CK, Overstreet JW. Sperm-immunobead binding decreases with in vitro incubation. Fertil Steril. 1994;62:167–71.
46. Grundy CE, Robinson J, Guthrie KA, Gordon AG, Hay DM. Establishment of pregnancy after removal of sperm antibodies in vitro. BMJ. 1992;304:292–3.
47. Verheyen G, Tournaye H, Laurier K, Devroey P, Van Steirteghem A. Auto-controlled study on in-vitro fertilization performance with 'antibody-free' spermatozoa selected by immunobead adsorption from semen of patients with anti-sperm antibodies. Hum Reprod. 1994;9:1119–26.
48. Junk SM, Matson PL, O'Halloran F, Yovich JL. Use of immunobeads to detect human antispermatozoal antibodies. Clin Reprod Fertil. 1986;4:199–206.
49. Hanson FM, Rock J. Artificial insemination with husband's sperm. Fertil Steril. 1951;2:162–74.
50. Shulman S, Harlin B, Davis P, Reyniak JV. Immune infertility and new approaches to treatment. Fertil Steril. 1978;29:309–13.
51. Adeghe AJ. Effect of washing on sperm surface autoantibodies. Br J Urol. 1987;60:360–3.
52. Shekarriz M, DeWire DM, Thomas AJ, Jr., Agarwal A. A method of human semen centrifugation to minimize the iatrogenic sperm injuries caused by reactive oxygen species. Eur Urol. 1995;28:31–5.
53. Bollendorf A, Check JH, Katsoff D, Fedele A. The use of chymotrypsin/galactose to treat spermatozoa bound with anti-sperm antibodies prior to intra-uterine insemination. Hum Reprod. 1994;9:484–8.
54. Bronson RA, Cooper GW, Rosenfeld DL, Gilbert JV, Plaut AG. The effect of an IgA1 protease on immunoglobulins bound to the sperm surface and sperm cervical mucus penetrating ability. Fertil Steril. 1987;47:985–91.
55. Kutteh WH, Kilian M, Ermel LD, Byrd EW, Mestecky J. Antisperm antibodies (ASAs) in infertile males: subclass distribution of IgA antibodies and the effect of an IgA1 protease on sperm-bound antibodies. Am J Reprod Immunol. 1994;31:77–83.
56. Pattinson HA, Mortimer D, Curtis EF, Leader A, Taylor PJ. Treatment of spermagglutination with proteolytic enzymes. I. Sperm

motility, vitality, longevity and successful disagglutination. Hum Reprod. 1990;5:167–73.
57. Pattinson HA, Mortimer D, Taylor PJ. Treatment of spermagglutination with proteolytic enzymes. II. Sperm function after enzymatic disagglutination. Hum Reprod. 1990;5:174–8.
58. Kiser GC, Alexander NJ, Fuchs EF, Fulgham DL. In vitro immune absorption of antisperm antibodies with immunobead-rise, immunomagnetic, and immunocolumn separation techniques. Fertil Steril. 1987;47:466–74.
59. Clarke GN, Hsieh C, Koh SH, Cauchi MN. Sperm antibodies, immunoglobulins, and complement in human follicular fluid. Am J Reprod Immunol. 1984;5:179–81.
60. Bronson RA. Antisperm antibodies: a critical evaluation and clinical guidelines. J Reprod Immunol. 1999;45:159–83.
61. Check JH, Bollendorf A, Katsoff D, Kozak J. The frequency of antisperm antibodies in the cervical mucus of women with poor postcoital tests and their effect on pregnancy rates. Am J Reprod Immunol. 1994;32:38–42.
62. Gregoriou O, Vitoratos N, Papadias C, Konidaris S, Maragudakis A, Zourlas PA. Intrauterine insemination as a treatment of infertility in women with antisperm antibodies. Int J Gynaecol Obstet. 1991;35:151–6.
63. Margalloth EJ, Sauter E, Bronson RA, Rosenfeld DL, Scholl GM, Cooper GW. Intrauterine insemination as treatment for antisperm antibodies in the female. Fertil Steril. 1988;50:441–6.
64. Ulstein M. Fertility of husbands at homologous insemination. Acta Obstet Gynecol Scand. 1973;52:5–8.
65. Galle PC, McRae MA, Colliver JA, Alexander JS. Sperm washing and intrauterine insemination for cervical factor, oligospermia, immunologic infertility and unexplained infertility. J Reprod Med. 1990;35:116–22.
66. Francavilla F, Romano R, Santucci R, Marrone V, Corrao G. Failure of intrauterine insemination in male immunological infertility in cases in which all spermatozoa are antibody-coated. Fertil Steril. 1992;58:587–92.
67. Check JH, Bollendorf A. Effect of antisperm antibodies on postcoital results and effect of intrauterine insemination on pregnancy outcome. Arch Androl. 1992;28:25–31.
68. Agarwal A. Treatment of immunological infertility by sperm washing and intrauterine insemination. Arch Androl. 1992;29:207–13.
69. Junk SM, Matson PL, Yovich JM, Bootsma B, Yovich JL. The fertilization of human oocytes by spermatozoa from men with antispermatozoal antibodies in semen. J In Vitro Fert Embryo Transf. 1986;3:350–2.
70. Ford WC, Williams KM, McLaughlin EA, Harrison S, Ray B, Hull MG. The indirect immunobead test for seminal antisperm antibodies and fertilization rates at in-vitro fertilization. Hum Reprod. 1996;11:1418–22.
71. Acosta AA, Van Der Merwe JP, Doncel G, Kruger TF, Sayilgan A, Franken DR, Kolm P. Fertilization efficiency of morphologically abnormal spermatozoa in assisted reproduction is further impaired by antisperm antibodies on the male partner's sperm. Fertil Steril. 1994;62:826–833.
72. Vujisic S, Lepej SZ, Jerkovic L, Emedi I, Sokolic B. Antisperm antibodies in semen, sera and follicular fluids of infertile patients: relation to reproductive outcome after in vitro fertilization. Am J Reprod Immunol. 2005;54:13–20.
73. Clarke GN. Association between sperm autoantibodies and enhanced embryo implantation rates during in vitro fertilization. Fertil Steril. 2006;86:753–4.
74. Clarke GN, Lopata A, McBain JC, Baker HW, Johnston WI. Effect of sperm antibodies in males on human in vitro fertilization (IVF). Am J Reprod Immunol Microbiol. 1985;8:62–6.
75. Lahteenmaki A. In-vitro fertilization in the presence of antisperm antibodies detected by the mixed antiglobulin reaction (MAR) and the tray agglutination test (TAT). Hum Reprod. 1993;8:84–8.
76. De Almeida M, Herry M, Testart J, Belaisch-Allart J, Frydman R, Jouannet P. In-vitro fertilization results from 13 women with antisperm antibodies. Hum Reprod. 1987;2:599–602.
77. Zini A, Lefebvre J, Kornitzer G, et al. Anti-sperm antibody levels are not related to fertilization or pregnancy rates after IVF or IVF/ICSI. J Reprod Immunol. 2011;88:80–4.
78. Yeh WR, Acosta AA, Seltman HJ, Doncel G. Impact of immunoglobulin isotype and sperm surface location of antisperm antibodies on fertilization in vitro in the human. Fertil Steril. 1995;63:1287–92.
79. Mardesic T, Ulcova-Gallova Z, Huttelova R, et al. The influence of different types of antibodies on in vitro fertilization results. Am J Reprod Immunol. 2000;43:1–5.
80. Clarke GN, Bourne H, Baker HW. Intracytoplasmic sperm injection for treating infertility associated with sperm autoimmunity. Fertil Steril. 1997;68:112–7
81. Check ML, Check JH, Katsoff D, Summers-Chase D. ICSI as an effective therapy for male factor with antisperm antibodies. Arch Androl. 2000;45:125–30.
82. Esteves SC, Schneider DT, Verza S Jr. Influence of antisperm antibodies in the semen on intracytoplasmic sperm injection outcome. Int Braz J Urol. 2007;33:795–802.
83. Nagy ZP, Verheyen G, Liu J, et al. Results of 55 intracytoplasmic sperm injection cycles in the treatment of male-immunological infertility. Hum Reprod. 1995;10:1775–80.
84. Ahmad K, Naz RK. Effects of human antisperm antibodies on development of preimplantation embryos. Arch Androl. 1992;29:9–20.
85. Naz RK. Involvement of fertilization antigen (FA-1) in involuntary immunoinfertility in humans. J Clin Invest. 1987;80:1375–83.
86. Menge AC, Christman GM, Ohl DA, Naz RK. Fertilization antigen-1 removes antisperm autoantibodies from spermatozoa of infertile men and results in increased rates of acrosome reaction. Fertil Steril. 1999;71:256–60.
87. Steures P, van der Steeg JW, Mol BW, et al. Prediction of an ongoing pregnancy after intrauterine insemination. Fertil Steril. 2004;82:45–51.
88. van Weert JM, Repping S, van der Steeg JW, Steures P, van der Veen F, Mol BW. IUI in male subfertility: are we able to select the proper patients? Reprod Biomed Online 2005;11:624–31.

Medication Strategies for the Male with Unexplained Infertility

24

Christopher L. Starks and Edmund S. Sabanegh

Introduction

Approximately 15 % of couples of reproductive age are affected by infertility [1]. Male factor contributes up to 50 % of these cases [2]. We preface this chapter with the statement that as our knowledge of genetics continues to improve at a rapid pace, we anticipate the role for empiric therapies for "unexplained infertility" to shift towards specific therapies for pinpointed abnormalities. Amongst men presenting with unexplained infertility, about 1.7 % of these patients will be found to have an identifiable endocrine diagnosis, for which there are specific treatments [3]. Their management will be discussed elsewhere.

Up to 25 % of infertile men will have no identifiable cause for their abnormal semen analyses [4]. We review in this chapter the use of empiric medical therapy (EMT) for men with unexplained male infertilty and idiopathic infertility. For men with normal and near normal sperm testing, at most empiric therapy is indicated; we further review the indications and use of EMT in a variety of scenarios.

In this review, we will discuss the potential indications and mechanisms of action as well as therapy choice for EMT. The major classes of medication are shown in Table 24.1, with potential sites of action reviewed in Fig. 24.1. We intentionally did not include steroid therapy for antisperm antibodies, for we believe this to be a specific etiology rather than an "unexplained infertilty" cause. Along the same lines, we did not include the use of antioxidant vitamin regimen because we would not consider these prescribed "medications" for inclusion into our chapter. Prior to administering any empiric medication therapy, we recommend a detailed conversation with patients. There are many considerations that factor into the recommendation of these agents, including baseline semen parameters, male physical examination, genetic and endocrine evaluation, female partner age, and female fertility issues. Many of these medications are not specifically approved by the Food and Drug Administration for male fertility, so it is incumbent upon the prescribing provider to thoroughly review the risks and benefits of the proposed therapy.

Antiestrogens

Selective estrogen receptor modulators are the most commonly used medical therapies for unexplained infertility. These medications competitively bind estrogen receptors, especially at the level of the hypothalamus and pituitary. The effect is to inhibit the negative feedback of estrogen on the system, which leads to increased endogenous gonadotropin-releasing hormone secretion. This results in increases in the production of follicle stimulating hormone (FSH) and luteinizing hormone (LH), ultimately promoting spermatogenesis. The most studied and prescribed medications of this type are clomiphene citrate and tamoxifen.

Clomiphene Citrate

Administration of clomiphene for idiopathic infertility varies in dosage, timing, and duration. Treatment doses range from clomiphene 25–100 mg daily or every other day. Common adverse effects of clomiphene therapy in men include nausea, headache, weight gain, alteration in libido, visual field changes, dizziness, gynecomastia, and allergic dermatitis; these side effects occur in less than 5 % of patients and are usually mild [5]. Clomiphene doses in excess of 200 mg/day can lead to suppression of spermatogenesis [7]. Serum gonadotropin and testosterone levels should be periodically monitored while on treatment. Additionally, a small number of patients may have decline in semen parameters, and as such, periodic semen analyses are indicated [5, 8].

C. L. Starks (✉)
The Urology Group of Virginia, Glickman Urologic and Kidney Institute, The Cleveland Clinic Foundation, 19415 Deerfield Ave., Suite 112 Leesburg 20176 20176 VA, USA
e-mail: christopherstrks2@gmail.com

E. S. Sabanegh
Department of Urology, The Cleveland Clinic, 9500, Euclid Ave, Q-10, Cleveland, OH 44120, USA

G. L. Schattman et al. (eds.), *Unexplained Infertility*, DOI 10.1007/978-1-4939-2140-9_24,

Table 24.1 Classes of medications used for empiric medical therapy

Antiestrogens
Clomiphene citrate
Tamoxifen
Aromatase inhibitors
Testolactone
Anastrazole
Gonadotropins
HCG
HMG
Recombinant human follicle stimulating hormone (FSH)
Androgens

One recent trial looked at a combination of clomiphene citrate and vitamin E in a prospective, randomized, placebo-controlled trial of 60 patients with idiopathic oligo-asthenospermia [9]. The trial showed this combination resulted in a significantly higher sperm count, increasing sperm count from a baseline of 10.2+/−4.14–18 million cells/ml+/−15 ($p=0.0025$). In placebo recipients, pretreatment concentration was 11.3+/−7.13–12 million cells/ml+/−8.6 ($p>0.05$). The progressive sperm motility also showed improvement in the treatment group. Additionally, the authors found a strong influence of this regimen on pregnancy rates, 36.7% in the combination versus 13.3% in the placebo group.

A second recent randomized trial showed a statistically significant increase in sperm count and motility for idiopathic infertility patients treated with clomiphene [10]. In this study, the treatment group had semen counts go from 20.38+/−16.2 to 42.51+/−29.4 million/ml ($p=0.01$). The motility percentage went from 23.78+/−17.5 to 43.38+/−20.1%, where $p=0.01$. Other placebo-controlled studies have also found a positive treatment effect for sperm counts and pregnancy rates for clomiphene [11–13].

However, the results from these trials are tempered with multiple other trials which have failed to show benefit from clomiphene therapy [14, 15]. A well-designed randomized and multicenter study by the WHO included 190 couples and showed no effect of clomiphene on pregnancy rates compared to placebo [16]. In a systematic meta-analysis, Cochrane review included ten studies involving 738 subfertile

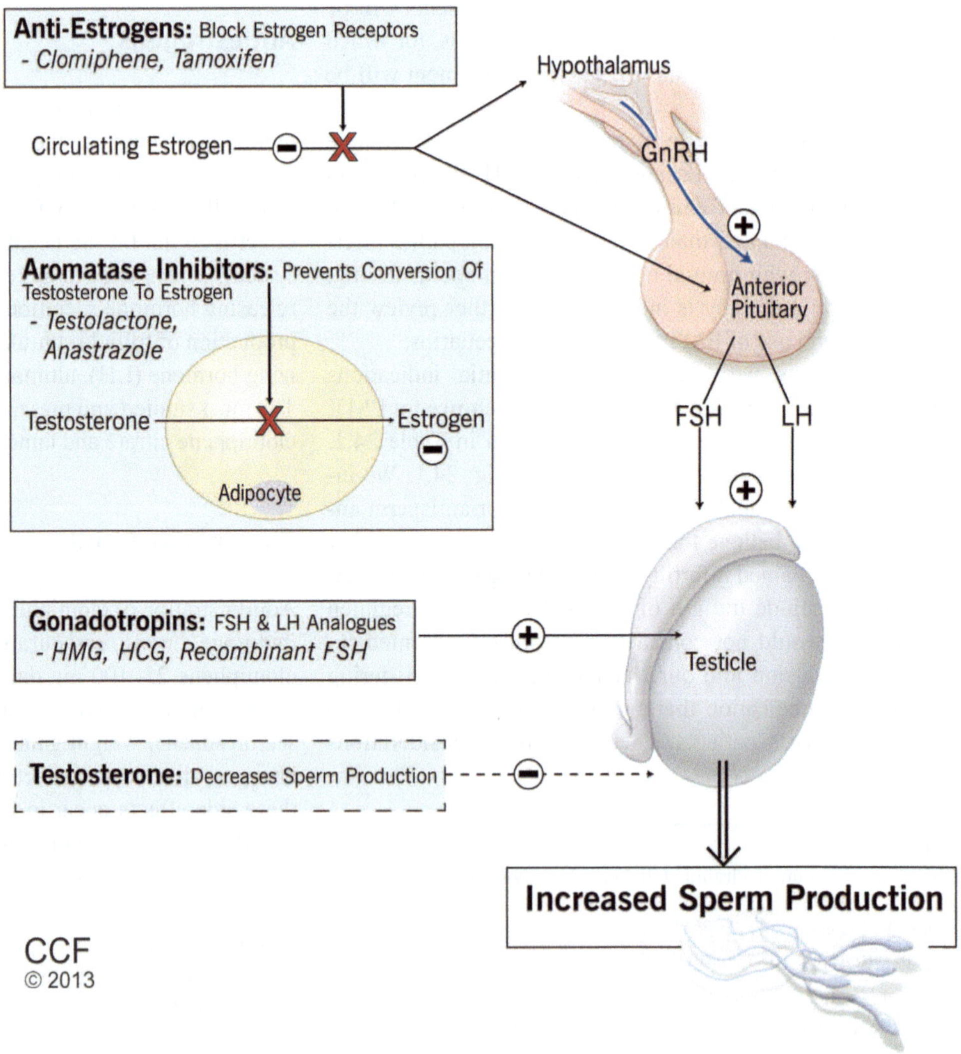

Fig. 24.1 Medications for male infertility. (Reprinted with permission from Cleveland Clinic Center for Medical Art & Photography © 2012. All Rights Reserved)

men with oligo-asthenozoospermia treated with at least 3 months of antiestrogen treatment [17]. They reported no difference in pregnancy rates with antiestrogen therapy.

Tamoxifen

Tamoxifen is known to have less estrogenic activity compared to clomiphene and has also been used as an oral agent to treat idiopathic male infertility. Treatment doses of tamoxifen range from 10 to 30 mg daily. The most common side effects are subjective flushing sensation (40–80 %) and risk of thrombus (1 %) [6]. Periodic lab analysis of liver function tests is recommended.

Initial uncontrolled trials reported improved sperm counts in men using tamoxifen [18, 19]. Subsequent controlled trials have all failed to show benefit from tamoxifen therapy for idiopathic male infertility [20, 21]. A meta-analysis of several randomized trials of tamoxifen demonstrated no significant treatment effect [22].

Additional evidence for the utilization of antiestrogens includes patients who will need intracytoplasmic sperm injection (ICSI) treatment. Hussein et al. looked at nonobstructive azoospermia patients who took antiestrogens for 3–9 months (mean duration of treatment 5.15 +/− 2.38 months). The authors found that 64 % of the patients responded to clomiphene and produced enough sperm in their ejaculate to allow for ICSI treatment, obviating the need for an extraction procedure [23]. It remains to be established which subpopulation of subfertile males will demonstrate the most benefit from these agents. Overall, antiestrogens are relatively inexpensive, well tolerated, and safe oral medications; however, there continues to be doubt about their efficacy and a lack of strong evidence to support their use.

Aromatase Inhibitors

Testolactone and Anastrazole

Aromatase is an enzyme which converts testosterone to estradiol and androstenedione to estrone. The peripheral aromatization of testosterone to an estrogen form has a negative feedback effect on gonadotropin production [24]. In 2001, Pavlovich et al. identified men with severe male factor infertility characterized by a decreased serum testosterone-to-estradiol ratio [25]. This physiology serves as the basis for the use of this class of agents as empiric therapy for male factor subfertility. Aromatase inhibitors have been used to treat idiopathic infertility by altering the inhibitory effects of estrogen; specifically, preventing the conversion of testosterone to estrogen will limit the estrogen-based inhibitory effects on spermatogenesis [24].

Testolactone and anastrazole are both aromatase inhibitors which have been prescribed for this purpose. Testolactone is a steroidal inhibitor, whereas anastrazole is a more selective nonsteroidal aromatase inhibitor. Testolactone is contraindicated in men with a previous history of male breast cancer. Anastrazole can increase the risk of developing osteoporosis (11 %) and joint disorders (17 %) [26]. Further, practitioners should consider checking serum liver function tests when administering anastrazole as up to 10 % of the patients may experience elevated liver enzymes.

Raman and Schlegel evaluated the effects of testolactone and anastrozole on a heterogeneous population of patients with abnormal testosterone to estradiol ratios (T/E_2 ratio < 10). The study included patients who were overweight, had Klinefelter's syndrome, and varicoceles. The authors found that both medications statistically demonstrated significant improvements in hormone profiles and semen parameters. In men treated with testolactone, the T/E2 ratio increased from 5.3 +/− 0.2 to 12.4 +/− 1.1 ($p < 0.001$). Additionally, there were improvements in sperm concentration, which increased from 5.5 to 11.2 million sperm per mL ($p < 0.01$), and sperm motility increased from 14.7 to 21.0 % ($p < 0.05$). For men treated with anastrazole, the T/E2 ratio increased from 7.2 +/− 0.3 to 18.1 +/− 1.0 ($p < 0.001$), and sperm concentration increased from 5.5 to 15.6 million per mL ($p < 0.01$) [27].

However, the Raman study was not specifically looking at idiopathic infertility patients, did not include a placebo group, and did not analyze pregnancy outcomes. Clark et al. performed a randomized, double blind, placebo-controlled trial looking at testolactone specifically in men with unexplained infertility [28]. These authors found no improvements in semen parameters or pregnancy rates compared to men taking placebo.

Gonadotropins

Human Chorionic Gonadotropin (HCG), Human Menopausal Gonadotropin (HMG), and Recombinant follicle stimulating hormone (FSH)

Human chorionic gonadotropin (HCG) and Human menopausal gonadotropin (HMG) have been used to treat idiopathic infertility. Recombinant FSH works via its primary mechanism, HCG works as an LH analog, and HMG displays both FSH and LH activity. All of these medications must be injected subcutaneously. Common side effects for these medications include pain at the injection site (6 %), nausea (2–3 %), fatigue (2 %), and gynecomastia (3 %). Serious venous and arterial thromboembolic events are rare but have been reported.

HCG and HMG

Multiple trials with varying methodology and populations have been conducted using these agents; two studies are noteworthy in trying to sort through this heterogeneous group of trials. Knuth et al. conducted the only randomized controlled study. Over a 3-month block, patients were administered 2500 IU of HCG twice per week and 150 IU of HMG three times a week or placebo [29]. They found there was no benefit in pregnancy or sperm parameters. Additionally, a Cochrane database review in 2006 states that gonadotropins may improve pregnancy rates, but there is not enough definitive evidence to support their use [30]. The authors note that the number of trials and participants are too few to power a final conclusion.

HMG used alone or in combination with HCG has not proven more effective than HCG alone [5, 31]. With a relatively high cost, need for frequent injections, and unproven efficacy of this treatment protocol, we do not currently recommend this therapy as an empiric treatment.

Recombinant FSH

Kamischke used recombinant FSH in their randomized, double blind, placebo-controlled trial of men with oligozoospermia and idiopathic infertility. Patients in this trial received placebo or 150 IU of rFSH daily for 12 weeks. They found no improvement of semen parameters or pregnancy rates in the rFSH group [32]. However, further studies need to be conducted to determine if there may be a role for FSH treatment to improve sperm quality and enhance fertilization by assisted reproductive technologies [22].

Androgens

Androgen administration is known to suppress spermatogenesis in the presence of an intact hypothalamic-pituitary-gonadal axis. Historically, the treatment of male infertility with androgens based upon theories of direct stimulation or a rebound effect has been used. However, continuous androgen administration has a contraceptive effect and diminishes spermatogenesis. Heller et al. in the 1950s were the first to describe the effect of exogenous testosterone on human testis [33]. After 10 weeks of androgen therapy, all patients became azoospermic. Many, but not all patients, had a return of their sperm counts to baseline levels within 6–18 months.

In the only placebo-controlled study of testosterone therapy to treat idiopathic oligozoospermia, Wang et al. showed no semen parameter improvement and no pregnancies [11]. Unfortunately, there is still evidence of widespread use of androgens among physicians who treat male infertility issues [34]. In a survey of practicing American Urological Association urologists, the authors found that 25 % of the respondents would give exogenous testosterone as an empiric treatment of an infertile male patient. Currently, there is no role for the use of testosterone in the treatment of idiopathic infertility. The bulk of available evidence suggests that testosterone therapy is in fact a potent inhibitor of spermatogenesis.

Conclusion

Of men who present with infertility, many will have an unexplained etiology. There is currently no consensus on the management of these men. Regarding the medical managements of such patients, within the practitioners' armamentarium exist estrogen receptor modulators, aromatase inhibitors, and gonadotropins. Exogenous androgens should not be used as an empiric treatment of the infertile patient. In this chapter, we have provided an overview and review of the evidence for and against these various treatments. The well-designed controlled studies remain to be performed in this area and will be critical to the proper selection and use of these agents to treat male factor infertility.

References

1. Sharlip I, Jarow J, Belker A, et al. Best practice policies for male infertility. Fertil Steril. 2002;77:873–82.
2. Nieschlag E. Classification of andrological disorders. In: Nieschlag E, Behre H, Nieschlag S, editors. Andrology: male reproductive health and dysfunction. 2nd edn. Berlin: Springer-Verlag; 1997 p 83–7.
3. Sigman M, Jarow JP. Endocrine evaluation of infertile men. Urology. 1997;50(5):659–64.
4. Cocuzza M, Agarwal A. Nonsurgical treatment of male infertility: specific and empiric therapy. Biologics. 2007;1:259.
5. Siddiq F, Sigman M. A new look at the medical management of infertility. Urol Clin N Am. 2002;29:949–63.
6. Willets AE, Corbo JM, Brown JN. Clomiphene for the treatment of male infertility. Reprod Sci. 2013;20:739.
7. Heller C, Rowley M, Heller G. Clomiphene Citrate: a correlation of its effects on sperm concentration and morphology, total gonadotrophin and testicular cytology in normal men. J Clin Endocrinol Metab. 1969;29:638–49.
8. Gilbaugh JH, Lipshultz L. Non-surgical treatment of male infertility. Urol Clin N Am. 1994;21:531.
9. Ghanem H, Shaeer O, El-Segini A. Combination clomphene citrate and antioxidant therapy for idiopathic male infertility: a randomized controlled trial. Fertil Steril. 2010;93:2232–5.
10. Moradi M, Moradi A, Alemi M, et al. Safety and efficacy of clomiphene citrate and L-carnitine in idiopathic male infertility; a comparative study. Urol J. 2010;7:188–193.
11. Wang C, Chan C, Wong K, et al. Comparison of the effectiveness of placebo, clomiphene citrate, mesterolone, pentoxifylline, and testosterone rebound therapy for the treatment of idiopathic oligospermia. Fertil Steril. 1983;40:358.
12. Check JH, Chase JS, Nowroozi K, et al. Empirical therapy of the male with clomiphene in couples with unexplained infertility. Int J Fertil. 1989;34:120.

13. Micic S, Dotlic R. Evaluation of sperm parameters in clinical trial with clomiphene citrate of oligospermic men. J Urol. 1985;133:221.
14. Abel BJ, Carswell G, Elton R, et al. Randomised trial of clomiphene citrate treatment and vitamin C for male infertility. Br J Urol. 1982;54(6):780–4.
15. Sokol R, Steiner BS, Bustillo M, et al. A controlled comparison of the efficacy of clomiphene citrate in male infertility. Fertil Steril. 1988;49(5):865–70.
16. World Health Organization (WHO). A double blind trial of clomiphene citrate for the treatment of idiopathic male infertility. Int J Androl. 1992;15(4):299–307.
17. Vandekerckhove P, Lilford R, Vail A, Hughes E, Hafez M. Clomiphene or tamoxifen for idiopathic oligo-asthnospermia review. Cochrane Database Syst Rev. 2007;4:CD 000151.
18. Buvat J, Ardaens K, Lemaire A, et al. Increased sperm counts in 25 cases of idiopathic normogonadotropic oligospermia following treatment with tamoxifen. Fertil Steril. 1983;39:700.
19. Bartsch G, Scheiber K. Tamoxifen treatment in oligospermia. Eur Urol. 1981;7:283.
20. Krause W, Holland-Moritz H, Schramm P. Treatment of idiopathic oligozoospermia with tamoxifen: a randomized controlled study. Int J Androl. 1992;15:14.
21. Ainmelk Y, Belisle S, Carmel M, et al. Tamoxifen citrate therapy in male infertility. Fertil Steril. 1987;48:113.
22. Liu PY, Handelsman DJ. The present and future state of hormonal treatment for male infertility. Hum Reprod Update. 2003;9(1):9–23.
23. Hussein A, Ozgok Y, Ross L, Niederberger C. Clomiphene administration for cases of nonobstructive azoospermia: a multicenter study. J Androl. 2005;26:787–91.
24. Hayes FJ, Seminara SB, et al. Aromatase inhibition in the human male reveals a hypothalamic site of estrogen feedback. J Clin Endocrinol Metab. 2000;84:3027–35.
25. Pavlovich CP, King P, Goldstein M, Schlegel PN. Evidence of a treatable endocrinopathy in infertile men. J Urol. 2009;165:837–41.
26. Hamada AJ, Montgomery B, Agarwal A. Male infertility: a critical review of pharmacologic management. Expert Opin Pharmacother. 2012;13(17):2511–31.
27. Raman JD, Schlegel PN. Aromatase inhibitors for male infertility. J Urol. 2002;167(2):624–9.
28. Clark RV, Sherins RJ. Treatment of men with idiopathic oligozoospermic infertility using the aromatase inhibitor, testolactone. Results of a double blinded, randomized, placebo-controlled trial with crossover. J Androl. 1989;10(3):240–7.
29. Knuth UA, Honigl W, et al. Treatment of severe oligospermia with human chorionic gonadotropin/human menopausal gonadotropin: a placebo-controlled, double blind trial. J Clin Endocrinol Metab. 1987;65(6):1081–7.
30. Attia AM, Al-Inany HG. Gonadotrophins for idiopathic male factor subfertility. Cochrane Database Syst Rev. 2007;4:CD 005071
31. Bodner DR. Critical review of pharmacologic therapies. Semin Reprod Endocrinol. 1988;6:377.
32. Kamischke A, Behre HM, Bergmann M, et al. Recombinant human follicle stimulating hormone for treatment of male idiopathic infertility: a randomized double blind, placebo-controlled, clinical trial. Hum Reprod. 1998;13:596–603.
33. Heller C, Nelson W, Hill I, et al. Improvement in spermatogenesis following depression of the human testis with testosterone. Fertil Steril. 1950;1:415.
34. Ko EY, Siddiqi K, Brannigan RE, Sabanegh ES. Empirical medial therapy for idiopathic male infertility: a survey of the American urological association. J Urol. 2012;187:973–8.

Clomiphene Citrate for Women with Unexplained Infertility

25

Richard P. Dickey

Introduction

The rationale for using CC alone or with IUI is that it may increase the number of eggs ovulated and correct subclinical ovulatory dysfunction such as a "luteal phase defect" [1]. Clomiphene citrate (CC) alone and CC combined with intrauterine insemination (IUI) are cost-effective treatments for unexplained infertility [2–4]. The advantages of CC over gonadotropins for ovulation induction (OI) include: a low incidence of multiple pregnancies and ovarian hyperstimulation syndrome (OHSS), low cost, oral administration, and less need for cycle monitoring. Numerous reports exist of an improvement in pregnancy rates for women with unexplained infertility treated with CC in randomized studies [5–8] although some studies did not find an improvement in pregnancy rates with CC or CC–IUI [9–11].

Administration of CC or IUI alone for three cycles, followed by CC plus IUI for three cycles, followed by low doses (<75 IU) of gonadotropin plus IUI for three cycles and finally by controlled ovarian hyperstimulation (COH) using higher doses of gonadotropin plus IUI was the traditional protocol for the treatment of unexplained infertility [4]. During the 1980s the traditional protocol was modified to include in vitro fertilization (IVF) after three unsuccessful cycles of COH–IUI. An important reason for use of CC or CC–IUI before COH is that it reduces the risk of twins and triplets and higher order multiple pregnancies (HOMP) [12, 13]. A recent alternative to the traditional protocol is to eliminate COH–IUI and proceed directly to IVF when pregnancy does not occur after three cycles of CC–IUI [14].

This chapter will describe why CC may be effective in treating unexplained infertility: when IUI is necessary, when tamoxifen (TMX) an analog of CC might be substituted for CC, the prerequisites for CC use to obtain optimal results, how long to use CC before progressing to COH or IVF, and how to minimize the risk of multiple pregnancies.

R. P. Dickey (✉)
The Fertility Institute, 800 N Causeway Blvd, Ste 2C, Mandeville, LA 70448, USA
e-mail: finooo@charter.net

Structure and Pharmacokinetics of Clomiphene and Tamoxifen (TMX)

Effective use of CC and TMX is enhanced by knowledge of their chemical structure and pharmacokinetics. CC and TMX are triphenyl ethylene stilbene derivatives with estrogenic or antiestrogen properties depending on the target tissue. They have nearly identical chemical structures and are related to TACE (chlorotrianisene), a nonsteroidal synthetic selective estrogen receptor modulators (SERM) that was formerly used for the treatment of menopause. CC is an isomeric mixture of ~38% *cis* isomer (zuclomiphene) and 62% *trans* isomer (enclomiphene). Enclomiphene is a partial estrogen agonist with antiestrogen properties whereas zuclomiphene is mildly estrogenic. TMX has only the *trans* isomer; 30 mg of TMX is approximately equal to 50 mg of CC for the purpose of ovulation induction. Both CC and TMX are competitive antagonists at the hypothalamic and pituitary estradiol receptor [15]. They also exhibit antiestrogenic activity at high doses and weak estrogenic activity at lower doses at peripheral receptor sites in the endometrium and cervical glands [15]. The antiestrogenic activity of CC is approximately three times greater than TMX.

The half life of CC in the plasma is 12 days [16]. Serum levels of zuclomiphene remain at least 10% of peak levels 28 days after ingestion of a single 50 mg tablet and small amounts of zuclomiphene continue to be excreted for at least 6 weeks [16]. When a single 50 mg tablet of CC is taken at 28-day intervals, basal levels of zuclomiphene increase by 50% per month [16]. The pharmacokinetics of TMX may be assumed to be similar to zuclomiphene. Because of its prolonged retention in the body CC may be more effective in inducing ovulation in the second and later cycles of treatment and in our experience, pregnancies due to CC may occur for up to two cycles after treatment has ended. It is also

G. L. Schattman et al. (eds.), *Unexplained Infertility*, DOI 10.1007/978-1-4939-2140-9_25,

possible that the antiestrogenic effect on the endometrium and cervical mucus may be intensified during the second and later cycles of treatment.

Blockade of estradiol receptors in the hypothalamus and pituitary increases gonadotropin-releasing hormone (GnRH) pulse frequency and pituitary sensitivity to GnRH [17, 18]. The net effect of these actions is that serum levels of FSH and LH increase three to fourfold during CC administration and for a few days after discontinuing CC [19]. In the ovary, multiple follicular developments are attenuated compared to COH due to lower levels of endogenous FSH in the early follicular phase because rising levels of estradiol suppress GnRH during the late follicular phase, similar to the occurrence in natural cycles.

Adverse Effects

The adverse effects of CC in addition to estrogen receptor blockade in endometrial and cervical tissues include hot flashes and scintillating scotoma. The reported increase in ovarian cancer after CC use was limited to women who took drugs for > 12 cycles without becoming pregnant [20]. That risk should be balanced against a 2.4-fold increased risk of ovarian cancer in women with a history of PCOS or nulliparity compared to controls [21]. The side effects of TMX when taken continuously for 5 years by women < 50 years of age for the prevention of breast cancer include a small (relative risk (RR)1.19) for endometrial cancer, an RR of 2.30 for deep vein thrombosis and an RR of 1.16 for pulmonary embolism [22]. There is no reason to believe that taking TMX for 5 days even when repeated for six cycles could result in an increased risk for these conditions.

How Clomiphene May Be Effective in the Treatment of Unexplained Infertility

The possibility of pregnancy and risk of multiple pregnancies are related to a woman's age, weight, the number of follicles that are 12 mm or larger at the time of spontaneous LH surge or hCG trigger and "fecundity per follicle." Fecundity per follicle is related to estradiol production per follicle which is a reflection of follicle development/size reflecting granulosa cell quantity and possibly quality. Because CC increases the number of preovulatory follicles, it also increases the quantity of granulosa cells in the late proliferative phase and progesterone levels are subsequently increased in the postovulatory luteal phase. Other factors positively or negatively related to CC effectiveness are endometrial receptivity, cervical mucus, and patient's weight.

Age

The effects of age on rates of single and multiple pregnancies in the authors' clinic are shown in Fig. 25.1a. For CC–IUI, pregnancy rates per cycle declined slowly from <28 to 41 years of age, and then more rapidly by 50% from age 42 to 44 [23]. Compared to CC–IUI, pregnancy rates per cycle were twice as high before age 32, for COH–IUI (human menopausal gonadotropin (hMG) IUI) and for CC + hMG – IUI (CC for 5 days followed by hMG for 3–4 days) but declined sharply thereafter and were identical to pregnancy rates for CC–IUI after age 37. However, these results may apply only to women with high antral follicle counts, e.g., PCOS. The incidence of multiple implantations in CC–IUI pregnancies was 15% before age 30 and 8–10% after age 30. No triplet implantations occurred after age 33 in CC–IUI cycles. The effectiveness of CC–IUI in unexplained infertility up to and including age 42 is also seen in Table 25.1 [24, 25]. Pregnancy rates per cycle through the first four cycles averaged 14.6% for age <35 and were still 12.1% for patients aged 38–42 when patients with endometriosis, tubal adhesions and < 5 million motile sperm were excluded.

Follicle Number and Size

The success of CC for unexplained infertility is in direct relationship to the number of preovulatory follicles > 10–12 mm at the time of LH surge or hCG trigger [23,

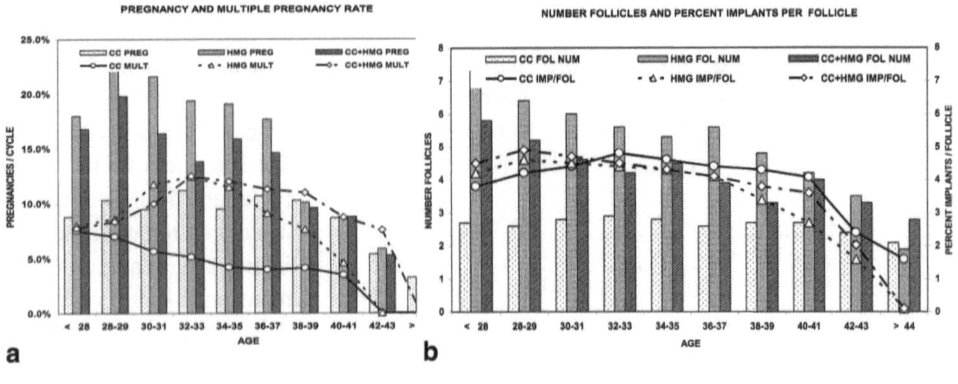

Fig. 25.1 Relationship to age. **a** Pregnancy rate (*horizontal bars*) and multiple implantation rates (*lines*) per cycle. **b** Number of follicles > 12 mm (*horizontal bars*) implants per follicle (*lines*) [24]

Table 25.1 Patient factors: Mean pregnancy rate cycles 1–4 ([24] with permission from Elsevier)

	Cycles	Pregnancies (%)	Odds ratio (95 % CI)
Diagnosis[a]			
Ovulatory dysfunction	1075	157 (14.6)	1.01 (0.86–1.44)
Polycystic ovaries	884	118 (13.3)	–
Luteal insufficiency	191	39 (20.4)	1.67 (1.12–2.49)*
Endometriosis	1102	89 (8.1)	0.57 (0.43–0.76)**
Tubal factor	279	16 (5.7)	0.39 (0.27–0.59)**
Other	354	37 (10.4)	0.76 (0.51–1.12)
Age[b]			
<30	431	63 (14.6)	–
30–34	604	84 (13.9)	0.94 (0.66–1.34)
35–37	221	26 (11.8)	0.78 (0.48–1.27)
38–42	173	21 (12.1)	0.81 (0.48–1.37)
≥ 43	53	2 (3.8)	0.29 (0.07–1.23)
Semen quality and source[c]			
WHO	410	53 (12.9)	–
IUI threshold	527	60 (11.4)	0.86 (0.58–1.28)
Sub-IUI threshold	186	6 (3.2)	0.22 (0.10–0.53)**
Donor	492	81 (16.5)	1.32 (0.91–1.93)
Number follicles >15 mm[d]			
1	377	37 (9.8)	–
2	286	41 (14.3)	1.54 (0.96–2.47)
≥3	215	38 (17.7)	1.97 (1.21–3.12)**

[a] Patients' age ≥43 and cycles with total initial motile sperm count <5 million or motility <30 % excluded
[b] Patients with endometriosis, tubal impairment, and cycles with total initial motile sperm count <5 million or motility <30 % excluded
[c] Patients' age ≥43, and patients with endometriosis and tubal factor excluded
[d] Patients' age ≥43, patients with endometriosis and tubal factor, and cycles with total initial motile sperm count <5 million or motility <30 % excluded

Table 25.2 Pregnancy results per cycle: clomiphene vs. HMG/FSH [49]

	Clomiphene[b,c]	HMG/FSH[b,d]
Number follicles ≥12 mm	2.7	6.4
Pregnancy rate	8–12 %	16–24 %
Twin births	10%	20 %
Triplets or more	0.07%	4 %[a]

[a] 20 % if age <32 and ≥7 follicles >10 mm
[b] Dickey et al. 2001
[c] Dickey et al. 2002
[d] Dickey et al. 2005

24]. CC increases the number of preovulatory follicles. The number of preovulatory follicles ≥12 mm averaged 2.7 in CC–IUI cycles and 6.4 in COH–IUI cycles from three combined studies (Table 25.2). The average pregnancy rates per cycle, 10–12 % for CC–IUI and 16–24 % for COH–IUI were proportional to the number of preovulatory follicles. The rate of twin pregnancy was 10 % for CC–IUI and 20 % for COH–IUI, and triplet and higher order rates per pregnancy were also proportional to the number of follicles ≥12 mm.

There was no difference in implantation rates per larger follicle between CC–IUI and COH–IUI (Fig. 25.1b). In a retrospective study of 1333 CC–IUI cycles that also included 803 COH–IUI cycles and 594 CC + hMG − IUI cycles, the number of follicles ≥12 mm and implantation rate per follicle ≥12 mm remained constant in CC–IUI cycles (average 2.7) from age <28 until age 41 [23]. In contrast, in COH–IUI cycles the number of follicles decreased from a mean of 7.3 before age 28 to 3.5 for ages 42–43 and was less than CC–IUI for women >44 years. This study demonstrated that follicle number may be the most important predictor of outcome in age-matched patients. Those who develop two, four, six, or more preovulatory follicles in CC–IUI cycles have the same chance of becoming pregnant or having multiple pregnancies as patients who develop two, four, six, or more preovulatory follicles in COH–IUI cycles.

Preovulatory Estradiol

Serum estradiol levels in the late proliferative phase are significantly higher during CC cycles than during control cycles [26]. Serum estradiol levels on the day of hCG trigger parallel the number of follicles ≥12 mm and reflect granulosa cell quantity and possibly quality [23]. The average estradiol level on the day of hCG trigger was 613 pg/ml in 524 CC–IUI cycles and 1194 pg/ml in 60 COH–IUI cycles performed for unexplained or male factor infertility, but the estradiol level per follicle ≥12 mm was similar, 254 pg/ml per follicle in patients using CC and 278 pg/ml per follicle in patients using gonadotropins [27]. The implantation rate per follicle was doubled when estradiol levels were ≥400 pg/ml compared to ≤200 pg/ml in both groups.

Luteal Phase Progesterone and Estradiol

One rationale for using CC in unexplained infertility and possibly an explanation of how it may work is that it increases mid-luteal phase progesterone levels. Several studies have shown that luteal phase deficiency, whether characterized by low peak progesterone levels, short luteal phase, or delayed endometrial development is corrected by CC [28–31]. In one randomized placebo controlled study, CC increased mid-luteal progesterone levels 66 % (from 43 to 71 nmol/l) and 3-month cumulative pregnancy rates 53 % (from 14.6 to 22.3 %) [7]. The definition of normal progesterone in the luteal phase is a subject of controversy since progesterone is secreted in a pulsatile fashion in relation to pituitary LH release. Wide fluctuations of serum progesterone levels are possible within the same patient depending on whether the blood is drawn during the peak or nadir of the pulse. Progesterone levels after hCG trigger and pregnancy should be more consistent since hCG has a longer half life than LH. Progesterone levels in the mid-luteal phase of spontaneous cycles that result in term pregnancies average 2200 ng/dL (22 pg/ml). According to this author's experience, progesterone levels in the mid-luteal phase, less than 1800 ng/dL (18 pg/ml) are evidence of possible luteal insufficiency, levels less than 1500 ng/dL (15 pg/ml) are infrequently associated with ongoing pregnancy [32].

Progesterone levels in CC cycles that result in term pregnancies average 3700 ng/dL (37 pg/ml) [33, 34]. The increased progesterone levels in response to CC persist throughout the first trimester of pregnancy. During the first 6 gestational weeks (4 weeks postovulation) serum progesterone levels are 200–300 % higher in CC pregnancies than in natural cycle pregnancies [33]. After the sixth gestational week levels decrease gradually but remain 50–70 % higher than in natural cycle pregnancies through at least the 14th gestational week.

Serum estradiol levels average 66 % higher in CC than in natural cycle pregnancies during the first to second week postovulation and remain so until at least the 14th gestational week. The increases in estradiol and progesterone levels in CC pregnancies are accompanied by an average 25 % increase in uterine artery (UA) blood flow volume during the first 8 weeks of pregnancy [33, 34]. Crown rump length during the first 8 weeks in IVF pregnancies that resulted in a live birth is positively related to UA blood flow [35].

Endometrium Thickness and Pattern

Endometrial thickness and pattern on the day of the spontaneous LH surge or hCG administration are associated with implantation success or failure [27, 36, 37]. Conception rarely occurs in CC and CC–IUI cycles when endometrial thickness is <6 mm on the day of spontaneous LH surge or hCG to trigger ovulation (Table 25.3 [27, 37]). Estradiol receptor content in the endometrium is 45 % lower during the late proliferative cycle in patients using CC compared to controls [26]. Endometrial glands in biopsies from patients treated with CC are described as narrower, less tortuous than normal, and having a decreased gland-to-stroma ratio [37–39].

The effect of CC on the endometrium is paradoxical. Studies of the effect of CC on the mid-luteal phase endometrium are suggestive of both an antiestrogen effect and progesterone deficiency. In the early proliferative phase of CC cycles, average endometrial thickness is decreased compared to natural cycles whereas one day after the LH surge, endometrial thickness is increased compared to natural cycles [31, 40]. The thinner endometrium in the early and late proliferative phases and thicker endometrium in the luteal phase of CC cycles may be explained by the declining levels of CC at the level of the estrogen receptors in the endometrium and by the rising levels of estradiol displacing CC from those receptors.

The luteal phase endometrial pattern seen on ultrasound (US) during CC cycles is less likely to be totally hyperechoic and more likely to show a center stripe (triple line pattern) compared to controls [26]. Conception rates in CC cycles are highest in patients who retained a central lumen and less than 50 % hyperechoic pattern in the mid-secretory phase which

Table 25.3 Endometrial thickness vs. outcome in OI– IUI cycles [27, 37]

			Pregnancy outcome		
Thickness (mm)	*Percent of total cycles* (%)	*Pregnancy rate* (%)	*Biochemical* (%)	*Miscarriage* (%)	*Term* (%)
<6	9.1	0	0	0	0
6–8	42.6	8.1	21.4	15.4	62.5
≥9	47.2	14.0	0	12.2	87.8

Table 25.4 Effect of switching patients from clomiphene to tamoxifen because of thin endometrium. (Based on data from Fertility Institute of New Orleans, unpublished)

	Clomiphene 100 mg	Tamoxifen 60 mg
Estradiol pg/ml	1231	840
Progesterone ng/mL	21.3	26.3
Follicles ≥ 18 mm	1.1	0.8
Follicles ≥ 10 mm	3.0	1.3
Total follicles	10.1	14.0
Endometrium mm	7.4	9.2
Endometrium < 8.0 mm	73 %	21 %

suggests delayed transformation to a typical secretory phase pattern.

In patients who were switched from CC to TMX because of a thin endometrium, average endometrial thickness increased by 23 % despite the fact that estradiol levels were 32 % lower (Table 25.4).

Cervical Mucus

Sperm penetration and passage through the mucus are necessary for conception to occur with intercourse. Alterations of cervical mucus during CC use have been identified in up to 60 % of cycles [41–48]. While the validity of a postcoital test (PCT) has been questioned, cervical factor infertility, diagnosed by the failure to find any motile sperm on a PCT performed 12–18 h after intercourse during the mid- to late follicular phase and repeated 1–2 days later if abnormal was identified as the primary cause for failure to conceive after three or more cycles of CC and timed intercourse in 39 % of patients referred for COH–IUI [49]. Less than 20 directionally motile sperm is associated with moderately decreased possibility of pregnancy in the same cycle. Less than 5 motile sperm or no motile sperm is associated with markedly decreased possibility of pregnancy in the same cycle [50]. In a randomized comparative study of the effect of CC and TMX on cervical mucus, quantity, viscosity, ferning, spinnbarkeit and cellularity were all significantly decreased in the CC group compared to controls, while quantity, viscosity, and spinnbarkeit were significantly increased compared to controls in the TMX group [48]. The number of directionally motile sperm decreased from 6.7 per high-powered field (hpf) in the control cycle to 3.2 in the CC cycle. An increase from 11.0 motile sperm/HPF in the control cycle to 12.2 in the TMX cycle was not significant. Other studies showed no difference between cervical mucous alterations with either CC or TMX [47, 51, 52] or a decrease in mucus score for TMX compared to placebo [53].

The hostile effect of CC on cervical mucus was unrelated to serum estradiol levels in cycles in which 150 mg CC was given cycle days 3 through 7 [54]. Another study found no difference in unfavorable cervical mucus scores in patients receiving CC doses of 50, 100, and 150–200 mg [55]. Based on these results, it would appear that the empirical use of supplemental estrogen and use of a lower dose of CC would have little effect on improving cervical mucus or poor sperm penetration. However, a dose of 25 mg CC, which would be approximately equal to 20 mg TMX, was not tested.

One approach to potentially improve cervical mucus in the face of unsatisfactory cervical mucus identified during a CC cycle is to start CC earlier. In women with regular ovulatory cycles, CC may be started on the third cycle day to obviate the antiestrogenic effects of CC which diminishes with each day after finishing the 5-day course of CC [16]. Other methods that have been evaluated in an effort to improve cervical mucus in natural as well as OI cycles are the use of guaifenesin and an alkaline douche [56, 57].

Despite some differences of opinion, the consensus opinion is that sperm penetration of cervical mucus is significantly decreased in a large enough proportion of women who take CC that pregnancy rates may be less than expected. Although the value of a PCT has been questioned to identify cervical mucus–sperm interaction abnormalities, it could be argued that one should be performed during the first cycle of CC. Rather than perform a PCT to determine if IUI is needed, some practitioners choose to perform IUI in all CC cycles. Whether the slight additional cost and inconvenience to the infertile couple of performing a PCT to determine if performance or referral to a more costly and inconvenient IUI is indicated is a decision for the physician. Some clinicians reserve IUI for patients who fail to conceive after two or three CC cycles with timed intercourse.

Weight

Elevated BMI as well as ovulatory disorders in obese women have been implicated in infertility. Overweight women often need higher doses of CC to become pregnant. The dose of CC needed for conception was related to weight in a retrospective study in which CC was started at 50 mg for 5 days and increased by 50 mg each cycle until a satisfactory ovarian response was evident by both a biphasic basal temperature and a mid-luteal progesterone ≥2000 ng/dL, or conception occurred, to a maximum dose of 250 mg a day [34]. CC (100 mg) was used during the cycle of conception in 48 % of patients who weighed ≥ 90 kg (> 198 lb), 45 % who weighed 75–89 kg (165–197 lbs), 37 % who weighed 60–74 kg (132–164 lbs), and 31 % who weighed between 45–60 kg (100–132 lbs). Amounts of CC > 100 mg were used during the cycle of conception in 27 % of patients who weighed ≥90 kg (198 lb), 18 % who weighed 75–89 kg (165–197 lbs), 17 % who weighed 60–74 kg (132–164 lbs), and 11 % who weighed 45–60 kg (100–132 lbs).

Achieving Optimal Results with CC in Unexplained Infertility

Failure of CC to improve pregnancy rates may be due to the presence of other endocrine abnormalities, fertilization failure due to functional sperm or oocyte abnormalities, tubal dysfunction or cervical mucus abnormalities or other unidentified factors. Failure may also be due to improper timing of intercourse or IUI. Endocrine abnormalities that cause suboptimal ovulation may adversely affect mother or baby during pregnancy. TSH and fasting insulin and glucose in anovulatory patients and in selected ovulatory patients should be measured. Dehydroepiandrosterone sulfate (DHEAS), testosterone, and 17 OH progesterone should be measured for clinical evidence of excess androgen. If no or insufficient sperm are present in a well-timed PCT with a normal mucus specimen taken from within the cervical canal, IUI should be performed for up to three cycles. In order to achieve optimal results with CC and to avoid HOMP, US and hormone monitoring should be performed to find the lowest ovulatory dose of CC and to identify patients with ≥3 preovulatory follicles.

Cycle Days 3–5: Ultrasound and Hormone Measurement

US should be performed before starting OI to rule out ovarian cysts and endometrial or uterine pathology and to determine an antral follicle count. The number of antral follicles at the start of OI is related to the average number of preovulatory follicles ≥12 mm and oocytes retrieved and fertilized in IVF cycles; however, the number of preovulatory follicles developing in response to CC is often only a small fraction of the total depending on the dose used and sensitivity of the follicles [58].

Serum estradiol levels need to be ≥50 pg/ml for CC to be effective. This level of estradiol is ordinarily attained by the third cycle day in normally cycling young women but may not be reached until the fifth day or later in older women and women with polycystic ovarian syndrome (PCOS). Serum progesterone levels ≥90 ng/dL are related to continuing activity of the corpus luteum which may inhibit or delay follicle development. Starting CC before these levels are attained may result in reduced numbers or no follicles developing as well as endometrial alterations. Delaying the start of CC until early follicular hormone levels are in the desired range will increase the chance of successful stimulation and outcome.

Preovulation (Days 10–12) Ultrasound and Hormone Measurement

A US performed 5–7 days after the last CC dose will show the number of follicles with the potential for ovulation, how soon ovulation is likely to occur, and the condition of the endometrium. Development of a single follicle ≥12 mm occurs in 21 %, one or two follicles ≥12 mm in 53 %, and three or more follicles ≥12 mm in 47 % of CC cycles [23]. If more than two follicles are ≥12 mm in women less than 31 years, there is a risk of triplet or higher order pregnancy. Lead follicles normally grow 2.0 mm/day in the late follicular phase. Overall, the risk of twin births with CC is 8–10 % and triplets 0.2 %.

Estradiol levels should be ≥200 ± 50 pg/ml per follicle ≥14 mm. Lower levels suggest decreased granulosa cell numbers or quality. Endometrial thickness should be ≥8 mm and should have a triple line pattern. A completely hyperechoic endometrial pattern and serum progesterone levels > 100 ng/dL indicate premature lutenization.

Mid-luteal Phase (5–7 Days After Ovulation) Ultrasound and Hormone Measurement

According to the authors' experience, a single progesterone level less than 1800 ng/dL (18 pg/ml) is evidence of a possible luteal insufficiency. Estradiol levels in the mid-luteal phase should be ≥180 pg/ml when progesterone is 1800 ng/dL or 18 pg/ml (1/10 or 10/1 ratio). Low levels of both estradiol and progesterone indicate deficient granulosa cell numbers or activity. If only progesterone is low and estradiol is ≥180 pg/ml, the problem could be a hemorrhagic, otherwise impaired corpus luteum or the possibility that progesterone was measured at the nadir. In either case, progesterone supplementation in the current cycle is indicated and the dose of CC should be increased in 50 mg increments in subsequent cycles. The frequency of progesterone supplementation is equally important as the dose and depends on the route of administration: if IM daily, if vaginal twice daily, if oral 3–4 times a day [59]. Endometrial thickness <9 mm may be corrected by adding supplemental estrogen in an ongoing cycle, and by switching to TMX or decreasing the dose of CC in subsequent cycles. However, a retrospective analysis of patients who were taking 25–250 mg CC the cycle of conception found no relationship between the dose of CC and thickness of the endometrial lining on the day of hCG trigger or spontaneous LH surge [34].

Adjunctive Treatment

Human Chorionic Gonadotropin

Human chorionic gonadotropin (hCG) to trigger ovulation is rarely necessary in CC cycles but can be used to time IUI or intercourse (TI) for the convenience of the couple. Ovulation normally occurs 36–40 h after hCG injection. Use of hCG does not increase multiple pregnancies [60].

Addition of Dexamethasone

Adding dexamethasone to CC cycles in patients with and without evidence of adrenal androgen excess (increased DHEAS concentrations) significantly improves ovulation and pregnancy rates compared to CC alone; however, it also increased multiple pregnancy rates [61]. In addition to suppressing adrenal androgen, dexamethasone may partially negate the antiestrogen effect of CC on the endometrium [62]. Dexamethasone is administered as a single 0.5 mg tablet at bedtime from cycle day one until 6 days after ovulation. Addition of dexamethasone should be considered when the number of preovulatory follicles developed in response to CC is fewer than desired and when DHEAS levels are > 180.

Addition of Metformin

Metformin improves ovulation in women with insulin resistance and hyperandrogenism associated with PCOS resistant to CC according to a systematic review of multiple small prospective randomized studies [63]. However, in a large randomized prospective study of anovulatory infertile women who were not CC resistant metformin alone at a maximum dose of 1000 mg per day was less effective in inducing ovulation (7 % live births) compared to CC alone (23 % live births) or the combination of metformin and CC (27 % live births) [64]. Despite conflicting results, the combination of metformin and CC may be tried in patients who are resistant to CC before switching to gonadotropins because of its low incidence of multiple pregnancies.

Treatment Results

The European Society of Human Reproduction and Endocrinology (ESHRE) workshop concluded that ovarian stimulation with CC doubled the pregnancy rate in women with unexplained infertility [65]. An analysis by the Practice Committee of the American Society of Reproductive Medicine in 1998 of the effectiveness of different empiric regimens for unexplained infertility reported in 45 studies found the clinical pregnancy rate per cycle to be 5.6 % for CC alone and 8.3 % for CC–IUI compared to 1.3–3.4 % for no treatment [3]. A Cochrane systemic review in 1996 found that CC increases the likelihood of ovulation tenfold and pregnancy sixfold compared to placebo in oligo-amenorrhic women [66]. A meta-analysis of CC with and without IUI for treatment of unexplained infertility found a 2.5-fold increase in pregnancies for CC [8]. A later 2010 Cochrane review by the same authors found that CC and CC–IUI were no more effective than no treatment or placebo for women with regular ovulatory cycles [10]. A 2011 study of 580 women in Scotland with unexplained infertility found no advantage for CC alone or IUI alone compared to expectant management [11]. In sum these studies indicate that the efficacy of CC alone unexplained infertility may be limited to women with ovulation defects.

A possible cause of the discrepancies between older and newer studies was the failure to detect ovulation defects when the finding was a low mid-luteal phase progesterone and the failure to detect defective sperm-cervical mucus penetration by not performing a PCT (Chap. 21). These two infertility factors for which CC and CC–IUI have been shown to be effective may together account for more than 60 % of unexplained infertility (Chap. 21). The results of CC–IUI at the Fertility Institute of New Orleans arranged according to diagnosis, age, sperm source and quality, and number of preovulatory follicles are shown in Table 25.1. The average pregnancy rate was 9.2 % per cycle through the first four cycles of CC–IUI and ranged from a low 3.2 % per cycle for male factor infertility to 20.4 % per cycle for patients diagnosed with luteal insufficiency. [24]. The pregnancy rate for "Other," mostly poor PCT averaged 10.4 % through four cycles for patients with age < 43 with normal semen analysis, normal cycles including progesterone levels ≥ 1800 ng/dL before CC, and absence of findings of endometriosis or tubal adhesions/obstruction.

In oligo-ovulatory and anovulatory women with no known tubal disease and partners with normal semen analysis, TMX and CC are equally effective with respect to pregnancies per cycle (OR 1.06) but achieve equal effectiveness in different ways [67]. Mean preovulation follicle numbers per cycle are fewer for TMX than for CC (OR 0. 76), but pregnancies per cycle are greater for TMX (OR 1.16).

Length of Treatment

The number of cycles that CC or CC–IUI should be continued with a good possibility of success before switching to COH–IUI or recommending IVF depends on the patients' age, the number of preovulatory follicles and the presumptive diagnosis. Cumulative pregnancy rates through six cycles of CC–IUI at the Fertility Institute of New Orleans are shown

(Fig. 25.2a–d; [24]). Cumulative pregnancy rates after six cycles reached 65 % for patients with ovulatory dysfunction and 38 % for "Other" (unexplained infertility the majority of which were related to abnormal cervical mucus); however, no pregnancies occurred after the fourth cycle for patients in the other/unexplained infertility category. In patients >43 years of age pregnancies did not occur after three cycles. Patients ages 30-42 continued to become pregnant through six cycles, but at a lower rate per cycle after cycle four. Patients with persistent mono-follicular cycles did not become pregnant after the fourth cycle. Most patients with age <30, unless they had other undiscovered problems, will become pregnant during the first four cycles of CC or CC–IUI.

Based on results from 3381 cycles, CC and/or CC–IUI may be continued for a minimum of four cycles in appropriate patients with some exceptions (severe sperm factor, age ≥43) before recommending COH–IUI, and may be continued longer than four cycles if the diagnosis is ovulatory dysfunction. In agreement with this recommendation, the authors of a 2008 multicenter retrospective cohort analysis of 15,303 cycles of IUI, 51 % of which were CC–IUI cycles, and a 5.6 % ongoing pregnancy rate per cycle, concluded that there was no rationale for stopping IUI before nine cycles had been completed [68].

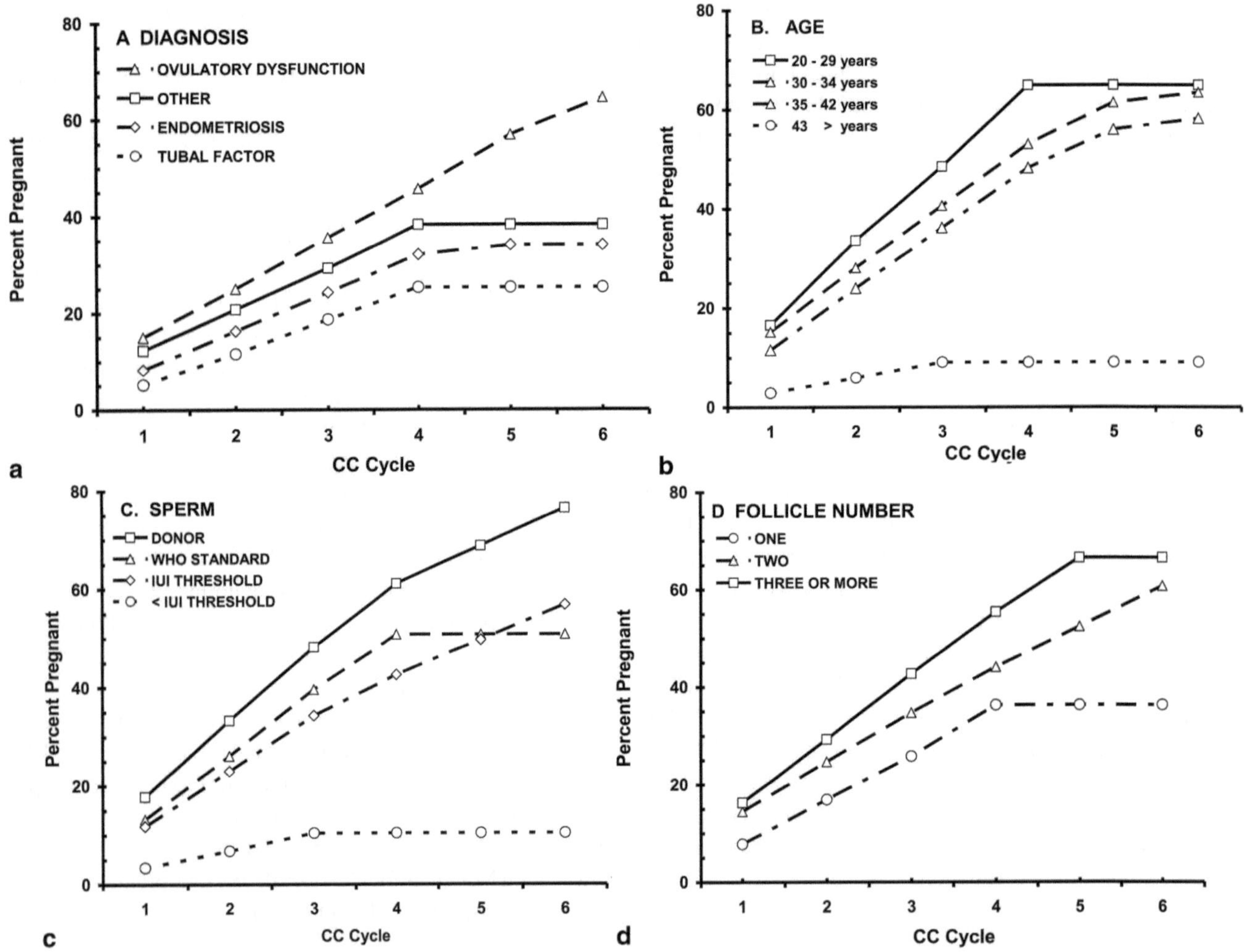

Fig. 25.2 Cumulative pregnancy rate: **a** Diagnosis: ovulatory dysfunction = anovulatory, polycystic ovaries, or luteal insufficiency; endometriosis = with or without tubal involvement; tubal factor = unilateral tubal obstruction or tubal adhesions without endometriosis; other = cervical factor, male factor, or unexplained infertility and normal cycles without endometriosis or tubal factor. Patients, age >43 and cycles with total initial motile sperm count <5 million or motility <30 % excluded. **b** Age, patients with endometriosis, tubal impairment, and cycles with total initial motile sperm count <5 million or motility <30 % excluded. **c** Cumulative pregnancy rate: sperm, WHO; initial sperm quality >World Health Organization (1992) criteria of 20 million concentration, 40 million total count, 50 % progressive motility, 30 % normal forms. IUI threshold; initial sperm quality less than WHO criteria but >5 million total motile sperm and >30 % initial motility (the threshold for recommending IUI rather than IVF. Dickey Fertil Steril 1999;71:684–9) Sub IUI—threshold; initial motile sperm count <5 million or motility <30 %. Patients age >43, and patients with endometriosis and tubal factor excluded. **d** Follicle number, patients age >43, and patients with endometriosis and tubal factor, and cycles with total initial motile sperm count <5 million or motility <30 % excluded ([24]; with permission from Elsevier)

Avoidance of Multiple Pregnancies

A common misconception left over from early abdominal US studies of spontaneous cycles in which a single dominant follicle was present is that only follicles >18–20 mm containing a mature egg can result in pregnancy. In a prospective observational study of 4062 COH–IUI cycles, follicles as small as 10 mm on the day of spontaneous LH surge or hCG trigger contributed to triplet pregnancies [69]. It is necessary to count all follicles >10 mm to assess the risk of triplet and higher order pregnancies (Table 25.5). Triplet and higher order pregnancies occurred in 15% of cycles when there were fewer than 3 follicles >12 mm, 45% of cycles with fewer than three follicles >14 mm, 72% of cycles with fewer than three follicles >16 mm, and 92% of cycles with fewer than three follicles >18 mm. Development of a single follicle >12 mm occurs in 21%, one or two follicles >12 mm in 53%, and three or more follicles >12 mm in 47% of CC cycles [23]. Failure to count follicles smaller than 16 mm is the principal reason why attempts to prevent all HOMP were made by canceling cycles [70].

Because of the higher risk of complications during pregnancy with a twin gestation, twin pregnancies should be avoided if possible, especially in women at increased risk for preterm birth due to obesity, small stature, uterine anomalies, and previous preterm birth [71]. In the USA, 11% of twins are born before completion of 32 weeks and 54% of infant deaths occur in infants born at <32 weeks of gestation [72, 73]. The use of CC alone and CC–IUI increases the risk of multiple pregnancies; primarily of twins (Table 25.2 [23, 24, 69]). Twin births occur in 10% of CC–IUI and 20% of COH–IUI cycles. Triplet and higher orders births occurred in .07% of CC and 4% of COH–IUI cycles. However, for women age <31 and treated with COH–IUI, triplet birth increased to 20% if they developed seven or more preovulatory follicles >10 mm. Twin and higher order pregnancies can be prevented when using OI to treat unexplained infertility by use of CC for four or more cycles before COH and by not performing IUI and cautioning couples not to have sexual intercourse when one or more than two preovulatory follicles are present. COH–IUI only doubles the average pregnancy rate per cycle compared to CC–IUI but greatly increases the risk of triplets and HOMPs. Because the difference in pregnancies can be made up by two or three additional cycles of CC–IUI, using COH–IUI is a high price to pay in order to achieve pregnancy more rapidly.

Table 25.5 Follicle size and prediction of triplet and higher order pregnancies ([69]; with permission from Elsevier)

Percentage of triplet pregnancies		
Follicle size (mm)	<3 follicles (%)	≥3 follicles (%)
≥10	0	100
≥12	15	85
≥14	45	55
≥16	72	18
≥18	92	8

Summary

Successful use of CC for treatment of unexplained infertility is a contradiction because it is only successful if the cause of infertility is suboptimal ovulation (insufficient preovulation stimulation of follicle and oocyte development) identifiable by low estradiol levels per follicle or inadequate endometrial development which can be discovered by US evaluation of endometrial thickness and pattern or histology, assisted by mid-luteal progesterone and estradiol levels. Likewise, if sperm count and motility are normal, IUI is only successful if motile sperm cannot pass through the cervical mucus which can be gleaned by a PCT. Nonetheless, ovulation induction with CC alone or with IUI, is an effective and relatively inexpensive first line treatment when a semen analysis is normal, tubal patency is confirmed, and menstrual cycles are regular. It can also be used before confirmation of tubal patency when there is no history or findings to suggest past sexually transmitted disease, pelvic surgery, or endometriosis. Its use should be limited to three or at most four cycles with some exceptions based on age and number of preovulation follicles that develop during treatment, before moving on to more aggressive treatment with gonadotropins. The American Society for Reproductive Medicine recommends moving rapidly to more aggressive therapy for women nearing the end of their reproductive years. Pregnancy rates may be improved and the risk of multiple pregnancies reduced by US and hormone monitoring.

References

1. Dickey RP, Holtkamp D. Development, pharmacology, and clinical experience with clomiphene citrate. Hum Reprod Rev. 1996;2:485–506.
2. Karande VC, Korn A, Morris R, Rao R, Balin M, Rinehart J, et al. Prospective randomized trial comparing the outcome and cost of in vitro fertilization with that of a traditional treatment algorithm as first-line therapy for couples with infertility. Fertil Steril. 1999;71:468–75.
3. Guzick DS, Sullivan MW, Adamson GD, Cedars MI, Falk RJ, Peterson EP, Strinkampf MP. Efficacy of treatment for unexplained infertility. Fertil Steril. 1998;70:207–13.
4. Practice Committee of the American Society for Reproductive Medicine. Effectiveness and treatment for unexplained infertility. Fertil Steril. 2006;86(Suppl 4):S111–4.
5. Deaton JL, Nakajima ST, Gibson M, Badger GJ, Blackmer KM, Brumsted JR. A randomized, controlled trial of clomiphene citrate and intrauterine insemination in couples with unexplained infertility or surgically corrected endometriosis. Fertil Steril. 1990;54:1083–8.

6. Collins JA, Milner RA, Rowe TC. The effect of treatment on pregnancy among couples with unexplained infertility. Int. J. Fertil. 1991;36:140–52.
7. Glazner CMA, Coulson C, Lambert PA, Watt EM, Hinton RA, Kelly NG, et al. Clomiphene treatment for women with unexplained infertility: placebo-controlled study of hormonal responses and conception rates. Gynecol Endocrinol. 1990;4:75–83.
8. Hughes EG, Vandekerckhove P. Clomiphene citrate vs placebo or no treatment. In Unexplained subfertility. Oxford: BMJ Publishing Group, Cochrane Library; 1996. (Review number 0002).
9. Fujii S, Fukui A, Kagiya A, Sato S, Saito Y. The effects of clomiphene citrate on normally ovulatory women. Fertil Steril. 1997;68:997–9.
10. Hughes EG, Brown J, Collins JJ, Vandekerckhove P. Clomiphene citrate for unexplained infertility in women. Cochrane Database Syst Rev. 2010;20(CD000057):1–29.
11. Wordsworth S, Buchanan J, Mollison J, Harrild K, Robertson L, Tay C, et al. Clomiphene citrate and intrauterine insemination as first line treatments for unexplained infertility: are they cost-effective? Hum Reprod. 2011;36:369–75.
12. Dickey RP, Taylor NN, Lu PY, Sartor MM, Pyrzak, R. Clomiphene citrate intrauterine insemination (IUI) before gonadotropin IUI affects the pregnancy rate and high order multiple pregnancy. Fertil Steril. 2004;81:545–50.
13. Dickey RP. Strategies to reduce multiple pregnancies due to ovulation stimulation. Modern trends. Fertil Steril. 2009;91:1–17.
14. Reindollar RH, Regan MM, Neumann PJ, et al. A randomized clinical trial to evaluate optimal treatment for unexplained infertility: the fast tract and standard treatment (FASTT) trial. Fertil Steril. 2010;94:888–9.
15. Furr BJA, Jordan VC. The pharmacology and clinical uses of tamoxifen. Pharmacol Ther. 1984;25:127–205.
16. Mikkelson TJ, et al. Single-dose pharmacokinetics of clomiphene citrate in normal volunteers. Fertil Steril. 1986;46:392–6.
17. Kerin JF, Liu JH, Phillipou G, Yen SSC. Evidence for a hypothalamic site of action of clomiphene citrate in women. J Clin Endocrinol Metab. 1985;61:265–8.
18. Hsueh AJW, Erickson GF, Yen SSC. Sensitization of pituitary cells to luteinizing hormone releasing hormone by clomiphene citrate in vitro. Nature. 1978;273:57–9
19. Dickey RP, Vorys N, Stevens VC, Hamwi G, Ullery JC. Observations on the mechanism of action of clomiphene (MRL 41). Fertil Steril. 1965;16:485–94.
20. Rossing MA, Daling JR, Weiss NS, et al. Ovarian tumors in a cohort of infertile women. N Engl J Med. 1994;331:771–6.
21. Schildkraut JM, Schwingle PJ, Bastos E, et al. Epithelial ovarian cancer risk among women with polycystic ovary syndrome. Obstet Gynecol. 1996;88:554–9.
22. Iqbal J, Ginsburg OM, Wijeratne D, Howekk A, Evans G, Sestak I, et al. Endometrial cancer and venous thromboembolism in women under age 50 who take tamoxifen for prevention of breast cancer: a systematic review. Cancer Treat Rev. 2012;38:318–28.
23. Dickey RP, Taylor SN, Lu PY, Sartor BM, Rye PH, Pyrzak R. Relationship of follicle numbers and estradiol concentrations to multiple implantation of 3608 intrauterine insemination cycles. Fertil Steril. 2001;75:69–78
24. Dickey RP, Taylor NN, Lu PY, Sartor MM, Rye PH, Pyrzak R. Effect of diagnosis, age, sperm quality, and number of preovulatory follicles on the outcome of multiple cycles of clomiphene citrate-intrauterine insemination. Fertil Steril. 2002;78;1088–95.
25. Dickey RP, Taylor SN, Rye PH, Lu PY, Pyrzak R. Comparison of sperm quality resulting in successful intrauterine insemination to world health organization threshold values for normal sperm. Fertil Steril. 1999;71:684–9.
26. Nakamura Y, Sugino N, Ono M, Ueda K, Yoshida Y, Kato H. Effects of clomiphene citrate on the endometrial thickness and echogenic pattern of the endometrium. Fertil Steril. 1997;67:256–60.
27. Dickey RP, Olar TT, Taylor SN, Curole DN, Harrigill K. Relationship of biochemical pregnancy to preovulatory endometrial thickness and pattern in patients undergoing ovulation induction. Hum Reprod. 1993;8:327–30.
28. Vuorento T, Rarsula K, Hovatta O, Huhtaniemi I, Kurunmäki H. Measurements of salivary progesterone throughout the menstrual cycle in women suffering from unexplained infertility revel high frequency of luteal phase defects. Fertil Steril. 1990;54:211–6.
29. Finn MM, Goling JP, Tallon DF, Meehan FP, Fottrell PF. Follicular growth and corpus luteum function in women with unexplained infertility, monitored by ultrasonography and measurement of daily salivary progesterone. Gynecol Endocrinol. 1989;3:297–308.
30. Rodin DA, Fisher AM, Clayton RN. Cycle abnormalities in infertile women with regular menstrual cycles: effects of clomiphene citrate treatment. Fertil Steril. 1994;62:42–7.
31. Randall JM, Templeton AT. Transvaginal sonographic assessment of follicular and endometrial growth in spontaneous and clomiphene citrate cycles. Fertil Steril. 1991;56:208–12.
32. Dickey RP. Evaluation and management of threatened and habitual first trimester abortion. In: Osofsky H, editor. Advances in clinical obstetrics and gynecology, vol. 2, Chap. 2. Chicago: Yearbook Medical Publishers; 1984. pp. 329–88.
33. Dickey RP, Hower JF. Effect of ovulation induction on uterine blood flow and oestradiol and progesterone concentrations in early pregnancy. Hum Reprod. 1995;10:2875–9.
34. Dickey RP. Doppler ultrasound investigation of uterine and ovarian blood flow in infertility and early pregnancy. Hum Reprod Rev. 1997;3:467–503
35. Dickey RP, Gasser RF, Hower JF, Matulich EM, Brown GT. Relationship of uterine blood flow to chorionic and embryo growth rates. Hum Reprod. 1995;10:2676–9.
36. Strowitzki T, Germeyer A, Popovici R, von Wolff M. The human endometrium as a fertility-determining factor. Hum Repro Update. 2006;12:617–30.
37. Dickey RP, Olar TT, Taylor SN, Curole DN, Matulich EM. Relationship of endometrial thickness and pattern to fecundity in ovulation induction cycles: effect of clomiphene citrate alone and with human menopausal gonadotropin. Fertil Steril. 1993;59:756–60.
38. Benda JA. Clomiphene's effect on endometrium in infertility. Int J Gynecol Path. 1992;11:273–82.
39. Bonhoff AJ, Naether OGJ, Johannisson E. Effects of clomiphene citrate stimulation on endometrial structure in infertile women. Hum Reprod. 1996;11:844–9
40. Randall JM, Templeton A. The effects of clomiphene citrate upon ovulation and endocrinology when administered to patients with unexplained infertility. Hum Reprod. 1991;6:659–64
41. Lamb EJ, Guderian AM. Clinical effects of clomiphene in anovulation. Obstet Gynecol. 1966:28:505–12.
42. Graff G. Suppression of cervical mucus during clomiphene therapy. Fertil Steril. 1971;22:209–12.
43. Diamond MP, Maxon WS, Vaughn WK, Osteen KG, Wentz AG. Antioestrogen effect of clomiphene citrate in a multiple follicular stimulation protocol. J In Vitro Fertil Embryo Transfer. 1986;3:106–9.
44. Check JH, Davis E, Adelson H. A randomized prospective study comparing pregnancy rates following clomiphene citrate and human menopausal gonadotrophin therapy. Hum Reprod. 1992;7:801–5.
45. Randall JM, Templeton A. Cervical mucus score and in vitro sperm mucus interaction in spontaneous and clomiphene citrate cycles. Fertil Steril. 1991;56:465–8.
46. Thompson LA, Burratt CLR, Thornton SJ, Bolton AE, Cooke ID. The effects of clomiphene citrate and cyclofenil on cervical

mucous volume and receptivity over the periovulatory period. Fertil Steril. 1993;59:125–9.
47. Acharya U, Irvine DS, Hamilton MPR, Templeton AA. The effect of three anti-oestrogen drugs on cervical mucus quality and in-vitro sperm-cervical mucus interaction in ovulatory women. Hum Reprod. 1993;8:437–41.
48. Annapurna V, Dhaliwal LK, Gopalan S. Effect of two anti-estrogens, clomiphene citrate and tamoxifen, on cervical mucus and sperm-cervical mucus interaction. Int J Fertil. 1997;42:215–8.
49. Dickey RP, Brinsden PR, Pyrzak R, editors. Manual of intrauterine insemination and ovulation induction. Cambridge: Cambridge University Press; 2010. p. 19–30.
50. Oei SG, Helmerhost EM, Kerise MJN. When is the postcoital test normal? A critical appraisal. Hum Reprod. 1995;10:1711–4.
51. Roumen JME, Desbur WH, Rolland R. Treatment of infertile women with a deficient post coital test with two antiestrogens, clomiphene and tamoxifen. Fertil Steril. 1984;41:237–43.
52. Buvat J, Buvat Herbaut M, Marcolin G, Ardaens Boulier K. Antiestrogens as treatment of female and male infertilities. Horm Res. 1987;28:219–29.
53. Tepper R, Luenfeld B, Shalev J, Ovadia J, Blankstein J. The effect of clomiphene citrate and tamoxifen on the cervical mucus. Acta Obstet Gynecol Scand. 1988;67:311–4.
54. Maxson WS, Pittaway DE, Hebert CM, Garner CH, Wentz AC. Antiestrogenic effect of clomiphene citrate: correlation with serum estradiol concentrations. Fertil Steril. 1984;41:356–9.
55. Gelert TJ, Buyalos RP. The effect of clomiphene citrate and menopausal gonadotropins on cervical mucus in ovulatory cycles. Fertil Steril. 1993;60:471–6.
56. Blasco L. Clinical approach to the evaluation of sperm cervical interactions. Fertil Steril. 1977;28:1133.
57. Check JH, Adelson HG, Wu CH. Improvement of cervical factor with guaifenesin. Fertil Steril. 1982;37:707–8
58. Dickey RP, Taylor SN, Lu PY, Sartor BM, Dunaway HE. Can the number of antral follicles before the start of gonadotropin stimulation predict the number of preovulation follicles and total oocytes in IVF cycles? P-600. Fertil Steril. 2010;97:S266.
59. Dickey RP, Bordson BL, Taylor SN, Curole DN, Dunaway HE. Micronized oral progesterone for luteal phase support in IVF. Abstracts of the scientific paper and poster session. The American Fertility Society; 1986:53.
60. Fisch P, Collins JA, Casper RE, Reid RL, Brown SE, Simpson C, et al. Unexplained infertility: evaluation of treatment with clomiphene and human chorionic gonadotropin. Fertil Steril. 1989;51:828–33.
61. Beck JI, Boothroyd C, Proctor M, Farquhar C, Hughes E. Oral anti-oestrogens and medical adjuncts for subfertility associated with anovulation. Cochrane Database Syst Rev. 2005;25(1):CD002249.
62. Parsanezhad ME, Albozi S, Motazedian S, Omrani G. Use of dexamethasone and clomiphene citrate in the treatment of clomiphene citrate-resistant patients with polycystic ovary syndrome and normal dehydroepiandrosterone sulfate levels; a prospective, double-blind, placebo-controlled trial. Fertil Steril. 2002;78:1001–4.
63. Siebert TI, Kruger TF, Steyn DW, Nosarka S. Is the addition of metformin efficacious in the treatment of clomiphene citrate-resistant patients with polycystic ovary syndrome? A structured literature review. Fertil Steril. 2006;78:1001–4.
64. Legro RS, Barnhart HX, Schlaff WD, Carr BR, Diamond MP, Carson SA, et al. Clomiphene, metformin or both for infertility in the polycystic ovary syndrome. N Engl J Med. 2007;356:551–6.
65. Crosignani PG, Collins J, Cooke ID, Diczfalusy E, Rubin B. Unexplained infertility. Hum Reprod. 1993;8(6):977–80.
66. Hughes E, Brown J, Collins JJ, Vanderkerchove P. Clomiphene citrate vs. placebo for ovulation induction in oligo-amenorrhoeic women. Cochrane Database Syst Rev. 1996;22(1):CD000056.
67. Steiner AZ, Terplan M, Paulson RJ. Comparison of tamozifen and clomiphene citrate for ovulation induction: a meta-analysis. Hum Reprod. 2005;20:1511–5.
68. Custers IM, Steures P, Hompes P, Flierman P, van Kasteren Y, van Dop PA, van der Veen F, Mol Ben WJ. Intrauterine insemination: how many cycles should we perform? Hum Reprod. 2008; 23:885–8.
69. Dickey RP, Taylor SN, Lu PY, Sartor BM, Rye PH, Pyrzak R. Risk factors for high-order multiple pregnancy and multiple birth after controlled ovarian hyperstimulation: results of 4,062 intrauterine insemination cycles. Fertil Steril. 2005;83:671–83.
70. Dickey RP. A year of inaction on high-order multiple pregnancies due to ovulation induction. Fertil Steril. 2003;79:14–6
71. Dickey RP, Xoing X, Gee RE, Pridjian G. Effect of maternal height and weight on risk of preterm birth in singleton and twin births resulting from IVF: a retrospective cohort study using SART-CORS. Fertil Steril. 2012;97:249–54.
72. Martin JA, Hamilton BE, Sutton PD, Ventura SJ, Mathews TJ, Osterman MJ. Births: final data for 2009. Natl Vital Stat Rep. 2011;60:1.
73. Mathews TJ, MacDorman MF. Infant mortality statistics from the 2007 period linked birth/infant death data set. Natl Vital Stat Rep. 2011;59:6. (Table D).

Aromatase Inhibitors in the Treatment of Unexplained Female Infertility

26

Lucky H. Sekhon, Patricia Rekawek and Lawrence Grunfeld

Unexplained infertility (UI) is thought to affect 10–30% of infertile couples [1, 2]. After failure of expectant management, which may involve untreated observation for a duration of 12 months or less, proposed treatment regimens include ovulation induction with oral or injectable medications with or without subsequent intrauterine insemination (IUI). Patients with UI are directed to in vitro fertilization (IVF) only after the failure of these therapies [3]. IUI is considered the first-line approach because of its simplicity, noninvasiveness, and reduced cost. Although IVF is known to be more effective on a per cycle basis than IUI, studies have shown that ovulation induction with IUI yields higher cumulative pregnancy rates in patients with idiopathic infertility, which may be attributable to a lower drop-out rate [4]. It is well established that ovulation induction in conjunction with IUI in patients with UI significantly increases pregnancy rates compared with natural cycle IUI [5–8] with reported pregnancy rates per cycle between 8 and 22% [9–11].

Ovulation Induction in Unexplained Infertility

A large proportion of unexplained infertility is thought to be related to alterations in ovulatory function that may not produce detectable hormonal changes [2]. The use of exogenous gonadotropins to achieve controlled ovarian hyperstimulation has been widely demonstrated [3, 12, 13]. Historically, ovulation induction for infertility was reserved for treatment of anovulatory women. It was expanded to treat suspected luteal phase defects and unexplained infertility in the 1980s. The rationale for use of ovulation induction in women with unexplained infertility, who by definition have regular ovulatory menstrual cycles, is to augment the probability of pregnancy by targeting subtle defects in follicle development that cannot be elucidated by a standard infertility workup. Increasing follicle stimulating hormone (FSH) stimulation would promote granulosa cell development and might enhance both oocyte health and the number of oocytes ovulated. Oral ovulation induction agents are typically administered on days 3 to 7 of the menstrual cycle. When used in conjunction with IUI to increase the density of motile sperm available to these oocytes, the likelihood of pregnancy may be further increased. Over the years, oral medications such as clomiphene citrate (CC) and aromatase inhibitors (AI) or injectable gonadotropin treatment have been used. Comparisons of the efficacy of oral agents with different types of gonadotropins in IUI programs have led to conflicting results in the literature [14–19].

CC is a nonsteroidal triphenylethylene derivative with both estrogenic and antiestrogenic effects with well-established efficacy in ovulation induction. The antiestrogenic effects of CC create the perception of an estrogen deficit at the level of the hypothalamus, triggering an increase in GnRH and gonadotropins with stimulation of follicular growth [20–23]. Up to 15–20% of patients with unexplained infertility fail to conceive after stimulation with CC [24]. This may be attributable to prolonged estrogen receptor depletion in the endometrium and the cervix, which may lead to endometrial thinning and poor cervical mucus in 15–50% of patients [24–26]. Additional potential negative effects on uterine blood flow [27], embryo development [28], and the coagulation system [29] have been proposed. Based on this, it has been argued that CC use may be associated with lower pregnancy rates and increased incidence of miscarriage. However, while some studies have suggested that fecundity may relate to endometrial thickness, others have failed to demonstrate any significant correlation [30, 31]. Combining CC with gonadotropins results in high estrogen and progesterone levels, which are hypothesized to neutralize the adverse effects on estrogen responsive tissues, if they exist. However,

L. H. Sekhon (✉)
Mount Sinai Medical Center, Klingenstein Pavilion,
1176 5th Ave, KP-9, New York, NY 10129, USA
e-mail: Lucky.Sekhon@mountsinai.org

P. Rekawek · L. Grunfeld
Department of Obstetrics, Gynecology, & Reproductive Medicine,
Icahn School of Medicine at Mount Sinai, 1245 Park Avenue, Apt. 5D,
New York, NY 10128, USA

G. L. Schattman et al. (eds.), *Unexplained Infertility*, DOI 10.1007/978-1-4939-2140-9_26,

the antiestrogenic effects of CC on the endometrium may counterbalance the benefit of increased endogenous FSH stimulation. AI, on the other hand, lead to a transient decline in estrogen production and do not cause estrogen receptor downregulation like CC. Therefore, these compounds stimulate gonadotropin production and follicular growth but do not interfere with estrogen levels in peripheral tissues such as the endometrium and cervix. Based on this fundamental difference and the experience gained with CC, AI have been examined for the purpose of ovulation induction in unexplained infertility [32].

Letrozole is a third-generation AI that was originally developed for the treatment of breast cancer. Aromatase is a cytochrome P-450 hemoprotein-containing enzyme complex that catalyzes the conversion of androstenedione and testosterone into estrogens [33, 34]. Letrozole blocks estrogen production by its selective, competitive, reversible inhibition of the aromatase enzyme. These compounds have a high oral bioavailability and relatively long half-life of 45 h [35]. AI have been shown to decrease estradiol production, with approximately 50% diminution in the amount of estradiol per mature follicles in peripheral blood on the day of human chorionic gonadotropin (HCG) administration [22, 32, 36]. As the luteinizing hormone (LH) surge is induced by a late follicular rise in estradiol concentrations that feeds back positively on the hypothalamic–pituitary axis [37], it is anticipated that letrozole delays the rise in LH. Letrozole is thought to not only lower estradiol but also the follicular proteins that antagonize the LH surge [22]. Studies have shown that in spite of estradiol levels per maturing follicles being nearly half the level seen in other ovarian stimulation regimens, a spontaneous LH surge occurs in up to 50% of patients receiving letrozole with FSH, with markedly reduced LH triggering levels of estradiol [22]. This indicates that letrozole may induce ovarian effects beyond merely reducing estrogen production; however, these effects are not well elucidated.

A preliminary study by Mitwally and Casper [32] illustrated the utility of letrozole, an AI as an ovulation induction agent in patients with polycystic ovarian syndrome (PCOS) and ovulatory infertility. Letrozole was given orally in a dose of 2.5 mg on days 3–7 after menses. In the PCOS group, ovulation was achieved in 9 of 12 cycles and pregnancy was achieved in three patients. A cohort study by Cortinez et al. [38] demonstrated the feasibility of letrozole in treating unexplained infertility, in that it was shown to induce moderate ovarian hyperstimulation in ovulatory infertile patients with estrogen levels similar to spontaneous cycles and higher midluteal progesterone, leading to both a normal endometrial histology and development of pinopodes, which are viewed as markers of endometrial receptivity. According to the prospective trial published in 2002, patients were randomized to receive either CC or letrozole and it compared the effect of either treatment to the outcome of the natural cycle that immediately preceded either treatment cycle [39]. In both groups, one follicle reached maturity during the menstrual cycle preceding the intervention. The number of growing follicles was 2.2 in the CC group, which was slightly higher than the finding of 1.7 in the AI group, both of which were statistically greater than the preceding natural cycle. Like CC, AI increase the stimulus to recruit follicles as well as the ovulatory surge as evidenced by a larger number of follicles reaching maturity. This study provided the basis for the use of AI for inducing controlled ovarian hyperstimulation in women who ovulate regularly.

Baysoy et al. [40] conducted a study in which 80 patients with unexplained infertility were randomized to receive letrozole or human menopausal gonadotropin (HMG). Low estradiol concentrations and small numbers of mature follicles were obtained at the time of the LH surge in the letrozole group. Despite this, the pregnancy rate per cycle was highest in the letrozole group, although this difference was not statistically significant. In addition, the financial burden was significantly higher in the HMG stimulation cases and no injections were required in the letrozole group. The findings of this study shed light on letrozole as a simple, convenient, and cost-effective treatment regimen in ovarian stimulation for IUI.

When administered in the early follicular phase, AI induce a hypoestrogenic state that releases the hypothalamic–pituitary axis from estrogenic negative feedback, which in turn increases FSH secretion and the development of ovarian follicles. Peripherally, inhibition of the aromatase-mediated conversion of androgens into estrogens may lead to temporary accumulation of androgens. Androgens have been shown to increase follicular sensitivity to FSH through amplification of the FSH receptor gene expression either directly or through other mediators such as the insulin-like growth factor system [41, 42]. As such, aromatase inhibition and estradiol suppression may allow for ovarian stimulation to be achieved with lower doses of FSH, improve ovarian response to FSH in poor responders, terminate the positive-feedback loop, and improve ovarian response to stimulation. In addition, aromatase inhibition may result in a better implantation rate and lower estrogen concentrations compared to CC [43]. AI, such as letrozole and anastrozole, have been tested successfully as alternative ovulation-inducing agents with a much lower average cost per cycle than FSH [32]. A low-cost adjuvant may eliminate the need for costly high doses of gonadotropins. Healey et al. [44] retrospectively analyzed results in patients using letrozole and FSH versus FSH alone in IUI cycles. The authors concluded that the addition of letrozole to gonadotropins decreased gonadotropin requirements and increased the number of preovulatory follicles, and despite thinner endometrial development, no effect on pregnancy rate was seen. Lack of endometrial development may have been attributable to the daily-administered dose of letrozole being twice as high as typical dose administered in other studies. Mitwally and Casper [36] examined whether adding letrozole to FSH for ovarian stimulation in patients undergoing ovulation induction with IUI could improve outcomes in patients that had previous FSH stimulated cycles demonstrating a poor response. This was an observational cohort study performed on 12 patients by using 2.5 mg letrozole daily and FSH ranging from 50 to 225 IU per day. Patients in the combined regimen group demonstrated improved ovarian response compared with FSH alone group as evidenced by a reduced gonadotropin dose requirement as well as a higher number of mature follicles. The cost benefit of letrozole was further proven in a study by Bedaiwy et al. [45] in which patients with anovulation, male factor infertility, unexplained infertility, or endometriosis underwent IUI cycles with FSH with and without letrozole as an oral adjunct. The FSH dose required for ovarian stimulation was shown to be significantly lower when letrozole was used. Although a significantly higher number of follicles greater than 16 mm size and endometrial thickness at the day of HCG administration was observed in the group receiving FSH alone, pregnancy rate was comparable in both groups. Furthermore, the IUI cancellation rate, an expression of excessive or poor response, was significantly lower with combined FSH and letrozole treatment.

Aromatase Inhibitors Versus Clomiphene Citrate

CC is the standard first-line treatment for ovulation induction for many decades. Some women (~15%) are resistant to even maximal doses (250 mg/day for 5–7 days) or demonstrate a suboptimal response to CC and require additional treatment using gonadotropins. There are clinical scenarios in which AIs may demonstrate an advantage over ovulation induction with CC. AI may be a better choice when a limited number of follicles are required [46]. Due to significantly lower estradiol levels, letrozole may be considered for empirical ovulation induction in infertile patients with estrogen-dependent neoplasms. As no hypothalamic–pituitary downregulation occurs during the late follicular phase, no adverse effects on peripheral targets such as the endometrium are expected. Letrozole treated patients have been shown to have endometrial thickness with an estrogenic triple-line pattern [22, 32, 36, 47, 48]. Peripheral effects on the endometrium have traditionally been hypothesized to contribute to lower pregnancy rates and higher miscarriage rates in patients stimulated with CC [49]. Controlled ovarian hyperstimulation with AI may avoid the theorized undesirable effects of CC on the endometrium. Letrozole is also thought to have a more favorable side-effect profile compared with CC, likely because of the difference in pharmacodynamics between the two drugs. AI have a reduced half-life (40–48 h) compared with clomiphene [50]. Clomiphene has been hypothesized to result in prolonged central estrogen receptor depletion because of its greater half-life, leading to supraphysiologic levels of estrogen without central suppression of FSH as the normal estrogen receptor-mediated feedback mechanisms are blocked. Persistent CC mediated downregulation of estrogen receptors may also result in bothersome symptoms such as hot flushes, premenstrual symptoms, and visual scotomata in addition to poor cervical mucus and thin endometrium. Vasomotor symptoms are also reported in patients using letrozole for ovulation induction, along with other idiosyncratic side effects, which may include mild headache or muscle and joint pain. These side effects have also been reported in long-term breast cancer studies of letrozole [51].

Mitwally and Casper [32] evaluated the efficacy of AI for ovulation induction in women that had previously failed CC treatment with unsuccessful ovulation or suboptimal endometrial thickness. This study included anovulatory women with PCOS and ovulatory women with other causes of infertility including male factor, endometriosis, or unexplained infertility. A higher proportion of PCOS patients (75%) were ovulatory with letrozole in comparison to their previous cycle with CC (44%). The mean number of mature follicles in letrozole and CC-stimulated cycles was similar in the ovulatory infertility patients. Pregnancy rates were 25 and 10% in patients with PCOS and ovulatory infertility, respectively. The mean endometrial thickness at the time of HCG administration was significantly higher in both patient groups compared with their previous CC-stimulated cycle. Although limited by a small sample size and selection bias in the patients who failed CC treatment were used as their own controls, the findings suggested that letrozole may be beneficial in patients with failed CC cycles and who demonstrate a thin endometrium with CC use. The endometrium sparing effect of letrozole was also demonstrated in a trial by Bayar et al. [30] in which 46 patients with unexplained infertility, early stage endometriosis and borderline male factor infertility were randomized to receive letrozole or CC for ovulation induction. The letrozole group was seen to have a significantly lower median estradiol level on the day of HCG administration. The rates of ovulation and median endometrial thickness were comparable in both groups. However, in six of the CC cycles the endometrium was found to be less than 5 mm, in contrast to patients undergoing letrozole stimulation who all demonstrated endometrial thickness greater than 5 mm.

Despite a number of studies that suggest letrozole has a positive influence on ovarian response and the endometrium, there are many conflicting reports in the literature showing no evidence of a beneficial effect of letrozole in ovarian stimulation cycles. In a pilot study, Fatemi et al. [43] compared the efficacy of 100 mg of CC versus 2.5 mg of letrozole daily in patients undergoing IUI and demonstrated lower estradiol concentration and follicle count in the AI group. Badawy et al. [52] conducted a randomized controlled trial in which 412 infertile women with unexplained infertility, undergoing IUI, were randomized to pretreatment with 100 mg of CC daily or 5 mg of letrozole daily for 5 days starting on day 3 of menses. Both groups had similar endometrial thickness before treatment and at the time of HCG administration, but differed in that serum estradiol and progesterone concentrations were statistically significantly higher in the CC group. The total number of follicles during stimulation was also significantly greater in the CC group. There was no statistically significant difference in pregnancy rates between both groups. Of note, there were two twin pregnancies achieved in the CC group. No higher order pregnancies or cases of ovarian hyperstimulation syndrome occurred in either group. The results of this study provided evidence that the antiestrogenic effects of CC did not adversely affect outcomes in the majority of treated women. The findings failed to demonstrate superiority of either letrozole or CC for inducing ovulation and achieving pregnancy in women with unexplained infertility. Furthermore, the rate of pregnancy loss after ovarian stimulation, with either AI or CC was not higher than after spontaneous pregnancy. Similarly, a randomized trial by Al-Fozan et al. [53] comparing 7.5 mg of letrozole with 100 mg of CC per day demonstrated similar ovarian response, endometrial thickness, and pregnancy rates after IUI. However, the patients treated with letrozole were seen to have a lower miscarriage that was not statistically significant.

Recent meta-analyses reviewed six randomized controlled studies comparing ovulation induction with letrozole versus CC in patients with PCOS [54, 55]. The reviews concluded that the pregnancy and live birth rates were comparable in both treatment groups. Of note, letrozole use was associated with significantly fewer mature follicles and significantly lower estrogen concentrations per cycle [54]. The multiple pregnancy rates were not significantly different between letrozole and CC treated subjects. The majority of studies was limited by small sample sizes, with the exception of the study by Badawy et al. [52] which included more than 50% of the study subjects analyzed in the meta-analysis, therefore having a large, disproportionate impact on all of the analyzed outcomes.

Aromatase Inhibitors and Clomiphene as Adjuncts to Gonadotropins

When gonadotropins are used alone for ovarian hyperstimulation the cost of treatment, incidence of multiple pregnancies, and probability of significant ovarian hyperstimulation syndrome are increased [16–18]. As such, combining oral ovulation induction agents with gonadotropin therapy to decrease the gonadotropin dose required for optimum stimulation has been explored as a method of ovarian induction [26, 56–58]. In a randomized trial by Badawy et al. [59], letrozole was shown to have no advantage over CC when either agent was combined with FSH in the treatment of unexplained female infertility. No difference between either regimens with respect to endometrial thickness or pregnancy rates was identified. However, the total number of follicles and serum estradiol and progesterone concentrations were significantly greater in the CC + gonadotropin group. Supraphysiological estradiol is thought to contribute to dyssynchrony between the development of the endometrium and early embryo development which can hinder implantation [60]. In conjunction with having higher estradiol levels, the CC group exhibited a nonstatistically increase in the rate of multiple follicles without a corresponding significant increase in multiple pregnancy or miscarriage rates. In a prospective nonrandomized study, Mitwally and Casper compared three ovulation induction regimens in women with unexplained infertility, consisting of letrozole combined with FSH, CC combined with FSH, or FSH alone [22]. The authors concluded that similar to CC, aromatase inhibition with letrozole reduced the required FSH dose for ovulation induction without the undesirable antiestrogenic effects sometimes observed with CC. Endometrial thickness was significantly lower in the CC group compared with the other treatment groups. The pregnancy rate was also significantly lower in the combined CC-FSH group (10.5%) as compared to the combined letrozole-FSH group (19.1%) and the FSH-only group (18.7%). Aromatase inhibition allowed a reduction in FSH dose similar to that seen with CC while maintaining the high pregnancy rate encountered with FSH-only regimens. The observation of a thicker endometrium in the letrozole-FSH group compared to the CC-FSH group supports the inference that the effect of CC on peripheral tissues can significantly contribute to a decrease in pregnancy rates. Estradiol levels were markedly lower in letrozole-FSH group as compared to both FSH-only and CC-FSH groups [22].

These findings have been confirmed by other studies, including a randomized blinded clinical trial by Barroso et al. [61] in which letrozole and CC were compared as adjuncts to FSH for the purpose of controlled ovarian hyperstimulation in women with unexplained infertility. Letrozole with FSH was shown to achieve similar number of mature follicles compared with CC with FSH, with lower peak serum estradiol levels, which were associated with increased endometrial thickness. The total dose of recombinant FSH was similar between groups. However, in this study, the differential effects of letrozole and CC on the endometrium did not translate into a significant difference in pregnancy rate between both groups, with pregnancy rates of 23.8 and 20% in letrozole/FSH and CC/FSH groups, respectively. This discrepancy may be attributable to a relatively small sample size resulting in poor statistical power for assessing this secondary outcome. There was no difference in the miscarriage rate or the proportion of multiple pregnancies in the groups treated with letrozole and CC.

Optimal Dosages of Aromatase Inhibitor Therapy

Despite several studies that have shown letrozole to be efficacious for ovarian stimulation, there is a paucity of studies examining the optimal dose. When deciding on the ideal oral ovulation induction agent to use alone or as an adjunct to gonadotropin stimulation with IUI, it is important to consider that the cost of letrozole per cycle is much higher than CC, especially when higher doses of letrozole are required. Through the inhibition of aromatase activity, letrozole prevents the conversion of androgens to estrogen, thereby increasing testosterone concentrations [62]. Although there is data to suggest that testosterone may increase follicular FSH-receptor expression in primates and promote follicular growth by amplifying FSH effects [41, 42, 62]. It has been hypothesized that higher concentrations of testosterone are produced with higher doses of letrozole, potentially causing an adverse effect on the endometrium. Most investigators have studied letrozole using a 2.5 mg dose for duration of 5 days during early stimulation [63–65], whereas others have used a range from 2.5 to 7 mg [54, 64]. In a study by Al-Fadhli et al. [66], patients assigned to receive 5 mg of letrozole produced an overall greater number of follicles, with higher pregnancy rates as compared to subjects that received 2.5 mg.

Badawy et al. [67] conducted a parallel-group randomized controlled trial comparing the efficacy of letrozole at doses of 2.5, 5, and 7.5 mg in 179 women undergoing ovulation induction and timed intercourse for treatment of unexplained infertility. The demographics of study groups were similar except for the fact that patients receiving the 7.5 mg dose tended to have a significantly longer duration of prior infertility compared with the 2.5 mg group. There was no significant difference between the three groups regarding the pretreatment endometrial thickness, pregnancy, or miscarriage rates. The findings showed a significant dose-dependent increase in the total number of follicles greater than 14 mm on the day of HCG administration, with the most follicles yielded following the 7.5 mg dose. The number of days needed to achieve a mature follicle also showed a significant dose-dependent decrease with increasing doses of letrozole. The increase in the number of mature follicles was not paralleled by a similar increase in pregnancy rate between the three groups. This is in contrast with the findings of Al-Fadhli et al. [66], who found no significant difference in the days needed for stimulation (11.4 versus 11.7 days) for patients receiving 2.5 versus 5 mg of letrozole, but demonstrated that a higher dosage was associated with a higher pregnancy rate. The mean endometrial thickness achieved was 7.5 (+/−0.3) mm in the group receiving the 2.5 mg dose and 7.8 (+/−0.3) mm in the group receiving the 5 mg dose. One might assume that the increased concentrations of midluteal progesterone and endometrial thickness in patients receiving higher doses of letrozole would optimize the luteal phase and lower miscarriage rates. Conversely, a slightly higher miscarriage rate was observed with the use of the 5 and 7.5 mg doses compared with the 2.5 mg dose, although this finding was not statistically significant. These conflicting findings from various studies may be attributed to recruitment of different patient populations.

A systematic review of five randomized controlled trials examining outcomes found that although gonadotropin/IUI was associated with a higher pregnancy rate, no significant differences between the various regimens with regard to live birth rates per couple were seen [20]. Injectable gonadotropins have some drawbacks which include the high cost of medication and the expense of the extra monitoring required, inconvenience, and a higher probability of high-order multiple gestations and ovarian hyperstimulation syndrome [21]. Although pregnancy rates with oral agents are lower, they are less expensive to use and have a more favorable side effect profile. Furthermore, studies have demonstrated that the combined use of oral agents along with gonadotropins enhances follicular recruitment while reducing the gonadotropin dose needed for optimal stimulation, ultimately reducing the cost of the cycle without a demonstrable effect on treatment outcome [22, 23]. Despite this knowledge, there continues to be a lack of consensus regarding the most favorable ovarian stimulation protocol for women with unexplained infertility.

Side Effects and Safety Concerns

Concern about the safety of letrozole and potential teratogenic effects was raised after an abstract presented at the 2005 American Society for Reproductive Medicine (ASRM) meeting of a follow-up of 150 babies born to women who underwent fertility treatment involving the use of letrozole or letrozole plus gonadotropin injections compared with 36,000 natural conceptions delivered in a community hospital [68]. The authors reported that the incidences of cardiac and bone anomalies were higher in the letrozole group than in the control group. The cardiac anomalies comprised of two cases of aortic stenosis in the 150 babies, which the authors calculated to be statistically higher than the rate of cardiac anomalies in the 36,000 babies born from low-risk pregnancies. Similarly, there were three different bone abnormalities in the letrozole babies. They also found that women with gestational diabetes given letrozole delivered infants with significantly lower birth weight than controls ($p<0.002$; 95% CI = 11.3–136.6). The overall rate of congenital anomalies was in the 3–4% range, similar to the general population. The study was fundamentally flawed in that the pregnancy outcome of infertility patients was being compared with pregnancy outcome in younger, fertile women with natural conceptions. The study was never published in a peer-reviewed journal. As a result of this report, the use of letrozole for ovulation induction in premenopausal women was discouraged owing to the potential for maternal and fetal toxicity and fetal malformations [69]. The manufacturer of letrozole distributed a letter to practicing physicians recommending that the drug not be used for fertility treatments.

Given the fact that AI are typically administered for approximately 5 days early in stimulation and stopped well before the time of ovulation, deleterious effects on a pregnancy achieved days to weeks later are highly unlikely. The exposure of oocytes to AI has not been shown to increase birth defects in early animal studies. Toxicology studies have shown that anastrozole is well tolerated at 1 and 6 months. Oral administration of anastrozole to pregnant rats and rabbits was not shown to cause any teratogenic effects [70]. Furthermore, in vitro exposure of mouse follicles to anastrozole did not increase meiotic spindle defects in oocytes and birth anomalies [71]. Luthra et al. treated aromatase-overexpressing mice with high doses of letrozole for 6 weeks and demonstrated that pregnancies conceived 2 weeks later were no different in outcome compared with controls in terms of litter size, birth weight, and anomalies [72]. Mitwally et al. [48] reported on pregnancy outcome for patients from three referral centers receiving letrozole for ovarian stimulation. They concluded that pregnancies conceived after letrozole had similar miscarriage and ectopic pregnancy rates compared with other modalities of ovarian stimulation. In addition, patients on letrozole had lower multiple gestation rates. A multicenter retrospective study by Tulandi et al. provided further evidence that the concern about letrozole use for ovulation induction may be unfounded [73]. The study was completed in 2006 and included 911 babies born to infertility patients treated in five Canadian centers, 514 conceived after letrozole treatment and 397 after CC treatment. The findings showed that the overall congenital malformation and chromosomal abnormality rates were 2.4% in the letrozole group and 4.8% in the CC group. The rate of major malformations in letrozole group was 1.2% versus 3% in the CC group; however, these differences were not statistically different. Ventricular septal defects occurred in 1.8% of the CC group compared with 0.2% of the letrozole group, which is slightly lower than the 1 in 400 rate quoted in the general population [74]. Similar to concerns regarding the possible teratogenicity of letrozole if administered during pregnancy [75], CC is listed by the FDA as a pregnancy category X drug [76]. No further studies in the literature have supported an increased risk of birth defects with the use of letrozole for ovulation induction, although the number of pregnancies is small in comparison to those resulting from CC treatment over the past 40 years.

Badawy et al. [77] conducted a prospective randomized trial comparing the safety and efficacy of AI and CC. All ovulation induction agents were shown to improve pregnancy outcomes with miscarriage rates comparable to that of the general population. There were no significant differences in terms of mean gestational age at delivery, premature deliveries, birth weight, growth restriction or 5 min Apgar scores between the stimulated and naturally conceived pregnancies. There was one case of complete cleft palate and one case of major congenital heart problem, which ended in early neonatal death in the letrozole group. However, maternal diabetes may have contributed largely to the development of a cardiac anomaly in this case. No congenital anomalies were reported in the anastrozole group.

Another major safety concern regarding ovulation induction is the potential risk for supraphysiological estradiol levels to promote the growth of estrogen sensitive tumors. AI have been used in conjunction with gonadotropins to safely induce ovulation for the purpose of oocyte and embryo freezing for fertility preservation in patients with endometrial and breast cancer [78]. This combined regimen is thought to be the safest strategy as it has been shown to achieve peak estradiol levels closer to that observed in natural cycles. In a prospective controlled trial which included 60 patients with breast cancer, letrozole or tamoxifen combined with low-dose FSH was shown to yield a greater number of successfully fertilized embryos than in the subject group treated with tamoxifen alone. Peak estradiol levels in letrozole with FSH and tamoxifen alone treatment groups were lower than levels seen in the tamoxifen with FSH group [79]. Azim et al. [80] conducted a prospective study in which 79 patients with breast cancer underwent ovulation induction with a combined letrozole with FSH regimen and compared with 136 control subjects with breast cancer. The hazard ratio for post-IVF recurrence of breast cancer was reported as 0.56 (95% CI 0.17–1.9), demonstrating that disease progression and prognosis was not compromised as a result of ovarian hyperstimulation.

Directions for Future Research

A review of the existing literature suggests that letrozole appears to be at least as effective as CC in induction of ovulation and in achievement of live births, with some potential advantages over CC. The outcome of ongoing multicenter trials may provide definitive evidence of the efficacy and safety of AI compared with CC for infertility treatment. There is currently a lack of robust, reliable data with many studies having been performed using different patient populations from various countries where key principles of clinical practice may differ. This heterogeneity could affect demographic factors that have a significant impact on pregnancy outcome, such as decreased maternal age in populations in which women may commence a fertility work up earlier. As the use of letrozole evolves from its initial indication as breast cancer adjuvant therapy to an ovulation induction agent, the drug's pharmacodynamics properties and teratogenic potential have been the focus of investigation. The short half-life and rapid clearance of letrozole prevents accumulation of the drug with repeated cycles of use and is reassuring regarding birth defects. It is unknown whether the higher concentrations of testosterone produced with higher doses of letrozole have an adverse effect on the endometrium and hormonal milieu of conception and pregnancy. Further studies examining endometrial receptivity and androgen profiles with letrozole treatment are needed. Also, prospective studies examining the long-term follow-up of children born as a result of ovulation induction using either CC or AI are warranted in order to establish safety profiles for both drugs. Anecdotal reports of low multiple pregnancy rates with the use of letrozole alone have yet to be well supported with much of the current evidence providing conflicting findings. Controlled ovarian stimulation with IUI continues to account for more than 50% of multiple pregnancies (twins) and the majority of high-order multiple pregnancies (triplets or greater) and demonstrates an increased risk of ovarian hyperstimulation syndrome with gonadotropin use. If the multiple pregnancy risk with letrozole use is reduced compared with CC or gonadotropin treatment, while maintaining equivalent pregnancy and live birth rates, this could form the basis for a major shift towards letrozole use for ovulation induction.

References

1.. Evers JL. Female subfertility. Lancet. 2002;360(9327):151–9.
2. Collins JA, Crosignani PG. Unexplained infertility: a review of, prognosis, treatment efficacy and management. Int J Gynecol Obstet. 1992;39(4):267–75.
3. Homburg R, Insler V. Ovulation induction in perspective. Hum Reprod Update. 2002;8(5):449–62.
4. Goverde AJ, McDonnell J, Vermeiden JP, Schats R, Rutten FF, Schoemaker J. Intrauterine insemination or in-vitro fertilisation in idiopathic subfertility and male subfertility: a randomised trial and cost-effectiveness analysis. Lancet. 2000;355(9197):13–8.
5. Hughes, EG. The effectiveness of ovulation induction and intrauterine insemination in the treatment of persistent infertility: a meta-analysis. Hum Reprod. 1997;12(9):1865–72.
6. Arici A, Byrd W, Bradshaw K, Kutteh WH, Marshburn P, Carr BR. Evaluation of clomiphene citrate and human chorionic gonadotropin treatment: a prospective, randomized, crossover study during intrauterine insemination cycles. Fertil Steril. 1994;61(2):314–8.
7. Cohlen BJ, Vandekerckhove P, te Velde ER, Habbema JD. Timed intercourse versus intra-uterine insemination with or without ovarian hyperstimulation for subfertility in men. Cochrane Database Syst Rev. 2000;2:CD000360.
8. Guzick DS, Carson SA, Coutifaris C, Oversheet JW, Factor-Litvak P, Steinkampf MP, et al. Efficacy of superovulation and intrauterine insemination in the treatment of infertility. National cooperative reproductive medicine network. N Engl J Med. 1999;340(3):177–83.
9. Sunde A, Kahn JA, Molne K. Intrauterine insemination: a European collaborative report. Hum Reprod. 1988;3(Suppl 2):69–73.
10. Dodson WC, Haney AF. Controlled ovarian hyperstimulation and intrauterine insemination for treatment of infertility. Fertil Steril. 1991;55(3):457–67.
11. Cohlen BJ, te Velde ER, van Kooij RJ, Looman CW, Habbema JD. Controlled ovarian hyperstimulation and intrauterine insemination for treating male subfertility: a controlled study. Hum Reprod. 1998;13(6):1553–8.
12. Dodson WC, Whitesides DB, Hughes CL Jr, Easley HA 3rd, Haney AF. Superovulation with intrauterine insemination in the treatment of infertility: a possible alternative to gamete intrafallopian transfer and in vitro fertilization. Fertil Steril. 1987;48(3):441–5.
13. Aboulghar M, Mansour R, Serour G, Abdrazek A, Amin Y, Rhodes C. Controlled ovarian hyperstimulation and intrauterine insemination for treatment of unexplained infertility should be limited to a maximum of three trials. Fertil Steril. 2001;75(1):88–91.
14. Karlstrom PO, Bergh T, Lundkvist O. A prospective randomized trial of artificial insemination versus intercourse in cycles stimulated with human menopausal gonadotropin or clomiphene citrate. Fertil Steril. 1993;59(3):554–9.
15. Balasch J, Ballesca JL, Pimentel C, Creus M, Fabregues F, Vanrell JA. Late low-dose pure follicle stimulating hormone for ovarian stimulation in intra-uterine insemination cycles. Hum Reprod. 1994;9(1):1863–6.
16. Hannoun A, Abu-Musa A, Kaspar H, Khalil A. Intrauterine insemination IUI: the effect of ovarian stimulation and infertility diagnosis on pregnancy outcome. Clin Exp Obstet Gynecol. 1998;25(4):144–6.
17. Ecochard R, Mathieu C, Royere D, Blache G, Rabilloud M, Czyba JC. A randomized prospective study comparing pregnancy rates after clomiphene citrate and human menopausal gonadotropin before intrauterine insemination. Fertil Steril. 2000;73(1):90–3.
18. Matorras R, Diaz T, Corcostegui B, Ramon O, Pijoan JI, Rodriguez-Escudero FJ. Ovarian stimulation in intrauterine insemination with donor sperm: a randomized study comparing clomiphene citrate in fixed protocol versus highly purified urinary FSH. Hum Reprod. 2002;17(8):2107–11.
19. Gregoriou O, Vlahos NF, Konidaris S, Papadias K, Botsis D, Creatsas GK. Randomized controlled trial comparing superovulation with letrozole versus recombinant follicle-stimulating hormone combined with intrauterine insemination for couples with unexplained infertility who had failed clomiphene citrate stimulation and intrauterine insemination. Fertil Steril. 2008;90(3):678–83.
20. Athaullah N, Proctor M, Johnson NP. Oral versus injectable ovulation induction agents for unexplained subfertility. Cochrane Database Syst Rev. 2002;3:CD003052.
21. Olivennes F. Patient-friendly ovarian stimulation. Reprod Biomed Online. 2003;7(1):30–4.
22. Mitwally MF, Casper RF. Aromatase inhibition reduces gonadotropin dose required for controlled ovarian stimulation in women with unexplained infertility. Hum Reprod. 2003;18:1588–97.
23. Mitwally MF, Casper RF. Aromatase inhibition reduces the dose of gonadotropin required for controlled ovarian hyperstimulation. J Soc Gynecol Investig. 2004;11(6):406–15.
24. Gonen Y, Casper RF. Sonographic determination of a possible adverse effect of clomiphene citrate on endometrial growth. Hum Reprod. 1990;5(6):670–4.

25. Yagel S, Ben-Chetrit A, Anteby E, Zacut D, Hochner-Celnikier D, Ron M. The effect of ethinyl estradiol on endometrial thickness and uterine volume during ovulation induction by clomiphene citrate. Fertil Steril. 1992;57(1):33–6.
26. Dickey RP, Olar TT, Taylor SN, Curole DN, Matulich EM. Relationship of endometrial thickness and pattern to fecundity in ovulation induction cycles: effect of clomiphene citrate alone and with human menopausal gonadotropin. Fertil Steril. 1993;59(4):756–60.
27. Hsu CC, Kuo HC, Wang ST, Huang KE. Interference with uterine blood flow by clomiphene citrate in women with unexplained infertility. Obstet Gynecol. 1995;86(6):917–21.
28. Laufer N, Pratt BM, DeCherney AH, Naftolin F, Merino M, Markert CL. The in vivo and in vitro effects of clomiphene citrate on ovulation, fertilization, and development of cultured mouse oocytes. Am J Obstet Gynecol. 1983;147(6):633–9.
29. Lox C, Canez M, DeLeon F, Dorsett J, Prien S. Hyperestrogenism induced by menotropins alone or in conjunction with leuprolide acetate in in vitro fertilization cycles: the impact on hemostasis. Fertil Steril. 1995;63(3):566–70.
30. Bayar U, Tanriverdi HA, Barut A, Ayoglu F, Ozcan O, Kaya E. Letrozole vs. clomiphene citrate in patients with ovulatory infertility. Fertil Steril. 2006;85(4):1045–8.
31. Badawy A, Abdel All I, Abu Elatta M. Clomiphene citrate or letrozole for ovulation induction in women with polycystic ovarian syndrome? A prospective randomized trial. Fertil Steril Online. 2007;02:062.
32. Mitwally MF, Casper RF. Use of an aromatase inhibitor for induction of ovulation in patients with an inadequate response to clomiphene substrate. Fertil.Steril. 2001;75(2):305–9.
33. Cole PA, Robinson CH. Mechanism and inhibition of cytochrome P-450 aromatase. J Med Chem. 1990;33(11):2933–42.
34. Akhtar M, Njar VC, Wright JN. Mechanistic studies on aromatase and related C–C bond cleaving P-450 enzymes. J Steroid Biochem Mol Biol. 1993;44(4–6):375–87.
35. Sioufi A, Gauducheau N, Pineau V, Marfil F, Jaouen A, Cardot JM, et al. Absolute bioavailability of letrozole in healthy post-menopausal women. Biopharm Drug Dispos. 1997;18(9):779–89.
36. Mitwally MF, Casper RF. Aromatase inhibition improves ovarian response to follicle-stimulating hormone in poor responders. Fertil Steril. 2002;77(4):776–80.
37. Hoff JD, Quigley ME, Yen SS. Hormonal dynamics at midcycle: a reevaluation. J Clin Endocrinol Metab. 1983;57(4):792–6.
38. Cortinez A, De Carvalho I, Vantman D, Gabler F, Iniguez G, Vega M. Hormonal profile and endometrial morphology in letrozole-controlled ovarian hyperstimulation in ovulatory infertile patients. Fertil Steril. 2005;83(1):110–5.
39. Fisher SA, Reid RL, Van Vugt DA, Casper RF. A randomized double-blind comparison of the effects of clomiphene citrate and the aromatase inhibitor letrozole on ovulatory function in normal women. Fertil Steril. 2002;78(2):280–5.
40. Baysoy A, Serdaroglu H, Jamal H, Karatekeli E, Ozornek H, Attar E. Letrozole versus human menopausal gonadotropin in women undergoing intrauterine insemination. Reprod Biomed Online. 2006;13(2):208–12.
41. Vendola KA, Zhou J, Adesanya OO, Weil SJ, Bondy CA. Androgens stimulate early stages of follicular growth in the primate ovary. J Clin Invest. 1998;101(12):2622–9.
42. Weil SJ, Vendola K, Zhou J, Adesanya OO, Wang J, Okafor J, Bondy CA. Androgen receptor gene expression in the primate ovary cellular localization, regulation, and functional correlations. J Clin Endocrinol Metab. 1998;83(7):2479–85.
43. Fatemi HM, Kolibianakis E, Tournaye H, Camus M, Van Steirteghem AC, Devroey P. Clomiphene citrate versus letrozole for ovarian stimulation: a pilot study. Reprod Biomed Online. 2003;7(5):543–6.
44. Healey S, Tan SL, Tulandi T, Biljan MM. Effects of letrozole on superovulation with gonadotropins in women undergoing intrauterine insemination. Fertil Steril. 2003;80(6):1325–9.
45. Bedaiwy MA, Forman R, Mousa NA, Hesham G, Al Inany HG, Casper RF. Cost-effectiveness of aromatase inhibitor co-treatment for controlled ovarian stimulation. Hum Reprod. 2006;21(11):2838–44.
46. Badawy A, Abdel Aal I, Abulatta M. Clomiphene citrate or anastrozole for ovulation induction in women with polycystic ovarian syndrome? A prospective controlled trial. Fertil Steril. 2009;92(3):860–3.
47. Mitwally MF, Casper RF. Aromatase inhibition for ovarian stimulation: future avenues for infertility management. Curr Opin Obstet Gynecol. 2002;14(3):255–63.
48. Mitwally MF, Biljan MM, Casper RF. Pregnancy outcome after the use of an aromatase inhibitor for ovarian stimulation. Am J Obstet Gynecol. 2005;192(2):381–6.
49. Adashi EY. Clomiphene citrate: mechanisms and sites of action a hypothesis revisited. Fertil Steril. 1984;42(3):331–44.
50. Santen RJ. Inhibition of aromatase: insights from recent studies. Steroids. 2003;68(7–8):559–67.
51. Goss PE, Ingle JN, Martino S, Robert NJ, Muss HB, Piccart MJ, et al. A randomized trial of letrozole in postmenopausal women after five years of tamoxifen therapy for early-stage breast cancer. N Engl J Med. 2003;349(19):1793–802.
52. Badawy A, Elnashar A, Totongy M. Clomiphene citrate or aromatase inhibitors for superovulation in women with unexplained infertility undergoing intrauterine insemination: a prospective randomized trial. Fertil Steril. 2009;92(4):1355–9.
53. Al-Fozan H, Al-Khadouri M, Tan SL, Tulandi T. A randomized trial of letrozole versus clomiphene citrate in women undergoing superovulation. Fertil Steril. 2004;82(6):1561–3.
54. He D, Jiang F. Meta-analysis of letrozole versus clomiphene citrate in polycystic ovary syndrome. Reprod Biomed Online. 2011;23(1):91–6.
55. Misso ML, Wong JL, Teede HJ, Hart R, Rombauts L, Melder AM, et al. Aromatase inhibitors for PCOS: a systematic review and meta-analysis. Hum Reprod Update. 2012;18(3):301–12.
56. Kemmann E, Jones JR. Sequential clomiphene citrate-menotropin therapy for induction or enhancement of ovulation. Fertil Steril. 1983;39(6):772–9.
57. Rose BI. A conservative, low-cost superovulation regimen. Int J Fertil. 1992;37(6):339–42.
58. Lu PY, Chen AL, Atkinson EJ, Lee SH, Erickson LD, Ory SJ. Minimal stimulation achieves pregnancy rates comparable to human menopausal gonadotropins in the treatment of infertility. Fertil Steril. 1996;65(3):583–7.
59. Badawy A, Elnashar E, Totony M. Clomiphene citrate or aromatase inhibitors combined with gonadotropins for superovulation in women undergoing intrauterine insemination: a prospective randomized trial. J Obstet Gynaecol. 2010;30(6):617–21.
60. Simon C, Cano F, Valbuena D, Remohi J, Pellicer A. Clinical evidence for detrimental effect on uterine receptivity of high serum oestradiol concentrations in high and normal responder patients. Hum Reprod. 1995;10(9):2432–7.
61. Barroso G, Menocal G, Felix H, Rojas-Juiz JC, Arslan M, Oehninger S. Comparison of the efficacy of the aromatase inhibitor letrozole and clomiphene citrate as adjuvants to recombinant follicle-stimulating hormone in controlled ovarian hyperstimulation: a prospective, randomized, blinded clinical trial. Fertil Steril. 2006;86(5):1428–31.
62. Bayar U, Basaran M, Kiran S, Coskun A, Gezer S. Use of an aromatase inhibitor in patients with polycystic ovary syndrome: a prospective randomized trial. Fertil Steril. 2006;86(5):1447–51.
63. Mitwally MF, Casper RF. Single-dose administration of an aromatase inhibitor for ovarian stimulation. Fertil Steril. 2005;83(1):229–31.
64. Atay V, Cam C, Muhcu M, Cam M, Karateke A. Comparison of letrozole and clomifene citrate in women with polycystic ovaries undergoing ovarian stimulation. J Int Med Res. 2006;34(1):73–6.

65. Begum MR, Quadir E, Begum A, Begum RA, Begum M. Role of aromatase inhibitor in ovulation induction in patients with poor response to clomifene citrate. J Obstet Gynaecol Res. 2006;32(5):502–6.
66. Al-Fadhli R, Sylvestre C, Buckett W, Tan SL, Tulandi T. A randomized trial of superovulation with two different doses of letrozole. Fertil Steril. 2006;85(1):161–4.
67. Badawy A, Metwally M, Fawzy M. Randomized controlled trial of three doses of letrozole for ovulation induction in patients with unexplained infertility. Reprod Biomed Online. 2007;14(5):559–62.
68. Biljan MM, Hemmings R, Brassard N. The outcome of 150 babies following the treatment with letrozole or letrozole and gonadotropins. Fertil Steril. 2005;84(Suppl 1):S95.
69. Fontana PG, Leclerc JM. Contraindication of Femara (letrozole) in premenopausal women. http://www.napra.ca/pdfs/advisories/Femara.pdf. Dec 2013. Accessed: 21 June 2014.
70. Physicians Desk Reference PDR. 55th ed. Anastrozole. Montvale: Medical Economics Company Inc.; 2001. p. 662–85.
71. Hu Y, Cortvrindt R, Smitz J. Effects of aromatase inhibition on in vitro follicle and oocyte development analyzed by early preantral mouse follicle culture. Mol Reprod Dev. 2002;61(4):549–59.
72. Luthra R, Kirma N, Jones J, Tekmal RR. Use of letrozole as a chemopreventive agent in aromatase overexpressing transgenic mice. J Steroid Biochem Mol Biol. 2003;86(3–5):461–7.
73. Tulandi T, Martin J, Al-Fadhli R, Kabli N, Forman R, Hitkari J, et al. Congenital malformations among 911 newborns conceived after infertility treatment with letrozole or clomiphene citrate. Fertil Steril. 2006;85(6):1761–5.
74. Hoffman JI. Incidence of congenital heart disease: I. Postnatal incidence. Pediatr Cardiol. 1995;16(3):103–13.
75. Tiboni GM. Aromatase inhibitors and teratogenesis. Fertil Steril. 2004;81(4):1158–9.
76. Drugs.com. Clomid (clomiphene citrate tablets USP). http://www.drugs.com/pro/clomid.html. 2014. Accessed 21 June 2014.
77. Badaway A, Shokeir T, Allam AF, Abdelhady H. Pregnancy outcome after ovulation induction with aromatase inhibitors or clomiphene citrate in unexplained infertility. Acta Obstet Gynecol Scand. 2009;88(2):187–91.
78. Azim A, Oktay K. Letrozole for ovulation induction and fertility preservation by embryo cryopreservation in young women with endometrial carcinoma. Fertil Steril. 2007;88(3):657–64.
79. Oktay KH. Options for preservation of fertility in women. N Engl J Med. 2005;353(13):1418–20.
80. Azim AA, Costantini-Ferrando M, Oktay K. Safety of fertility preservation by ovarian stimulation with letrozole and gonadotropins in patients with breast cancer: a prospective controlled study. J Clin Oncol. 2008;26(16):2630–5.

Gonadotropins for Women with Unexplained Infertility

27

Anupa Nandi and Roy Homburg

Introduction

Unexplained infertility refers to a diagnosis (or lack of diagnosis) made in couples in whom all the standard investigations such as tests of ovulation, tubal patency, and semen analysis are normal. It is seen to exist in as many as 30–40% of infertile couples [1]. Treatment generally is indicated when the duration of infertility is more than three years or the female partner is >35 years of age [2]. Though the place of ovarian stimulation in these ovulatory women is debatable, over the past 15 years, there has been a marked increase in the use of ovarian stimulation for the treatment of unexplained infertility. Ovarian stimulation significantly improves the fecundity in couples with unexplained infertility [3, 4, 5]. This could be achieved by correcting subtle deficiencies in the ovulation process, improving the endocrine environment, and/or endometrial receptivity. Ovarian stimulation with gonadotropins has been shown to produce better pregnancy rates than either clomiphene citrate (CC) or intrauterine insemination (IUI) alone [6, 7]. Various agents available for ovarian stimulation are gonadotropins, CC, aromatase inhibitors (AI), and pulsatile gonadotropin releasing hormone (GnRH).

While CC and AI are dealt with in detail in the preceding chapters, our aim in this chapter is to evaluate the use of gonadotropins in couples with unexplained infertility.

Use of Gonadotropins in Unexplained Infertility

Various factors influence the choice of treatment options in couples with unexplained infertility—age of the female partner, duration of infertility, Anti-Mullerian Hormone (AMH) level and other ovarian reserve markers (AFC, day 3 FSH, etc.), past obstetric history such as recurrent miscarriage and endometriosis [3]. Traditional treatment options for these couples have included expectant management (EM), IUI with or without controlled ovarian hyperstimulation (COH) or in-vitro fertilization (IVF).

With less than 2 years of unexplained infertility and in women <35 years of age, the prognosis is shown to be good even without therapy and over time they have a similar chance of achieving pregnancy even without treatments such as IUI or IVF [8, 9]. In fact the new National Institute for Health and Care Excellence (NICE) clinical guideline 2012 suggested that couples with unexplained infertility should be encouraged to try for natural conception for 2 years before they are offered treatment and they recommended offering IVF treatment to them after 2 years of EM with the exclusion of the COH + IUI option [10].

However, unexplained infertility adds considerable stress and further EM may not be acceptable to the majority of couples and hence they look for more active intervention [11]. Superovulation with or without IUI has frequently been used as first line option for these couples.

Types of Gonadotropins

Gonadotropins used in clinical practice in ovarian stimulation are follicle-stimulating hormone (FSH), Luteinizing Hormone (LH) and human chorionic gonadotropin (hCG). Human pituitary gonadotropins were first used successfully in clinical practice in 1958 [12]. Since then they have been used extensively and various preparations are now available for clinical use.

Urinary Human Menopausal Gonadotropins

The first preparations of gonadotropins available for clinical use were derived from urine of postmenopausal women. Human menopausal gonadotropin (hMG) has both FSH (75 IU) and LH (75 IU) activity in equal amount. The initial

R. Homburg (✉) · A. Nandi
Fertility Centre, Homerton University Hospitals NHS Trust, Homerton Row, Homerton, London E9 6SR, UK
e-mail: r.homburg@vumc.nl

A. Nandi
e-mail: anupa.nandi@gmail.com

G. L. Schattman et al. (eds.), *Unexplained Infertility*, DOI 10.1007/978-1-4939-2140-9_27,

preparations were rather crude and contained a significant amount of other non-gonadotropin proteins. These proteins were antigenic and were responsible for occasional allergic reactions observed in some patients. While initial preparations were only available for intramuscular administration, subsequently refinements removing the non-gonadotropin proteins made it suitable for subcutaneous injection.

Purified and Highly Purified FSH

Since the 1980s, purified FSH preparations have been produced by removing LH and non-gonadotropin proteins by monoclonal antibody techniques. Purified FSH has < 1 IU of LH activity per 75 IU of FSH activity but still has significant amounts of other proteins and requires intramuscular injection. Subsequently, highly purified FSH (HP-FSH) has been produced which contains <0.001 IU of LH per 75 IU of FSH and negligible amounts of other non-characterized proteins and can be administered subcutaneously. Reducing the non-gonadotropin proteins in these products also reduces the chance of allergic reactions.

Recombinant FSH

Reduced availability of postmenopausal urine made it difficult to produce urinary FSH in the quantities needed to meet increasing demand. Thanks to recombinant technology, production of recombinant FSH (rFSH) was made possible in virtually unlimited quantity. Recombinant FSH has similar amino acid sequence and in vitro biological activity as urinary FSH with no LH activity. rFSH has been available for clinical use since 1990. Recombinant LH is also available and has similar pharmacokinetics to native pituitary LH. However, most of the LH activity in hMG preparations comes from pituitary hCG which has a different pharmacodynamic profile and the physiologic impact of co-administering rLH remains to be determined.

Human Chorionic Gonadotropin (hCG)

hCG, readily available and cheap to manufacture is used to simulate the LH surge and induce final oocyte maturation and ovulation once follicular development is achieved with FSH. Capitalizing on the homology between LH and hCG and the longer half-life of hCG, it has also been used to augment follicle growth in LH-deficient individuals as well as poor responder patients and stimulate progesterone production post-LH surge for luteal phase support. Both urinary and recombinant hCGs are available for clinical use.

Which Preparation to Use?

Many studies have compared the different FSH preparations available. While some studies suggest that the addition of LH activity results in better outcomes (pregnancy rates) compared to rFSH [13–15], others studies have not confirmed this and find similar outcomes with rFSH being more cost-effective, compared to hMG [16–18]. In the latest Cochrane review, there was no difference seen between rFSH and hMG with respect to live birth rate [19].

Physiological Principles of Gonadotropins—the Threshold/Window Theory

The aim of ovulation induction with gonadotropins is monofollicular growth. To achieve that it is of utmost importance to understand the basic physiological principles of the pituitary–ovarian interaction. The initial follicular recruitment from the primordial pool is independent of FSH and is thought to take about 70–80 days. The follicles undergo changes from primary, secondary to small antral follicles until they become responsive to FSH. During the luteo-follicular transition the FSH level rises and it has been suggested that the FSH needs to increase above a certain level to induce follicular growth. This has led to the *threshold theory* [20]. If the FSH level increases much higher than the threshold level and is sustained, then excessive stimulation can occur in patients with ample follicular reserve. Also, it has been suggested that the recruited follicles exhibit different degrees of FSH sensitivity [21] and this FSH sensitivity changes under the influence of various growth factors [21].

Towards the late follicular phase, the level of FSH drops due to negative feedback from rising estradiol and inhibin B levels. Only the follicle that has maximum sensitivity to FSH will continue to grow in the climate of decreasing FSH levels and others with less sensitivity will become atretic, thus leading to the development of only one dominant follicle [21]. This gives rise to the *FSH window* concept. That means raised FSH level above threshold is needed for a short period to ensure growth of a single dominant follicle [22].

Therefore, if FSH is given in a dose that exceeds the threshold level for a longer period (i.e. widening the window), it will induce growth of multiple follicles by rescuing the follicles that were destined to undergo atresia. This forms the basis of super ovulation with gonadotropins. Also, these principles will help us to formulate various protocols of gonadotropin administration to avoid ovarian hyperstimulation.

Gonadotropins Compared to Clomiphene Citrate

For 50 years CC has held a strong position as a first line option for couples with unexplained infertility. It acts by increasing endogenous FSH by its antiestrogenic effect. It has been used for ovarian stimulation both alone and with IUI. It has been particularly popular due to its low cost, minimal monitoring [23], and it is well tolerated [24]. Though initial studies supported the use of clomiphene and showed it to be equally effective as gonadotropins in achieving live birth

[25], subsequent studies showed the opposite to be true [7, 26]. Recently its effectiveness in ovulatory women with unexplained infertility has been refuted showing that the use of clomiphene is no better than EM [27]; this was later confirmed by a subsequent systematic review [28] and shown not to be cost-effective [29].

Gonadotropins Compared to Aromatase Inhibitors

Due to the antiestrogenic effects of clomiphene on the endometrium and cervical mucus, it has a deleterious effect on endometrial development and hence pregnancy rates [30]. Recently, there has been a lot of interest in the use of AI. This is because, although AI suppress estrogen production and increase endogenous FSH, they do not have an antiestrogenic effects on the endometrium in the late follicular phase [31]. In addition to this, AI induce increased intraovarian androgen levels that may synergize with the central effects of decreased estrogen to enhance follicular recruitment and ovarian response to gonadotropin stimulation [32]. There have been only two studies so far, which have compared AI with gonadotropins for ovulation induction in unexplained infertility and both have shown AI to be comparable to gonadotropins in this regard. In the first randomized controlled trial (RCT), letrozole 5 mg from day 3 to day 7 was compared to 75–150 IU of hMG in 80 women aged 20–35 years with unexplained infertility undergoing IUI. Pregnancy rates between the two groups were not statistically different; 18.4% in the letrozole group and 15.7% for the gonadotropin group, although cost was significantly higher in the gonadotropin group [33]. In the second RCT, 50 couples with unexplained infertility were randomized to take letrozole 5 mg for 5 days or 150 IU of rFSH daily. Again the pregnancy rates per cycle were found to be comparable between the two groups with 8.9% in the letrozole group and 14% in the gonadotropin group. Letrozole was associated with significantly less cost and more patient convenience [34].

The Use of Combined Treatments with Gonadotropins

Letrozole has also been used together with gonadotropins. The first study was a preliminary report of 12 patients who had poor response with FSH alone in previous cycles. These patients were given letrozole 5 mg from day 3 to day 7 along with 50–225 IU of FSH daily with IUI. Letrozole was associated with a significantly higher number of mature follicles and lower FSH dose requirement [35]. Subsequent to this, several controlled and uncontrolled studies have been conducted comparing letrozole and clomiphene in combination with gonadotropins. Letrozole was shown to improve the follicular sensitivity to FSH, leading to better follicular recruitment/growth, reduced dose requirement of FSH and hence was more cost-effective [36]. When letrozole 5 mg for 5 days was compared to clomiphene 100 mg for 5 days along with gonadotropins prior to IUI, no significant difference was noted between the two groups, demonstrating that both letrozole and clomiphene were equally effective in this regard [37, 38].

Gonadotropins Along with IUI

Gonadotropins are frequently used either alone or with IUI for ovulation induction in couples with unexplained infertility. When IUI is performed along with gonadotropins, higher live birth rates were seen compared to IUI alone or EM [5]. The success of ovarian stimulation with gonadotropins and IUI varies widely in the literature ranging from 8 to 18% [4, 39]. This wide variation is due to differences in patient populations, duration of infertility, protocol for ovarian stimulation, method of insemination, sperm preparation and total motile sperm inseminated.

Dose of Gonadotropins

The aim of gonadotropin therapy for unexplained infertility in ovulatory women is to induce multifollicular development, which will in turn improve cycle fecundity [40]. Hence, strict ultrasound monitoring and dose adjustment may be required to decrease the risk of ovarian hyperstimulation syndrome (OHSS). Though the standard starting dose of FSH ranges between 75 and 150 IU for ovarian stimulation with IUI, the optimum dose is difficult to decide as every patient's individual threshold to respond (follicle sensitivity, body weight, FSH receptor polymorphisms, ovarian reserve, etc.) to a specific dose of gonadotropin is different. While some patients respond to lower dose of gonadotropin, others with similar ovarian reserve will require higher doses to initiate a response. This is due to the FSH receptor polymorphism that might exist in some individuals [41]. The latest Cochrane review suggested using the lowest possible dose of gonadotropins as the pregnancy rates are comparable to high-dose protocols and are associated with a lower risk of OHSS [42].

Premature LH Surge

One of the problems faced when performing ovulation induction designed to cause multi-follicular recruitment (superovulation) is a higher incidence of premature LH surges due to supraphysiologic estradiol (E2) levels before oocyte maturity. This leads to an increased rate of cycle cancellation, lower implantation rates, and frustration [43]. It can happen in up to 24% of IUI cycles [44]. CC, GnRH agonists, and antagonists have been used clinically to prevent a premature LH surge [45–47]. Initial studies showed improved pregnancy rates with GnRH antagonists in gonadotropin-stimulated IUI cycles [48], but subsequent multicentre trials failed to show any increased pregnancy rate with GnRH antagonists [47, 49]. However, these latter studies did show a lower incidence of LH surge and premature luteinization on adding GnRH antagonist. GnRH agonist and antagonist have been compared in women with unexplained infertility undergoing stimulated IUI. In one RCT, there was no difference between the two in regard to pregnancy rates, but GnRH antagonists offered a shorter and simpler option [50]. GnRH antagonists appear to be useful in women with previous premature LH surge during COH or to delay insemination for personal reasons.

Trigger for Ovulation Induction

In ovarian stimulation with gonadotropin and IUI cycles, it is of utmost importance that the insemination is performed around the time of ovulation. This is because both sperm and oocyte have a limited life span. Sperm survive for ~48 h and the oocyte may be fertilized for up to 12 h post LH surge. The usual practice is to trigger final oocyte maturation and ovulation with hCG. However, the use of hCG along with COH has been linked to OHSS [51]. GnRH agonist or waiting for a spontaneous LH surge may be used instead. A recent Cochrane review has analyzed ten studies comparing all these options and has shown that there is no significant difference in live birth rates between them and concluded that the choice should depend on a patient's choice, hospital facility and cost [52].

Luteal Phase Support

For a successful pregnancy outcome, it is essential to have a good luteal phase with sufficient progesterone support from the corpus luteum. One of the main problems of COH is a higher possibility of luteal phase deficiency leading to poor pregnancy outcome. This is because, in COH, multiple follicles produce multiple corpora lutea. This in turn produces supra-physiological levels of progesterone which exert a negative feedback on pituitary LH and reduce LH support for the corpus luteum. This results in premature luteolysis and hence luteal phase deficiency [53]. This is more relevant in IVF cycles using GnRH agonists or antagonists. How far this applies to IUI cycles is controversial as the number of follicles in stimulated IUI is limited. The hCG used for ovulation trigger has been shown to have a beneficial effect on the luteal phase [54]. Another agent frequently used for luteal phase support is progesterone, administered vaginally, rectally, orally or by intramuscular administration. Several studies have looked into the prospect of luteal phase support with vaginal progesterone in IUI. The two most recent systematic reviews and meta-analyses analysed 5 RCTs and have concluded that vaginal progesterone supplementation significantly improves live birth rates in IUI cycles stimulated with gonadotropins [55, 56].

Complications Associated with Gonadotropin Therapy and How to Avoid Them

The main complications of COH with gonadotropins are OHSS and multiple pregnancies—both caused by multiple follicular development. It is not possible to avoid either complication entirely since the goal of treatment is the development of more than a single follicle. However, while high-order multiple pregnancies (triplets or more) can be significantly reduced by conservative treatment protocols and avoiding pregnancy when more than 2 or 3 follicles develop, severe OHSS, a potentially life-threatening condition, is to be avoided at all costs.

OHSS

OHSS is a condition characterized by a shift of fluid from the intracellular compartment to the extracellular spaces leading to hypovolemia and hemoconcentration. While the exact mechanism is still being debated, hCG remains the catalyst that allows it to occur. The hCG causes an inflammatory milieu in the preovulatory follicle and the release of vasoactive substances from the ovaries which increases vascular permeability [57]. There are two types of OHSS. The first, early onset, is caused by the hCG trigger given to induce final oocyte maturation. The second, late onset, occurs if the patient becomes pregnant and secretes hCG into the maternal circulation. High estrogen levels from multiple follicles act as a mediator of hCG on the vascular system [40]. Limiting the number of follicles by careful monitoring and dose adjustments [42], withholding hCG [58], and/or cancelling the cycle avoiding pregnancy altogether remains the most commonly used methods to prevent OHSS. Other methods used are coasting (withholding gonadotropins until estradiol falls to <3000 pg/ml before administering hCG for follicle maturation) [59], follicular reduction by aspirating some of the developing follicles prior to hCG [60], administering a GnRH agonist to induce an LH surge for final oocyte maturation [61], converting to IVF and cryopreserving embryos with delayed transfer in a non-stimulated cycle or postponing embryo transfer and evaluating for signs of early OHSS with cryopreservation of all embryos for patients at high risk [62]. All these measures reduce but do not eliminate the possibility of experiencing OHSS.

Multiple Pregnancies

While many people associate IVF with the problem of twins or high-order multiple pregnancy, in fact superovulation with or without IUI in women with unexplained infertility accounts for most of these pregnancies [63]. IVF, with restrictions on the maximum number of embryos to be transferred in some countries and less restrictive guidelines in others, is associated with far fewer high-order multiple pregnancies. Furthermore, recent technological advances such as extended embryo culture to the blastocyst stage and preimplantation aneuploidy screening have increased the use of elective single embryo transfer, which has further reduced the number of multiple pregnancies in women undergoing IVF cycles [64, 65].

While it is impossible to eliminate the risk of multiple pregnancy in superovulation + IUI, the aim should be to reduce the risk to as low as possible with low-dose gonadotropin treatment and close ultrasound monitoring to monitor for risk factors and adjust gonadotropin dose or cancel cycles.

Is Gonadotropin Treatment for Superovulation a Thing of the Past?

Recently, the role of ovarian stimulation and IUI in couples with unexplained infertility has been questioned and the recent NICE guideline recommends not offering controlled ovarian stimulation and/or IUI for these couples [10]. As per the NICE guideline, these women should be offered IVF after 2 years of EM [10].

The effectiveness of IUI in unexplained infertility has been questioned by a multicenter randomized clinical study [8]. In this study, 253 couples with women aged <39 years and having an estimated probability of spontaneous pregnancy of 30–40 % were randomized to either COH + IUI for 6 months or EM for 6 months and showed similar pregnancy rates in both groups. The authors concluded that COH + IUI are no better than EM. However, this small study is not conclusive and the results may be questioned as the success rate of COH + IUI per cycle in the participating centers was <10 % and the insemination was performed irrespective of the total motile sperm count (TMS) after preparation. This approach may have lowered outcomes as there is evidence that lower TMS affects the success of IUI [66].

Another prospective trial randomized women into either a conventional arm (followed by up to three cycles of FSH/IUI and finally up to 6 cycles of IVF if not successful) or an accelerated arm (CC/IUI for up to 3 cycles followed by up to 6 cycles of IVF if not successful, omitting the FSH/IUI cycles). An increased pregnancy rate was observed in the accelerated arm compared to the conventional arm and was also found to be more cost-effective [67].

However, a recent Cochrane review has failed to prove effectiveness of IVF over EM or IUI in unexplained infertility due to inadequate data from RCTs. Regardless, they have concluded that IVF may be more effective than COH + IUI [68].

In theory, increasing the number of ovulatory follicles should increase pregnancy rates and gonadotropin + IUI has long been a popular standard approach to treat patients with unexplained infertility, as it has fewer dropouts compared to IVF due to its less invasive and less time-consuming nature [69].

Conclusion

A diagnosis of unexplained infertility is associated with dissatisfaction, frustration, stress, helplessness, and a sense of failure. Although these couples are tolerant of a short period of EM, the majority seek more active treatment especially if unsuccessful within a given time period. Although for women >35 years of age and those with poor ovarian reserve and long duration infertility, IVF seems a reasonable first line option, the use of gonadotropins for COH is presently widely accepted for patients with unexplained infertility. Prior to the use of gonadotropins with IUI, a frank discussion with the couple regarding success rates, costs, risks and alternatives is warranted. This discussion should be documented in the patient's medical record. Until additional, well-designed studies are performed, the best initial approach to treatment in couples with unexplained infertility will remain a matter of debate. Ovulation induction with gonadotropins in ovulatory patients with patent fallopian tubes as well as normal semen parameters will most likely remain in our list of acceptable treatment alternatives.

References

1. Smith S, Pfiefer SM, Collins J. Diagnosis and management of female infertility. JAMA. 2003;290:1767–70.
2. Collins JA, Burrows EA, Willan AR. The prognosis for live birth among untreated infertile couple. Fertl Steril. 1995;64:22–8.
3. Nuojua-Huttunen S, Tomas C, Bloigu R, Tuomivaara L, Martikainen H. Intrauterine insemination treatment in subfertility: an analysis of factors affecting outcome. Hum Reprod. 1999;14(3):698–703 (0268–1161).
4. Guzick DS, Carson SA, Coutifaris C, Overstreet JW, Factor-Litvak P, Steinkampf MP, Hill JA, Mastroianni L, Buster JE, Nakajima ST, Vogel DL, Canfield RE. Efficacy of superovulation and intrauterine insemination in the treatment of infertility. National Cooperative Reproductive Medicine Network. N Engl J Med. 1999 Jan 21;340(3):177–83.
5. Veltman-Verhulst SM, Cohlen BJ, Hughes E, Heineman MJ. Intra-uterine insemination for unexplained subfertility. Cochrane Database Syst Rev. 2012;9: CD001838. doi:10.1002/14651858.CD001838.pub4.
6. Karlström PO, Bergh T, Lundkvist O. A prospective randomized trial of artificial insemination versus intercourse in cycles stimu-

lated with human menopausal gonadotropin or clomiphene citrate. Fertil Steril. 1993 Mar;59(3):554–9.
7. Costello MF. Systematic review of the treatment of ovulatory infertility with clomiphene citrate and intrauterine insemination. Aust N Z J Obstet Gynaecol. 2004 Apr;44(2):93–102 (0004–8666).
8. Steures P, van der Steeg JW, Hompes PG, Habbema JD, Eijkemans MJ, Broekmans FJ, Verhoeve HR, Bossuyt PM, van der Veen F, Mol BW, Collaborative Effort on the Clinical Evaluation in Reproductive Medicine. Intrauterine insemination with controlled ovarian hyperstimulation versus expectant management for couples with unexplained subfertility and an intermediate prognosis: a randomised clinical trial. Lancet. 2006 Jul;368(9531):216–21.
9. Brandes M, Hamilton CJ, van der Steen JO, de Bruin JP, Bots RS, Nelen WL, Kremer JA. Unexplained infertility: overall ongoing pregnancy rate and mode of conception. Hum Reprod. 2011;26(2):360–68.
10. NICE Guideline. Fertility: assessment and treatment for people with fertility problems. NICE clinical guideline (CG 156). 2013;1.8.1: 3–4
11. Nadeem R. Unexplained infertility: an exploration of women's perceptions of diagnosis, treatment and decision-making. J Obstet Gynaecol. 2010 Jan;30(1):83–84 (0144–3615).
12. Gemzell CA, Diczfalusy E, Tillinger KG. Clinical effects of human pituitary follicle stimulating hormone (FSH). J Clin Endocrinol Metab. 1958;18:138–48.
13. European and Israeli Study group on highly purified Menotropin versus Recombinant Follicle Stimulating Hormone. Efficacy and safety of highly purified menotropin versus recombinant follicle-stimulating hormone in in vitro fertilization/intracytoplasmic sperm injection cycles: a randomised. Comparative trial. Fertil Steril. 2002;78(3):520–8.
14. Anderson AN, Devroey P, Arce JC. Clinical outcome following stimulation with highly purified hMG or recombinant FSH in patients undergoing IVF: a randomised assessor- blind controlled trial. Hum Reprod. 2006;21(12):3217–27.
15. Coomarasamy A, Afnan M, Cheema D, van der Veen F, Bossuyt PM, van Wely M. Urinary hMG versus recombinant FSH for controlled ovarian hyperstimulation following an agonist long down-regulation protocol in IVF or ICSI treatment: a systematic review and meta-analysis. Hum Reprod. 2008;23(2):310–5.
16. Trew GH, Brown AP, Gillard S, Blackmore S, Clewlow C, O''Donohoe P, Wasiak R. In vitro fertilisation with recombinant follicle stimulating hormone requires less IU usage compared with highly purified human menopausal gonadotrophin: results from a European retrospective observational chart review. Reprod Biol Endocrinol. 2010;8:(137). doi:10.1186/1477-7827-8-137 (1477–7827).
17. Demirol A, Gurgan T. Comparison of different gonadotrophin preparations in intrauterine insemination cycles for the treatment of unexplained infertility: a prospective randomized study. Hum Reprod. 2007 Jan;22(1):97–100 (Epub 2006 Sep 5).
18. Ravelli A, Poso F, Gennarelli G, Moffa F, Grassi G, Massobrio M. Recombinant versus highly-purified, urinary follicle stimulating hormone (r-FSH vs HP-uFSH) in ovulation induction: a prospective, randomized study with cost-minimization analysis. Reprod Biol Endocrinol. 2006 Jul;4:38.
19. Van Wely M, Kwan I, Burt AL, et al. Recombinant versus urinary gonadotrophin for ovarian stimulation in assisted reproductive technology cycles. Cochrane Database Syst Rev. 2011;2:CD005354.
20. Brown JB. Pituitary control of ovarian function–concepts derived from gonadotrophin therapy. Aust N Z J Obstet Gynecol. 1978 Feb;18(1):46–54.
21. Scheele F, Schoemaker J. The role of follicle-stimulating hormone in the selection of follicles in human ovaries: a survey of the literature and a proposed model. Gynaecol Endocrinol. 1996;10:55–66.
22. Fauser BC, Van Heusden AM. Manipulation of human ovary function: physiological concepts and clinical consequences. Endocr Rev. 1997;18:71–106.
23. Practice Committee of the American Society for Reproductive Medicine. Effectiveness and treatment for unexplained infertility. Fertil Steril. 2006;86:S111–4.
24. Pittman JH, Hammoud A, Keye WR, Gurtcheff SE, Czajkowski L, Gibson M. Psychological and physical symptoms in women undergoing superovulation with clomiphene citrate: a double-blind, placebo-controlled, crossover study. Fertil Steril. 2011 Sept;96(3):S153 (0015–0282).
25. Dankert T, Kremer JA, Cohlen BJ, Hamilton CJ, Pasker-de Jong PC, Straatman H, van Dop PA. A randomized clinical trial of clomiphene citrate versus low dose recombinant FSH foe ovarian hyperstimulation in intrauterine insemination cycles for unexplained and male subfertility. Hum Reprod. 2007 Mar;22(3):792–7 (Epub 2006 Nov 16).
26. Berker B, Kahraman K, Taskin S, Sukur YE, Sonmezer M, Atabekoglu CS. Recombinant FSH versus clomiphene citrate for ovarian stimulation in couples with unexplained infertility and male subfertility undergoing intrauterine insemination: a randomized trial. Arch Gynecol Obstet. 2011 Dec;284(6):1561–6 (0932–0067;1432–0711).
27. Bhattacharya S, Harrild K, Mollison J, Wordsworth S, Tay C, Harrold A, McQueen D, Lyall H, Johnston L, Burrage J, Grossett S, Walton H, Lynch J, Johnstone A, Kini S, Raja A, Templeton A. Clomifene citrate or unstimulated intrauterine insemination compared with expectant management for unexplained infertility: pragmatic randomised controlled trial. BMJ (Clinical research ed.). 2008;337:a716 (1468–5833).
28. Hughes E, Brown J, Collins JJ, Vanderkerchove P. Clomiphene citrate for unexplained subinfertility in women. Cochrane Database Syst Rev 2010;(1):CD000057. doi:10.1002/14651858.CD000057.pub2.
29. Wordsworth S, Buchanan J, Mollison J, Harrild K, Robertson L, Tay C, Harrold A, McQueen D, Lyall H, Johnston L, Burrage J, Grossett S, Walton H, Lynch J, Johnstone A, Kini S, Raja A, Templeton A, Bhattacharya S. Clomifene citrate and intrauterine insemination as first-line treatments for unexplained infertility: are they cost-effective? Hum Reprod. 2011 Feb;26(2):369–75 (0268–1161; 1460–2350).
30. Massai MR, de Ziegler D, Lesobre V, Bergeron C, Frydman R, Bouchard P. Clomiphene citrate affects cervical mucus and endometrial morphology independently of the changes in plasma hormone levels induced by multiple follicular recruitment. Fertil Steril. 1993;59(6):1179–86.
31. Holzer H, Casper R, Tulandi T. A new era in ovulation induction. Fertil Steril. 2006;85(2):277–84.
32. Pritts AE. Letrozole for ovulation induction and controlled ovarian stimulation. Curr Opin Obstet Gynaecol. 2010;22:289–94.
33. Baysoy A, Serdaroglu H, Jamal H, Karatekali E, Ozornek H, Attar E. Letrozole versus human menopausal gonadotropin in women undergoing intrauterine insemination. Reprod Miomed Online. 2006;13(2):208–12.
34. Gregoriou O, Vlahos NF, Konidaris S, Papadias K, Botsis D, Creatsas GK. Randomized controlled trial comparing superovulation with letrozole versus recombinant follicle-stimulating hormone combined with intrauterine insemination for couples with unexplained infertility who had failed clomiphene citrate stimulation and intrauterine insemination. Fertil Steril. 2008 Sep;90(3):678–83 (Epub 2007 Oct 25).
35. Mitwally MF, Casper RF. Aromatase inhibition improves ovarian response to follicle-stimulating hormone in poor responders. Fertile Steril. 2002;77(4):776–80.
36. Bedaiwy MA, Forman R, Mousa NA, Al Inany HG, Casper RF. Cost-effectiveness of aromatase inhibitor co-treatment for controlled ovarian stimulation. Hum Reprod. 2006;21(11):2838–44.
37. Barroso G, Menocal G, Felix H, Rojas-Ruiz JC, Arslan M, Oehninger S. Comparison of the efficacy of the aromatase inhibitor letrozole and clomiphene citrate as adjuvants to recombinant

follicle-stimulating hormone in controlled ovarian stimulation: a prospective, randomized, blinded clinical trial. Fertil Steril. 2006;86(5):1428–31.
38. Badawy A, Elnashar A, Totongy M. Clomiphene citrate or aromatase inhibitors combined with gonadotropins for superovulation in women undergoing intrauterine insemination: a prospective randomised trial. J Obstet Gynaecol. 2010;30(6):617–21.
39. Goverde AJ, McDonnell J, Vermeiden JP, Schats R, Rutten FF, Schoemaker J. Intrauterine insemination or in-vitro fertilisation in idiopathic subfertility and male subfertility: a randomised trial and cost effectiveness analysis. Lancet. 2000;355:13–8.
40. Amer S. Gonadotropin induction of ovulation. Obstetrics, Gynaecology and Reproductive medicine Med. 2007;17(7):205–10.
41. Simoni M, Nieschlag E, Gromoll J. Isoforms and single nucleotide polymorphisms of the FSH receptor gene: implications for human reproduction. Hum Reprod Update. 2002;8(5):413–21.
42. Cantineau AEP, Cohlen BJ, Heineman MJ. Ovarian stimulation protocols (anti-oestrogens, gonadotrophins with and without GnRH agonists/antagonists) for intrauterine insemination (IUI) in women with subfertility. Cochrane Database Syst Rev. 2007;2:CD005356. (10.1002/14651858.CD005356.pub2).
43. Manzi D, Dumez S, Scott LB, Nulsen JC. Selective use of leuprolide acetate in women undergoing superovulation with intrauterine insemination results in significant improvement in pregnancy outcome. Fert Steril. 1995;63:866–73.
44. Cohlen BJ, te Velde ER, van Kooij RJ, Looman CW, Habbema JD. Controlled ovarian hyperstimulation and intrauterine insemination for treating male subfertility: a controlled study. Hum Reprod. 1998;13:1553–8.
45. Al-Inany H, Azab H, El-Khayat W, NadaA, El-Khattan E, Abou-Serra AM. The effectiveness of clomiphene citrate in LH surge suppression in women undergoing IUI: a randomized controlled trial. Fertil Steril. 2010 Nov; 94(6):2167–71.
46. Garliardi CL, Emmi AM, Weiss G, Schmidt CL. Gonadotropin-releasing hormone agonist improves the efficiency of controlled ovarian hyperstimulation/intrauterine insemination. Fertil Steril. 1991;55(5):939–44.
47. Lambalk CB, Leader A, Olivennes F, Fluker MR, Andersen AN, Ingerslev J, Khalaf Y, Avril C, Belaisch-Allart J, Roulier R, et al. Treatment with the GnRH antagonist ganirelix prevents premature LH rises and luteinization in stimulated intrauterine insemination: results of a double-blind, placebo-controlled, multicentre trial. Hum Reprod. 2006;21:632–9.
48. Gomez-Palomares JL, Julia B, Acevedo-Martin B, Martinez-Burgos M, Hernandez ER, Ricciarelli E. Timing ovulation for intrauterine insemination with a GnRH antagonist. Hum Reprod. 2005;20:368–72.
49. Crosignani PG, Somigliana E, Intrauterine Insemination Study Group. Effect of GnRH antagonists in FSH mildly stimulated intrauterine insemination cycles: a multicentre randomized trial. Hum Reprod. 2007 Feb;22(2):500–5 (Epub 2006 Oct 24).
50. Zikopoulos K, Kaponis A, Adonakis G, Sotiriadis A, Kalantaridou A, Georgiou I. A prospective randomized study comparing gonadotropin-releasing hormone agonists or gonadotropin-releasing hormone antagonists in couples with unexplained infertility and/or mild oligozoospermia. Fertil Steril. 2005;83(5):1354–62.
51. Schenker J, Weinstein D. Ovarian hyperstimulation syndrome: a current survey. Fertil Steril. 1978;30:255–68.
52. Cantineau AE, Janssen MJ, Cohlen BJ. Synchronised approach for intrauterine insemination in subfertile couples. Cochrane Database Syst Rev. 2010;14(4):CD006942.
53. Fauser BC, Devroey P. Reproductive biology and IVF: ovarian stimulation and luteal phase consequences. Trends Endocrinol Metab. 2003;14:236–42.
54. Olson JL, Reprod RW, Schreiber JR, Vaitukaitis YL. Shortened luteal phase after ovulation induction with human menopausal gonadotropin and chorionic gonadotropin. Fertil Steril. 1983;39:284–91.
55. Miralpeix E, González-Comadran M, SolÃ I, Manau D, Carreras R, Checa MA. Efficacy of luteal phase support with vaginal progesterone in intrauterine insemination: a systematic review and meta-analysis. J Assist Reprod Genet. 2014 Jan;31(1):89–100.
56. Hill MJ, Whitcomb BW, Lewis TD, Wu M, Terry N, DeCherney AH, Levens ED, Propst AM. Progesterone luteal support after ovulation induction and intrauterine insemination: a systematic review and meta-analysis. Fertil Steril. 2013 Nov;100(5):1373–80.
57. Gómez R, Soares SR, Busso C, Garcia-Velasco JA, Simón C, Pellicer A. Physiology and pathology of ovarian hyperstimulation syndrome. Semin Reprod Med. 2010;28:448–57. doi:10.1055/s-0030–1265670.
58. Delvigne A, Rozenberg S. Epidemiology and prevention of ovarian hyperstimulation syndrome (OHSS): a review. Hum Reprod Update. 2002;8:559–77.
59. Waldenstrom U, Kahn J, Marsk L, Nilsson S. High pregnancy rate and successful prevention of severe ovarian hyperstimulation syndrome by prolonged coasting of very hyperstimulated patients: a multicentre study. Human Reprod. 1999;14:294–7.
60. Egbase PE, Makhsee M, Alsharhan M, Grudzinskas JG. Timed unilateral ovarian follicular aspiration prior to administration of human chorionic gonadotrophin for the prevention of severe ovarian hyperstimulation syndrome in in-vitro fertilization: a prospective randomized study. Hum Reprod. 1997;12:2603–6.
61. Gonen Y, Balakier H, Powell W, Casper RF. Use of gonadotrophin releasing hormone agonist to trigger follicular maturation for in-vitro fertilization. J Clin Endocrinol Metab. 1990;71:918–22.
62. Awonuga AO, Pittrof RJ, Zaidi J, Dean N, Jacobs HS, Tan SL. Elective cryopreservation of all embryos in women at risk of developing ovarian hyperstimulation syndrome may not prevent the condition but reduces the live birth rate. J Assist Reprod Genet. 1996;13:401–6.
63. Ozturk O, Templeton A. In-vitro fertilisation and risk of multiple pregnancy. Lancet. 2002 Jan;359(9302):232.
64. Heitmann RJ, Burney RO, Klein N, Chow GE. Elective single embryo transfer vs. double embryo transfer: evaluation of pregnancy and multiple gestation rates. Fertil Steril. 2011 Mar;95(4):S27 (0015–0282).
65. Min JK, Hughes E, Young D, Gysler M, Hemmings R, Cheung AP, Goodrow GJ, Senikas V, Wong BC, Sierra S, Carranza-Mamane B, Case A, Dwyer C, Graham J, Havelock J, Lee F, Liu K, Vause T. Elective single embryo transfer following in vitro fertilization. J Obstet Gynaecol Can. (Journal d''obstetrique et gynecologie du Canada). 2010 Apr;32(4):363–77 (1701–2163).
66. Wainer R, Albert M, Dorion A, Bailly M, Bergère M, Lombroso R, Gombault M, Selva J. Influence of the number of motile spermatozoa inseminated and of their morphology on the success of intrauterine insemination. Hum Reprod. 2004 Sep;19(9):2060–5 (Epub 2004 Jul 8).
67. Reindollar RH, Regan MM, Neumann PJ, Levine B-S, Thornton KL, Alper MM. A randomized clinical trial to evaluate optimal treatment for unexplained infertility: the fast track and standard treatment (FASTT) trial. Fertil steril. 2010;94(3):888–899 (0015–0282).
68. Pandian Z, Gibreel A, Bhattacharya S. In vitro fertilisation for unexplained infertility. Cochrane Database Syst Rev. 2012;4:CD003357 (1469–493X).
69. Land JA, Courtar DA, Evers JLH. Patient drop out in an assisted reproductive technology programme: implications for pregnancy rates. Fertil Steril. 1997;68:278–81.

Part VI

Assisted Reproductive Techniques and Future Perspectives

Gonadotropin in Assisted Reproduction: An Evolution Perspective

28

Rogério B. F. Leão and Sandro C. Esteves

Introduction

Gonadotropin therapy has a central role in ovarian stimulation. Its introduction in medical practice dates from almost one century ago, and represented a major upgrade in infertility treatments.

Follicle stimulation hormone (FSH) was originally derived from animal (pregnant mare serum) or human (postmortem pituitary glands) sources, but these preparations were abandoned because of safety concerns [1–3]. Gonadotropins were first extracted from urine in the 1940s: human chorionic gonadotropin (hCG) in 1940 and human menopausal gonadotropin (hMG) in 1949. Over a decade later, the first urinary forms of hCG and hMG became commercially available [2, 3]. Treatment of anovulatory women with exogenous gonadotropin administration started in the 1960s and expanded to ovulatory women to promote multifollicular development in the 1980s [1–3].

Further improvements in the purification methods led to the production of FSH-only products in the 1980s, followed by the highly purified urinary FSH (HP-hFSH), which became available 10 years later, in 1993 [2–3]. In the 1970s and 1980s, advances in DNA technology enabled the development of recombinant human FSH (rec-hFSH), which became commercially available in 1995 [2–4]. In 2000, recombinant human luteinizing hormone (rec-hLH) became available and, with the launch of recombinant human hCG (rec-hCG) in 2001, the complete recombinant gonadotropin portfolio was launched [2, 3]. The most recent developments have been (i) the introduction of the filled-by-mass (FbM) rec-hFSH formulation in 2004, which improved batch-to-batch consistency when compared with products quantified by the standard rat in vivo bioassay, (ii) the combination of rec-hFSH and rec-hLH in the same formulation in 2007, (iii) the long-acting FSH gonadotropin in 2010, and (iv) the novel family of pen injectors that deliver recombinant gonadotropins in 2011 [5–11].

The purposes of this chapter are (1) to review the glycoproteic structure and actions of gonadotropins, (2) to describe the discovery landmarks of exogenous gonatropin preparations, from earlier animal extracts to current products manufactured by recombinant technology, (3) to examine the quality, safety, and clinical efficacy of commercially available gonadotropins, (4) to examine the rationale of using luteinizing hormone (LH) supplementation during ovarian stimulation and the differences in LH activity between rec-hLH and hMG preparations, and lastly (5) to present the future perspectives on novel pharmaceutical preparations for follicular stimulation.

Physiology of Endogenous Gonadotropins: A Brief Overview

Gonadotropins comprise a category of glycoproteic hormones including FSH, LH, and hCG. FSH and LH are synthesized and secreted by gonadotrophs of the anterior pituitary gland under stimulation of pulsatile secretion of gonadotropin-releasing hormone (GnRH) from the hypothalamus [12]. Human chorionic gonadotropin is synthesized during pregnancy by syncytiotrophoblast cells and also by the pituitary in perimenopause and menopause women [13, 14].

FSH and LH bind to G protein-coupled receptors and stimulate the production of cyclic adenosine monophosphate (cAMP) by activation of protein kinase A pathway [15]. In males, FSH is essential for Sertoli cell function and spermatogenesis whereas in females it stimulates recruitment and growth of early antral follicles (2–5 mm in diameter) [16]. FSH receptors are expressed only in the granulosa cells (GC) while LH/hCG receptors are expressed in both GC and

S. C. Esteves (✉) · R.B.F. Leão
ANDROFERT, Andrology and Human Reproduction Clinic, Referral Center for Male Reproduction, Avenida Dr. Heitor Penteado, 1464, Campinas, SP 13075-460, Brazil
e-mail: s.esteves@androfert.com.br

G. L. Schattman et al. (eds.), *Unexplained Infertility*, DOI 10.1007/978-1-4939-2140-9_28,

theca cells. Although LH/hCG receptors expression is at its maximum in GC of preovulatory follicles, antral follicles with 3–10 mm in diameter already express these receptors at approximately 10 % of the maximum [17]. While FSH acts as the main antral follicular growth regulator, LH plays a key role in promoting steroidogenesis and development of the leading follicle and has different functions in different stages of the cycle [18]. During the early follicular phase, LH stimulates the production of androgens by theca cells. Androgens are then transferred to the GC and transformed into estrogens via aromatization [19]. Lastly, LH promotes final follicular maturation via its direct effects on the GC in the late follicular phase [20].

Follicular Recruitment and Growth During Menacme

The primordial follicle comprises the oocyte, arrested at the diplotene stage of the meiotic prophase, and a single layer of spindle-shaped GC. Primordial follicles undergo growth and atresia at all times, not interrupted by pregnancy, ovulation, or periods of anovulation. This dynamic process continues at all ages, including infancy and around menopause [22]. It is a continuous phenomenon driven by unknown mechanisms, but it appears to be independent of pituitary gonadotropins [16]. The early development of follicles occurs over the time span of several menstrual cycles. In ovulatory women, it has been estimated that follicle growth from primordial to large preantral stages takes approximately 150 days [23]. Most of this time span (up to the late developmental stage) involves responses independent of hormonal regulation. In vitro studies indicate that activin stimulates granulosa cell division in preantral follicles, which, in turn, are influenced by other growth factors including TGF-β, bone morphogenetic proteins and growth and differentiation factor 9. In addition, GC of preantral follicles are responsive to estrogens, androgens, insulin, and insulin-like growth factor-1. Despite that, translation of these findings in vivo is yet to be fully confirmed [24].

Preantral folliculogenesis thus provides a continuous source of early antral follicles from the primordial pool [24]. Studies on human folliculogenesis have shown that FSH receptor gene expression is halted until primordial follicles begin to grow [25]. The early antral follicles become FSH responsive and will constitute the pool of available follicles that can be stimulated to develop [16]. As a result of corpus luteum demise and subsequent decrease in estrogen production during the luteo–follicular transition, FSH serum concentrations start to rise before menses and continue to increase during the first 6 days of the follicular phase [16, 18, 22, 24]. FSH rise is crucial to rescue antral follicles from atresia. A threshold concentration of FSH must be achieved to initiate follicular development otherwise the cohort of follicles available to grow is doomed to apoptosis [16, 26]. Under FSH influence at the beginning of the menstrual cycle, a group of 3–11 follicles per ovary is propelled to grow in a process named "recruitment" [12, 27].

Upon FSH binding to its receptor, adenylate cyclase-mediated signal is activated, which is followed by the expression of multiple mRNAs that encode proteins responsible for cell proliferation, differentiation, and function. FSH stimulates the proliferation and growth of granulosa cells (mitogenic action) and induces aromatase activity via P450 activation [22]. Concomitantly, there is an increase in the number of FSH receptors as GC respond to FSH. The regulation of GC's FSH receptor activity is complex and involves not only the direct cAMP-mediated FSH influence on its own receptor gene but also estrogen and other inhibitory agents including epidermal growth factor, fibroblast growth factor and GnRH-like protein. Inhibin and activin, also produced by granulosa cells in response to FSH, have autocrine activity and stimulate the production of FSH receptors thus enhancing FSH action [18, 22].

Ovarian Steroidogenesis

The two-cell system, first proposed by Falck in 1959, is a logical explanation for the events involved in ovarian steroidogenesis [22, 28]. This system is based on the assumption that while FSH receptors are present only in the GC, LH receptors are present in the theca cells and absent in the GC during the early follicular stages [18, 22]. Theca cells are characterized by exhibiting steroidogenic activity in response to LH stimulation. Specifically, cholesterol is converted in androgens, that is, testosterone and androstenedione, by transcription activities of cholesterol side-chain cleavage enzyme (P450scc), P450c17 and 3β-hydroxysteroid dehydrogenase (3β-HSD) genes. The starting point of steroid biosynthesis is cholesterol, a carbon 27 (C27) steroid [18, 29, 30]. Cholesterol is converted to pregnenolone (C21) by P450scc (CYP11A—cytochrome P450, family 11, subfamily A, polypeptide 1), whose regulation is mediated by steroidogenic acute regulatory protein (StAR). StAR facilitates the influx of cholesterol into the mitochondria where P450scc is located. StAR expression is enhanced by cAMP and by stimulation of GC with FSH, LH and hCG [30].

The primary route of pregnenolone metabolism is via the delta-5 pathway, the first two steps of which are driven by the same enzyme, CYP17 (P450c17). The hydroxylation of pregnenolone at the C17a position forms 17-hydroxypregnenolone, and the subsequent removal of the acetyl group forms the androgen precursor dehydroepiandrosterone (DHEA). Accordingly, CYP17 has both hydroxylase and lyase activity. Lastly, DHEA is converted to androstenedione by 3β-HSD (Fig. 28.1; [18, 29, 30]). A secondary route of

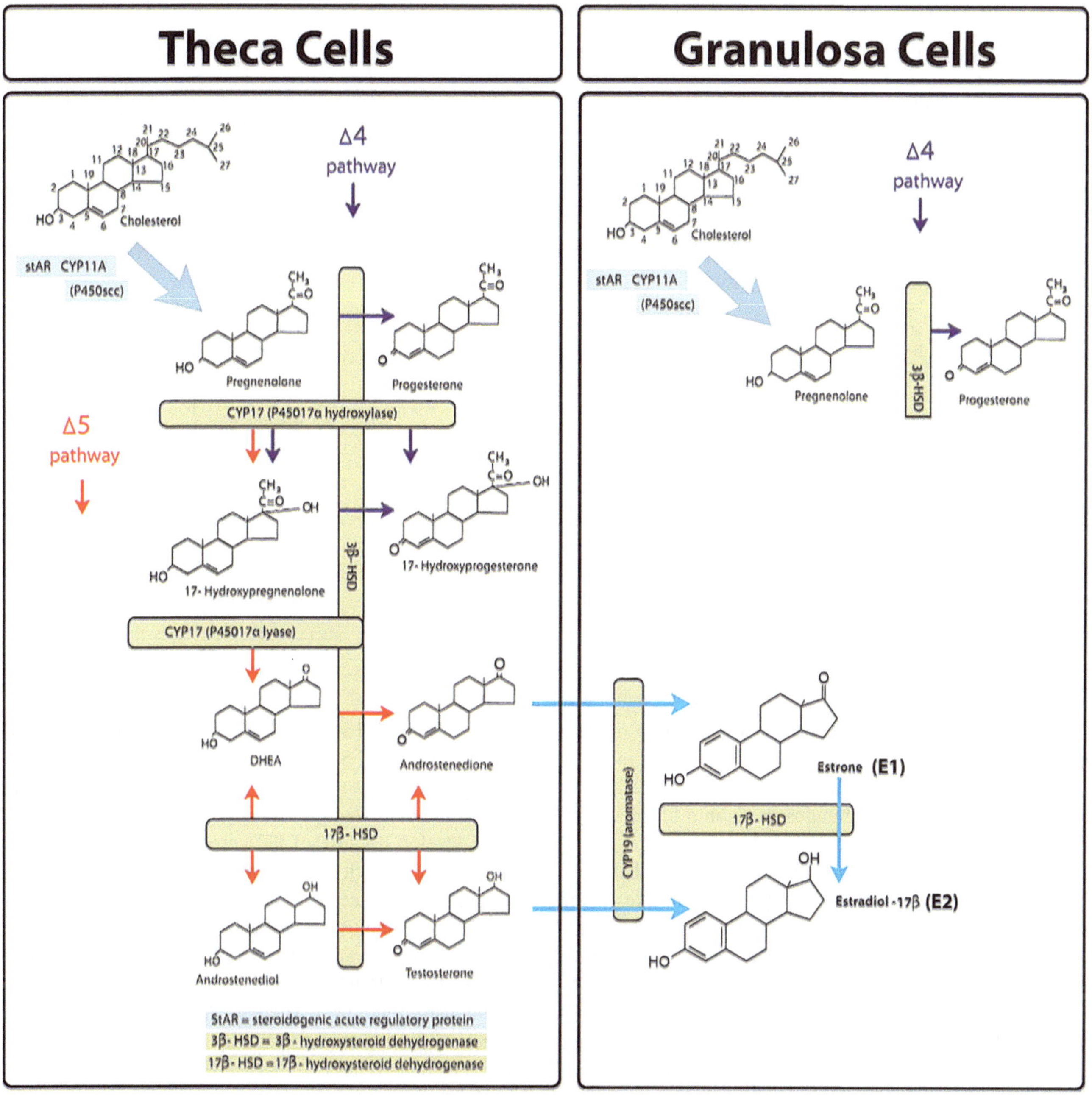

Fig. 28.1 Human ovarian steroidogenesis. The starting point for steroid biosynthesis is the conversion of cholesterol in pregnenolone by P450scc. One route of pregnenolone metabolism is the delta-5 pathway (*red arrows*) by action of CYP17 (P450c17). Hydroxylation of pregnenolone at the C17a position forms 17-hydroxypregnenolone, and subsequent removal of the acetyl group forms the androgen precursor dehydroepiandrosterone (*DHEA*). Another route of pregnenolone metabolism is the delta-4 pathway (*purple arrows*) in which pregnenolone is converted to progesterone by the action of 3b-HSD (an irreversible conversion). Progesterone is then converted to 17-hydroxyprogesterone by CYP17. In humans, 17-hydroxyprogesterone cannot be further metabolized. Aromatization of androgens to estrogens is a distinct activity within the granulosa layer induced by FSH via activation of the P450 aromatase (P450arom) gene

metabolism involves the conversion of pregnenolone to progesterone by the action of 3β-HSD via the delta-4 pathway. Progesterone is then converted to 17-hydroxyprogesterone by CYP17 (Fig. 28.1; [30]).

Importantly, CYP17 is located exclusively in thecal and interstitial cells, the extrafollicular compartment of the ovary, whereas CYP19 (aromatase), that converts androgens to estrogens, is expressed exclusively in GC, the intrafollicular compartment [31, 32]. Thus, aromatization of androgens to estrogens is a distinct activity within the granulosa layer induced by FSH via activation of the P450 aromatase (P450arom) gene. Androgens produced in the theca layer

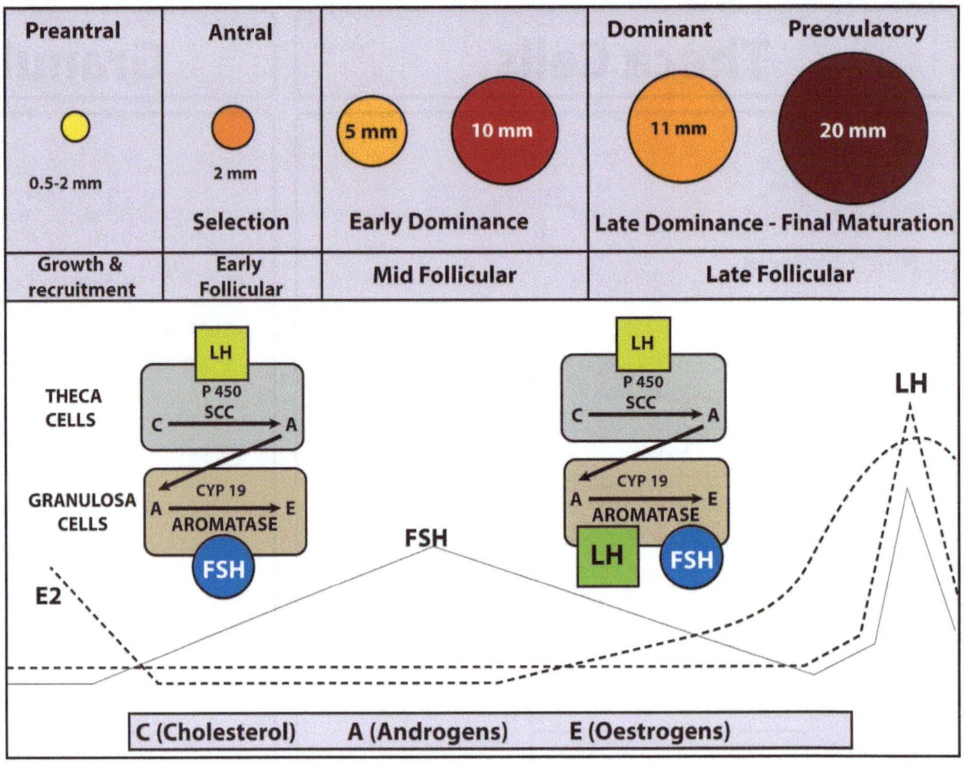

Fig. 28.2 The "two-cell" system. FSH receptors are present only in the granulosa cells. LH receptors are present in the theca cells and initially absent in the granulosa cells. In response to LH, theca cells convert cholesterol to androgens (testosterone and androstenedione). CYP17 is located exclusively in thecal cells whereas CYP19 (aromatase) is expressed only in the granulosa. Thus, androgens must diffuse into the granulosa layer to be converted to estrogen via aromatization induced by FSH. Both FSH and LH act via AMPc production. In the late follicular phase, FSH induces LH receptor formation in the granulosa cells, which acquire LH responsiveness. In the granulosa, LH enhances FSH action (increasing estrogen production)

must therefore diffuse into the granulosa layer to be converted to estrogens. Hence, increasing levels of estradiol in the peripheral circulation during follicular phase reflect the release of estrogen from granulosa cells into blood vessels (Fig. 28.2; [18, 22]).

Theca and granulosa cells also secrete peptides that act as both autocrine and paracrine factors [33]. Insulin-like growth factor (IGF) is secreted by theca cells and enhances LH-mediated androgen production within the thecal compartment as well as FSH-mediated aromatization in granulosa cells. Inhibin and activin are produced in the granulosa cells in response to FSH, and modulate the expression of steroidogenic enzymes, especially P450c17 in theca cells. While inhibin enhances androgen synthesis, activin has an opposite effect. Activin also has the important autocrine role of enhancing FSH action mainly by increasing the expression of FSH receptors [18].

In conclusion, estrogen secretion by the follicle prior to ovulation is the result of combined LH and FSH stimulation of the two cell types, theca and granulosa, influenced by autocrine and paracrine factors (Fig. 28.3; [18, 22]).

Follicular Selection

The enzymatic activity within both granulosa and theca cells leads to estradiol rise (and inhibin), and as a consequence FSH serum concentration progressively falls due to inhibition of GnRH synthesis in the hypothalamus [16, 18]. The mid-follicular FSH fall causes atresia of less mature follicles that are unable to grow without adequate FSH stimulation. On the other hand, a maturing selected follicle continues to develop because of its increased sensitivity to FSH that in turn makes it less dependent to FSH itself [16]. In addition, FSH induces LH receptor expression in preovulatory follicle granulosa cells [34]. The action of LH on its receptors also activates adenyl cyclase leading to the production of cAMP, which represents an additional stimulus to follicular growth [35]. Thereby, the maturing follicle also reduces its dependency on FSH by acquiring LH receptors and LH responsiveness [16, 34, 36, 37].

LH acts in GC to stimulate steroidogenesis, ultimately leading to an increase in estrogen production (Figs. 28.2 and 28.3) [22]. At first, estrogen levels rise slowly during the late follicular phase. It is then followed by a rapid rise that reaches its peak approximately 24–36 h prior to ovulation [38]. The LH surge occurs when the peak of estradiol is achieved [39]. Under physiologic conditions, an estradiol threshold of 200 pg/mL for at least 2 days is needed for LH surge [40].

Most circulating progesterone (~ 95 %) is produced in the intrafollicular compartment by the granulosa cells via the action of 3β-HSD that catalyzes the conversion of pregnonolone (delta-4 pathway) under LH influence (Fig. 28.1; [22, 29]). Despite a marked increase in progesterone levels measured at the veins of the active ovary in the mid-follicular phase, peripheral concentrations increase only slightly probably

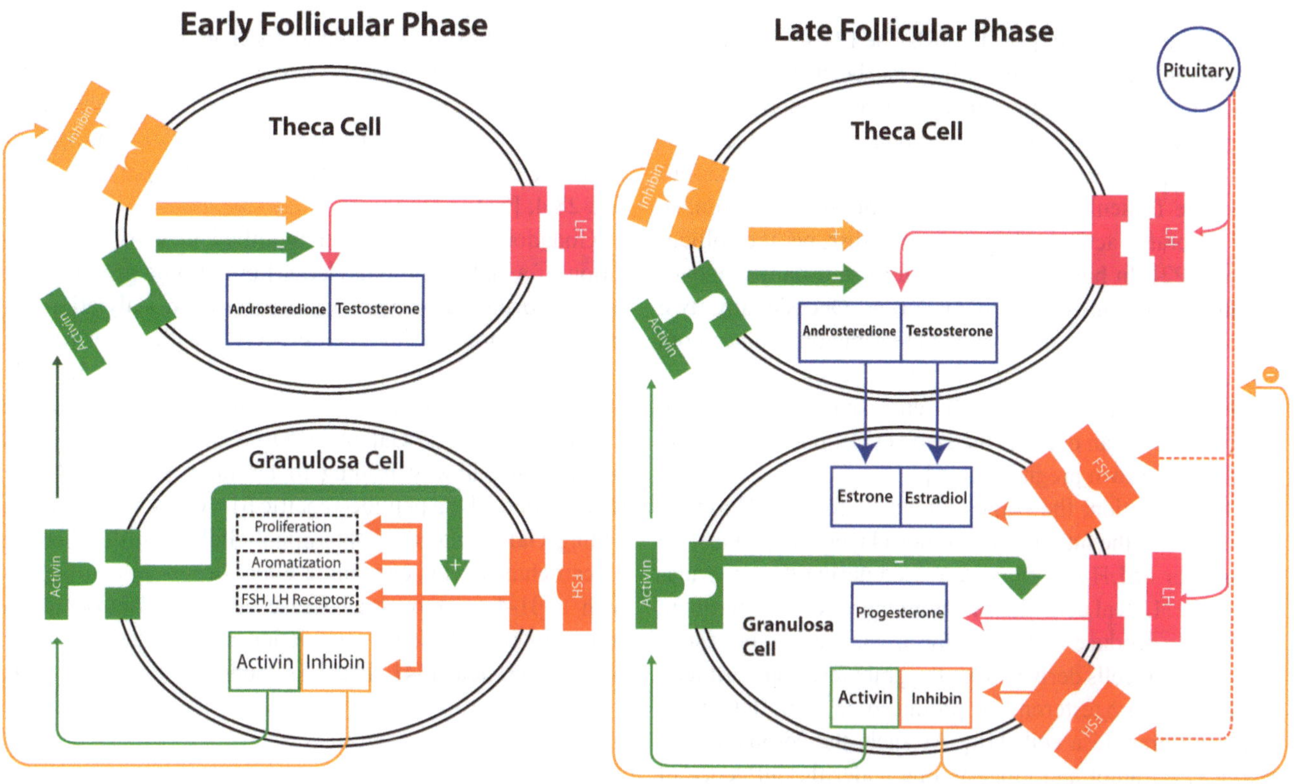

Fig. 28.3 Modulation of steroidogenic enzymes. In the early follicular phase inhibin and activin are produced by the granulosa cells in response to FSH. They have important paracrine functions to modulate the expression of steroidogenic enzymes, especially P450c17 in theca cells. Inhibin enhances LH function thus stimulating androgen synthesis to latter aromatization to estrogen in the granulosa, whereas activin suppresses androgen synthesis. Activin has also an important autocrine role of enhancing FSH action especially by increasing the production of FSH receptors. Production of inhibin by the granulosa cells is increased in the late follicular phase while activin is decreased, with a positive effect on androgen production by theca cells. FSH induces LH receptor formation in the granulosa cells, which acquire LH responsiveness and thus, less FSH dependence. In granulosa, LH enhances FSH action which in turn increase estrogen production, initiates progesterone production (negatively modulated by activin), and control granulosa production of inhibin. The increase in inhibin, in turn, suppresses FSH secretion by the pituitary, important to ensure the dominance of a single follicle

due to active liver metabolism [42]. Progesterone can be further converted to 17-hydroxyprogesterone by CYP17 (via delta-4 pathway). However, very little 17-hydroxyprogesterone is converted to androstenedione since human CYP17 catalyses this reaction at only 3 % of the rate for the conversion of 17-hydroxypregnenolone to DHEA [29, 21, 41]. Hence, 17-hydroxyprogesterone is basically the final product of the delta-4 pathway in humans. Moreover, progesterone cannot be metabolized in the GCs because CYP17 is not expressed within this cell compartment; as such, progesterone is the final product of the delta-4 pathway in the intrafollicular compartment and cannot be further converted to estradiol within the GC under the effect of LH (or hCG) [31].

The preovulatory rise in progesterone facilitates the positive feedback action of estrogen on the pituitary; the latter is the key factor to induce the midcycle LH peak. Progesterone also stimulates a midcycle FSH surge, important to support the full expression of LH receptors in the granulosa layer [22, 44]. In experimental studies, it has been demonstrated that elevated levels of estradiol per se can elicit simultaneous surges of LH and FSH, thus indicating that progesterone is not mandatory although it certainly enhances estradiol action [22, 45].

Ovulation

The LH surge triggers resumption of oocyte meiosis that had been halted at prophase I (germinal vesicle stage). Also, it promotes luteinization of granulosa cells and the synthesis of prostaglandins and other eicosanoids that are essential for follicle rupture. The LH surge is characterized by three phases: (i) a rapidly ascending phase lasting for 14 h, (ii) a plateau of approximately 14 h, and (iii) a descending phase of about 20 h [46]. During the LH surge, intrafollicular levels of progesterone continue to rise up to the time of ovulation. FSH, LH, and progesterone stimulate the activity of proteolytic enzymes, such as matrix metalloproteinases, disintegrin, and metalloproteinase with thrombospondin-like repeats (adamts), which digest collagen in the follicular wall and increase its distensibility [22, 47, 48]. The LH surge also triggers the release of histamine, which has been shown to fully support follicle rupture in some experimental models [22].

Granulosa and theca cells also produce plasminogen activator in response to the LH surge, which activates plasminogen in the follicular fluid to produce plasmin. Plasmin, in turn, generates active collagenase that disrupts the follicular wall [22]. In humans, only one follicle usually achieves dominance and grows up to ovulation. Occasionally, two follicles reach the 10 mm stage at the same time; since both are equally sensitive to FSH, they survive and grow in this relatively low physiological FSH environment. As a result, two ovulations can occur in the same cycle, possibly leading to a dizygotic twin pregnancy [16].

After ovulation, the corpus luteum is formed. Hormone production by the luteinized granulosa layer is dependent on the number of LH receptors expressed during the preovulatory phase. Luteal cells derived from the theca compartment continue to produce androgens for aromatization into estrogens by luteal cells derived from the granulosa compartment. In addition, progesterone is produced in both luteinized theca and granulosa cells [18]. As such, the corpus luteum produces estradiol and progesterone under the influence of endogeneous LH activity. As the luteal phase progresses, progesterone inhibits LH release via negative feedback. During the luteal-follicular transition, the LH decline causes the corpus luteum to involute and demise [49]. If implantation occurs, the syncytiotrophoblast cells start to produce hCG, which binds to LH/hCG receptors. In early pregnancy, hCG rescues the corpus luteum and maintains luteal function until placental steroidogenesis is well established [22].

Structure and Function of Endogenous Gonadotropins

Gonadotropins (FSH, LH, and hCG) are proteins covalently linked to a carbohydrate (glycoproteins). They are composed of two noncovalently linked protein subunits, the alpha and beta. The three-dimensional structure and the active conformation of the subunits are maintained by internal disulfide bonds [50]. The alpha subunit contains 92 amino acids and is identical in FSH, LH, and hCG. In contrast, beta subunits are distinct and confer unique receptor specificity as well as differential biological and immunological properties [51]. Protein subunits alone have no biologic activity; the latter is provided by the attachment of carbohydrate moieties forming heterodimers [3]. In general, protein glycosylation plays a very important regulatory role in determining protein activity and function. The extent and pattern of glycosylation convey the differential spectrum of charges, bioactivities and half-lives of each glycoprotein [52]. Glycoproteins have two basic types of glycosylation patterns, the O-linked and N-linked. O-linked glycosylation is characterized by attachment of the carbohydrate N-acetylgalactosamine (GalNAc) to the hydroxyl group of an amino acid, serine, or threonine. N-linked glycosylation involves attachment of N-acetyl glucosamine (GlcNAc) to the amide group of asparagine (Asn; Fig. 28.4; [53]).

Gonadotropins are further modified in vivo by the addition of a sialic acid (sialylation) or sulfonic group (sulfonation) to the carbohydrate moieties. Both sialylation and sulfonation are physiological processes with major roles in gonadotropin biological activity modulation [54, 55]. The oligosaccharides often terminate with sialic acid and/or sulfonated β1-4-linked GalNAc (SO_3-4GalNAc) [54, 56]. The sulfonation pathway leading to terminal SO_3-4GalNAc is first regulated by a peptide-specific β1-4GalNAc-transferase adding GalNAc to the subterminal GlcNAc residue on the glycan chains. This enzymatic effect occurs in competition with a β1-4-galactosyltransferase adding galactose to the subterminal GlcNAc in a sialylation pathway leading to terminal sialic acid [54]. There are some elements that must

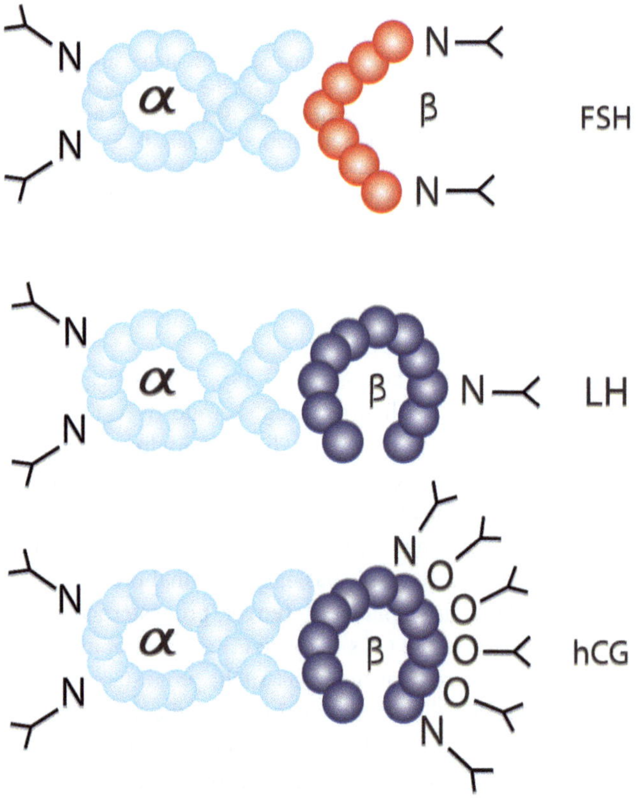

Fig. 28.4 Glycosylation patterns of FSH, LH, and hCG. The alpha subunits of each hormone are identical in amino acid sequence and contain two sites of N-linked glycosylation. The beta subunit confers hormone specificity and contains variable amounts of N-linked glycosylation. LH beta subunit contains a single site of N-linked glycosylation, while FSH and hCG beta subunits contain two sites of N-linked glycosylation. In addition, hCG has an extended C-terminal that contains four sites of O-linked glycosylation

be recognized by GalNAc-transferase [57]. For example, a Pro-Leu-Arg tripeptide motif in the beta subunit of LH and a cluster of cationic amino acids (Pro-Leu-Arg-Ser-Lys-Lys) in the corresponding alpha subunit are recognized by the β1-4GalNAc-transferase leading to a considerably increased rate of GalNAc transfer to the LH molecule. Unlike LH, the tripeptide motif is not present in the beta subunit of FSH thus resulting in a low-enzymatic activity of the peptide-specific β1-4GalNAc-transferase. Therefore, sulfonation plays a considerably lower role in the clearance of FSH compared with LH. On the other hand, sialylation pathway dominates the FSH molecule [54]. The extent and pattern of glycosylation also seem to be under hormonal influence, most likely from a combination of steroidal feedback and GnRH [55, 58].

Molecules with increased number of sulfonated Gal-NAc disappear faster from the circulation than less sulfonated isoforms, due to their affinity to specific SO_3-4GalNAc receptors in the liver [54, 59]. On the other hand, increased number of sialic acids enhances half-life [54, 60]. While removal of the carbohydrate moieties of either subunit diminishes gonadotropic activity, experimental data indicate that carbohydrate chains have no role in gonadotropins binding to their receptors [61]. However, carbohydrate components affect the biologic activity of the hormone-receptor complex after binding, thus playing a critical role in activation (coupling) of the adenylate cyclase system [62].

Follicle-Stimulating Hormone (FSH)

Likewise LH and hCG, the alpha subunit of FSH has 92 amino acids (AA). The beta subunit is composed of 111 amino acids with four N-linked glycosylation sites, two on the alpha subunit, added to Asn52 and Asn78, and two on the beta subunit (Asn7 and Asn24) [53, 63]. Thereby, each subunit is attached to two carbohydrate moieties with variable compositions that, in turn, create different isoforms (Fig. 28.5; [3, 53]). These multiple isoforms of FSH differ in their plasma half-lives (ranging from 3 to 4 h) and bioactivity [3].

Although both sialic acid and sulfonated GalNAc residues modulate the half-lives of human gonadotropins, sialic acid residues are much more common in FSH than sulfonated residues [60]. Increased sialylation enhances FSH metabolic stability by decreasing both glomerular filtration and clearance by sialoglycoprotein receptors in the liver, which is the major site for gonadotropin clearance [64, 65]. It means that the greater the sialic acid content, the longer the hormone remains in circulation [54–56, 60, 64, 65].

Production of different isoforms is controlled by a combination of steroidal feedback and GnRH [55, 66]. The higher the estradiol levels, the lower the FSH sialylation (Table 28.1; [3, 67]). Therefore, the pattern of circulating

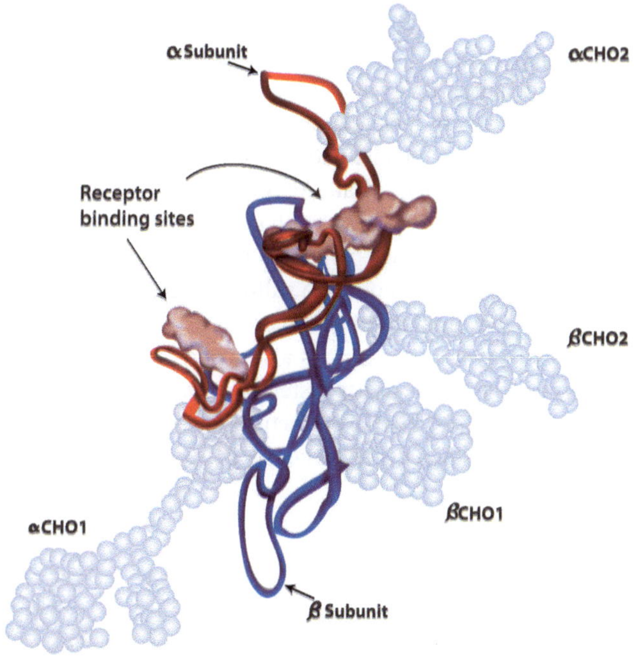

Fig. 28.5 Follicle-stimulating hormone molecule. FSH is a glycoprotein consisted of two subunits, the alpha subunit (*red*) and the beta subunit (*blue*). There are four carbohydrate attachment sites, two in each subunit. The carbohydrate chains are represented by the *light blue balls*

Table 28.1 Characteristics of native FSH isoforms

Isoform	Sialic acid content	Biologic activity	In vivo half-life	Predominance
Acid	High	Low	Long	Early/mid-follicular and luteal phase
Basic	Low	High	Short	Late follicular/preovulatory phase

FSH during the menstrual cycle is dynamic with respect not only to its quantity (concentration) but also to isoform distribution (quality) [58]. The isoform profile is more acidic during early follicular to midfollicular phase, and become more basic shortly before ovulation [3, 58, 68]. These dynamic changes in sialylation are not mimicked by exogenous gonadotropin formulations, and it is unknown whether the absence of such fluctuations during controlled ovarian stimulation (COS) would affect oocyte quality [3].

Luteinizing Hormone

Although the LH alpha subunit is identical to that of FSH, the beta subunit contains more amino acids (121 AA) than FSH, a difference that confers its specific biologic activity and is responsible for its interaction with the LH receptor [3].

Elimination of LH from circulation is modulated by the number of both SO3-GalNAc and sialic acid residues attached to the carbohydrate moieties [64]. LH β-subunits contain a single site of N-linked glycosylation (Asn 30) and less sialic acid residues (only 1 or 2); as such, LH has a short initial half-life of only 20–30 min (Fig. 28.6; [64]). Furthermore, LH molecules with increased number of SO3-4GalNAc disappear faster from the circulation due to binding of sulfonic groups to specific SO3-4GalNAc receptors at the hepatic endothelial cells [54, 59]. In rats, it has been demonstrated that the aforesaid hepatic receptors bind bovine LH with highest affinity only when two or more sulfonated GalNAc residues are present on multiple oligosaccharides. Because this particular carbohydrate structure is also found on human LH, it seems possible that a similar system operates in humans [60].

Likewise FSH, LH shows fluctuations in isoform profile during the menstrual cycle. More basic LH isoforms are seen

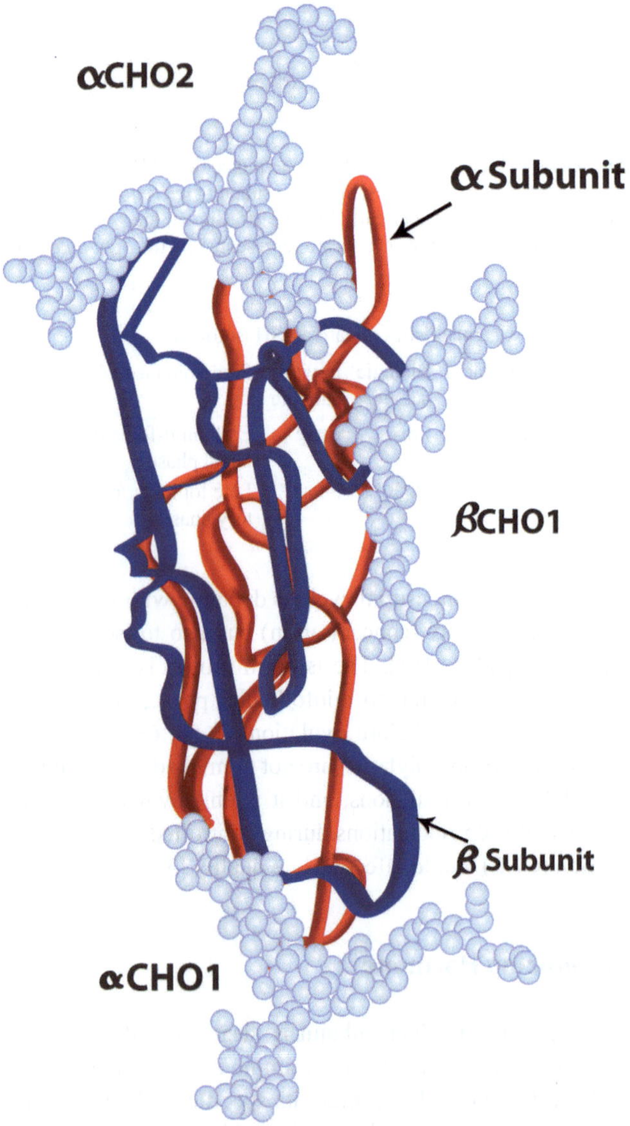

Fig. 28.6 Luteinizing hormone molecule. LH is a glycoprotein with two subunits, the alpha subunit (*red*), similar to that of FSH and hCG with two carbohydrate attachment sites, and the beta subunit (*blue*), with only one carbohydrate attachment site. The carbohydrate chains are represented by the *light blue balls*

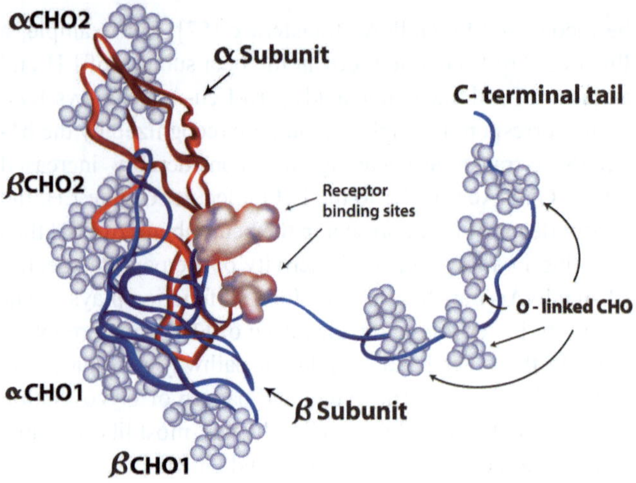

Fig. 28.7 Human chorionic gonadotropin molecule. hCG is similar in its structural attributes to LH. A notable exception is the presence of a long carboxy-terminal segment that is O-glycosylated (O-linked CHO), conferring longer half-life to hCG. The alpha and beta subunits are represented in *red* and *blue strands*, respectively, whereas the carbohydrate chains are represented by the *light blue balls*

at midcycle due to considerably decreased sulfonation concomitant with slightly increased sialylation. Both changes increase LH half-life in the circulation, thus explaining the increased levels of serum LH at this period. This change in isoform profile seems to be physiologically important for ovulation triggering [60].

Human Chorionic Gonadotropin

As already mentioned, the alpha subunit of hCG is identical to those of LH and FSH. Although hCG amino acid sequence is similar to that of LH, a notable difference is the presence of a long carboxyterminal segment with 24 AA containing four sites of O-linked oligosaccharides (Fig. 28.7; [3, 53]). In addition, hCG beta subunits contain two sites of N-linked glycosylation compared with a single site in LH. Due to the higher number of both glycosylation sites and sialic acid residues (approximately 20) than LH, native hCG exhibit a markedly longer terminal half-life in comparison with LH (Table 28.2; [64]).

Landmark Studies in the Development of Exogenous Gonadotropins

Early Understanding of the Hypothalamic–Pituitary–Ovarian Axis

The development of gonadotropin preparations began in 1910, when experimental evidence suggested that the pituitary had a role in the regulation of gonadal stems. Crowe

Table 28.2 Structural characteristics of endogenous FSH, LH, and hCG

	Alpha subunit	Beta subunit	N-linked glycosylation sites (alpha)	N-linked glycosylation sites (beta)	O-linked glycosylation sites (beta)	Carboxyl terminal segment	Half-life
FSH	92 AA	111 AA	2	2	–	Absent	3–4 h
LH	92 AA	121 AA	2	1	–	Absent	20–30 min
hCG	92 AA	145 AA	2	2	4	Present	24 h

$t\frac{1}{2}$=time that it takes for the concentration in blood plasma of a substance to reach one-half of its steady-state value
AA amino acids

et al. were the first to show that partial pituitary ablation resulted in gonadal atrophy in adult dogs and persistence of infantilism in puppies. Two years later, Aschner confirmed these findings and postulated that pituitary function depended upon the function of higher centers in the brain. This author was the first to suggest that the gonads were affected by pituitary extracts and that their use might have clinical applications [2].

In the late 1920s, numerous studies with different species showed that implantation of anterior pituitary tissue from sexually mature females into sexually immature counterparts induced precocious sexual maturity, marked enlargement of the ovaries and superovulation. In contrast, reproductive function was lost after complete pituitary ablation in both sexes [2, 3].

In 1929, Zondek proposed that two hormones were secreted by the pituitary and had stimulatory effects to the gonads. These hormones were named "Prolan A" and "Prolan B" which are now known as FSH and LH, respectively. These authors described the relationship between the pituitary and gonads and the cyclical secretory dynamics of the two gonadotropins in women [2, 3].

Discovery of hCG, PMSG, and Animal Pituitary Extracts

Zondek, in collaboration with Ascheim (1927), demonstrated that the blood and urine of pregnant women contained a gonad-stimulating substance capable of inducing both follicular maturation and ovarian stromal luteinization when injected into immature mice. They believed that this substance was produced by the anterior pituitary. Subsequently, it has been shown that this substance was human chorionic gonadotropin (hCG) being produced in the placental tissue of the syncytiotrophoblast [2, 3, 69]. In vitro production of hCG was then possible by culturing placental tissue. hCG was commercially launched in 1931 under the label of Pregnon®, later changed to Pregnyl® [2, 3].

In 1930, following the discovery of hCG, a substance found in the maternal–fetal interface of pregnant mares and extracted from their blood was purified, stabilized as a powder, and sterilized for use in laboratory and clinical studies. This substance was named "pregnant mare's serum gonadotropin" (PMSG; [3]). Early observations revealed that hCG administered alone in the follicular phase failed to promote follicular development and ovulation, indicating that hCG had no effect in the absence of FSH [2, 70]. In contrast, clinical trials demonstrated that PMSG was able to induce an ovarian response, but attempts to fully induce ovulation produced inconsistent results [71]. Concomitantly, researchers sought other gonadotropic animal extracts to be used in the treatment of infertile patients suffering from gonadotropin insufficiency. In the 1930s, gonadotropins extracted from swine and sheep pituitaries were tested clinically to treat such patients [2].

The concept of using PMSG, hog or sheep pituitary gonadotropins to stimulate follicular development and hCG to trigger ovulation (two-step protocol) was introduced in 1941 [72]. Pituitary animal extracts and PMSG were used in both Europe and the USA until the early 1960s, despite the findings that such treatments resulted in the production of neutralizing antibodies (antihormones), which rendered the ovaries unresponsive to repeated stimulation [2, 3, 73]. Due to the aforementioned effect, PMSG was withdrawn from the market in the early 1970s. Nevertheless, animal-derived gonadotropins were still available in some eastern European countries until 1998 [2].

Human Pituitary Gonadotropin

The recognition that animal gonadotropins induced the production of antihormone antibodies, which could neutralize not only the preparation administered but also endogenous gonadotropins, had been the driven forces of scientific and technological efforts to extract and purify gonadotropins from human sources. In this sense, a special interest group, named "G club," was formed in 1953 to coordinate and promote the development of specific assay procedures as well as bioassay standards and purification methods to obtain gonadotropin preparations suitable for therapeutic purposes [2].

Human pituitary gonadotropin (hPG) was first isolated in 1958 by Carl Gemzell. Between 1958 and 1988, hPG preparations were successfully used for ovulation induction worldwide [74, 75]. However, it soon became clear that the supply of human pituitaries was too limited to fulfill its constantly growing demand [1–3]. Pituitary glands from ten individuals were needed to yield sufficient quantities of gonadotropin to stimulate one patient for one cycle. In addition, there were constant problems with purification and dose standardization

[1]. By the mid—1980s, cases of dementia and death due to iatrogenic Creutzfeldt-Jacob disease (CJD) were identified in Australia, France, and the UK, and were linked to the use of hPG and human pituitary growth hormone. As a consequence, hPG was banned from the market approximately 20 years after its introduction [2, 3].

Gonadotropin Preparations Currently Available for Clinical Use

Human Menopausal Gonadotropin

hMG, or menotropin, was first extracted from the urine of postmenopausal women in 1949 [2]. Urine was originally obtained from an Italian nunnery, and early preparations contained varying amounts of FSH, LH, and hCG in only 5% pure forms [3]. Improvements in the purification techniques standardized FSH and LH activities to 75 IU for each type of gonadotropin in 1963, as measured by standard in vivo bioassays (Steelman–Pohley assay). The first hMG preparation was registered in Italy in 1950, but clinical trials only started 10 years later [3]. hMG preparations have both FSH and LH activity, but the latter is primarily derived from the hCG component present in postmenopausal urine and concentrated during purification [2, 13, 14]. Sometimes hCG is added to achieve the desired amount of LH-like biological activity [2]. In 1999, purified hMG gonadotropins were introduced, allowing its subcutaneous (SC) administration [3, 4]. At present, both conventional hMG and highly purified hMG (HP-hMG) are commercially available in a FSH:LH ratio of 1:1 [4].

Urinary FSH

In the 1980s, pure urinary FSH preparations were produced by removing LH with polyclonal antibodies. The production process was essentially passive since LH was separated from the bulk material, and FSH, together with some other urinary proteins, was collected and lyophilized. Despite being a biologically purer urinary gonadotropin, urofollitropin, or purified urinary follicle-stimulating hormone (hFSH-P) still contained high amounts of urinary proteins [76]. Further technological advances made it possible to use highly specific monoclonal antibodies to extract FSH and produce HP-hFSH. The latter became commercially available in 1993 and is available to date. Such preparations contain <0.1 IU of LH and <5% of unidentified urinary proteins. FSH specific activity is approximately 10,000 IU/mg protein compared to 100–150 IU/mg protein in the earlier urinary hMG preparations (Table 28.3). Likewise HP-hMG, the enhanced purity of HP-hFSH enabled SC delivery [3]. Subcutaneous gonadotropin administration represented an important gain for patients. Consistently better tolerability (lower pain at injection site) was reported with SC injections compared with the intramuscular route. More importantly, it allowed self-administration which is more convenient and less time-consuming, as patients need fewer visits to the clinic or hospital for injections [77, 78].

Recombinant FSH Preparations

Recombinant technology has met the need for a more reliable source of FSH. Under appropriate conditions, the genes coding for the human FSH alpha subunit and betasubunit have been incorporated into the nuclear DNA of a host cell via a plasmid vector, using spliced DNA strings containing the FSH gene and segments of bacterial DNA [2, 3, 79]. Early recombinant technology focused on producing biological molecules in bacterial cells, usually *Escherichia coli*, as for insulin production. However, due to the complex structure of human gonadotropins and the need of post-translational glycosylation, which define the degradation time and bioactivity, production of functional FSH was not possible using prokaryotes. Certain mammalian cell lines have been otherwise used to produce recombinant complex proteins, including erythropoietin and gonadotropins. The Chinese hamster ovary (CHO) cell line has been chosen to produce gonadotropins because it is genetically stable, fully characterized and easily transfected with foreign DNA. Furthermore, it can be grown in cell cultures on a large scale and produce adequate levels of biologically active rec-hFSH [2, 79].

In 1995, the first rec-hFSH (follitropin alfa) was licensed for clinical use in the European Union. One year later, a similar

Table 28.3 Differences between hMG and FSH gonadotropin formulations

	Purity (FSH content) (%)	Mean specific FSH activity (U/mg protein)	LH activity (IU/vial)	Injected protein per 75 IU (mcg)
hMG	<5	~100	75	~750
HP-hMG	<70	2000–2500	75	~33
rec-hFSH				
Follitropin beta	>99	7000–10,000	0	8.1
Follitropin alfa	>99	13,645	0	6.1

rec-hFSH recombinant human follicle-stimulating hormone, *hMG* human menopausal gonadotropin, *HP-hMG* highly purified human menopausal gonadotropin rec-hFSH (follitropin beta) was made available [2]. In the manufacturing process of follitropin alfa, two separate vectors, one for each subunit, are used to build the master cell bank of FSH-producing cell line, unlike follitropin beta in which a single vector contains the coding sequences of both subunit genes [79, 80]. The subsequent production steps are similar for both preparations (Fig. 28.8). First, a working cell bank is established by growing cells from a single vial that contains identical cell preparations. An aliquot from the selected clone of CHO cells is grown in T-flasks, then subcultured into roller bottles and allowed to expand for up to 36 days. The cells are then mixed with a suspension of microcarrier beads and transferred to a bioreactor vessel with continuous culture media infusion for an average of 34 days. The cell culture supernatant medium, containing the proteins secreted by the cells, is collected from the bioreactor. The harvested "crude FSH" is stored at 48 °C until purification [2]. Lastly, the protein is purified by chromatography, followed by ultrafiltration. The downstream purification process differs for the two commercially available recombinant FSH preparations. The follitropin beta process uses a series of anion and cation exchange chromatography steps, hydrophobic chromatography and size exclusion chromatography. A similar series of chromatography steps are used in the production of follitropin alfa, in addition to an immunoaffinity step with a specific monoclonal antibody that is similar to the one used in the production of HP-hFSH [2, 79]. Each purification step is rigorously controlled in order to ensure batch-to-batch consistency of the final purified product [2]. While the production of urine-derived gonadotropins is often performed in open, nonsterile environments, the production of rec-hFSH takes place in closed, sterile environments, such as the bioreactor. Both the production and the purification of rec-hFSH are subject to continuous quality control assessments, ensuring a pure, consistent and high-quality product [79]. These same concepts highlighted above are now used in the manufacturing process of other recombinant gonadotropins including LH and hCG [2, 3].

Both recombinant FSH preparations are structurally similar to native FSH. Despite being named follitropin alfa and follitropin beta, each one comprises alpha and beta glycoprotein chains [3]. However, due to the slight differences in their production and purification procedures the preparations are not identical, with variations in posttranslational glycosylation that result in different sialic acid residue compositions and different isoelectric coefficients [3, 81, 82]. Follitropins alfa and beta are similar to the native FSH isoforms found in the blood around mid-cycle (more basic isoforms), but

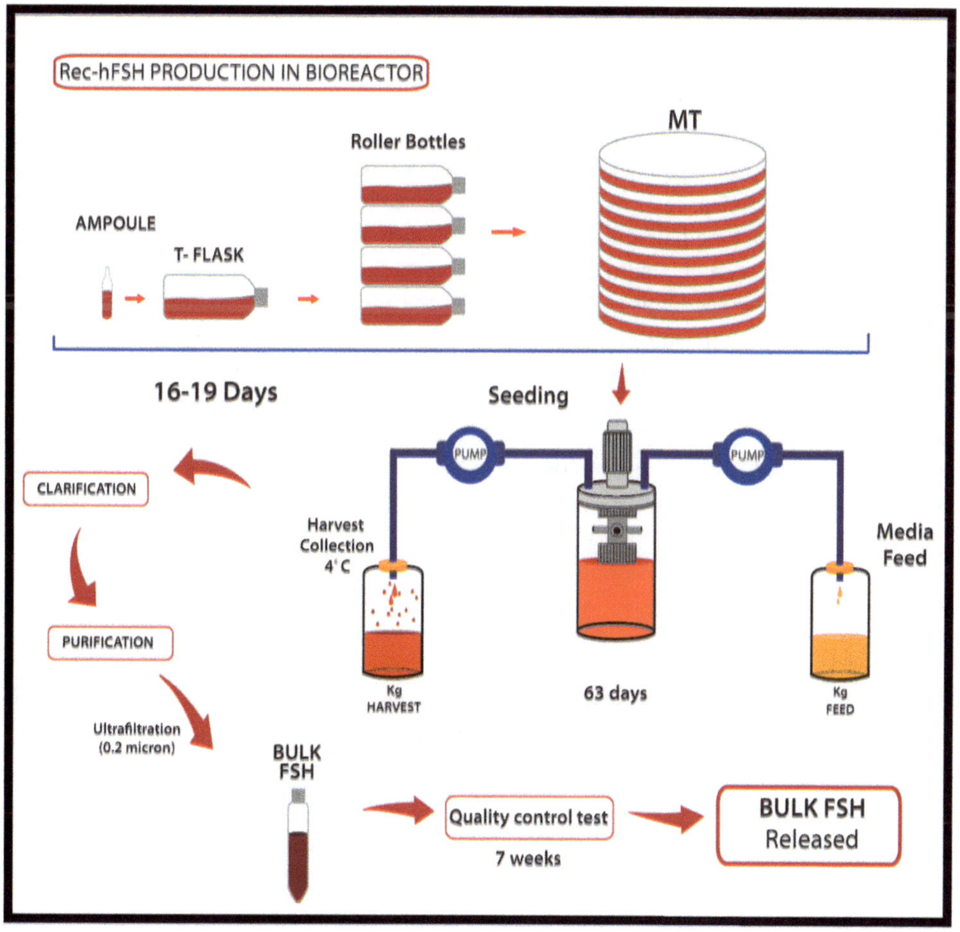

Fig. 28.8 Recombinant technology: how does it work? Chinese hamster ovary cells are first grown in T-flasks, then subcultured in roller bottles and allowed to expand for up to 36 days. Then, cells are mixed with a suspension of microcarrier beads and transferred to a bioreactor vessel perfused continuously with growth promoting medium for an average period of 34 days. The cell culture supernatant medium, containing "crude glycoprotein" is collected from the bioreactor and stored at 48 °C until purification. The protein is purified by chromatography, followed by ultrafiltration. The final product is released after extensive quality control testing over a period of 7 weeks

they differ slightly in the charge heterogeneity as follitropin alfa has slightly more acidic glycoforms than follitropin beta [58, 81]. Despite these differences, both preparations have equivalent immunopotency, in vitro biopotency and internal carbohydrate complexity. Immunoassay showed that initial and terminal half-lives after administration of 150 IU recombinant FSH were 2 and 17 h, respectively. Given their intrinsically similar structures, clinical efficacy is expected to be equally similar [3, 81, 83].

Long-Acting FSH Preparations

Due to the relatively short half-life of FSH (about 1 day), daily FSH injections are needed during the stimulation period to prevent the drop of serum FSH levels below the threshold which cause follicular growth arrest [84]. After each injection, peak serum FSH levels are reached within 10–12 h, and then FSH levels decline until the next injection. Steady state levels are reached only after 3–5 days of treatment, thus dose adjustments before day 5 of stimulation are not advised [85].

A number of technological approaches have been used to develop longer-acting FSH molecules, most of which have involved altering the structure of the FSH molecule itself [85]. Recently, a novel long-acting gonadotropin molecule has been developed by combining rec-hFSH with the C-terminal peptide of hCG using site-directed mutagenesis and gene transfer techniques. It is based on the principle that the highest half-life of hCG is given by the long carboxy terminal segment called C-terminal peptide (CTP) of the beta subunit. The hCG-CTP includes four additional O-linked carbohydrate side chains, each with two terminal sialic acid residues that confer long half-life to hCG [64, 86, 87]. The new molecule has been created using a chimeric gene containing the sequence encoding the CTP fused to the translated sequence of the human FSH beta subunit. The chimera was then transfected with the common glycoprotein alpha subunit and expressed in CHO cells. It has been demonstrated that the presence of the CTP sequence had no significant effect on the assembly or secretion of the intact dimer by stable cell lines. The chimeric recombinant molecule has shown to have similar in vitro receptor binding and steroidogenic activity compared with wild-type FSH, but with significantly enhanced in vivo activity and plasma half-life [85, 88].

The generation of a new CHO cell line expressing the aforementioned FSH hybrid molecule has led to the development of corifollitropin alfa, which was launched in the market in 2010. Corifollitropin alfa is devoid of LH activity. As such, it interacts exclusively with FSH receptors and has a plasma half-life of 65 h [9, 88]. The optimal corifollitropin dose has been calculated to be 100 mcg for women with a body weight ≤60 kg and 150 mcg for women with a body weight >60 kg. From phase II and III studies, it was concluded that a single injection of corifollitropin alfa would replace the first seven daily injections of standard gonadotropins, and that stimulation could be continued with daily FSH injections until the final oocyte maturation had been reached [89]. As the aim of corifollitropin alfa is to simplify treatment and reduce burden associated with multiple injections, it has been developed to be used in GnRH antagonist cycles [85].

Gonadotropin Preparations Containing LH Activity

Currently, there are three groups of commercially available gonadotropin preparations containing LH activity, that is, (i) urinary hMG, in which LH activity is dependent on hCG rather than on pure LH glycoprotein, (ii) pure LH glycoprotein produced by recombinant technology (lutropin alfa), and (iii) a combination of pure FSH and LH glycoproteins in a fixed ratio of 2:1 also manufactured by recombinant technology (Table 28.4; [3]).

While hMG has been used for ovarian stimulation since 1960, rec-hLH (lutropin alfa) was introduced in the market in the year 2000 for use in women with gonadotropin insufficiency. The manufacturing process of rec-hLH is similar to rec-hFSH. Lutropin alfa is highly pure and has high-biological activity (9000 IU/mg protein; [3]). It is intended to be used subcutaneously in daily injections. Up to date, lutropin alfa is the only recombinant form of human LH

Table 28.4 Differences in LH activity of gonadotropins commercially available

	Purity (LH content)	FSH activity (IU/vial)	LH activity (IU/vial)	hCG content (IU/vial)	Specific activity (LH/mg protein)
Lutropin alfa	>99%	0	75	–	9,000
Follitropin alfa + lutropin alfa 2:1	>99%	150	75	–	9,000
HP-hMG	Unknown[a]	75	75[a]	~8	–

1 μg of lutropin alfa = 22 IU

HP-hMG highly purified human menopausal gonadotropin

[a] derives primarily from the hCG component, which preferentially is concentrated during the purification process and sometimes was added to achieve the desired amount of LH-like biological activity

developed for use in ovarian stimulation. It is presented in vials of 82.5 IU lyophilized pure glycoprotein powder to be reconstituted with diluent before administration using a conventional syringe and needle (75 IU of lutropin alfa is delivered per vial) [90].

At present, rec-hLH is used not only to support follicular development during COS in hypogonadotropic hypogonadic woman but also in other categories of female infertility [2, 91, 92]. Recombinant LH has three major differences compared to urinary products. First, it has higher purity and specific activity because it is manufactured using recombinant technology. Second, it is associated with better dose precision due to FbM technology that virtually eliminates batch-to-batch variation and will be discussed later in this chapter [2, 6, 93]. Third, LH activity is derived directly from pure LH glycoprotein unlike hMG, in which hCG is concentrated during purification or added to achieve the desired amount of LH-like biological activity [2]. LH and hCG differ in the composition of their carbohydrate moieties which, in turn, affect bioactivity and half-life. As mentioned earlier, LH activity in serum is 30 times higher when hCG is used due to its higher binding affinity to LH receptors. After administration, recombinant human LH is eliminated with a terminal half-life of 9–12 h in contrast to 23–31 h of hCG [64, 94]. It has been shown that the expression of LH/hCG receptor gene, as well as genes involved in the biosynthesis of cholesterol and steroids in granulosa cells, are lower in patients treated with hMG preparations [95]. Such effects are caused by a constant ligand exposure during the follicular phase due to longer half-life and higher binding affinity of hCG compared with rec-hLH. In animal models, down-regulation of LH receptors is maintained for up to 48 h after hMG administration [96]. These findings indicate that the GCs have lower LH-induced cholesterol uptake, a decrease in the novo cholesterol synthesis and a decrease in steroid synthesis, thus explaining the observed lower serum progesterone levels achieved in patients treated with hMG [95, 97]. The clinical implications of these findings, however, have not been fully elucidated [98].

In 2007, a new fixed combination of rec-hFSH and rec-hLH at 2:1 ratio was launched (follitropin alfa + lutropin alfa) as an alternative for those women who need LH supplementation [8]. The 2:1 ratio of FSH and LH in a fixed dose combination was obtained by recombinant technology and vial filling using protein mass (FbM). The use of FbM as opposed of filled-by-bioassay was possible because the specific activity, isoform distribution and sialylation profile of both gonadotropins are highly consistent among manufactured batches [6]. The bioequivalence of rec-hFSH and rec-hLH administrated alone or in combination has been similar [8, 99].

Human Chorionic Gonadotropin Preparations

During controlled ovarian stimulation, hCG administration has been the gold standard for ovulation induction as a surrogate for the mid-cycle LH surge for several decades [100]. Due to structural and biological similarities, hCG and LH bind to and activate the same LH/hCG receptor [101]. However, the half-life of hCG is much longer than LH, and serum LH activity of hCG is 30 times higher than LH. Therefore, the luteotropic activity of hCG exerts is markedly higher than LH [94, 102]. After hCG administration, approximately 36 h is required for completion of the meiotic process. In the absence of oocyte retrieval, ovulation will ensue approximately 4 h later [103].

The first chorionic gonadotropin preparations were developed in 1931 from urine of pregnant women. At present, preparations of urinary hCG are marketed in lyophilized vials of 5000 or 10,000 IU to be used intramuscularly. Although improvements have been achieved in the purification process of urinary hCG, with highly purified presentations being introduced in 1976, urinary hCG is nowadays not recommended for subcutaneous administration. In 2001, hCG preparations using recombinant technology were launched (choriogonadotropin alfa). Recombinant hCG is available in prefilled syringes containing 250 mcg of pure hCG, which is equivalent to approximately 6750 IU of urinary hCG [3]. Recently, a new prefilled pen device has been introduced for administration of rec-hCG. Besides the benefits of higher purity, rec-hCG enables subcutaneous administration, unlike urinary hCG which requires intramuscular administration. Recombinant hCG is thus better tolerated and allows patient self-administration [104]. Nevertheless, the clinical efficacy of both urinary and recombinant preparations to induce final follicular maturation and resumption of oocyte meiosis does not seem to differ [105]. In a Cochrane meta-analysis including 11 randomized controlled trials (RCT) with a total of 1187 women, Youssef et al. compared rec-hCG versus urinary hCG for final oocyte maturation triggering in GnRH agonist down-regulated cycles for in vitro fertilization/intracytoplasmatic sperm injection (IVF/ICSI). There was no evidence of a statistically significant difference between rec-hCG and urinary regarding ongoing pregnancy/live birth rate (6 RCTs: odds ratio [OR] = 1.04, 95 % confidence interval [CI]: 0.79 to 1.37; $I^2 = 0\,\%$), incidence of ovarian hyperstimulation syndrome (OHSS; 3 RCTs: OR = 1.5, 95 % CI: 0.37 to 4.1; $I^2 = 0\,\%$) and number of retrieved oocytes (9 RCTs: Mean difference = −0.04, 95 % CI: −0.69 to 0.62; $I^2 = 18\,\%$; [105]).

A list of gonadotropin preparations currently available for clinical use is provided in Table 28.5.

Table 28.5 List of gonadotropins available for clinical use

Product	Technology	Brand name	Manufacturer
hMG	Urine-derived	Menogon®; Repronex®	Ferring
HP-hMG	Urine-derived	Menopur® Merional®	Ferring IBSA
HP-hFSH	Urine-derived	Fostimon® Bravelle® Fertinex®	IBSA Ferring Serono
u-hCG	Urine-derived	Choragon® Brevactid® Choriomon®, Gonasi HP® A.P.L® Biogonadyl® Primogonyl® Profasi® Pregnyl®; Predalon® Endocorion® Corion®	Ferring Ferring IBSA Wyeth Biomed-Lublin Schering Serono Organon Elea Win-Medicare
rec-hFSH (follitropin beta)	Recombinant	Puregon®; Follistim®	MSD
rec-hFSH (follitropin alfa)	Recombinant	GONAL-f®	MerckSerono
long-acting FSH (corifollitropin alfa)	Recombinant	Elonva®	Schering-Plough
rec-hLH (lutropin alfa)	Recombinant	Luveris®	MerckSerono
rec-hFSH + rec-hLH 2:1 (follitropin alfa + lutropin alfa)	Recombinant	Pergoveris®	MerckSerono
rec-hCG	Recombinant	Ovidrel®; Ovitrelle®; Ovidrelle®	MerckSerono

hMG human menopausal gonadotropin, *HP-hMG* highly purified human menopausal gonadotropin, *u-hCG* urinary hCG, *rec-hFSH* recombinant human follicle-stimulating hormone, *rec-hLH* recombinant LH, *rec-hCG* recombinant hCG

Quality and Safety Profile of Urinary and Recombinant Gonadotropins

Urine-derived gonadotropins require large amounts of human urine as a primary source for manufacturing. In the 1960s and 1970s, when the demand for gonadotropins was still low, most urine was collected in Italy and the Netherlands, and the quality of the source material was somehow controlled. However, the development of new clinical indications for gonadotropins combined with the expansion of infertility treatment on a worldwide basis led to a rapid increase in demand. Urine collection was expanded to countries such as Spain, China, Brazil, and Argentina. As the demand for gonadotropins began to rise exponentially in the 1980s, the ability to control the source material became more difficult. Unlike blood collection, human urine collection is not subject to specific regulations regarding collection. Moreover, urine is collected at home from tens of thousands of individual donors and pooled. A medical questionnaire is usually the only source of health information. Because urine is pooled, the donor source cannot be traced. As the pool is constantly changing, standardization is difficult to ascertain. Transportation (from urine collection sites to processing facility) is poorly monitored and therefore quality cannot be checked throughout all manufacturing steps [76, 106, 107].

Although sophisticated purification techniques are currently available, which allow the safe clinical use of urinary formulations, extraneous urinary proteins may account for more than 30% of the protein content in highly purified hMG products, as demonstrated by high-performance liquid chromatography analysis (Table 28.3; [93]). Following two-dimensional sodium dodecyl sulfate-polyacrylamide gel electrophoresis (SDS-PAGE) and mass spectrometry protein identification, a total of 23 non-gonadotropin-related proteins have been identified at variable levels in different batches of the urine-derived preparations [107]. In other studies, two-dimensional gel analysis demonstrated that protein impurities were composed of leukocyte elastase inhibitor, protein C inhibitor and zinc-α_2-glycoprotein. These proteins are involved in receptor activity, immune response, protein metabolism, and cell growth. Tumor necrosis factor-binding protein I, transferrin and immunoglobulin-related proteins were also present in both hMG and urinary FSH preparations. Lastly, recent data has shown that some of these impurities are prion proteins, which are a matter of great concern for health regulatory agencies because of their association with transmissible spongiform encephalopathy (TSE) diseases [108]. A prion is a mis-folded isoform of a normal cellular protein found in the brain (PrPc). When a prion comes into contact with another normal version of this protein, it induces the normal protein to adopt the mis-folded shape. The body is unable to recognize and break down the abnormally folded protein. As a result, prions accumulate in the central nervous system, interfering with normal brain function. Conversion of PrPc into the abnormal form can occur spontaneously or following infection. Abnormal prions include PrPsc, the protein associated with scrapie, and PrPres, the protein resistant to enzyme degradation found in patients with CJD [109]. Inactivation of prions in urine-derived material may denature proteins, including FSH. For instance, urea, a commonly used denaturant, destroys the dimeric structure of proteins. This is one reason why urine-derived gonadotropins cannot be as pure as recombinant ones. Cross-contamination is another concern in urine-derived products. A rogue element in one individual donation of urine may spread through a complete batch and potentially cause problems in the final product. Quality control is only possible through the stringent donor collection, transportation, and production. In fact, several regulatory agencies have set limitations to urine-derived products [76, 106].

Although the clinical significance of most protein contamination from urinary gonadotropins is unknown, it is certain that these contaminants are not needed to induce optimal follicle development. More importantly, these findings underscore the poor quality of urinary sources and stress the need for more reliable proteins [76, 106]. Many of the risks associated with biologically extracted proteins are avoided when the protein is produced synthetically. This is the case with recombinant preparations, which contain pure glycoprotein as demonstrated by SDS-PAGE and western blot analysis [110].

Given its high purity, each product batch of recombinant gonadotropin is routinely characterized and controlled using physicochemical techniques, including size exclusion high performance liquid chromatography (SE-HPLC), which allows assessment of both the integrity and the amount of glycoproteins; and isoelectric focusing (IEF) and glycan mapping, which characterize protein glycoforms present in each preparation [111, 112].

Quantification and Filling Method of Urinary and Recombinant Gonadotropins

The conventional method used to quantify the glycoprotein activity in gonadotropin products is the Steelman–Pohley assay, which is an in vivo rat bioassay. As well as being costly and subject to ethical concerns related to the use of animals, this technique has an inherent variability of up to 20 % [6, 113]. In 2003, Driebergen and Baer demonstrated the batch-to-batch consistency of follitropin alfa in terms of specific activity, isoform pattern and sialylation profile. The authors showed that there was a constant relationship between FSH mass and its biological activity. Following these observations, a new method was developed to calibrate each batch of follitropin alfa using SE-HPLC, which measures glycoprotein content by protein mass [6]. This technique has enabled follitropin alfa to be filled and released on the basis of mass (75 IU of FSH assessed by the Steelman-Pohley assay corresponds to between 5.0 and 5.5 μg of follitropin alfa), with dose variability of only 2 % [3, 6]. Follitropin alfa FbM was commercially available in 2004 and has progressively replaced follitropin alfa filled-by-bioassay [7]. To ensure an optimal response to controlled ovarian stimulation, it is essential that the FSH dose administered is accurate. If the FSH dose is too low, the ovaries will not be sufficiently stimulated and the cycle may be cancelled. On the other hand, if the dose is too high, the ovaries may be over stimulated, what may increase the risks of OHSS. In this sense, the FbM method seems to be advantageous over in vivo bioassyas to reduce the fluctuations among gonadotropin batches and the risks associated with poorly controlled dose precision [3, 4].

Route of Administration and Injection Devices of Gonadotropin Preparations

The pharmaceutical presentation of urinary gonadotropins consists of a freeze-dried lyosphere containing either 75 IU of FSH/hMG or 5000/10,000 IU of hCG that have to be dissolved in sterile water before injection [4]. Intramuscular administration is the route of choice for most urinary gonadotropins. Nevertheless, the higher the gonadotropin purity the higher its specific activity, and therefore less material has to be injected to achieve its desired effect. Such characteristics made it possible to apply highly purified urine-derived gonadotropins as well as recombinant ones subcutaneously and in small volumes (Table 28.3; [93]).

Moreover, given the highest specific activity of recombinant gonadotropins, novel injection devices have been developed. In 2001, follitropin beta has been made available as a ready-to-use solution with a cartridge presentation for administration with a pen device [78]. This injector was an adapted insulin pen, which has been better accepted by diabetes patients in comparison with conventional syringes [114, 115]. Importantly, the injector was reusable and allowed follitropin beta self-administration in precise individualized dosing ranging from 25 to 450 IU [78]. Earlier studies have shown that drug delivery by pen devices was bioequivalent to those of conventional syringe injections. However, due to unavoidable losses during syringe filling and/or removing excess air, 18 % of the FSH amount was lost in conventional syringe application when compared to a ready-for-use solution with a pen device [78]. This finding may explain the results of a RCT including 200 patients, in which delivery of follitropin beta using a pen device was compared with delivery of follitropin alfa using conventional syringe. The authors of this aforementioned study noted that the group of patients receiving the medication by pen injector needed significantly lower amount of rec-hFSH ($p<0.01$) to promote follicular development and had shorter duration of stimulation ($p=0.001$). Additionally, the overall patient satisfaction was significantly better ($p<0.001$) whereas pain complaint at the injection site was significantly decreased ($p=0.027$) in the follitropin beta/pen group compared with the follitropin alfa/syringe group [78]. These results corroborate the findings of an earlier RCT with 60 women in which pain complaint was significantly lower when follitropin beta was administered by a pen device compared with when follitropin alfa was administered with a conventional syringe. It should be noted that a microneedle was used to inject FSH in very small volumes of fluid in the pen group compared with tuberculin needles and larger volume in conventional injections [116].

With the availability of FbM technology, a novel prefilled pen device was introduced in 2004 for follitropin alfa. Unlike the follitropin beta device that used follitropin beta filled-by-bioassay, it was a disposable prefilled injector that provided precise and accurate dosing with minimal batch-to-batch variability and enabling FSH dosing in relatively small increments of 37.5 UI [6, 93]. In a RCT including 100 women, the efficacy, convenience and local reactions after the administration of follitropin alfa were compared either using the pen device or the conventional syringe. Outcomes including self-administration and patient satisfaction ($p<0.001$), the overall incidence of local reactions ($p=0.047$), overall pain score ($p<0.001$), and burning sensation at the injection site ($p=0.041$) clearly favored the pen device group [117]. Later, in 2007, patients and their partners received nurse-led training on three gonadotropin presentations: (i) powdered urofollitropin with conventional needles and syringes for administration, (ii) follitropin beta in a premixed and prefilled cartridge with a reusable injection device, and (iii) follitropin alfa in a disposable, premixed and prefilled injection device. A total of 123 participants attended the training and were asked to complete a post-training questionnaire. More participants expressed a preference for using pen injectors compared with conventional syringes (84.6% versus 5.7%; $p<0.0001$). Of the 94 participants who preferred a particular device, more preferred the follitropin alfa prefilled pen (68.1%) than the follitropin beta cartridge and pen (24.5%; $p<0.0001$) or urofollitropin with needle-free reconstitution device and conventional syringe (7.4%; $p<0.0001$; [118]).

Recently in 2011, a new family of pen devices has been approved in the European Union, Canada, and Australia, which include follitropin alfa, lutropin alfa, and chorigonadotropin alfa [10, 11]. In conclusion, the introduction of recombinant technology, filling method by mass, and pen devices for gonadotropin administration represented an important advancement to make infertility treatments more patient-friendly ([78, 116, 117]; Fig. 28.9).

Studies on the Clinical Efficacy of Gonadotropins

Meta-Analyses Comparing Urinary and Recombinant Gonadotropins Used for COS in Assisted Reproductive Technology (ART)

A number of meta-analyses have compared the efficacy of different gonadotropin products, with conflicting results (Table 28.6; [119–122]). Coomarasamy et al., including seven randomized trials and 2159 women, compared hMG versus rec-hFSH following a long down-regulation protocol in IVF/ICSI cycles. The authors found that hMG preparations yielded a significantly higher clinical pregnancy (relative risk [RR] = 1.17, 95% CI: 1.03 to 1.34) and live birth rate (RR = 1.18, 95% CI: 1.02 to 1.38; $p=0.03$). No significant differences were noted for spontaneous abortion, multiple pregnancy, cycle cancellation and OHSS rates. The observed difference represented a 4% increase in live birth rate with hMG when compared with rec-hFSH. However, the lower confidence interval limit has been just 1% [119]. In 2009, Al-Inany et al. pooled six randomized trials including 2371 participants and compared HP-hMG versus rec-hFSH. The authors could not find a difference between gonadotropin preparations in either clinical pregnancy or ongoing pregnancy/live birth rate. However, after grouping the treatment cycles by method, the ongoing pregnancy/live birth rate favored the HP-hMG group (OR = 1.31, 95% CI: 1.02 to 1.68; $p=0.03$; [120]). Like the meta-analytic study of Coomarasamy et al., the lower confidence interval limit was below 1% [119, 120].

In 2010, Jee et al. compared HP-hMG and follitropin alfa by pooling five prospective RCTs ($n=2299$), and found no difference in ongoing pregnancy rate per started cycle (RR = 1.10; 95% CI: 0.96 to 1.26) or per embryo transfer (RR = 1.13; 95% CI: 0.99 to 1.29), as well as in the live birth rates per embryo transfer (RR = 1.14; 95% CI: 0.98 to 1.33; [122]). In a meta-analysis of Van Wely et al., including 28 trials and 7339 couples, FSH (both urinary and recombinant) was compared to hMG. Overall, the authors have not observed any differences in live birth or OHSS rates. Comparing only hMG/HP-hMG to rec-hFSH, however, significantly fewer clinical pregnancies (OR = 0.85; 95% CI: 0.74 to 0.99; $I^2=0\%$; 12 trials, $n=3775$; $p=0.03$) and live births/ongoing pregnancies (OR = 0.84; 95% CI: 0.72 to 0.99; $I^2=0\%$; 11 trials, $n=3197$; $p=0.04$) were obtained with rec-hFSH compared to hMG. Subgroup analyses grouping the treatment cycles by an individual sponsor suggested that live birth and clinical pregnancy favored hMG in trials sponsored by hMG manufacturers. However, further analysis of hMG-sponsored trials and non-sponsored trials revealed comparable summary OR and confidence intervals that overlapped. Hence, though a bias could not be completely ruled out, its effect on

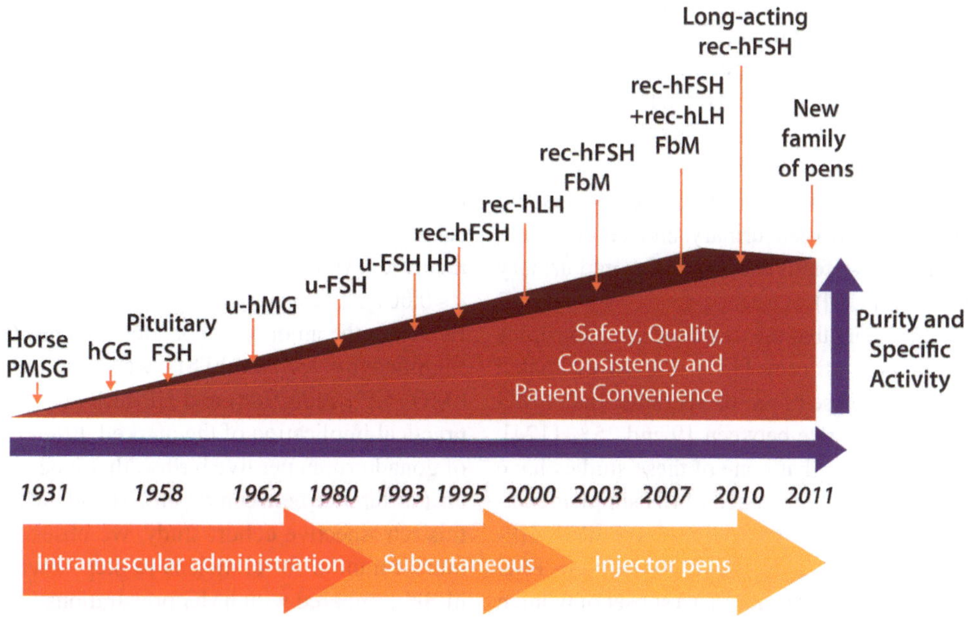

Fig. 28.9 Historical evolution of gonadotropins. FSH was originally derived from animal (pregnant mare serum) or human (postmortem pituitary glands) sources, but these preparations were abandoned because of safety concerns. Gonadotropins were first extracted from urine in the 1940s; human chorionic gonadotropin (*hCG*) in 1940 and then human menopausal gonadotropin (*hMG*) in 1949. Over a decade later, the first urinary forms of hCG and hMG became commercially available. Further improvements in purification methods led to the production of follicle-stimulating hormone (*FSH*)-only products in the 1980s, and the subsequent development of highly purified FSH (*HP-hFSH*), which became available 10 years later, in 1993, allowing the use of subcutaneous injections. In the 1970s and 1980s, advances in DNA technology enabled the development of recombinant human FSH (*rec-hFSH*), which became commercially available in 1995. In 2000, recombinant human luteinizing hormone (*rec-hLH*) became available and, with the launch of recombinant human hCG (*rec-hCG*) in 2001, the complete recombinant gonadotropin portfolio was available. The most recent developments have been the introduction of filled-by-mass (*FbM*) follitropin alfa formulation, fixed combination of follitropin alfa + lutropin alfa, long-acting FSH gonadotropin, and a new family of prefilled pen injector devices

Table 28.6 Meta-analyses comparing pregnancy rates in ART cycles using urinary and recombinant gonadotropins

Authors	Year	Gonadotropins	Number of RCTs included	Number of participants	Conclusions
Coomarasamy et al.	2008	rec-hFSH vs. hMG	7	2159	Higher clinical pregnancy and live birth rates when hMG was used for COS; No significant differences in spontaneous abortion, multiple pregnancy, cycle cancellation and OHSS rates
Al Inany et al.	2009	rec-hFSH vs. hMG/HP-hMG	6	2371	No significant differences in clinical, ongoing pregnancy or live birth rates
Jee et al.	2010	rec-hFSH vs. HP-hMG	5	2299	No significant differences in ongoing pregnancy and live birth rates
Van Wely et al.	2010	rec-hFSH vs. hFSH-P/HP-hFSH/hMG/HP-hMG	28	7339	Insufficient evidence of a difference in the odds of clinical pregnancy, live birth or OHSS
Van Wely et al.	2012	rec-hFSH vs. hMG/HP-hMG	12	3197	Fewer clinical pregnancies and live birth with rec-hFSH
Gerli et al.	2013	rec-hFSH vs. hFSH-P/HP-hFSH	8	955	No significant differences in the number of oocytes retrieved, number of mature oocytes, days of stimulation, clinical pregnancy and live birth rate

RCT randomized controlled trial, *rec-hFSH* recombinant human follicle-stimulating hormone, *hMG* human menopausal gonadotropin, *HP-hMG* highly purified human menopausal gonadotropin, *hFSH-P* purified urinary follicle-stimulating hormone, *HP-hFSH* highly purified urinary follicle-stimulating hormone, *COS* controlled ovarian stimulation, *OHSS* ovarian hyperstimulation syndrome the outcomes appeared to be limited [121]. Lastly, in 2013, Geri et al. compared HP-hFSH and rec-hFSH by including six trials involving 955 participants. The authors found no difference in live birth rates (OR = 0.84; 95 % CI: 0.63–1.11), clinical pregnancy rate (OR = 0.85, 95 % CI: 0.68 to 1.07), number of oocytes retrieved, number of mature oocytes and duration of stimulation between urinary and recombinant preparations, but the cost-effectiveness ratio favored urinary FSH (€ 2056 vs. 7174; [123]).

In conclusion, it appears that the available gonadotropins have comparable clinical efficacy [121]. For an estimated live birth rate of 25 %, the use of rec-hFSH rather than hMG would result in a live birth rate between 19 and 25 % [124]. It should be noted, however, that none of these studies have stratified patients according to the need of LH supplementation during COS. As such, results tend to favor hMG/HP-hMG preparations since rec-hFSH shows exclusively FSH activity, and recent evidence indicates that a subset of women clearly benefit by LH supplementation during COS [93].

Studies Comparing the Potency of Different Gonadotropin Formulations

Hompes et al., in a randomized controlled trial, compared 312 IVF/ICSI cycles with HP-hMG and 317 using rec-hFSH, all of them associated with a GnRH agonist for pituitary suppression. The authors showed that significantly more oocytes were retrieved in the group of patients treated with rec-hFSH (7.8 and 10.6, respectively; $p < 0.001$), with no differences in pregnancy rates [125]. In another RCT involving 280 women, Bosch et al. compared the aforementioned gonadotropins in association with GnRH antagonists. A significantly higher number of oocytes was obtained from patients who received rec-hFSH compared with hMG (14.4 ± 8.1 vs. 11.3 ± 6.0, respectively; $p < 0.001$). No significant differences were observed in the ongoing pregnancy rate per started cycle (35.0 vs. 32.1 %, respectively; RR = 1.09; 95 % CI: 0.78–1.51; risk difference [RD] = 2.9 %; [97]). Recently, Devroey et al. in another RCT involving more than 700 patients compared HP-hMG ($n = 374$) with rec-hFSH ($n = 375$) in antagonist cycles with single blastocyst transfer. Again, more oocytes were retrieved in the group treated with rec-hFSH (10.6 ± 5.8 vs. 9.1 ± 5.2; $p < 0.001$), and ongoing pregnancy and live birth rates did not differ [126].

Recently, we examined the clinical efficacy of different gonadotropin products for ovarian stimulation in one of the largest observational studies to date. In this study, we compared follitropin alfa FbM ($n = 236$), hMG ($n = 299$), and HP-hMG ($n = 330$) in normogonadotropic down-regulated women undergoing ICSI. Overall, women who received the different gonadotropin preparations achieved comparable pregnancy results. The clinical pregnancy rate per initiated cycle was 34.7, 35.5, and 40 % for rec-hFSH, hMG, and HP-hMG, respectively while the live birth rate per initiated cycle was 30.1, 24.4, and 32.4 %, respectively. However, the total dose of gonadotropin used for ovarian stimulation was significantly lower in the group of women who received rec-hFSH (2268 ± 747 IU) compared with those who received hMG (2685 ± 720 IU) or HP-hMG (2903 ± 867 IU; $p < 0.001$). The difference in favor of rec-hFSH was also reflected in the amount of gonadotropin needed per live birth. Significantly less rec-hFSH was required compared with hMG (52 % reduction) and HP-hMG (21 % reduction). One practical implication of the marked difference in the amount of gonadotropin per live birth is that it neutralizes part of the cost difference between rec-hFSH and hMG preparations. In this retrospective cohort study, we observed that it was far more common for clinicians to step down the dose of rec-hFSH compared with hMG preparations [4].

In summary, there is fair evidence to support the concept that recombinant FSH is more potent than hMG.

Studies Comparing Follitropin Alfa and Follitropin Beta

Four studies directly compared the two forms of recombinant FSH formulations, follitropin alfa and follitropin beta, in women undergoing COS under pituitary GnRH agonist suppression for IVF (Table 28.7; [127–130]). Tupalla et al. evaluated 344 women in a double-blind RCT and found that pregnancy rates per cycle did not differ between follitropin alfa (33.5 %) and follitropin beta (32.9 %) groups. In addition, the authors of the aforementioned study did not find any differences in the number of oocytes retrieved, fertilization rate, cleavage rate, and incidence of OHSS [127]. Birsden et al., in an assessor-blind RCT involving 44 women, compared the same formulations and found higher clinical pregnancy rates with the use of follitropin alfa (31.8 %) compared with follitropin beta (18.2 %), albeit nonstatistically significant. In this study, no differences were observed in the cumulative dose of FSH, duration of ovarian stimulation, number of follicles ≥ 14 mm on the day of hCG, number of oocytes retrieved, number of viable embryos and incidence of systemic adverse events. However, the authors reported that local reactions at the injection site were more often observed with the use of follitropin beta (28 %) than with follitropin alfa (17.5 %; $p < 0.05$; [128]). Harlin et al., in another prospective study including 296 IVF cycles, reported similar pregnancy rates per transfer with follitropin alfa (29.1 %) and beta (28.1 %). No differences were found in the endometrial thickness, estradiol levels, number of follicles > 15 mm on the day of hCG as well as in the number of oocytes retrieved, fertilized, and cleaved. Of note, serum progesterone

Table 28.7 Prospective-designed in vitro fertilization (IVF) trials comparing follitropin alfa and follitropin beta in terms of clinical efficacy and safety

Authors, year	Number of participants	Main findings
Tuppala et al., 1999	344	No differences in number of oocytes, fertilization rate, cleavage rate, clinical pregnancy and OHSS rates
Brinsden et al., 2000	44	No differences in cumulative dose of FSH, duration of ovarian stimulation, number of follicles ≥14 mm on the day of hCG, number of oocytes retrieved, number of viable embryos, clinical pregnancy rate, and incidence of systemic adverse events; Significantly more local reactions at the injection site with follitropin beta compared with follitropin alfa
Harlim et al., 2000	396	No differences in endometrial thickness, estradiol levels, number of >15 mm follicles on the day of hCG, number of retrieved oocytes, number of fertilized oocytes, number of cleaved embryos, and clinical pregnancy rate; Lower serum progesterone levels on oocyte retrieval day in cycles stimulated with follitropin beta
Harlim et al., 2002	812	No differences in endometrial thickness, estradiol levels on hCG day, pregnancy and delivery rates; Significantly higher total dose of FSH, lower number of treatment days, higher number of fertilized oocytes and cleaved embryos, and higher levels of progesterone on oocyte retrieval day with the use of follitropin alfa

levels on the day of oocyte retrieval were lower in the follitropin beta group (30.3±1.8 nmol/L) compared with the follitropin alfa group (37.7±1.5 nmol/L; $p=0.005$; [129]). Subsequently, the same group of authors conducted an open, semi-randomized trial evaluating 812 initiated cycles. Despite using higher gonadotropin total dose (2233±45 IU vs. 2090±52 IU; $p<0.05$), the group of women that received follitropin alfa had shorter treatment duration (11.8±0.11 vs. 12.5±0.18 days; $p<0.005$) and higher number of fertilized oocytes (4.9±0.15 vs. 4.3±0.17; $p<0.05$) as well as cleaved zygotes (4.7±0.14 vs. 4.1±0.16; $p<0.01$). In the aforementioned study, neither the number of retrieved oocytes (7.3±0.19 vs. 7.0±0.22) nor the clinical pregnancy (26 vs. 28%) and delivery rates (22% vs. 22%) differed between the follitropin alfa and the beta groups, respectively. Furthermore, no differences were found in endometrial thickness and estradiol levels on the day of hCG, but the serum progesterone levels on the day of oocyte retrieval were lower with follitropin beta (29.1±0.95 nmol/L) than follitropin alfa (35.3±0.98 nmol/L; $p<0.001$; [130]). It should be noted, however, that all mentioned studies were performed before the introduction of FbM technology and novel injector devices by the manufacturer of follitropin alfa [6].

Recombinant Gonadotropins Filled-by-Mass and Filled-by-Bioassay

A meta-analysis including four RCTs involving 1055 women and two case-control studies with 272 patients have compared the efficacy and safety of ovarian stimulation using follitropin alfa FbM compared with follitropin alfa filled by bioassay. The average rec-hFSH dose per patient was lessened by 230 IU with the administration of follitropin alfa FbM compared with the one filled-by-bioassay (Weighted mean difference [WMD]=−230.3; 95% CI: −326 to −134.5; $p<0.001$), and the number of treatment days was reduced by 0.48 (WMD=−0.48; 95% CI: −0.69 to −0.27, $p<0.001$). In addition, the peak levels of estradiol on the day of hCG administration (WMD=613.1 pmol/L; 95% CI: 142.4 to 1083.7 pmol/L; $p=0.01$), number of oocytes retrieved (WMD=0.84; 95% CI: 0.18 to 1.51; $p<0.013$) and number of embryos obtained (WMD=0.88; 95% CI: 0.40 to 1.37; $p<0.001$) were higher in the patients undergoing ovarian stimulation with follitropin alfa FbM. However, statistically significant differences were not observed in clinical pregnancy (OR = 1.3; 95% CI: 0.91 to 1.82) and ovarian hyperstimulation syndrome (OR = 0.78; 95% CI: 0.45 to 1.36) rates between the two groups [131].

Recently, a prospective study compared eleven egg donors in two different cycles in which the same dose (150–225 IU) of follitropin alfa was used. In one cycle patients received follitropin alfa FbM whereas in the other the filled-by-assay presentation was administered. No differences were demonstrated regarding the duration of ovarian stimulation (9.9±1.6 and 10.1±1.2 days, respectively), total dose of follitropin alfa used (2464±966 and 2345±858 IU), estradiol peak levels (2405±568 and 3123±1165 pg/mL), and number of developed blastocysts (5.1±3.0 and 5.4±3.1). Significantly higher number of follicles >14 mm (17.9±5.7) and number of oocytes retrieved (23.8±8.7) have been obtained in the group of patients treated with follitropin alfa FbM compared with the group treated with rec-hFSH filled-by-bioassay (13.2±3.7 follicles, $p=0.004$; 17.1±8.5 oocytes retrieved, $p=0.01$; [7]).

Long-Acting and Conventional rec-hFSH

A recent meta-analysis of four pharmaceutical industry-sponsored RCTs including 2377 participants evaluated the effectiveness, safety, and tolerance of corifollitropin alfa compared with rec-hFSH (follitropin beta) in IVF and ICSI cycles using GnRH antagonists. The results favored corifollitropin alfa with regard to the number of oocytes retrieved (WMD = 1.99; 95 % CI: 1.02 to 2.97; $p<0.0001$), number of mature oocytes (WMD = 1.92; 95 % CI: 1.25 to 2.59; $p<0.001$), and number of embryos formed (WMD = 1.09; 95 % CI: 0.68 to 1.49; $p<0.0001$). Clinical pregnancy, ongoing pregnancy, live birth and miscarriage rates were not different regardless of the drug used for COS. The median duration of ovarian stimulation was 9 days in both treatment groups, thus indicating that two additional single daily injections of rec-hFSH were needed to complete the treatment regimen in the group of women who received corifollitropin alfa. Controlled ovarian stimulation with corifollitropin resulted in significantly higher cycle cancellations due to excessive response compared with daily rec-hFSH injections (OR = 5.67; 95 % CI: 1.07 to 30.13; $p=0.04$), although the incidence of OHSS was not statistically significant between the groups (OR = 1.29; 95 % CI: 0.78 to 2.26; [132]). These results were further corroborated by a Cochrane review of the same aforementioned studies [133].

The main shortcoming of corifollitropin alfa is that no dose adjustments can be made in patients with either low response or excessive response after the initial injection. From the limited data available, it seems that corifollitropin alfa is efficacious and safe for COS in normal responders but more data are needed for other subgroups of patients [132].

Luteinizing Hormone Supplementation During COS: Rationale and Results

Rationale of LH Supplementation: To Whom and Why?

The "LH window" concept, as outlined by Shoham in 2002, proposes that in the absence of a threshold level of serum LH, estradiol production will be insufficient for follicular development, endometrial proliferation and corpus luteum formation. However, exposure of the developing follicle to excessive LH results in the suppression of granulosa cells proliferation, follicular atresia (nondominant follicles), premature luteinization, and impairment of oocyte development [134]. This concept can be clearly observed in patients with hypogonadotrophic hypogonadism who do not achieve adequate steroidogenesis by stimulation with FSH alone, but resume sufficient estradiol production by LH supplementation [135]. Evidence therefore suggests that in reproductive cycles optimal follicular development occurs within a "LH window," that is, above a LH threshold of 1.1 and below a LH ceiling of 5.1 IU/L [134, 135].

Even after pituitary suppression, still widely used in association with COS, residual circulating levels of endogenous LH are usually adequate to support multiple follicular growth and oocyte development in COS with gonadotropins devoid of LH activity [136, 137]. In fact, only 1 % of LH receptors need to be occupied to drive adequate ovarian steroidogenesis. The general consensus regarding LH supplementation during COS is that most women have sufficient levels of endogenous LH and do not require supplementation (Table 28.8). Four meta-analyses, all of them published in 2007, concluded that the indiscriminate use of LH supplementation in IVF cycles was not beneficial [138–141].

Nevertheless, ovarian response to COS with FSH only-containing gonadotropins has been poor in a subset of normogonadotropic women including those in advanced reproductive age (≥ 35 years old; [92, 142]), diminished ovarian reserve [91, 140], and highly suppressed levels of endogenous LH, in whom LH activity falls below the LH threshold [143–147]. In addition, early studies identified a subgroup of normogonadotropic patients who had normal estimated ovarian reserve but suboptimal responses to FSH stimulation [148–151]. Such women expressed ovarian resistance to FSH which was restored by using LH supplementation during COS, as demonstrated by Ferraretti and colleagues. These authors selected 126 women undergoing COS with a fixed dose of rec-hFSH in a GnRH agonist down-regulation protocol for IVF/ICSI with suboptimal initial follicular recruitment. Hypo-responsiveness to rec-hFSH was defined by the observation of steady follicular growth (> 10 antral follicles ≥ 8 mm in diameter) and estradiol levels (≥ 100 pg/mL) between stimulation days 7 to 10 despite continuous rec-hFSH administration. Upon reaching this stage, patients were randomized to receive (i) increased rec-hFSH dose alone ($n=54$), (ii) rec-hLH (75 or 150 IU/day) in addition to increased FSH dose ($n=54$), and (iii) hMG in addition to increased rec-hFSH ($n=26$). Fifty-four age-matched women with normal responses to COS were included as a control group. The group receiving rec-hLH achieved a higher pregnancy rate (54.4 %) compared with both the patients receiving rec-hFSH alone (24.4 %; $p<0.05$) and hMG (11 %; $p<0.05$). Pregnancy rates in the group of women receiving rec-hLH supplementation were not different from controls (41 %). Live birth rates in both rec-hLH (40.7 %) and control (37 %) groups were two times higher than in the other two groups (22 and 18 %, respectively). However, the difference did not reach statistical significance [151]. The results of the aforementioned study were corroborated by de Placido et al., who also studied patients hypo-responsive to COS, defined by the presence of low serum estradiol levels (below 180 pg/mL) and no follicles over 10 mm on stimulation day

Table 28.8 Meta-analyses of clinical ART studies comparing COS with rec-hFSH with and without rec-hLH supplementation

Author and year	Patient selection	GnRH analogue	No. RCTs included	No. participants	Primary outcomes	Secondary outcomes
Mochtar et al., 2007	Unselected	Agonist	11	2396	CPR[a]: OR = 1.15; (95 % CI: 0.91 to 1.45) OPR[a]: OR = 1.22 (95 % CI: 0.95 to 1.56)	No differences in OHSS rates, total rec-hFSH dose, estradiol levels and number of oocytes retrieved
	Unselected	Antagonist	3	216	CPR[a]: OR = 0.79 (95 % CI: 0.26 to 2.43) OPR[a]: OR = 0.83 (95 % CI: 0.39 to 1.8)	
	Poor responders	Agonist	3	310	OPR[a]: OR = 1.85 (95 % CI: 1.1 to 3.11)	–
Oliveira et al., 2007	Unselected	Agonist	4	1227	CPR[b]: OR = 1.1 (95 % CI: 0.85 to 1.42)	Fewer days of stimulation, lower total dose of rec-hFSH used and higher estradiol levels on hCG day in the rec-hLH group. No difference in number of oocytes, number of mature oocytes, IR and miscarriage rates
Baruffi et al., 2007	Unselected	Antagonist	5	434	CPR[b]: OR = 0.89 (95 % CI: 0.57 to 1.39)	No difference in total rec-hFSH dose used, duration of stimulation, no. oocytes, IR and miscarriage rates. Higher E2 level and mature oocytes with the rec-hLH use
Kolibianakis et al., 2007	Unselected	Agonist/antagonist	7	701	LBR[a]: OR = 0.92 (95 % CI: 0.65 to 1.31) CPR[a]: OR = 0.86 (95 % CI: 0.61 to 1.20)	No difference in total rec-hFSH dose used, duration of stimulation, number of oocytes, number of mature oocytes and fertilization rates
Hill et al., 2012	≥35 year	Agonist/antagonist	7	603	CPR[a]: OR 1.37 (95 % CI: 1.03 to 1.83)	Higher IR in the rec-hLH group. No difference in estradiol levels.
Bosdou et al., 2012	Poor responders	Agonist/antagonist	7	902	CPR[a]: RD = 6 %, (95 % CI: − 0.3 to + 13 %) LBR[a]: RD = + 19 % (95 % CI: + 1 to + 36 %)	No difference in the no. oocytes retrieved, total dose of rec-hFSH and duration of stimulation
Fan et al., 2013	Poor responders	Agonist	3	458	OPR: OR = 1.30 (95 % CI: 0.80 to 2.11)	No difference in the no. oocytes retrieved, total dose of rec-hFSH, duration of stimulation, number of MII oocytes and cycle cancellation

CPR clinical pregnancy rate, OPR: ongoing pregnancy rate, *LBR* live birth rate, *IR* implantation rate, *RD* risk difference, *OR* odds ratio, *OHSS* ovarian hyperstimulation syndrome, *rec-hFSH* recombinant human follicle-stimulation hormone

[a] per randomized women

[b] per oocyte retrieval

8. Patients were randomized to receive either daily injections of 75 UI rec-hLH starting on stimulation day 8 (n=65) or increased daily doses (step-up by 150 UI) of rec-hFSH (n=65). Both aforesaid groups were compared to normal responders who received no LH supplementation (n=130). The number of oocytes retrieved was significantly higher in the patients who received recombinant LH supplementation (9.0±4.3) compared with those to whom increased doses of rec-hFSH was administered (6.1±2.6; $p<0.01$), even though these values were lower than those obtained in the control group (10.49±3.7; $p<0.05$; [150]). Interestingly, it has been shown later that some of these hypo-responders harbored single nucleotide polymorphisms of FSH and LH receptors [152].

In summary, evidence indicates that a subset of women has less responsive ovaries to COS explained by a variety of factors, including reduced paracrine ovarian activity [153], LH receptor polymorphisms [152], reduced androgen secretory capacity [154], decreased number of functional LH receptors [155], and reduced LH bioactivity while LH imnunoreactivity is unchanged [156, 157]. Thus, it has been hypothesized that the aforementioned women would benefit from the use of LH-containing gonadotropin preparations [144, 146, 150, 158, 159]. The potential benefit of LH administration seems to be related to its action at the follicular level, which promotes an increase in androgen production for its later aromatization to estrogens, thus restoring the follicular milieu with a positive impact on oocyte quality.

Clinical Studies on LH Supplementation During COS in Selected Patients

A recent meta-analysis by Hill et al. demonstrated the beneficial effect of LH supplementation in down-regulated women over 34 years undergoing COS with rec-hFSH. The study included 7 RCTs (902 women) and compared COS using rec-hFSH alone or in combination with rec-hLH. GnRH-agonist down-regulation was used in five trials while GnRH antagonist and GnRH-agonist micro-flare were used in the remaining trials. The dose and day of starting rec-hLH supplementation varied among trials. In five of them a fixed dose of 150 IU rec-hLH, which started either on the sixth or seventh stimulation day, was used. One trial used a fixed 2:1 ratio of rec-hFSH and rec-hLH while another used a fixed dose of 75 IU rec-hLH regardless of the FSH dose; in both of them LH supplementation was given from the first day of stimulation on. Implantation (OR =1.36; 95% CI: 1.05 to 1.78, I^2=12%) and clinical pregnancy rates (OR =1.37; 95% CI: 1.03 to 1.83, I^2=28%) were significantly higher for women who received rec-hLH in addition to rec-hFSH compared with those in whom rec-hFSH was administered alone [92].

Along the same lines, Mochtar et al., specifically evaluating poor responders, have also demonstrated the usefulness of adding rec-hLH to COS. These authors pooled three RCTs including 310 participants, and showed that higher ongoing pregnancy rates (OR =1.85; 95% CI: 1.1 to 3.11) were obtained in patients treated with the combination of rec-hFSH and rec-hLH compared with rec-hFSH alone [140]. In another meta-analysis by Bosdou et al., which included 7 RCTs and 603 poor responders, differences in clinical pregnancy were not detected in the group of patients receiving LH supplementation. Notwithstanding, the definition of poor responders was not uniform and two of the included RCTs, in fact, evaluated slow/hypo-responders rather than poor responders. The protocols of stimulation also varied as GnRH antagonists and agonists were used in two trials each, and GnRH-agonist short protocol was applied in three studies. The way rec-hLH supplementation was given also varied as daily doses of either 75 or 150 IU were used, and the starting day differed or was not described. Rec-hLH was added to rec-hFSH from the first stimulation day on in one trial, at stimulation day 7 in three studies, at day 8 in one RCT and on the day of the first GnRH antagonist injection in another one. Although statistical significance was not reached, the magnitude of the effect size and the width of the 95% CI regarding the clinical pregnancy rates (RD=+6%; 95% CI: −0.3 to +13%; p=0.06) suggested a potential clinical benefit of LH supplementation. Nevertheless, the authors of the aforesaid meta-analyses did find benefit in the use of rec-hLH supplementation in terms of live birth rates after IVF (RD=+19%; CI: +1 to +36%), but their results derived from a single RCT [91]. Lastly, Fan et al. also studying poor responders in 3 RCTs reported no differences in ongoing pregnancy rates with LH supplementation (OR=1.30; 95% CI: 0.80 to 2.11). Furthermore, there was no significant difference in the number of oocytes retrieved, total dose of rec-hFSH used, total duration of stimulation, number of retrieved metaphase II oocytes and cycle cancellation rate between the study and control groups [160].

Despite the aforementioned evidence suggesting a beneficial effect of LH supplementation in selected patients, results should be interpreted with caution due to the several limitations from the studies included in these meta-analyses (Table 28.8). First, definition of poor ovarian response was not uniform across studies. Second, ovarian stimulation protocols differed in terms of dosing, onset of LH supplementation and duration of stimulation. Third, in most cases a definite conclusion has not been reached due to the limited number of included studies [91]. At present, the role of LH supplementation during COS is still debatable, and it is certain that more studies are needed until a definitive conclusion is reached. Among many questions, what clinicians want to know is to which subgroups to offer LH supplementation, and what is the best protocol for LH supplementation.

In this sense we still do not know how much LH is needed and when to start LH supplementation, and if the LH dose should be flexible or fixed [91, 146, 160].

Clinical Studies on COS with a Fixed Combination of 2:1 Ratio Follitropin Alfa + Lutropin Alfa

The clinical experience with this novel recombinant gonadotropin presentation is still limited. An open-label RCT in 2012 compared this new formulation with HP-hMG in 35 women with hypogonadotropic hypogonadism. The proportion of patients reaching ovulation did not differ between the groups (70 vs. 88 % respectively), but the pregnancy rate was significantly higher in the rec-hLH group (55.6 vs. 23.3 %; $p=0.01$; [161]). In a RCT involving 106 women with low baseline endogenous LH levels (<1.2 IU/L) in the presence of normal FSH levels undergoing IVF, fewer days of stimulation (10.9 ± 1.1 vs. 14.1 ± 1.6; $p=0.013$) and higher number of retrieved oocytes (7.8 ± 1.1 vs. 4.1 ± 12; $p=0.002$) were noted in the group that received follitropin alfa + lutropin alfa 2:1 compared with the group who received hMG. However, differences were not observed in estradiol levels on hCG day (1987 ± 699 pg/mL vs. 2056 ± 560 pg/mL), pregnancy rates per cycle (28.3 vs. 29.3 %) and implantation rates (12.1 vs. 12.2 %), despite a higher cancellation rates due to excessive response was noted in women receiving follitropin + lutropin alfa (11.1 vs. 1.7 %; $p=0.042$; [162]).

Recently, a large matched case-control study involving 4719 patients undergoing COS in a long down-regulation GnRH-agonist protocol using either hMG or a fixed combination of rec-hFSH and rec-hLH at a 2:1 ratio favored the latter with respect to the probability of achieving a clinical pregnancy in IVF (32 vs. 26 %; $p=0.02$; [163]). Lastly, in 2013, a crossover study evaluated 33 patients using HP-hMG in their first IVF cycle and 2:1 rec-hFSH plus rec-hLH in their second IVF attempt. Estradiol levels on the day of hCG (2633 ± 871 vs. 2101 ± 816; $p<0.05$) and the number of oocytes retrieved (9.8 ± 3.3 vs. 7.3 ± 3.1; $p<0.01$) were higher in the group that received the 2:1 rec-hFSH plus rec-hLH formulation. Despite of that, implantation and clinical pregnancy rates per started cycle were not different between the groups (29.6 and 48.4 %, respectively, for hMG and 28.4 % and 48.4 for rec-hFSH plus rec-hLH; [164]).

At present, there is insufficient clinical evidence to confirm the superiority of the fixed rec-hFSH plus rec-hLH recombinant combination over hMG. However, it seems sound to assume that LH activity driven by the two formulations is not equivalent. Unlike rec-hLH, LH activity in hMG derives from hCG which has markedly longer half-life and higher binding affinity to LH/hCG receptors compared to LH [94]. Down-regulation of LH receptors for up to 48 h has been reported in animal models after hCG administration [96]. In fact, there is a consistent lower expression of LH/hCG receptor gene and genes involved in the biosynthesis of cholesterol and steroids in granulosa cells in patients treated with hMG compared to those treated with rec-hFSH [95]. The lower gene expression may reflect down-regulation of LH/hCG receptors caused by a constant ligand exposure to hCG during the follicular phase. These findings indicate that granulosa cells of patients treated with hMG have lower LH-induced cholesterol uptake, a decrease in de novo cholesterol synthesis and a decrease in steroid synthesis. This would also explain the lower progesterone levels reported in these patients. In conclusion, the choice of preparations used for COS might be important for granulosa cell function and may influence the developmental competence of the oocyte and function of the corpus luteum [95].

Clinical Impact of Progesterone Rise During COS with Gonadotropins

In a normal menstrual cycle, there is a progressive increase in progesterone levels as follicles develop [165]. Granulosa cells grow and express LH receptors under FSH influence [22, 34]. In the late follicular phase, LH acts on granulosa LH receptors and stimulates progesterone production [22]. In the event of COS, multiple follicular growth is achieved. Recombinant FSH has higher FSH bioactivity compared to urinary FSH and hMG, thus leading to the development of more follicles and granulosa cells [97, 125, 126, 166–168]. Furthermore, FSH induces up-regulation of LH receptors in granulosa cells, unlike hMG [22, 96]. In accordance with the number of follicles and FSH drive, progesterone output to the periphery will be magnified. Endogenous (and exogenous) LH binds to LH receptors in the GC and induces progesterone (P4) synthesis; most circulating P4 (95 %) is produced in the intrafollicular compartment by the granulosa cells. Thereby, serum progesterone levels are usually higher in rec-hFSH stimulated-cycles compared with hMG, and it merely reflects the presence of a larger number of developing follicles, and possibly higher levels of endogenous LH present [95, 97, 169].

In recent years, increased attention has been given to the potential negative impact of premature progesterone elevation on embryo implantation [98, 170–172]. In the meta-analysis of Venetis et al., the authors included 12 eligible studies (10 of which were retrospective) and assessed 2624 patients undergoing COS in association with GnRH agonist and 109 with GnRH antagonist. A detrimental effect of progesterone rise, measured on the day of hCG administration, on the probability of achieving a clinical pregnancy was not confirmed (GnRH agonist group: OR = 0.86; 95 % CI: 0.59 to 1.25; GnRH antagonist: OR = 0.57; 95 % CI: 0.09 to 3.56; [98]). In 2012, Kobilianakis et al. in a small meta-analysis including five studies and 585 patients (all using GnRH antagonist) demonstrated that progesterone elevation on the day of hCG administration was associated with a significantly decreased probability of achieving a clinical pregnancy per initiated cycle (WMD = −9%; 95% CI: −17 to −2%; [170]). These conflicting data may be explained by the fact that both meta-analyses included mostly retrospective studies and the cutoff points to discriminate patients with elevated and normal progesterone levels were not uniform [98, 170].

In an attempt to establish a cutoff point for progesterone elevation that could be critical for IVF outcomes, Bosch et al. performed a retrospective analysis of 4032 patients undergoing IVF/ICSI cycles using GnRH agonists or antagonists. In this study, a significant ($p<0.001$) inverse association was observed between ongoing pregnancy and serum progesterone levels on the day of hCG administration irrespective of the GnRH analogue used for pituitary suppression. The odds-ratio of ongoing pregnancy was calculated for different progesterone intervals and results were compared. There was a significant difference in the probability of pregnancy only between the 1.26–1.50 and 1.51–1.75 ng/mL intervals, both for the overall study group ($p=0.003$) and the subgroups (GnRH agonist: $p=0.028$; GnRH antagonist: $p=0.024$). Patients with serum progesterone levels ≤1.5 ng/mL had higher ongoing pregnancy rates than those with progesterone levels >1.5 ng/mL (31.0 vs. 19.1%; $p=0.00006$; OR = 0.53; 95% CI: 0.38 to 0.72). Multivariate regression analysis showed that daily FSH dose, number of oocytes and estradiol values on the day of hCG administration were positively associated with progesterone levels ($p<0.0001$ for all). Progesterone levels were also significantly higher in women treated with GnRH agonists versus antagonists ($p=0.0003$). The authors of the aforementioned study concluded that the cutoff point of 1.5 ng/mL could represent the critical threshold level at which there would be a negative impact of progesterone on ongoing pregnancy rates [171].

In a large retrospective cohort study, Xu et al. evaluated a group of 11,055 women who had had fresh embryo transfers and a group including 4021 frozen embryo transfers (FET) after IVF/ICSI according to P4 levels. The ongoing pregnancy rate in fresh cycles was inversely associated with serum progesterone levels on the day of hCG administration. On the other hand, no such negative impact of elevated P4 levels was observed in FET. In contrast with the study of Bosch and colleagues, which defined a single P4 cutoff point, Xu et al. proposed that P4 cutoff points should be according to different ovarian response, that is, serum P4 level of 1.5 ng/mL as the threshold for poor responders (≤4 oocytes), 1.75 ng/mL for intermediate responders (5–19 oocytes), and 2.25 ng/mL for high responders (≥20 oocytes). Of note, elevated progesterone had no impact on the oocyte and embryo quality thus suggesting that its likely detrimental effect relates to the endometrial receptivity [172]. This hypothesis has been corroborated by data from oocyte donation programs, which indicates that pregnancy rates of the recipients are not influenced by progesterone levels of the donors measured at the day of hCG administration [166, 173, 174].

In conclusion, serum progesterone rise in COS is a direct effect of the number of developing follicles. Although current data suggest that elevated progesterone levels on the day of hCG administration may negatively impact embryo implantation in fresh transfers, prospective randomized trials are needed to confirm these results and to determine why, when and how much progesterone is detrimental for implantation rates [98].

Future Developments in Gonadotropin Preparations

Pharmaceutical companies have been working on the development of low-molecular weight (LMW) gonadotropins, that is, new non-peptide molecules with in vivo bioactivity to properly stimulate FSH and LH receptors when taken orally [175, 176]. FSH and LH receptors constitute a subgroup of G protein coupled receptors with 7-transmembrane domains and a large N-terminal extracellular region, which is the predominant site of hormone binding (Fig. 28.10; [175, 177, 178]). Receptor activation requires that hormones bind to the N-terminal region, thus leading to intramolecular signal transduction from the ligand-receptor complex to the transmembrane domains. However,

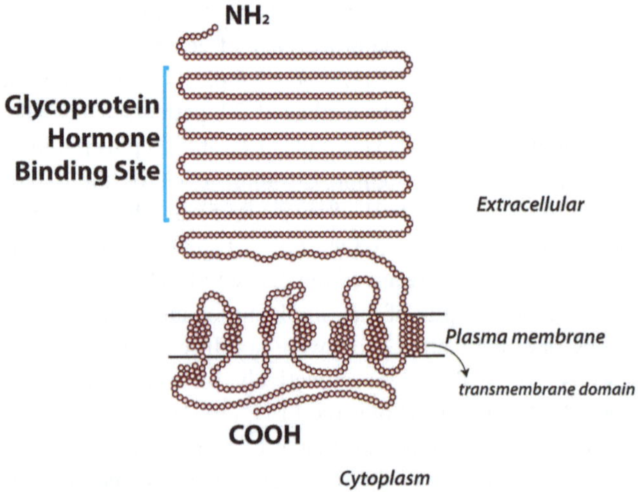

Fig. 28.10 FSH and LH receptors. FSH and LH receptors are included in the subgroup of G protein coupled receptors. Such receptors are characterized by having 7-transmembrane domains and a large N-terminal extracellular region, which is the predominant site of hormone binding. In contrast to FSH and LH, most low-molecular weight (*LMW*) FSH and LH receptor agonists (and antagonists) are allosteric compounds that interact with the transmembrane domains instead of the N-terminal region

the mechanism that underlies this intramolecular signaling pathway is poorly understood [175, 179]. The main signaling pathway of FSH receptors in granulosa cells appears to involve stimulation of adenylyl cyclase via coupling to Gs proteins [175, 177]. This pathway is responsible for granulosa cell differentiation and growth, aromatase expression and LH receptor induction [175].

The first LMW peptides with bioactivity to FSH receptors were described in 2002. In recent years, other compounds have been identified, including biaryl diketopiperazines, thienopyrimidines, dihydropyridines, and thiazolidinones. In the meantime, peptides with agonist activity to LH have been also identified [175, 176]. To date, oral bioavailability and/or oral efficacy of these earlier compounds have not been reported. In fact, most LMW FSH receptor agonists (and antagonists) are thought to be allosteric compounds presumably interacting with the transmembrane domains instead of the N-terminal region. As such, the signaling pathways induced by these molecules are different from those induced by the native, orthosteric ligands. Recently, a new developed LMW agonist to FSH (and LH) receptor has shown to be orally bioactive in animal studies [176, 177]. In the future, it seems possible that orally taking gonadotropins would replace the injectable presentations currently available [175, 176].

Conclusions

Gonadotropin therapy has a central role for ovarian stimulation in infertility treatments. Efforts have been made to improve gonadotropin preparations over the last century. Undoubtedly, current gonadotropins have better quality and safety profile as well as clinical efficacy than the earlier ones. In this sense, a major achievement has been the introduction of recombinant technology in the manufacturing process of FSH, LH, and hCG. Recombinant gonadotropins are purer than urinary-derived gonadotropins, and the introduction of FbM technology virtually eliminated batch-to-batch variations and enabled accurate dosing in relatively smaller increments thus refining COS. Recombinant and FbM technologies combined have been the driven forces for the introduction of prefilled pen devices that made ovarian stimulation more patient-friendly. Recently, a novel FSH preparation with long-lasting activity has been introduced, but clinical results are still limited. The next step in gonadotropin development, that is, orally bioactive molecules with either agonist or antagonist actions on FSH and LH receptors, is already on its way.

Although FSH is the key gonadotropin to promote follicular recruitment and growth during COS, the importance of LH has been revisited. At present, the general consensus is that most women have sufficient levels of endogenous LH to support ovarian stimulation with FSH alone. However, a subgroup comprising approximately 15–20 % of women undergoing ART have less sensitive ovaries and fair evidence suggests that LH supplementation to FSH would be beneficial during COS. These categories include older patients (≥35 years), poor and slow/hypo responders to COS, and those with deeply suppressed endogenous LH. Currently, three gonadotropin formulations are commercially available to deliver LH activity: hMG (with LH activity originated from hCG), rec-hLH and a newly released fixed combination of rec-hFSH and rec-hLH at 2:1 ratio. Research has indicated that the choice of preparations used for COS is important for granulosa cell function and may influence the developmental competence of the oocyte and function of the corpus luteum. Such findings have been gradually translated to the clinical field.

Acknowledgment The authors are grateful to Mrs. Fabiola C. Bento for language revision.

References

1. Beall SA, DeCherney A. History and challenges surrounding ovarian stimulation in the treatment of infertility. Fertil Steril. 2012;97(4):785–801.
2. Lunenfeld B. Historical perspectives in gonadotrophin therapy. Human Reprod Update. 2004;10(6):453–67.
3. Practice Committee of American Society for Reproductive Medicine, Birmingham, Alabama. Gonadotropin preparations: past, present, and future perspectives. Fertil Steril. 2008;90(Suppl 5):S13–S20.
4. Howles CM. Genetic engineering of human FSH (Gonal-F). Hum Reprod Update. 1996;2(2):172–91.
5. Esteves SC, Schertz JC, Verza S Jr, Schneider DT, Zabaglia SF. A comparison of menotropin, highly-purified menotropin and follitropin alfa in cycles of intracytoplasmic sperm injection. Reprod Biol Endocrinol. 2009;7:111.
6. Driebergen R, Baer G. Quantification of follicle stimulating hormone (follitropin alfa): is in vivo bioassay still relevant in the recombinant age? Curr Med Res Opin. 2003;19(1):41–6.
7. Martinez G, Sanguineti F, Sepulveda J, Dorey J, Arici A, Patrizio P. A comparison between follitropin α filled by mass and follitropin a filled by bioassay in the same egg donors. Reprod Biomed Online. 2011;22(Suppl 1):S20–2.
8. Bosch E. Recombinant human follicular stimulating hormone and recombinant human luteinizing hormone in a 2:1 ratio combination. Pharmacological characteristics and clinical applications. Expert Opin Biol Ther. 2010;10(6):1001–9.
9. Verbost P, Sloot WN, Rose UM, de Leeuw R, Hanssen RG, Verheijden GF. Pharmacologic profiling of corifollitropin alfa, the first developed sustained follicle stimulant. Eur J Pharmacol. 2011;651(1–3):227–33.
10. Christen M, Schertz JC, Arriagada P, Keitel J, Müller H. The redesigned follitropin α pen injector for infertility treatment. Expert Opin Drug Deliv. 2011;8(6):833–9.
11. Saunders H, Schertz JC, Hecker C, Lang B, Arriagada P. The recombinant human chorionic gonadotropin prefilled pen: results of patient and nurse human factors usability testing. Expert Opin Drug Deliv. 2012;9(8):893–900.

12. Speroff L, Fritz MA. Neuroendocrinology. In: Speroff L, Fritz MA, editors. Clinical gynecologic endocrinology and infertility. Philadelphia: Lippincott Williams & Wilkins; 2005. pp. 295–6.
13. Cole LA, Khanlian SA, Muller CY. Detection of perimenopause or postmenopause human chorionic gonadotropin: an unnecessary source of alarm. Am J Obstet Gynecol. 2008;198(3):275. e1–7.
14. Cole LA, Khanlian SA, Muller CY. Normal production of human chorionic gonadotropin in perimenopausal and menopausal women and after oophorectomy. Int J Gynecol Cancer. 2009;19(9):1556–9.
15. Hsueh AJ, Adashi EY, Jones PB, Welsh TH Jr. Hormonal regulation of the differentiation of cultured ovarian granulosa cells. Endocr Rev. 1984;5(1):76–127.
16. Vegetti W, Alagna F. FSH and folliculogenesis: from physiology to ovarian stimulation. Reprod Biomed Online. 2006;12(6):684–94.
17. Jeppesen JV, Kristensen SG, Nielsen ME, et al. LH-receptor gene expression in human granulosa and cumulus cells from antral and preovulatory follicles. J Clin Endocrinol Metab. 2012;97(8):E1524–31.
18. Speroff L, Fritz MA. Hormone biosynthesis, metabolism, and mechanisms of action. Stereidogenesis. In: Speroff L, Fritz MA, editors. Clinical gynecologic endocrinology and infertility. Philadelphia: Lippincott Williams & Wilkins; 2005. pp. 109–16.
19. Young JM, McNeilly AS. Theca: the forgotten cell of the ovarian follicle. Reproduction. 2010;140(4):489–504.
20. Alviggi C, Mollo A, Clarizia R, De Placido G. Exploiting LH in ovarian stimulation. Reprod Biomed Online. 2006;12(2):221–33.
21. Speroff L, Fritz MA. Regulation of the menstrual cycle. In: Speroff L, Fritz MA, editors. Cinical gynecologic endocrinology and infertility. Philadelphia: Lippincott Williams & Wilkins; 2005. pp. 348–83.
22. Gougeon A. Dynamics of human follicular growth: morphologic, dynamic and functional aspects. In: Leung PKC, Addashi EY, editors. The ovary. San Diego: Elsevier Academic; 2004. pp. 25–43.
23. Zeleznik AJ. The physiology of follicle selection. Reprod Biol Endocrinol. 2004;16(2):31.
24. Oktay K, Briggs DA, Gosden RG. Ontogeny of follicle-stimulating hormone receptor gene expression in isolated human ovarian follicles. J Clin Endocrinol Metab. 1997;82(11):3748–51.
25. Brown JB. Pituitary control of ovarian function-concepts derived from gonadotrophin therapy. Aust N Z J Obstet Gynaecol. 1978;18(1):46–54.
26. Pache TD, Wladimiroff JW, de Jong FH, Hop WC, Fauser BC. Growth patterns of nondominant ovarian follicles during the normal menstrual cycle. Fertil Steril. 1990;54(4):638–42.
27. Falck B. Site of production of oestrogen in rat ovary as studied in microtransplants. Acta Physiol Scand Suppl. 1959;47(163):1–101.
28. Miller WL. Steroidogenic enzymes. Endocr Dev. 2008;13:1–18.
29. Wickenheisser JK, Nelson-DeGrave VL, McAllister JM. Human ovarian theca cells in culture. Trends Endocrinol Metab. 2006;17(2):65–71.
30. Smyth CD, Miró F, Whitelaw PF, Howles CM, Hillier SG. Ovarian thecal/interstitial androgen synthesis is enhanced by a follicle-stimulating hormone-stimulated paracrine mechanism. Endocrinology. 1993;133(4):1532–8.
31. Whitelaw PF, Smyth CD, Howles CM, Hillier SG. Cell-specific expression of aromatase and LH receptor mRNAs in rat ovary. J Mol Endocrinol. 1992;9(3):309–12.
32. Kol S, Adashi EY. Intraovarian factors regulating ovarian function. Curr Opin Obstet Gynecol. 1995;7(3):209–13.
33. Zeleznik AJ, Hillier SG. The role of gonadotropins in the selection of the preovulatory follicle. Clin Obstet Gynecol. 1984;27(4):927–40.
34. Goff AK, Armstrong DT. Stimulatory action of gonadotropins and prostaglandins on adenosine-3′,5′-monophosphate production by isolated rat granulosa cells. Endocrinology. 1977;101(5):1461–7.
35. Campbell BK, Dobson H, Baird DT, Scaramuzzi RJ. Examination of the relative role of FSH and LH in the mechanism of ovulatory follicle selection in sheep. J Reprod Fertil. 1999;117(2):355–67.
36. Sullivan MW, Stewart-Akers A, Krasnow JS, Berga SL, Zeleznik AJ. Ovarian responses in women to recombinant follicle-stimulating hormone and luteinizing hormone (LH): a role for LH in the final stages of follicular maturation. J Clin Endocrinol Metab. 1999;84(1):228–32.
37. Pauerstein CJ, Eddy CA, Croxatto HD, Hess R, Siler-Khodr TM, Croxatto HB. Temporal relationships of estrogen, progesterone, and luteinizing hormone levels to ovulation in women and infrahuman primates. Am J Obstet Gynecol. 1978;130(8):876–86.
38. Fritz MA, McLachlan RI, Cohen NL, Dahl KD, Bremmer WJ, Soules MR. Onset and characteristics of the midcycle surge in bioactive and immunoactive luteinizing hormone secretion in normal women: influence of physiological variations in periovulatory ovarian steorid hormone secretion. J Clin Endocrinol Metab. 1992;75(2):489–93.
39. Young JR, Jaffe RB. Strength-duration characteristics of estrogen effects on gonadotropin response to gonadotropin-releasing hormone in women. II. Effects of varying concentrations of estradiol. J Clin Endocrinol Metab. 1976;42(3):432–42.
40. Coutts JRT, Gaukroger JM, Kader AS, et al. Steroidogenesis by the Human Graafian Follicle. In: Coutts JRT, editor. Functional morphology of the human ovary. Lancaster: MTP; 1981. pp. 56–72.
41. Filicori M, Cognigni GE, Taraborrelli S, et al. Luteinizing hormone activity supplementation enhances follicle-stimulating hormone efficacy and improves ovulation induction outcome. Clin Endocrinol Metab. 1999;84(8):2659–63.
42. Couzinet B, Brailly S, Bouchard P, Schaison G. Progesterone stimulates luteinizing hormone secretion by acting directly on the pituitary. J Clin Endocrinol Metab. 1992;74(2):374–8.
43. Liu JH, Yen SSC. Induction of midcycle gonadotropin surge by ovarian steroids in women: a critical evaluation. J Clin Endocrinol Metab. 1983;57(4):797–802.
44. Hoff JD, Quigley ME, Yen SS. Hormonal dynamics at midcycle: a reevaluation. J Clin Endocrinol Metab. 1983;57(4):792–6.
45. McCord LA, Li F, Rosewell KL, Brännström M, Curry TE. Ovarian expression and regulation of the stromelysins during the periovulatory period in the human and the rat. Biol Reprod. 2012;86(3):78.
46. Peluffo MC, Murphy MJ, Baughman ST, Stouffer RL, Hennebold JD. Systematic analysis of protease gene expression in the rhesus macaque ovulatory follicle: metalloproteinase involvement in follicle rupture. Endocrinology. 2011;152(10):3963–74.
47. Speroff L, Fritz MA. The ovary: embryology and development. In: Speroff L, Fritz MA, editors. Clinical gynecologic endocrinology and infertility. Philadelphia: Lippincott Williams & Wilkins; 2005. pp. 215–16.
48. Lapthorn AJ, Harris DC, Littlejohn A, et al. Crystal structure of human chorionic gonadotropin. Nature. 1994;369(6480):455–61.
49. Vaitukaitis JL, Ross GT, Braunstein GD, Rayford PL. Gonadotropins and their subunits: basic and clinical studies. Recent Prog Horm Res. 1976;32:289–331.
50. Ulloa-Aguirre A, Espinoza R, Damian-Matsumura P, Chappel SC. Immunological and biological potencies of the different molecular species of gonadotrophins. Hum Reprod. 1988;3(4):491–501.
51. Rozell TG, Okrainetz RJ. FSH: one hormone with multiple forms, or a family of multiples hormones. In: Chedrese PJ, editor. Reproductive endocrinology: a molecular approach. New York: Springer Science + Business Media; 2009. pp. 145–60.
52. Wide L, Naessén T, Sundström-Poromaa I, Eriksson K. Sulfonation and sialylation of gonadotropins in women during the menstrual cycle, after menopause, and with polycystic ovarian syndrome and in men. J Clin Endocrinol Metab. 2007;92(11):4410–7.
53. Ulloa-Aguirre A, Midgley AR Jr, Beitins IZ, Padmanabhan V. Follicle-stimulating isohormones: characterization and physiological relevance. Endocr Rev. 1995;16(6):765–87.

54. Green ED, Baenziger JU. Asparagine-linked oligosaccharides on lutropin, follitropin, and thyrotropin. I. Structural elucidation of the sulfated and sialylated oligosaccharides on bovine, ovine, and human pituitary glycoprotein hormones. J Biol Chem. 1988;263(1):25–35.
55. Smith PL, Baenziger JU. Molecular basis of recognition by the glycoprotein hormone-specific N-acetylgalactosamine-transferase. Proc Natl Acad Sci U S A. 1992;89(1):329–33.
56. Anobile CJ, Talbot JA, McCann SJ, Padmanabhan V, Robertson WR. Glycoform composition of serum gonadotrophins through the normal menstrual cycle and in the post-menopausal state. Mol Hum Reprod. 1998;4(7):631–9.
57. Fiete D, Srivastava V, Hindsgaul O, Baenziger JU. A hepatic reticuloendothelial cell receptor specific for SO4-4GalNAc beta 1,4GlcNAc beta 1,2Man alpha that mediates rapid clearance of lutropin. Cell. 1991;67(6):1103–10.
58. Wide L, Eriksson K, Sluss PM, Hall JE. Serum half-life of pituitary gonadotropins is decreased by sulfonation and increased by sialylation in women. J Clin Endocrinol Metab. 2009;94(3):958–64.
59. Combarnous Y. Molecular basis of the specificity of binding of glycoprotein hormones to their receptors. Endocr Rev. 1992;13(4):670–91.
60. Galway AB, Hsueh AJ, Keene JL, Yamoto M, Fauser BC, Boime I. In vitro and in vivo bioactivity of recombinant human follicle-stimulating hormone and partially deglycosylated variants secreted by transfected eukaryotic cell lines. Endocrinology. 1990;127(1):93–100.
61. Fox KM, Dias JA, Van Roey P. Three-dimensional structure of human follicle-stimulating hormone. Mol Endocrinol. 2001;15(3):378–89.
62. Campbell RK. Molecular pharmacology of gonadotropins. Endocrine. 2005;26(3):291–6.
63. Morell AG, Gregoriadis G, Scheinberg IH, Hickman J, Ashwell G. The role of sialic acid in determining the survival of glycoproteins in the circulation. J Biol Chem. 1971;246(5):1461–7.
64. Padmanabhan V, Lang LL, Sonstein J, Kelch RP, Beitins IZ. Modulation of serum follicle-stimulating hormone bioactivity and isoform distribution by estrogenic steroids in normal women and in gonadal dysgenesis. J Clin Endocrinol Metab. 1988;67(3):465–73.
65. Zambrano E, Olivares A, Mendez JP, et al. Dynamics of basal and gonadotropin-releasing hormone-releasable serum follicle-stimulating hormone charge isoform distribution throughout the human menstrual cycle. J Clin Endocrinol Metab. 1995;80(5):1647–56.
66. Wide L, Bakos O. More basic forms of both human follicle-stimulating hormone and luteinizing hormone in serum at midcycle compared with the follicular or luteal phase. J Clin Endocrinol Metab. 1993;76(4):885–9.
67. Midgley AR Jr, Pierce GB Jr. Immunohistochemical localization of human chorionic gonadotropin. J Exp Med. 1962;115:289–94.
68. Hamblen EC, Davis CD, Durham NC. Treatment of hypo-ovarianism by the sequential and cyclic administration of equine and chorionic gonadotropins-so-called one-two cyclic gonadotropic therapy Summary of 5 years' results. Am J Obstet Gynecol. 1945;50:137–46.
69. Hamblen EC. The clinical evaluation of ovarian responses to gonadotropic therapy. Endocrinology. 1939;24(6):848–66.
70. Mazer C, Ravetz E. The effect of combined administration of chorionic gonadotropin and pituitary synergist on the human ovary. Am J Obstet Gynaecol. 1941;41:474–588.
71. Maddock WO, Leach RB, Tokuyama I, Paulsen CA, Roy WR. Effects of hog pituitary follicle-stimulating hormone in women: antihormone formation and inhibition of ovarian function. J Clin Endocrinol Metab. 1956;16(4):433–48.
72. Buxton CL, Hermann W. Induction of ovulation in the human with human gonadotropins. Yale J Biol Med. 1960;33:145–7.
73. Gemzell CA. Induction of ovulation with human pituitary gonadotrophins. Fertil Steril. 1962;13:153–68.
74. Giudice E, Crisci C, Eshkol A, Papoian R. Composition of commercial gonadotrophin preparations extracted from human postmenopausal urine: characterization of non-gonadotrophin proteins. Hum Reprod. 1994;9(12):2291–9.
75. Alviggi C, Revelli A, Anserini P, et al. A prospective, randomised, controlled clinical study on the assessment of tolerability and of clinical efficacy of Merional (hMG-IBSA) administered subcutaneously versus Merional administered intramuscularly in women undergoing multifollicular ovarian stimulation in an ART programme (IVF). Reprod Biol Endocrinol. 2007;5:45.
76. Platteau P, Laurent E, Albano C, et al. An open, randomized single-centre study to compare the efficacy and convenience of follitropin beta administered by a pen device with follitropin alpha administered by a conventional syringe in women undergoing ovarian stimulation for IVF/ICSI. Hum Reprod. 2003;18(6):1200–4.
77. Howles CM. Genetic engineering of human FSH (Gonal-F). Hum Reprod Update. 1996;2(2):172–91.
78. Olijve W, de Boer W, Mulders JW, van Wezenbeek PM. Molecular biology and biochemistry of human recombinant follicle stimulating hormone (Puregon). Mol Hum Reprod. 1996;2(5):371–82.
79. de Leeuw R, Mulders J, Voortman G, Rombout F, Damm J, Kloosterboer L. Structure-function relationship of recombinant follicle stimulating hormone (Puregon). Mol Hum Reprod. 1996;2(5):361–9.
80. Horsman G, Talbot JA, McLoughlin JD, Lambert A, Robertson WR. A biological, immunological and physico-chemical comparison of the current clinical batches of the recombinant FSH preparations Gonal-F and Puregon. Hum Reprod. 2000;15(9):1898–902.
81. Orvieto R, Nahum R, Rabinson J, Ashkenazi J, Anteby EY, Meltcer S. Follitropin-alpha (Gonal-F) versus follitropin-beta (Puregon) in controlled ovarian hyperstimulation for in vitro fertilization: is there any difference? Fertil Steril. 2009;91(Suppl 4):1522–5.
82. Fauser BC, van Heusden AM. Manipulation of human ovarian function: physiological concepts and clinical consequences. Endocr Rev. 1997;18(1):71–106.
83. Fauser BC, Mannaerts BM, Devroey P, Leader A, Boime I, Baird DT. Advances in recombinant DNA technology: corifollitropin alfa, a hybrid molecule with sustained follicle-stimulating activity and reduced injection frequency. Hum Reprod Update. 2009;15(3):309–21.
84. Birken S, Canfield RE. Isolation and amino acid sequence of COOH-terminal fragments from the beta subunit of human choriogonadotropin. J Biol Chem. 1977;252(15):5386–92.
85. Kessler MJ, Mise T, Ghai RD, Bahl OP. Structure and location of the O-glycosidic carbohydrate units of human chorionic gonadotropin. J Biol Chem. 1979;254(16):7909–14.
86. Fares FA, Suganuma N, Nishimori K, LaPolt PS, Hsueh AJ, Boime I. Design of a long-acting follitropin agonist by fusing the C-terminal sequence of the chorionic gonadotropin beta subunit to the follitropin beta subunit. Proc Natl Acad Sci U S A. 1992;89(10):4304–8.
87. Balen AH, Mulders AG, Fauser BC, et al. Pharmacodynamics of a single low dose of long-acting recombinant follicle- stimulating hormone (FSH-carboxy terminal peptide, corifollitropin alfa) in women with World Health Organization group II anovulatory infertility. J Clin Endocrinol Metab. 2004;89(12):6297–304.
88. Dhillon S, Keating GM. Lutropin alfa. Drugs. 2008;68(11):1529–40.
89. Bosdou JK, Venetis CA, Kolibianakis EM, et al. The use of androgens or androgen-modulating agents in poor responders undergoing in vitro fertilization: a systematic review and meta-analysis. Hum Reprod Update. 2012;18(2):127–45.
90. Hill MJ, Levens ED, Levy G, et al. The use of recombinant luteinizing hormone in patients undergoing assisted reproductive techniques with advanced reproductive age: a systematic review and meta-analysis. Fertil Steril. 2012;97(5):1108–14.

91. Bassett RM, Driebergen R. Continued improvements in the quality and consistency of follitropin alfa, recombinant human FSH. Reprod Biomed Online. 2005;10(2):169–77.
92. le Cotonnec JY, Porchet HC, Beltrami V, Munafo A. Clinical pharmacology of recombinant human luteinizing hormone: Part I. Pharmacokinetics after intravenous administration to healthy female volunteers and comparison with urinary human luteinizing hormone. Fertil Steril. 1998;69(2):189–94.
93. Grøndahl ML, Borup R, Lee YB, Myrhøj V, Meinertz H, Sørensen S. Differences in gene expression of granulosa cells from women undergoing controlled ovarian hyperstimulation with either recombinant follicle-stimulating hormone or highly purified human menopausal gonadotropin. Fertil Steril. 2009;91(5):1820–30.
94. Menon KM, Munshi UM, Clouser CL, Nair AK. Regulation of luteinizing hormone/human chorionic gonadotropin receptor expression: a perspective. Biol Reprod. 2004;70(4):861–6.
95. Bosch E, Vidal C, Labarta E, Simon C, Remohi J, Pellicer A. Highly purified hMG versus recombinant FSH in ovarian hyperstimulation with GnRH antagonists-a randomized study. Hum Reprod. 2008;23(10):2346–51.
96. Venetis CA, Kolibianakis EM, Papanikolaou E, Bontis J, Devroey P, Tarlatzis BC. Is progesterone elevation on the day of human chorionic gonadotrophin administration associated with the probability of pregnancy in in vitro fertilization? A systematic review and meta-analysis. Hum Reprod Update. 2007;13(4):343–55.
97. Picard M, Rossier C, Papasouliotis O, Lugan I. Bioequivalence of recombinant human FSH and recombinant human LH in a fixed 2:1 combination: two phase I, randomised, crossover studies. Curr Med Res Opin. 2008;24(4):1199–208.
98. Humaidan P, Kol S, Papanikolaou EG. Copenhagen GnRH agonist triggering workshop group. GnRH agonist for triggering of final oocyte maturation: time for a change of practice? Hum Reprod Update. 2011;17(4):510–24.
99. Kessler MJ, Reddy MS, Shah RH, Bahl OP. Structures of N-glycosidic carbohydrate units of human chorionic gonadotropin. J Biol Chem. 1979;254(16):7901–8.
100. Yen SS, Llerena O, Little B, Pearson OH. Disappearance rates of endogenous luteinizing hormone and chorionic gonadotropin in man. J Clin Endocrinol Metab. 1968;28(12):1763–7.
101. Steptoe P, Edwards RG. Laparoscopic recovery of preovulatory human oocytes after priming of ovaries with gonadotrophins. Lancet. 1970;1(7649):683–9.
102. Driscoll GL, Tyler JP, Hangan JT, Fisher PR, Birdsall MA, Knight DC. A prospective, randomized, controlled, double-blind, double-dummy comparison of recombinant and urinary HCG for inducing oocyte maturation and follicular luteinization in ovarian stimulation. Hum Reprod. 2000;15(6):1305–10.
103. Youssef MA, Al-Inany HG, Aboulghar M, Mansour R, Abou-Setta AM. Recombinant versus urinary human chorionic gonadotrophin for final oocyte maturation triggering in IVF and ICSI cycles. Cochrane Database Syst Rev. 2011;13(4):CD003719.
104. van de Weijer BH, Mulders JW, Bos ES, Verhaert PD, van den Hooven HW. Compositional analyses of a human menopausal gonadotrophin preparation extracted from urine (menotropin). Identification of some of its major impurities. Reprod Biomed Online. 2003;7(5):547–57.
105. Kuwabara Y, Mine K, Katayama A, Inagawa T, Akira S, Takeshita T. Proteomic analyses of recombinant human follicle-stimulating hormone and urinary-derived gonadotropin preparations. J Reprod Med. 2009;54(8):459–66.
106. Bassett R, Lispi M, Ceccarelli D, et al. Analytical identification of additional impurities in urinary-derived gonadotrophins. Reprod Biomed Online. 2009;19(3):300–13.
107. Johnson RT, Gibbs CJ Jr. Creutzfeldt-Jakob disease and related transmissible spongiform encephalopathies. N Engl J Med. 1998;339(27):1994–2004.
108. Bassett R, Lispi M, Ceccarelli D, et al. Analytical identification of additional impurities in urinary-derived gonadotrophins. Reprod Biomed Online. 2009;19(3):300–13.
109. Gervais A, Hammel YA, Pelloux S, et al. Glycosylation of human recombinant gonadotrophins: characterization and batch-to-batch consistency. Glycobiology. 2003;13(3):179–89.
110. Hugues JN, Barlow DH, Rosenwaks Z, et al. Improvement in consistency of response to ovarian stimulation with recombinant human follicle stimulating hormone resulting from a new method for calibrating the therapeutic preparation. Reprod Biomed Online. 2003;6(2):185–90.
111. Steelman SL, Pohley FM. Assay of follicle stimulating hormone based on the augmentation with human chorionic gonadotropin. Endocrinology. 1953;53(6):604–16.
112. Bohannon NJ. Insulin delivery using pen devices. Simple-to-use tools may help young and old alike. Postgrad Med. 1999;106(5):57–8, 61–4, 68.
113. Kadiri A, Chraibi A, Marouan F et al. Comparison of NovoPen 3 and syringes/vials in the acceptance of insulin therapy in NIDDM patients with secondary failure to oral hypoglycaemic agents. Diabetes Res Clin Pract. 1998;41(1):15–23.
114. Craenmehr E, Bontje PM, Hoomans E, Voortman G, Mannaerts BM. Follitropin-beta administered by pen device has superior local tolerance compared with follitropin-alpha administered by conventional syringe. Reprod Biomed Online. 2001;3(3):185–9.
115. Aghssa MM, Azargoon A, Ramezanzadeh F, Bagheri M. A comparison of the efficacy, tolerability, and convenience of two formulations of follitropin-alpha in Iranian woman undergoing intracytoplasmic sperm injection cycles. Fertil Steril. 2008;90(4):1043–8.
116. Weiss N. Gonadotrophin products: empowering patients to choose the product that meets their needs. Reprod Biomed Online. 2007;15(1):31–7.
117. Coomarasamy A, Afnan M, Cheema D, van der Veen F, Bossuyt PM, van Wely M. Urinary hMG versus recombinant FSH for controlled ovarian hyperstimulation following an agonist long down-regulation protocol in IVF or ICSI treatment: a systematic review and meta-analysis. Hum Reprod. 2008;23(2):310–5.
118. Al-Inany HG, Abou-Setta AM, Aboulghar MA, Mansour RT, Serour GI. Highly purified hMG achieves better pregnancy rates in IVF cycles but not ICSI cycles compared with recombinant FSH: a meta-analysis. Gynecol Endocrinol. 2009;25(6):372–8.
119. van Wely M, Kwan I, Burt AL, et al. Recombinant versus urinary gonadotrophin for ovarian stimulation in assisted reproductive technology cycles. Cochrane Database Syst Rev. 2011;16(2): CD005354.
120. Jee BC, Suh CS, Kim YB, Kim SH, Moon SY. Clinical efficacy of highly purified hMG versus recombinant FSH in IVF/ICSI cycles: a meta-analysis. Gynecol Obstet Invest. 2010;70(2):132–7.
121. Gerli S, Bini V, Favilli A, Di Renzo GC. Clinical efficacy and cost-effectiveness of HP-human FSH (Fostimon®) versus rFSH (Gonal-F®) in IVF-ICSI cycles: a meta-analysis. Gynecol Endocrinol. 2013;29(6):520–9.
122. van Wely M, Kwan I, Burt AL, et al. Recombinant versus urinary gonadotrophin for ovarian stimulation in assisted reproductive technology cycles. A Cochrane review. Hum Reprod Update. 2012;18(2):111.
123. Hompes PG, Broekmans FJ, Hoozemans DA, Schats R, FIRM group. Effectiveness of highly purified human menopausal gonadotropin vs. recombinant follicle-stimulating hormone in first-cycle in vitro fertilization-intracytoplasmic sperm injection patients. Fertil Steril. 2008;89(6):1685–93.
124. Devroey P, Pellicer A, Nyboe Andersen A, Arce JC, Menopur in GnRH antagonist cycles with single embryo transfer trial group. A randomized assessor-blind trial comparing highly purified hMG

and recombinant FSH in a GnRH antagonist cycle with compulsory single-blastocyst transfer. Fertil Steril. 2012;97(3):561–71.
125. Tulppala M, Aho M, Tuuri T, et al. Comparison of two recombinant follicle-stimulating hormone preparations in in-vitro fertilization: a randomized clinical study. Hum Reprod. 1999;14(11):2709–15.
126. Brinsden P, Akagbosu F, Gibbons LM, et al. A comparison of the efficacy and tolerability of two recombinant human follicle-stimulating hormone preparations in patients undergoing in vitro fertilization-embryo transfer. Fertil Steril. 2000;73(1):114–6.
127. Harlin J, Csemiczky G, Wramsby H, Fried G. Recombinant follicle stimulating hormone in in-vitro fertilization treatment-clinical experience with follitropin alpha and follitropin beta. Hum Reprod. 2000;15(2):239–44.
128. Harlin J, Aanesen G, Csemiczky G, Wramsby H, Fried G. Delivery rates following IVF treatment, using two recombinant FSH preparations for ovarian stimulation. Hum Reprod. 2002;17(2):304–9.
129. Saz-Parkinson Z, López-Cuadrado T, Bouza C, Amate JM. Outcomes of new quality standards of follitropin alfa on ovarian stimulation: meta-analysis of previous studies. BioDrugs. 2009;23(1):37–42.
130. Mahmoud Youssef MA, van Wely M, Aboulfoutouh I, El-Khyat W, van der Veen F, Al-Inany H. Is there a place for corifollitropin alfa in IVF/ICSI cycles? A systematic review and meta-analysis. Fertil Steril. 2012;97(4):876-85. (Erratum in: Fertil Steril 2012;97(6):1479).
131. Pouwer AW, Farquhar C, Kremer JA. Long-acting FSH versus daily FSH for women undergoing assisted reproduction. Cochrane Database Syst Rev. 2012;6:CD009577.
132. Shoham Z, Smith H, Yeko T, O'Brien F, Hemsey G, O'Dea L. Recombinant LH (lutropin alfa) for the treatment of hypogonadotrophic women with profound LH deficiency: a randomized, double-blind, placebo-controlled, proof-of-efficacy study. Clin Endocrinol (Oxf). 2008;69(3):471–8.
133. European Recombinant Human LH Study Group. Recombinant human luteinizing hormone (LH) to support recombinant human follicle-stimulating hormone (FSH)-induced follicular development in LH-and FSH-deficient anovulatory women: a dose-finding study. J Clin Endocrinol Metab. 1998;83(5):1507–14.
134. Loumaye E, Engrand P, Howles CM, O'Dea L. Assessment of the role of serum luteinizing hormone and estradiol response to follicle-stimulating hormone on in vitro fertilization treatment outcome. Fertil Steril. 1997;67(5):889–99.
135. Sills ES, Levy DP, Moomjy M, et al. A prospective, randomized comparison of ovulation induction using highly purified follicle- stimulating hormone alone and with recombinant human luteinizing hormone in in-vitro fertilization. Hum Reprod. 1999;14:2230–5.
136. Baruffi RL, Mauri AL, Petersen CG, et al. Recombinant LH supplementation to recombinant FSH during induced ovarian stimulation in the GnRH-antagonist protocol: a meta-analysis. Reprod Biomed Online. 2007;14(1):14–25.
137. Kolibianakis EM, Kalogeropoulou L, Griesinger G, et al. Among patients treated with FSH and GnRH analogues for in vitro fertilization, is the addition of recombinant LH associated with the probability of live birth? A systematic review and meta-analysis. Hum Reprod Update. 2007;13(5):445–52.
138. Mochtar MH, Van der V, Ziech M, van Wely M. Recombinant Luteinizing Hormone (rLH) for controlled ovarian hyperstimulation in assisted reproductive cycles. Cochrane Database Syst Rev. 2007;18(2): CD005070.
139. Oliveira JB, Mauri AL, Petersen CG, et al. Recombinant luteinizing hormone supplementation to recombinant follicle-stimulation hormone during induced ovarian stimulation in the GnRH-agonist protocol: a meta-analysis. J Assist Reprod Genet. 2007;24(2–3):67–75.
140. Marrs R, Meldrum D, Muasher S, Schoolcraft W, Werlin L, Kelly E. Randomized trial to compare the effect of recombinant human FSH (follitropin alfa) with or without recombinant human LH in women undergoing assisted reproduction treatment. Reprod Biomed Online. 2004;8(2):175–82.
141. Esposito MA, Barnhart KT, Coutifaris C, Patrizio P. Role of periovulatory luteinizing hormone concentrations during assisted reproductive technology cycles stimulated exclusively with recombinant follicle-stimulating hormone. Fertil Steril. 2001;75(3):519–24.
142. Westergaard LG, Laursen SB, Andersen CY. Increased risk of early pregnancy loss by profound suppression of luteinizing hormone during ovarian stimulation in normogonadotrophic women undergoing assisted reproduction. Hum Reprod. 2000;15(5):1003–8.
143. Humaidan P, Bungum L, Bungum M, Andersen CY. Ovarian response and pregnancy outcome related to mid-follicular LH levels in women undergoing assisted reproduction with GnRH agonist down-regulation and recombinant FSH stimulation. Hum Reprod. 2002;17(8):2016–21.
144. Laml T, Obruca A, Fischl F, Huber JC. Recombinant luteinizing hormone in ovarian hyperstimulation after stimulation failure in normogonadotrophic women. Gynecol Endocrinol. 1999;13(2):98–103.
145. Nakagawa K, Ohgi S, Nakashima A, Horikawa T, Sugiyama R, Saito H. The ratio of late-follicular to mid-follicular phase LH concentrations efficiently predicts ART outcomes in women undergoing ART treatment with GnRH-agonist long protocol and stimulation with recombinant FSH. J Assist Reprod Genet. 2008;25(8):359–64.
146. De Placido G, Mollo A, Alviggi C, et al. Rescue of IVF cycles by HMG in pituitary down-regulated normogonadotrophic young women characterized by a poor initial response to recombinant FSH. Hum Reprod. 2001;16(9):1875–79.
147. De Placido G, Alviggi C, Mollo A et al. Effects of recombinant LH (rLH) supplementation during controlled ovarian hyperstimulation (COH) in normogonadotrophic women with an initial inadequate response to recombinant FSH (rFSH) after pituitary downregulation. Clin Endocrinol (Oxf). 2004;60(5):637–43.
148. De Placido G, Alviggi C, Perino A, et al. Recombinant human LH supplementation versus recombinant human FSH (rFSH) step-up protocol during controlled ovarian stimulation in normogonadotrophic women with initial inadequate ovarian response to rFSH. A multicentre, prospective, randomized controlled trial. Hum Reprod. 2005;20(2):390–6.
149. Ferraretti AP, Gianaroli L, Magli MC, D'angelo A, Farfalli V, Montanaro N. Exogenous luteinizing hormone in controlled ovarian hyperstimulation for assisted reproduction techniques. Fertil Steril. 2004;82(6):1521–6.
150. Alviggi C, Clarizia R, Pettersson K, et al. Suboptimal response to GnRHa long protocol is associated with a common LH polymorphism. Reprod Biomed Online. 2009;18(1):9–14.
151. Hurwitz JM, Santoro N. Inhibins, activins, and follistatin in the aging female and male. Semin Reprod Med. 2004;22(3):209–17.
152. Piltonen T, Koivunen R, Ruokonen A, Tapanainen JS. Ovarian age-related responsiveness to human chorionic gonadotropin. J Clin Endocrinol Metab. 2003;88(7):3327–32.
153. Vihko KK, Kujansuu E, Mörsky P, Huhtaniemi I, Punnonen R. Gonadotropins and gonadotropin receptors during the perimenopause. Eur J Endocrinol. 1996;134(3):357–61.
154. Marrama P, Montanini V, Celani MF, et al. Decrease in luteinizing hormone biological activity/immunoreactivity ratio in elderly men. Maturitas. 1984;5(4):223–31.
155. Mitchell R, Hollis S, Rothwell C, Robertson WR. Age related changes in the pituitary-testicular axis in normal men; lower serum testo- sterone results from decreased bioactive LH drive. Clin Endocrinol. 1995;42(5):501–7.

156. Fleming R, Rehka P, Deshpande N, Jamieson ME, Yates RW, Lyall H. Suppression of LH during ovarian stimulation: effects differ in cycles stimulated with purified urinary FSH and recombinant FSH. Hum Reprod. 2000;15(7):1440–5.
157. Lévy DP, Navarro JM, Schattman GL, Davis OK, Rosenwaks Z. The role of LH in ovarian stimulation: exogenous LH: let's design the future. Hum Reprod. 2000;15(11):2258-65. (Review. Erratum in: Hum Reprod 2001;16(3) 598).
158. Fan W, Li S, Chen Q, Huang Z, Ma Q, Wang Y. Recombinant luteinizing hormone supplementation in poor responders undergoing IVF: a systematic review and meta-analysis. Gynecol Endocrinol. 2013;29(4):278–84.
159. Carone D, Caropreso C, Vitti A, Chiappetta R. Efficacy of different gonadotropin combinations to support ovulation induction in WHO type I anovulation infertility: clinical evidences of human recombinant FSH/human recombinant LH in a 2:1 ratio and highly purified human menopausal gonadotropin stimulation protocols. J Endocrinol Invest. 2012;35(11):996–1002.
160. Pacchiarotti A, Sbracia M, Frega A, Selman H, Rinaldi L, Pacchiarotti A. Urinary hMG (Meropur) versus recombinant FSH plus recombinant LH (Pergoveris) in IVF: a multicenter, prospective, randomized controlled trial. Fertil Steril. 2010;94(6):2467–9.
161. Bühler KF, Fischer R. Recombinant human LH supplementation versus supplementation with urinary hCG-based LH activity during controlled ovarian stimulation in the long GnRH-agonist protocol: a matched case-control study. Gynecol Endocrinol. 2012;28(5):345–50.
162. Fábregues F, Creus M, Casals G, Carmona F, Balasch J. Outcome from consecutive ICSI cycles in patients treated with recombinant human LH and those supplemented with urinary hCG-based LH activity during controlled ovarian stimulation in the long GnRH-agonist protocol. Gynecol Endocrinol. 2013;29(5):430–5.
163. Fanchin R, Righini C, Olivennes F, de Ziegler D, Selva J, Frydman R. Premature progesterone elevation does not alter oocyte quality in in vitro fertilization. Fertil Steril. 1996;65(6):1178–83.
164. Ziebe S, Lundin K, Janssens R, Helmgaard L, Arce JC; MERIT (Menotrophin vs Recombinant FSH in vitro Fertilisation Trial) Group. Influence of ovarian stimulation with HP-hMG or recombinant FSH on embryo quality parameters in patients undergoing IVF. Hum Reprod. 2007;22(9):2404–13.
165. Petanovski Z, Dimitrov G, Aydin B, et al. Recombinant FSH versus HP-HMG for controled ovarian stimulation in intracytoplasmic sperm injection cycles. Med Arh. 2011;65(3):153–6.
166. Ye H, Huang G, Pei L, Zeng P, Luo X. Outcome of in vitro fertilization following stimulation with highly purified hMG or recombinant FSH in downregulated women of advanced reproductive age: a prospective, randomized and controlled trial. Gynecol Endocrinol. 2012;28(7):540–4.
167. Hugues JN, Massé-Laroche E, Reboul-Marty J, Boîko O, Meynant C, Cédrin-Durnerin I. Impact of endogenous luteinizing hormone serum levels on progesterone elevation on the day of human chorionic gonadotropin administration. Fertil Steril. 2011;96(3):600–4.
168. Kolibianakis EM, Venetis CA, Bontis J, Tarlatzis BC. Significantly lower pregnancy rates in the presence of progesterone elevation in patients treated with GnRH antagonists and gonadotrophins: a systematic review and meta-analysis. Curr Pharm Biotechnol. 2012;13(3):464–70.
169. Bosch E, Labarta E, Crespo J, et al. Circulating progesterone levels and ongoing pregnancy rates in controlled ovarian stimulation cycles for in vitro fertilization: analysis of over 4000 cycles. Hum Reprod. 2010;25(8):2092–100.
170. Xu B, Li Z. Zhang H, et al. Serum progesterone level effects on the outcome of in vitro fertilization in patients with different ovarian response: an analysis of more than 10,000 cycles. Fertil Steril. 2012;97(6):1321–7.
171. Hofmann GE, Bentzien F, Bergh PA, et al. Premature luteinization in controlled ovarian hyperstimulation has no adverse effect on oocyte and embryo quality. Fertil Steril. 1993;60(4):675–9.
172. Melo MA, Meseguer M, Garrido N, Bosch E, Pellicer A, Remohí J. The significance of premature luteinization in an oocyte-donation programme. Hum Reprod. 2006;21(6):1503–7.
173. van Koppen CJ, Verbost PM van de Lagemaat R, et al. Signaling of an allosteric, nanomolar potent, low molecular weight agonist for the follicle-stimulating hormone receptor. Biochem Pharmacol. 2013;85(8):1162–70.
174. van de Lagemaat R, Timmers CM, Kelder J, van Koppen C, Mosselman S, Hanssen RG. Induction of ovulation by a potent, orally active, low molecular weight agonist (Org 43553) of the luteinizing hormone receptor. Hum Reprod. 2009;24(3):640–8.
175. Yanofsky SD, Shen ES, Holden F, et al. Allosteric activation of the follicle-stimulating hormone (FSH) receptor by selective, nonpeptide agonists. J Biol Chem. 2006;281(19):13226–33.
176. Costagliola S, Urizar E, Mendive F, Vassart G. Specificity and promiscuity of gonadotropin receptors. Reproduction. 2005;130(3):275–81.
177. Jiang X, Liu H, Chen X, et al. Structure of follicle-stimulating hormone in complex with the entire ectodomain of its receptor. Proc Natl Acad Sci U S A. 2012;109(31):12491–6.

Intrauterine Insemination in Unexplained Female Infertility

29

Paolo Emanuele Levi Setti, Irene Zerbetto, Alberto Vaiarelli, Marcello Desgro and Pasquale Patrizio

Introduction

Infertility remains prevalent and problematic among couples worldwide [1, 2]. With an average monthly fecundity rate of only 20 %, humans are not as fertile as other mammals [3]. Infertility is defined as the inability to conceive after 12 months of unprotected sexual intercourse for couples where the woman is younger than 35 years old and after 6 months for women older than 35 years. However, there is no uniform definition for unexplained infertility (UI). An estimated 4–17 % of couples seek medical treatment in order to rectify their infertility, and it is reasonable to assume that this percentage is underestimated because many cases of infertility are not reported [4]. The etiology of infertility is unexplained in about 8–28 % of cases [1, 5]. UI is diagnosed when the standard work-up reveals normal semen analysis, normal uterus with bilateral tubal patency (evaluated with ultrasound and hysterosalpingogram), and regular ovulatory cycles (midluteal phase serum progesterone). Recently, a diagnostic laparoscopy (LPS) is no longer considered essential to reach the diagnosis of UI [6]. However, a laparoscopy is still accepted as gold standard for diagnosing tubal pathology or other pelvic reproductive diseases such as adhesions and "minimal or mild" endometriosis. In other instances, a completely normal pelvic anatomical survey and history of well-timed intercourse (TI) and infertility lasting for 2 or more years could justify the recommendation to proceed directly to in vitro fertilization (IVF) bypassing cycles of ovulatory stimulation with or without intrauterine inseminations (IUIs).

For the infertile couple, a diagnosis of UI may be very frustrating and is often interpreted as meaning that if there is no explanation for the cause of infertility and then there must be no effective treatment. The prognosis is worst when the duration of infertility exceeds 3 years and the female partner is >35 years of age [7]. It has been observed that the proportion of spontaneous pregnancies is higher in couples with UI thus suggesting an overall better fertility prognosis compared with couples with infertility of known causes. The treatment of UI, given the lack of a solid diagnosis, is empirical and many different regimens have been used.

Treatment options are expectant management (EM) after educating the couple about properly monitoring ovulation (with LH-kits for example) and timing intercourse, IUI, with or without controlled ovarian stimulation (COS), and IVF with or without intracytoplasmic sperm injection (ICSI). IUI cycles, with or without COS, are generally the first step in the treatment algorithm. Many authors recommend after three or six unsuccessful cycles of ovulation induction or IUI switching to assisted reproductive technologies (ART). However, in a recent paper, Bonneau et al. [8] have underlined that after three cycles of ovulation induction with or without IUI and no pregnancy, women should be offered a diagnostic LPS before ART. Laparoscopy might play an important role in choosing the strategy for the management of infertility when the patient is younger than 35 years and with a history of infertility not longer than 2–3 years. In this group of patient, diagnostic LPS should be strongly considered in UI work-up because predictive factors (as minimal endometriosis, adnexal adhesions, and tubal inefficiency) are usually found during this procedure.

Definition of UI

The fertility work-up consists of complete medical and sexual history for both partners; two semen analysis: cycle monitoring including ultrasonographic ovulation detection, mild-luteal progesterone, including Chlamydia antibody test, hystero/sonohysterosalpingography (HSG) or laparoscopy with dye test. The diagnosis of UI is confirmed when all the findings are normal.

P. E. L. Setti (✉) · I. Zerbetto · A. Vaiarelli · M. Desgro · P. Patrizio
Department of Gynecology and Division of Gynecology and Reproductive Medicine, IRCCS Istituto Clinico Humanitas, Via Manzoni 56, 20086 Rozzano (Milano), Italy
e-mail: Paulo.levi_setti@humanitas.it

G. L. Schattman et al. (eds.), *Unexplained Infertility*, DOI 10.1007/978-1-4939-2140-9_29,

Couples with UI are defined as follows:

1. Couples who have tried to conceive for at least 1 year without success (if younger than 35 years or 6 months if older than 35 years).
2. No abnormality found during infertility investigation, with laboratory evidence of regular ovulation (normal levels of luteal progesterone), normal tubal patency and exclusion of other tubal or pelvic abnormalities by hystero/sonohystero-salpingography or laparoscopy or both.
3. Normal semen analysis according to the World Health Organization (WHO 2010): sperm concentration more than 15 million/mL, total motility (% motile) of at least 40 %, progressive motility 32 %, normal morphology of at least 4 % (strict criterion), vitality (% alive) 58 %, and no anti-sperm antibodies.

Patients with poor ovarian reserve, according to the European Society of Human Reproduction and Embryology criteria [9], are not considered as affected by UI.

The definition of UI may vary in women 40 years or older. In this group of patients reduced ovarian reserve may or may not be apparent, but oocyte quality is certainly a factor for their reduced chances of pregnancy and often they are classified as with UI [2]. This is an important point because the ability to conceive decreases with advancing maternal age either spontaneously or when treated with assisted reproductive technologies. Many women are still unaware of the age-related sharp decline in reproductive efficiency and for a variety of reasons postpone motherhood and seek treatment at the age of 40 or older [10].

Other patients with a known cause of infertility including a moderate male factor, moderate to severe endometriosis, tubal disease and a cervical factor are excluded from the diagnosis of UI.

Treatment of Unexplained Infertility

Guidelines from the Royal College of Obstetricians and Gynaecologists (RCOG, 1998) [11] have recommended that couples should have tried expectant treatment before assisted reproductive treatment. A recent study suggested that treatments like empirical clomiphene citrate (CC) and IUI do not offer superior live-birth rates (LBRs) compared with EM in UI [12]. The chance of achieving a pregnancy depends mainly on *patient's* age, duration of infertility, and history of any other pregnancy in the same relationship. The conventional approach starts with EM followed by CC alone with TI, followed by IUI in natural cycles, then CC with IUI before resorting to the use of injectable gonadotropins (FSH and LH) termed COS and IUI. When COS/IUI cycles fail, IVF and ICSI are recommended.

An observational study of 1236 couples with UI in the Netherlands noted that between 10 and 25 % conceived during 1 year while being on a waiting list to undergo IVF [13]. Overall, approximately 1 to 4 % of couples with UI will conceive spontaneously each month. Younger women with shorter durations of infertility are the ones most likely to conceive with EM. If a couple has been attempting to conceive for 2 or more years or if the woman is 35 years or older, a more aggressive approach is justified.

Intrauterine Insemination for Unexplained Infertility

IUI is a widely used, relatively simple, fertility treatment for couples with UI. The clinical pregnancy rate with IUI is 11–33 % for all causes of infertility. Semen is "processed" in the laboratory by either swim-up or filtration gradients methods and the final sample containing normal motile sperm in a small volume (about 0.4 to 0.5 mL) is inserted into the uterine cavity using a small catheter. In this way, the cervix is bypassed. IUI can be performed with or without medications. For the correct timing of the insemination, cycle's monitoring is carried out. This is usually done by ultrasound assessment of follicle growth or by monitoring the preovulatory luteinizing hormone rise in blood or urine. In COS cycles, ovulation is often induced by human chorionic gonadotropin (hCG) when at least one or two follicles are ≥ 18 mm and the endometrial thickness > 7 mm. There is no clear understanding on the optimal timing, i.e., whether the IUI should be carried out the day after hCG administration or 36 h later. Likewise, it is still debated whether one IUI per cycle is sufficient as opposed to two consecutive ones. Some data suggest that timing of insemination may be kept at 24 or 36 h after hCG injection to suit the convenience of the clinic or of the care provider [14]. A recent study examining single versus double IUI for UI has shown no clear benefit of double over single inseminations in couples with UI [15] .

The increased risk of multiple pregnancies is a logical consequence of stimulating the growth of multiple follicles. The incidence of multiple pregnancies after treatment with COS and IUI varies between 10 (CC cycles) and 40 % and the overall contribution of this treatment to multiple births is estimated to be around 30 % [16]. The question is whether this multiple pregnancy rate is acceptable or whether it can be reduced to acceptable numbers. Recently, more and more evidence is being collected that the strict monitoring of the patients [17, 18], but in particular the mild ovarian hyperstimulation [19] could reduce the incidence multiple pregnancies. Several trials using mild stimulation protocols for IUI have been published, showing promising results of acceptable pregnancy rates with very low multiple pregnancy rates [20].

The two most commonly used drugs for COS are CC, which is an oral treatment, and gonadotropins administered by subcutaneous injection. CC is a derivative of triphenylethylene steroids. CC is the most commonly used oral agent for the induction of ovulation. It is a nonsteroidal selective estrogen receptor modulator that has predominant antiestrogenic action resulting in long-lasting estrogen receptor depletion. CC was widely used during the early follicular phase of COH in the 1980s due to the ease of administration (oral route), low cost, and acceptable success rate. The incidence of multiple gestations with the use of CC is approximately 8 % and most of these are twins. Side effects include antiestrogenic effects systemically, on the endometrium and cervical mucus [21]. The most common side effect is vasomotor symptoms, which occur in approximately 10 % of women taking CC. Less common side effects include mood swings, breast tenderness, headaches, and nausea. Visual disturbances occur in less than 2 % but occasionally can be permanent. There is not an increase of congenital anomalies or birth defects in the children conceived by women taking CC. Although some retrospective studies have reported an increased risk of ovarian cancer [22], overall there does not seem to be an increase in the incidence of ovarian or breast cancer in infertile women who have taken CC [23, 24]. CC (50 mg) is taken once daily, beginning on day 3 or 5 of the cycle for 5 days. Follicle monitoring with transvaginal sonography aims at assessing follicular and endometrial development beginning from cycle day 11 or earlier depending on the women's cycle. The dose of CC can be increased to 100 mg in subsequent cycle up to a maximum of 150 mg if the ovarian response is suboptimal with standard doses.

In the event, the endometrial thickness is suboptimal or the ovarian response is insufficient or after 2–3 cycles of no pregnancy, it is recommend to proceed with the use of gonadotropins (FSH alone or FSH and LH). With gonadotropins patients must understand the expense of the medications and the need for a closer monitoring (more office visits), to check follicle number and growth serum and sometimes estradiol levels, so to minimize the risks of ovarian hyperstimulation and the risk of high-order multiple pregnancies (HOMP). The key is to start with lower dosages of medication, 50 to 100 IU of FSH daily from cycle day 2 or 3. Clinical judgment is necessary in dosing the medication and adjusting the dose throughout the cycle according to follicular number and growth. There are significant risks of twins (11 %) and high-order multiples (3.0–4.1 %) when using gonadotropins [25]. A meta-analysis of seven studies showed a significantly higher pregnancy rate for treatment with gonadotropins (28 %) compared to treatment with CC (19 %) when combined with IUI [26]. Usually, the cycles are cancelled if there are >4 developing follicles observed on sonography. The recent Cochrane review (2012) emphasized that IUI increases the chance of pregnancy compared to correct timing of intercourse and furthermore LBRs are higher in IUI cycles with COS. However, increased multiple pregnancy rates are concerning and further studies are needed to assess the magnitude of this problems.

The Cochrane database [1] for couples with UI showed that IUI improves the LBR compared with TI, both with and without COS. The individual trials were contradictory and often lacked sufficient power to draw firm conclusion. There were five trials included per comparison:

1. IUI versus TI or EM both in a natural cycle: there was no evidence of a significant difference in pregnancy rates (OR 1.53, 95 % CI 0.88 to 2.64) and LBRs (23 % with IUI versus 16 % in the EM group). There were no significant differences in side effects (multiple pregnancies, miscarriage, and ectopic pregnancies) between the IUI and TI groups.
2. IUI versus TI both in stimulated cycles: there was evidence of an increased chance of pregnancy after IUI (six RCTs, 517 women: OR 1.68, 95 % CI 1.13 to 2.50).
3. IUI in combination with COS compared to IUI in a natural cycle: a significant increase in LBR was found for women treated with IUI and COS compared to women treated with IUI only (four RCTs, 396 woman: OR 2.07, 95 % CI 1.22 to 3.50).
4. IUI in combination with COS was compared with TI in a natural cycle: there was no evidence of a difference in pregnancy rate (two RCTs, total 304 women: data not pooled).
5. IUI in a natural cycle versus TI in a stimulated cycle: it was observed that the LBRs were 23 and 13 % for women treated with IUI compared to TI in a stimulated cycle, respectively. There was a small but significant difference in favor of IUI in a natural cycle (OR 1.95, 95 % CI 1.10 to 3.44) for couples with UI.

However, the trials provided insufficient data to investigate the impact of IUI with or without COS on several important outcomes including live births, multiple pregnancies, miscarriage, and risk of ovarian hyperstimulation. The type of drug and dose, the treatment duration, and cancellation criteria may have influenced the outcomes. A reason for this could be that this study used the most aggressive stimulation methods, accepted a maximum of six dominant follicles and treated couples for up to five cycles.

We can, therefore, conclude that in couples with unexplained subfertility the combination of CO and IUI seems to be the most effective strategy.

For the purpose of this book chapter, we have considered useful to show some data from the Italian National ART database [27] in order to underline the role of IUI in Italy for the treatment of infertility and in particular in unexplained cases.

Table 29.1 describes IUI cycles carried out in 2010 in Italy from 302 ART clinics where this technique has offered.

Table 29.1 Assisted reproductive technologies (ART) in Italy in 2010—IUI cycles performed in 2010 as reported by the Italian ART Register in 2012

	Total numbers	Incidence (%)
Cycles IUI	32,069	
Pregnancies	3306	16.8
Live birth[a]	2465	7.6
Singleton	1989	89.6
Twin	2010	9.5
Triplet	21	0.9

[a] Five-hundred thirteen (15.5 %) pregnancies were lost to follow up and four-hundred ninety nine (20.5 %) of monitored pregnancies had a negative outcome

A total of 19,707 patients underwent 32,069 IUI cycles and 3,306 pregnancies were obtained. Five-hundred thirteen of these pregnancies (15.5 %) were lost for follow-up and from the remaining 2793 pregnancies, a total of 2465 children were born alive. Pregnancy rates per patients treated with IUI were 16.8 and 10.3 % per cycle. The percentage of twin births was 9.5 % while the triplet rate was 0.9 %. The overall rate of miscarriages, therapeutic abortions, intrauterine deaths, and ectopic pregnancy was 20.5 %. Considering patients age, the pregnancy rate for women under 34 was 14.5, 10.8 % in women between 35 and 39 years old, 8.2 % for women between 40 and 42 years old, and 3 % in patient 43 years or older (Table 29.2). These data confirmed how the age of the patient is highly relevant for a positive outcome when IUI procedure is implemented. Table 29.3 shows that the negative outcome of pregnancies achieved through IUI in relation to the age of the patients. The percentage ranges from 15.6 % in women with age "≤to 34 to 47.8 % in women with age >43 years.

Table 29.2 Assisted reproductive technologies (ART) in Italy in 2010—Outcome of IUI in relation to the age during cycles performed in 2010 as reported by the Italian ART Register in 2012

Female age (years)	Percentage of successful procedure	Live birth
≤34	14.5	1.604
35–39	10.8	1.329
40–42	8.2	321
≥43	3.0	52
Total		3.306

Table 29.3 Assisted reproductive technologies (ART) in Italy 2010—IUI monitored pregnancies negative outcomes in relation to the classes of female age in cycles performed in 2010 as reported by the Italian ART database in 2012

Female age (years)	Pregnancies	Negative outcome	Percentage
≤34	1.362	212	15.6
35–39	1.098	234	21.3
40–42	287	105	36.6
≥43	46	22	47.8
Total	2.793	573[a]	20.5

[a] Four-hundred ninety nine (17.9 %) spontaneous abortions, twenty three (0.8 %) therapeutic abortions, forty five (1.6 %) ectopic pregnancies, and six (0.2 %) intrauterine deaths

How Many IUI Cycles Should Be Performed in Patients with UI?

Data on the optimum number of IUI treatment cycles are inconsistent. Most authors recommend not to continue IUI after three to four cycles [28] whereas some others advise to continue with IUI even after six or more cycles [29, 30]. In this group of patients is very difficult to quantify the appropriate number of IUI before proceeding to ART. In general, after four to six cycles of IUI in young patients it is appropriate to resort to ART [31]. Prognostic factors related to a higher cumulative pregnancy rate are duration of infertility less than 2 years, a previous pregnancy with the same partner and female age <30 years. In these instances, couples could be encouraged to use less invasive treatments for up to 2–3 years because they have a similar chance of achieving pregnancy without treatment [32, 33]. ART (IVF or ICSI) is indicated as first treatment option when the duration of UI is at least 3 years. Some data suggest that each additional month of infertility reduces the chance of pregnancy by 2 %, or about 25 % year. Similarly, for each year of the female partner's age >30, the pregnancy rate is reduced by 9 % [2, 34].

Siam et al. [35] investigated the relationship between prevalence of antisperm antibodies and genital infection with *Chlamydia trachomatis* in women with UI. Infection with chlamydia is one of the most common sexually transmitted diseases and sperm-associated antibody could impair fertility through various mechanisms. The study, however, failed to find a positive correlation between current or past chlamydia infection and the level of antisperm antibodies in women suffering of UI. Antisperm antibodies were significantly higher in infertile women, but without a significant difference between infertile women with past or current *C. trachomatis* infection.

Another group of UI patients is those with "secondary UI" with the same or another partner. There are no clear data in the literature for these groups of patients. Good medical practice would suggest to do an extensive work-up to exclude conditions that could have altered the mechanisms of reproduction (e.g., a cesarean section with the prior delivery and the presence of pelvic adhesions) and then set up a therapeutic approach. Some authors have investigated the relationship between hyaluronan (HA)-binding assay and pregnancy rates in IUI cycles. The HA-binding evaluates the maturity and fertility potential of sperm and may be useful to discriminate between patients who would benefit from treatment with IUI if the binding is 80 % or higher [36]. Other authors have concluded that HA-binding test does not predict pregnancy rates in IUI cycle [37]. To our knowledge, there is no data about the effect of HA assay on IUI cycles in couples with UI.

IUI Versus in Vitro Fertilization for Unexplained Infertility

IVF is a widely accepted treatment for UI, with estimated LBRs per cycle varying from 33.1 % in women younger than 35 years old and 12.5 % in women between 40 and 42 years [38]. Two randomized trials compared gonadotropin stimulated IUI with IVF in cases of UI. Crosignani et al. [39] showed birth rate of 24.5 and 22.9 %, respectively, when two cycles of each treatment were being offered. Goverde et al. [40] evaluated a treatment plan involving six cycles of unstimulated and stimulated IUI or IVF. This trial showed low pregnancy rate/cycles with IVF and multiple pregnancy rates of 21 %. Withdrawal rate was higher in IVF cycles (42 %) than FSH/IUI cycles (16 %). The Cochrane [41] analyzed six RTCs: LBR per patient was significantly higher with IVF (45.8 %) than EM (3.7 %) (OR 22.00). There was no evidence of a significant different in LBR between IVF and IUI alone (OR 1.96, 95 % CI 0.88 to 4.36), 40.7 % with IVF versus 25.9 % with IUI. The clinical effectiveness between FSH/IUI and IVF treatment of UI was small. Cost effectiveness of primary offer of IVF versus primary offer of IUI followed by IVF in couples with unexplained or mild male factor subfertility has been evaluated [42, 43]. The Cochrane concluded the review, assessing that IVF may result in more births than other techniques for couples with UI, but the research is not conclusive.

Conclusion

Treatment of UI is very much dependent on availability of resources and patients' age and duration of infertility. The LBR for women > 40 years using COS with gonadotrophin/IUI is 2.6 % [44]. The standard protocol involves proceeding from low-tech to high-tech treatment options. A Cochrane review shows evidence that the addition of COS to IUI treatment improves LBRs in couples with UI. A smaller but statistical significant rise in pregnancy rate was found for IUI when compared with TI in stimulated cycles. The multiple pregnancy rates should be kept to a minimum by using mild stimulation protocols and strict cancellation criteria. Couples should be fully informed about the risks of IUI and COS and alternative treatment options should be offered. There is a definite need for multicenter randomized controlled trials to identify the best treatment option in UI. However, IVF may be more effective than the combination of IUI with ovarian stimulation, but results must be carefully interpreted. The perception of couples and their desire to achieve tangible results is also important. Adverse events and costs associated with the compared interventions have not been adequately assessed. Clinicians and couples should balance the invasive nature of IVF and related costs against chances of success with other treatment modalities. To best select an appropriate therapy, the patient's characteristics (age, duration of infertility, parity, primary or secondary infertility, and previous therapy) should be fully explored and known.

References

1. Veltman-Verhulst SM, Cohlen BJ, Hughes E, Heineman MJ. Intra-uterine insemination for unexplained subfertility. Cochrane Database Syst Rev. 2012;9:CD001838.
2. Ray A, Shah A, Gudi A, Homburg R. Unexplained infertility: an update and review of practice. Reprod Biomed Online. 2012;24(6):591–602.
3. Evers JL. Female subfertility. Lancet. 2002;360(9327):151–9.
4. Gnoth C, Godehardt E, Frank-Herrmann P, Friol K, Tigges J, Freundl G. Definition and prevalence of subfertility and infertility. Hum Reprod. 2005;20(5):1144–7.
5. NICE. Fertility: assessment and treatment for people with fertility problems. London: Royal College of Obstetric and Gynecology (RCOG); 2005. pp. 75–80.
6. Badawy A, Khiary M, Ragab A, Hassan M, Sherif L. Laparoscopy–or not–for management of unexplained infertility. J Obstet Gynaecol. 2010;30(7):712–5.
7. Collins JA, Burrows EA, Wilan AR. The prognosis for live birth among untreated infertile couples. Fertil Steril. 1995;64(1):22–8.
8. Bonneau C, Chanelles O, Sifer C, Poncelet C. Use of laparoscopy in unexplained infertility. Eur J Obstet Gynecol Reprod Biol. 2012;163(1):57–61.
9. Ferraretti AP, Goossens V, de Mouzon J, et al. Assisted reproductive technology in Europe, 2008: results generated from European registers by ESHRE. Hum Reprod. 2012;27(9):2571–84.
10. Wyndham N, Marin Figueira PG, Patrizio P. A persistent misperception: assisted reproductive technology can reverse the "aged biological clock". Fertil Steril. 2012;97(5):1044–7.
11. Royal College of Obstetricians and Gynaecologists. The management of infertility in secondary care. London: RCOG Press; 1998.
12. Bhattacharya S, Harrild K, Mollison J, et al. Clomifene citrate or unstimulated intrauterine insemination compared with expectant management for unexplained infertility: pragmatic randomised controlled trial. BMJ. 2008;337:a716.
13. Eijkemans MJ, Lintsen AM, Hunault CC, et al. Pregnancy chances on an IVF/ICSI waiting list: a national prospective cohort study. Hum Reprod. 2008;23(7):1627–32.
14. Rahman SM, Karmakar D, Malhotra N, Kumar S. Timing of intrauterine insemination: an attempt to unravel the enigma. Arch Gynecol Obstet. 2011;284(4):1023–7.
15. Bagis T, Haydardedeoglu B, Kilicdag EB, Cok T, Simsek E, Parlakgumus AH. Single versus double intrauterine insemination in multi-follicular ovarian hyperstimulation cycles: a randomized trial. Hum Reprod. 2010;25(7):1684–90.
16. Fauser BC, Devroey P, Macklon NS. Multiple birth resulting from ovarian stimulation for subfertility treatment. Lancet. 2005;365(9473):1807–16.
17. Dickey RP, Taylor SN, Lu PY, Sartor BM, Rye PH, Pyrzak R. Risk factors for high-order multiple pregnancy and multiple birth after controlled ovarian hyperstimulation: results of 4,062 intrauterine insemination cycles. Fertil Steril. 2005;83(3):671–83.

18. Tur R, Barri PN, Coroleu B, Buxaderas R, Parera N, Balasch J. Use of a prediction model for high-order multiple implantation after ovarian stimulation with gonadotropins. Fertil Steril. 2005;83(1):116–21.
19. te Velde ER Cohlen BJ. The management of infertility. N Engl J Med. 1999;340(3):224–6.
20. Balasch J. Gonadotrophin ovarian stimulation and intrauterine insemination for unexplained infertility. Reprod Biomed Online. 2004;9(6):664–72.
21. Check JH, Dietterich C, Lurie D. The effect of consecutive cycles of clomiphene citrate therapy on endometrial thickness and echo pattern. Obstet Gynecol. 1995;86(3):341–5.
22. Cetin I, Cozzi V, Antonazzo P. Infertility as a cancer risk factor—a review. Placenta. 2008;29(Suppl B):169–77.
23. Zreik TG, Ayoub CM, Hannoun A, Karam CJ, Munkarah AR. Fertility drugs and risk of ovarian cancer: dispelling the myth. Curr Opin Obstet Gynecol. 2008;20(3):313–9.
24. Sanner K, Conner P, Bergfeldt K, et al. Ovarian epithelial neoplasia after hormonal infertility treatment: long-term follow-up of a historical cohort in Sweden. Fertil Steril. 2009;91(4):1152–8.
25. Kaplan PF, Patel M, Austin DJ, Freund R. Assessing the risk of multiple gestation in gonadotropin intrauterine insemination cycles. Am J Obstet Gynecol. 2002;186(6):1244–7. (discussion 1247–1249).
26. Cantineau AE, Cohlen BJ, Heineman MJ. Ovarian stimulation protocols (anti-oestrogens, gonadotrophins with and without GnRH agonists/antagonists) for intrauterine insemination (IUI) in women with subfertility. Cochrane Database Syst Rev. 2007; 18(2):CD005356..
27. Italian National ART Database. IUI Cycles performed in 2010 from 302 ART Clinics. 2012. http://www.iss.it/rpma. Accessed 12 Feb. 2012.
28. Sahakyan M, Harlow BL, Hornstein MD. Influence of age, diagnosis, and cycle number on pregnancy rates with gonadotropin-induced controlled ovarian hyperstimulation and intrauterine insemination. Fertil Steril. 1999;72(3):500–4.
29. Campana A, Sakkas D, Stalberg A, et al. Intrauterine insemination: evaluation of the results according to the woman's age, sperm quality, total sperm count per insemination and life table analysis. Hum Reprod. 1996;11(4):732–6.
30. Berg U, Brucker C, Berg FD. Effect of motile sperm count after swim-up on outcome of intrauterine insemination. Fertil Steril. 1997;67(4):747–50.
31. van den Boogaard NM, Hompes PG, Barnhart K, et al. The prognostic profile of subfertile couples and treatment outcome after expectant management, intrauterine insemination and in vitro fertilisation: a study protocol for the meta-analysis of individual patient data. BJOG. 2012;119(8):953–7.
32. Stolwijk AM, Zielhuis GA, Hamilton CJ, et al. Prognostic models for the probability of achieving an ongoing pregnancy after in-vitro fertilization and the importance of testing their predictive value. Hum Reprod. 1996;11(10):2298–303.
33. Stolwijk AM, Wetzels AM, Braat DD. Cumulative probability of achieving an ongoing pregnancy after in-vitro fertilization and intracytoplasmic sperm injection according to a woman's age, subfertility diagnosis and primary or secondary subfertility. Hum Reprod. 2000;15(1):203–9.
34. Gnoth C, Godehardt D, Godehardt E, Frank-Herrmann P, Freundl G. Time to pregnancy: results of the German prospective study and impact on the management of infertility. Hum Reprod. 2003;18(9):1959–66.
35. Siam EM, Hefzy EM. The relationship between antisperm antibodies prevalence and genital chlamydia trachomatis infection in women with unexplained infertility. Afr J Reprod Health. 2011;15(3):93–101.
36. Huszar G, Ozenci CC, Cayli S, Zavaczki Z, Hansch E, Vigue L. Hyaluronic acid binding by human sperm indicates cellular maturity, viability, and unreacted acrosomal status. Fertil Steril. 2003;79(Suppl 3):1616–24.
37. Boynukalin FK, Esinler I, Guven S, Gunalp S. Hyaluronan binding assay does not predict pregnancy rates in IUI cycles in couples with unexplained infertility. Arch Gynecol Obstet. 2012;286(6):1577–80.
38. Human Fertilization Embryology Authority. Latest UK IVF figures. 2009–2010. http://www.hfea.gov.uk. Accessed 12 Feb. 2013.
39. Crosignani PG, Walters DE, Soliani A. The ESHRE multicentre trial on the treatment of unexplained infertility: a preliminary report. European Society of Human Reproduction and Embryology. Hum Reprod. 1991;6(7):953–8.
40. Goverde AJ, McDonnell J, Vermeiden JP, Schats R, Rutten FF, Schoemaker J. Intrauterine insemination or in-vitro fertilisation in idiopathic subfertility and male subfertility: a randomised trial and cost-effectiveness analysis. Lancet. 2000;355(9197):13–8.
41. Pandian Z, Gibreel A, Bhattacharya S. In vitro fertilisation for unexplained subfertility. Cochrane Database Syst Rev. 2012;4:CD003357.
42. Pashayan N, Lyratzopoulos G, Mathur R. Cost-effectiveness of primary offer of IVF vs. primary offer of IUI followed by IVF (for IUI failures) in couples with unexplained or mild male factor subfertility. BMC Health Serv Res. 2006;6:80.
43. Reindollar RH, Regan MM, Neumann PJ, et al. A randomized clinical trial to evaluate optimal treatment for unexplained infertility: the fast track and standard treatment (FASTT) trial. Fertil Steril. 2010;94(3):888–99.
44. Wiser A, Shalom-Paz E, Reinblatt SL, et al. Ovarian stimulation and intrauterine insemination in women aged 40 years or more. Reprod Biomed Online. 2012;24(2):170–3.

Role of In Vitro Fertilization in Unexplained Female Infertility

30

Hassan Sallam, Fathy Ezzeldin and Nooman Sallam

Abbreviations

CPR	Clinical pregnancy rate
FR	Fertilization rate
LBR	Live birth rate
OR	Odds ratio
Pre-Rx women	Pretreated women
RR	Relative risk
Rx-naïve women	Treatment-naïve women
TFF	Total fertilization failure

Introduction

As the name implies, "unexplained female infertility" should be diagnosed when the female partner of an infertile couple has been investigated, and no cause for her infertility was found assuming that the male partner is normal or has recently sired children. However, there is no established definition for unexplained infertility [1–5], and the diagnosis depends on the range of investigations to which the patient was subjected [6].

Notwithstanding this limitation, women diagnosed with unexplained infertility have been offered a number of alternative treatments with various claims of success [5, 7]. These include ovulation induction with clomiphene citrate (CC) [8], gonadotrophins (HMG) [9], or aromatase inhibitors [10], flushing the uterine cavity with various physiological solutions or radio-opaque medium [11], empirical use of bromocryptin [12] or danazol [13], intrauterine insemination (IUI) with or without controlled ovarian hyperstimulation (COH) [14–18], intraperitoneal insemination (IPI) [19], fallopian tube sperm perfusion [20], gamete intrafallopian transfer (GIFT), as well as in vitro fertilization (IVF) with or without intracytoplasmic sperm injection (ICSI) [16, 21–23]. This chapter will evaluate the role of IVF in unexplained female infertility in the light of evidence.

IVF for Unexplained Infertility

The birth of Louise Brown in July of 1978 opened a new era in the treatment of infertility due to various etiologies. Although the technique was first introduced for the treatment of tubal infertility, it has since been increasingly used in the treatment of infertile couples with mild oligospermia as well as unexplained infertility with various claims of success. In 1991, the European Society of Human Reproduction and Embryology (ESHRE) conducted a multicenter randomized controlled trial (RCT), involving 19 centers, comparing 5 modalities of treatment of unexplained infertility. They found that the mean clinical pregnancy rates for IUI, IPI, GIFT, and IVF were 27.4, 27, 28, and 25.7 %, respectively; compared to 15.2 % for patient treated with COH ($P = 0.058$) [19]. Subsequently, a combined report on national USA data of 2003 was published by the Centers for Disease Control and Prevention (CDC), the American Society for Reproductive Medicine (ASRM), and the Society for Assisted Reproductive Technology (SART). The live birth rate among women with unexplained infertility treated with IVF was 30.4 % [24].

IVF Versus Expectant Management in Unexplained Infertility

As pregnancy is a probabilistic concept and can occur spontaneously against many odds, proper evaluation of any therapeutic modality for the treatment of infertility necessitates its comparison with expectant management, ideally in a RCT. In 1998, Guzick et al. conducted a review of published reports on various modalities used in the treatment of

H. Sallam (✉)
Department of Obstetrics and Gynaecology, Alexandria University, 22 Victor Emanuel Square, 21615 Alexandria, Egypt
e-mail: hnsallam@link.net

F. Ezzeldin · N. Sallam
Assisted Reproduction Unit, Alexandria Fertility Center, 22 Victor Emanuel Square, 21615 Alexandria, Egypt

G. L. Schattman et al. (eds.), *Unexplained Infertility,* DOI 10.1007/978-1-4939-2140-9_30,

unexplained infertility. They found a combined pregnancy rate per initiated cycle of 3.8 % for patients treated with IUI, 5.6 % for those treated with CC, 8.3 % for those treated with both CC and IUI, 7.7 % for those treated with HMG, 17.1 % for those treated with both HMG and IUI, 20.7 % for those treated with IVF, and 27.0 % for those treated with GIFT. These data compared to a combined pregnancy rate of 1.3–4.1 % in patients who received no treatment [7].

Subsequent studies reported higher pregnancy and live birth rates in couples with unexplained infertility treated with IVF. In 2004, Hughes et al. conducted a multicenter RCT comparing IVF to expectant management (90 days) in patients with unexplained infertility, and reported a live birth rate of 29 % in patients treated with IVF versus 1 % for expected management. The number needed to treat (NNT) was 4 (95 % CI, 3–6) [25]. These results have recently been challenged by a cohort study conducted in the Netherlands by Brandes et al. The authors randomly assigned 446 couples with unexplained infertility to one of three treatment strategies: (a) expectant management (up to 2 years) followed by IUI (3–6 cycles) followed by IVF; (b) IUI followed by IVF; and (c) immediate IVF. The results showed that 81.5 % of the couples achieved an ongoing pregnancy. Most of the pregnancies (73.9 %) were conceived spontaneously; although, the ongoing pregnancy rate was 55.9 % in couples randomized to expectant management, 42.3 % in those treated with IUI, and 62.5 % in those treated with IVF [26]. The authors recommended that as most pregnancies were conceived spontaneously, if the pregnancy prognosis is good, expectant management should be the initial approach. They also suggested that prognosis criteria for treatment with IUI or IVF need to be investigated in RCTs.

To provide more clarity, Pandian et al. have published three Cochrane reviews on the subject [22, 27, 28]. In their most recent review, they concluded that in couples with unexplained infertility, IVF was associated with a significantly higher clinical pregnancy rate per woman randomized compared to expectant management (OR = 3.24; 95 % CI = 1.07–9.80). The live birth rate per woman randomized was also significantly higher (OR = 22.00; 95 % CI = 2.56–189.37) [22] (Table 30.1).

IVF Versus IUI for Unexplained Infertility

Although IVF has proven its benefit in the management of unexplained infertility, the technique is associated with high costs, multiple pregnancy, ovarian hyperstimulation (OHSS), and increased perinatal morbidity and mortality [29]. It has therefore been suggested that couples with unexplained infertility may similarly benefit from IUI with or without COH while avoiding these side effects. Numerous studies have been conducted comparing both techniques with various claims of success including some RCTs [30–33].

The updated Cochrane review published in 2012 by Pandian et al. analyzed these RCTs and concluded that there was no significant difference in the live birth rate between IVF and IUI (without COH) in the management of these patients (OR = 1.96; 95 % CI = 0.88–4.36) [22]. Similarly, there was no significant difference in the clinical pregnancy rate between patients treated with IVF and those treated with IUI + COH if these patients were treatment-naive women (OR = 1.10; 95 % CI = 0.60–2.03). However, in pretreated women, IVF was associated with a higher clinical pregnancy rate compared to IUI + COH (OR = 12.78; 95 % CI = 7.54–21.65) [22]. There was also no significant difference in the live birth rate between patients treated with IVF and those treated with IUI + COH if these patients were treatment-naive women (OR = 1.09; 95 % CI = 0.74–1.59), while in pretreated women, IVF was associated with a higher live birth rate compared to IUI + COH (OR = 2.66; 95 % CI = 1.94–3.63) [22]. However, all these data were based on small studies, and the authors suggested that further RCTs are needed before reaching firm conclusions [22] (Table 30.1).

IVF Versus ICSI in Unexplained Infertility

As total fertilization failure (TFF) may be encountered in patients with unexplained infertility treated with IVF due to unexpected problems in either the sperm or the ovum or both, it has been suggested that ICSI may be a more successful line of

Table 30.1 Odds ratios and relative risk of outcome measures in meta-analyses comparing techniques used in the management of unexplained infertility

Outcome measure	OR or RR (95 % CI)
IVF versus expectant management (CPR)	OR = 3.24 (95 % CI = 1.07–9.80)*
IVF versus expectant management (LBR)	OR = 22.00 (95 % CI = 2.56–189.37)*
IVF versus IUI (LBR)	OR = 1.96 (95 % CI = 0.88–4.36)
IVF versus IUI + COH (CPR) in Rx-naïve women	OR = 1.10 (95 % CI = 0.60–2.03)
IVF versus IUI + COH (CPR) in pre-Rx women	OR = 12.78 (95 % CI = 7.54–21.65)*
IVF versus IUI + COH (LBR) in Rx-naïve women	OR = 1.09 (95 % CI = 0.74–1.59)
IVF versus IUI + COH (LBR) in pre-Rx women	OR = 2.66 (95 % CI = 1.94–3.63)*
ICSI versus IVF (FR per injected oocyte)	RR = 1.49 (95 % CI = 1.35–1.65)*
ICSI versus IVF (FR per retrieved oocyte)	RR = 1.27 (95 % CI = 1.02–1.58)*
IVF versus ICSI (incidence of TFF)	RR = 8.22 (95 % CI = 4.44–15.23)*

* Statistically significant

treatment [21, 34–39]. It has also been suggested that in those couples, splitting the oocytes between IVF and ICSI may help in identifying the cause of infertility besides achieving pregnancy. By subjecting the sibling oocytes to IVF and ICSI, the presence or otherwise of TFF as well as its origin may be determined [40–44].

Many studies compared ICSI to IVF in treatment of unexplained infertility with controversial results. Some studies found that ICSI was associated with higher fertilization rates compared to IVF [35, 40, 41, 45–47], while others found no significant difference [48]. In an attempt to clarify matters, Johnson et al. conducted a meta-analysis of RCTs and found that ICSI increases the fertilization rate and decreases the risk of TFF in couples with well-defined unexplained infertility [23]. The pooled relative risk (RR) per injected oocyte was higher with ICSI than with conventional insemination (RR = 1.49; 95 % CI = 1.35–1.65). The pooled RR of fertilization per retrieved oocyte was also higher with ICSI than with conventional insemination (RR = 1.27; 95 % CI = 1.02–1.58). The authors also found that the pooled RR of TFF was significantly higher with conventional insemination than with ICSI (RR = 8.22; 95% CI = 4.44–15.23; Table 30.1). The number of subjects needed to be treated with ICSI to prevent one case of TFF was five [23]. Whether ICSI is superior to IVF in terms of clinical pregnancies necessitates RCTs comparing the techniques in two groups of unexplained infertility couples. For ethical reasons, such a study may never be done as no clinician would like to risk TFF in his patients just to conduct such a study.

Cost Effectiveness

The cost effectiveness of any medical procedure is important information both from the patient's and the service provider's point of view, and the procedures used in the management of couples with unexplained infertility are no exception. In the study of Guzick et al., the estimated cost per pregnancy in these couples was US$ 10,000 for CC and IUI, US$ 17,000 for HMG and IUI, and US$ 50,000 for IVF [7]. Karande et al. reported similar figures with each pregnancy achieved through immediate IVF costing US$ 57,161 compared to US$ 20,019 for patients undergoing their standard management protocol consisting of three CC cycles, followed by three HMG cycles followed by four IVF cycles [49]. The marginal cost was US$ 37,142 per pregnancy higher in the immediate IVF group. Similarly, in a Dutch study, Goverde et al. found that IUI was a more cost-effective treatment than IVF, with each pregnancy ending in a live birth costing US$ 4,511-5,710 for IUI compared to US$ 14,679 for IVF [30]. The marginal cost per live birth was US$ 10,168 greater in IVF than in IUI alone.

A recent study analyzed the cost-effectiveness of performing IVF and ICSI on sibling oocytes (split IVF-ICSI cycle) versus performing IVF only in couples with unexplained infertility [50]. The authors found that if a single cycle was needed to achieve the live birth, an all-IVF-cycle is preferred as the incremental cost-effectiveness ratio (ICER) of split IVF-ICSI or all ICSI (US$ 58,766) does not justify the increased live birth rate (3 %). If two cycles are needed, split IVF/ICSI is preferred as the increased cumulative live birth rate (3.3 %) is gained at an ICER of US$ 29,666 [50].

The cost of achieving one pregnancy by IVF in couples with unexplained infertility compares favorably with the cost of achieving pregnancy by IVF for other indications. In 2001, Collins estimated that the average cost per delivery arising from IVF cycles performed for all indications was US$ 56,419 in the USA and US$ 20,522 in eight other countries [51]. Finally, the high cost of achieving pregnancy through IVF should be considered in the light of the time taken to achieve this pregnancy, which is an important psychological landmark. In the study by Karande et al., the mean time taken to achieve a pregnancy (± SD) was 6.8 ± 3.8 months, 5.7 ± 5.0 months, and 5.8 ± 4.7 months, in patients treated with IVF, with the standard treatment protocol of the authors and for patients who refused to enter in the study, respectively [49].

Conclusion

IVF is an effective treatment for unexplained infertility. The clinical pregnancy and live birth rates are significantly higher than expectant management. It is also more effective than IUI in patients who received previous treatments. In unexplained infertility, ICSI is associated with higher fertilization rates compared to IVF and is more effective in eliminating TFF. IVF is less cost-effective than IUI but this should be seen in the context of time to pregnancy.

References

1. Aboulghar MA, Mansour RT, Serour GI, et al. Diagnosis and management of unexplained infertility: an update. Arch Gynecol Obstet. 2003;267:177–88.
2. Qoaas A, Dokras A. Diagnosis and treatment of unexplained infertility. Rev Obstet Gynecol. 2008;1:69–76.
3. Gnoth C, Godehardt E, Frank-Herrmann P, et al. Definition and prevalence of subfertility and infertility. Hum Reprod. 2005;20:1144–7.
4. Ray A, Shah A, Gudi A, et al. Unexplained infertility: an update and review of practice. Reprod Biomed Online. 2012;24:591–602.
5. Sallam HN. Unexplained infertility. In: Rizk BR, Sallam HN, editors. Clinical infertility and in-vitro fertilization. St. Louis: Jaypee Brothers Medical Publishers;2012:117–20.

6. Bradley RJ, Rosen MP. Subfertility and gastrointestinal disease: 'unexplained' is often undiagnosed. Obstet Gynecol Surv. 2004;59:108–17.
7. Guzick DS, Sullivan MW, Adamson GD, et al. Efficacy of treatment for unexplained infertility. Fertil Steril. 1998;70:207–13.
8. Hughes E, Brown J, Collins JJ, et al. Clomiphene citrate for unexplained subfertility in women. Cochrane Database Syst Rev. 2010;1:CD000057.
9. Athaullah N, Proctor M, Johnson NP. Oral versus injectable ovulation induction agents for unexplained subfertility. Cochrane Database Syst Rev. 2002;3:CD003052.
10. Polyzos NP, Tzioras S, Mauri D, et al. Treatment of unexplained infertility with aromatase inhibitors or clomiphene citrate: a systematic review and meta-analysis. Obstet Gynecol Surv. 2008;63:472–9.
11. Johnson NP. A review of the use of lipiodol flushing for unexplained infertility. Treat Endocrinol. 2005;4:233–43.
12. Hughes E, Collins J, Vandekerckhove P. Bromocriptine for unexplained subfertility in women. Cochrane Database Syst Rev. 2007;4:CD000044.
13. Hughes E, Brown J, Tiffin G, et al. Danazol for unexplained subfertility. Cochrane Database Syst Rev. 2007;1:CD000069.
14. Hughes EG. Stimulated intra-uterine insemination is not a natural choice for the treatment of unexplained subfertility. 'Effective treatment' or 'not a natural choice'? Hum Reprod. 2003;18:912–4.
15. Verhulst SM, Cohlen BJ, Hughes E, et al. Intra-uterine insemination for unexplained subfertility. Cochrane Database Syst Rev. 2006;4:CD001838
16. Tsafrir A, Simon A, Margalioth EJ, et al. What should be the first-line treatment for unexplained infertility in women over 40 years of age—ovulation induction and IUI, or IVF? Reprod Biomed Online. 2009;19(Suppl 4):4334
17. Veltman-Verhulst SM, Cohlen BJ, Hughes E, et al. Intra-uterine insemination for unexplained subfertility. Cochrane Database Syst Rev. 2012;9:CD001838.
18. Wolff EF, Vahidi N, Alford C, et al. Influences on endometrial development during intrauterine insemination: clinical experience of 2929 patients with unexplained infertility. Fertil Steril. 2013;100:194–9.
19. Crosignani PG, Walters DE, Soliani A. The ESHRE multicentre trial on the treatment of unexplained infertility: a preliminary report. European Society of Human Reproduction and Embryology. Hum Reprod. 1991;6:953–8.
20. Cantineau AE, Cohlen BJ, Heineman MJ. Intra-uterine insemination versus fallopian tube sperm perfusion for non-tubal infertility. Cochrane Database Syst Rev. 2009;2:CD001502.
21. Check JH, Yuan W, Garberi-Levito MC, et al. Effect of method of oocyte fertilization on fertilization, pregnancy and implantation rates in women with unexplained infertility. Clin Exp Obstet Gynecol. 2011;38:203–5.
22. Pandian Z, Gibreel A, Bhattacharya S. In vitro fertilisation for unexplained subfertility. Cochrane Database Syst Rev. 2012;4:CD003357.
23. Johnson LN, Sasson IE, Sammel MD, et al. Does intracytoplasmic sperm injection improve the fertilization rate and decrease the total fertilization failure rate in couples with well-defined unexplained infertility? A systematic review and meta-analysis. Fertil Steril. 2013;100:704–11.
24. ASRM Practice Committee of the American Society for Reproductive Medicine. Effectiveness and treatment for unexplained infertility. Fertil Steril. 2004;82(Suppl 1):160–3.
25. Hughes EG, Beecroft ML, Wilkie V, et al. A multicentre randomized controlled trial of expectant management versus IVF in women with fallopian tube patency. Hum Reprod. 2004;19:1105–9.
26. Brandes M, Hamilton CJ, van der Steen JO, et al. Unexplained infertility: overall ongoing pregnancy rate and mode of conception. Hum Reprod. 2011;26:360–8.
27. Pandian Z, Bhattacharya S, Nikolaou D, et al. In vitro fertilisation for unexplained subfertility. Cochrane Database Syst Rev. 2002;2:CD003357.
28. Pandian Z, Bhattacharya S, Vale L, et al. In vitro fertilisation for unexplained subfertility. Cochrane Database Syst Rev. 2005;2:CD003357.
29. Van Voorhis BJ. Outcomes from assisted reproductive technology. Obstet Gynecol. 2006;107:183–200.
30. Goverde AJ, McDonnell J, Vermeiden JPW, et al. Intrauterine insemination or in vitro fertilisation in idiopathic subfertility and male subfertility: a randomised trial and cost-effectiveness analysis. Lancet. 2000;355:13–8.
31. Reindollar RH, Regan MM, Neumann PJ, et al. A randomized clinical trial to evaluate optimal treatment for unexplained infertility: the fast track and standard treatment (FASTT) trial. Fertil Steril. 2009;94:888–99.
32. Chambers GM, Sullivan EA, Shanahan M, et al. Is in vitro fertilisation more effective than stimulated intrauterine insemination as a first-line therapy for subfertility? A cohort analysis. Aust N Z J Obstet Gynaecol. 2010;50:280–8.
33. Custers IM, van Rumste MM, van der Steeg JW, et al. Long-term outcome in couples with unexplained subfertility and an intermediate prognosis initially randomized between expectant management and immediate treatment. Hum Reprod. 2012;27:444–50.
34. Kamal A, Mansour R, Fahmy I, et al. Easily decapitated spermatozoa defect: a possible cause of unexplained infertility. Hum Reprod. 1999;14:2791–5.
35. Omland AK, Bjercke S, Ertzeid G, et al. Intracytoplasmic sperm injection (ICSI) in unexplained and stage I endometriosis-associated infertility after fertilization failure with in vitro fertilization (IVF). J Assist Reprod Genet. 2006;23:351–7.
36. Paz G, Yavetz H, Margalit M, et al. The involvement of the zona pellucida in unexplained infertile women. Harefuah. 2008;147:77–80. (Article in Hebrew).
37. Check JH, Summers-Chase D, Cohen R, et al. Artificial oocyte activation with calcium ionophore allowed fertilization and pregnancy in a couple with long-term unexplained infertility where the female partner had diminished EGG reserve and failure to fertilize oocytes despite intracytoplasmic sperm injection. Clin Exp Obstet Gynecol. 2010;37:263–5.
38. Combelles CM, Morozumi K, Yanagimachi R, et al. Diagnosing cellular defects in an unexplained case of total fertilization failure. Hum Reprod. 2010;25:1666–71.
39. Katsoff B, Check JH, Mitchell-Williams J. Defective oocytes are not a common cause of unexplained infertility as determined by evaluation of sharing oocytes between infertile donors and recipients. Clin Exp Obstet Gynecol. 2013;40:193–5
40. Aboulghar MA, Mansour RT, Serour GI, et al. Intracytoplasmic sperm injection and conventional in vitro fertilization for sibling oocytes in cases of unexplained infertility and borderline semen. J Assist Reprod Genet. 1996;13:38–42.
41. Ruiz A, Remohí J, Minguez Y, et al. The role of in vitro fertilization and intracytoplasmic sperm injection in couples with unexplained infertility after failed intrauterine insemination. Fertil Steril. 1997;68:171–3.
42. Jaroudi K, Al-Hassan S, Al-Sufayan H, et al. Intracytoplasmic sperm injection and conventional in vitro fertilization are complementary techniques in management of unexplained infertility. J Assist Reprod Genet. 2003;20:377–81.
43. Li Z, Lin H, Xiao W, et al. Fertilization of IVF/ICSI using sibling oocytes from couples with subfertile male or unexplained infertility. J Huazhong Univ Sci Technol Med Sci. 2004;24:365–8.

44. Shveiky D, Simon A, Gino H, et al. Sibling oocyte submission to IVF and ICSI in unexplained infertility patients: a potential assay for gamete quality. Reprod Biomed Online. 2006;12:371–4.
45. Khamsi F, Yavas Y, Roberge S, et al. Intracytoplasmic sperm injection increased fertilization and good-quality embryo formation in patients with nonmale factor indications for in vitro fertilization: a prospective randomized study. Fertil Steril. 2001;75:342–7.
46. Hershlag A, Paine T, Kvapil G, et al. In vitro fertilization/intracytoplasmic sperm injection split: an insemination method to prevent fertilization failure. Fertil Steril. 2002;77:229–32.
47. Bungum L, Bungum M, Humaidan P, et al. A strategy for treatment of couples with unexplained infertility who failed to conceive after intrauterine insemination. Reprod Biomed Online. 2004;8:584–9.
48. Check JH, Bollendorf A, Summers-Chase D, et al. Conventional oocyte insemination may result in a better pregnancy outcome than intracytoplasmic sperm injection (ICSI) for unexplained infertility. Clin Exp Obstet Gynecol. 2009;36:150–1.
49. Karande VC, Korn A, Morris R, et al. Prospective randomized trial comparing the outcome and cost of in vitro fertilization with that of a traditional treatment algorithm as first-line therapy for couples with infertility. Fertil Steril. 1999;71:468–75.
50. Vitek WS, Galárraga O, Klatsky PC, et al. Management of the first in vitro fertilization cycle for unexplained infertility: a cost-effectiveness analysis of split in vitro fertilization-intracytoplasmic sperm injection. Fertil Steril. 2013;100:1381–8.
51. Collins J. Cost-effectiveness of in vitro fertilization. Semin Reprod Med. 2001;19:279–89.

Role of Assisted Reproduction Techniques in the Management of Unexplained Male Infertility

31

Bhushan K. Gangrade, Zamip Patel and Sejal Dharia Patel

Introduction

Infertility is classically defined as the inability of couples to conceive after 12 months of unprotected intercourse. According to an estimate, more than 72 million women in the world are infertile and may require some form of infertility treatment to achieve pregnancy [1]. In the USA, approximately 6.7 million women constituting 11 % of the females in the reproductive age group (15–44 years) are estimated to have impaired fertility (Centers for Disease Control and Prevention, Atlanta, GA). Even though the statistical data and estimates record the incidence of infertility in women, the primary cause of infertility may be equally attributed to both the male and the female partner in majority (approximately 80 %) of the cases. In 10–20 % couples, both partners appear to have normal findings with no apparent explanation for infertility (unexplained infertility). In couples with unexplained infertility, suspicion often falls on undiagnosed female factors such as oocyte genetics, embryo grade secondary to poor oocyte quality, implantation failure, or other physiological/immunological causes. It is seldom that in such instances the primary cause of infertility is attributed to the male. The treatment of couples with unexplained infertility becomes rather difficult since at present time it is not possible to establish the relative contributions of the male partner. This is largely due to profound difficulties which exist in accurate diagnosis of male infertility. Conventional semen analysis broadly predicts the probability of male's contribution toward successful pregnancy. However, the lack of functional clinical diagnostic tests makes it difficult to assign the primary diagnosis of male infertility especially in men with normal semen parameters. Unfortunately, a number of shortcomings in the scheme of diagnosis further complicate the diagnosis of men. Marked interejaculate variations in semen parameters [2], subjective evaluation of sperm morphology and progression, and wide interlaboratory variations in sperm assessment proficiencies further complicate the evaluation. There is also evidence that excessive inter- and intraobserver variations in sperm morphology evaluation exist that make it difficult for healthcare providers to have confidence in assigning weight to semen parameters.

The World Health Organization (WHO) criteria for semen reference values [3] do not take into account functional or physiological defects in sperm and as a result men classified as normal according to semen parameters may be unable to impregnate their partners. Likewise in a population of men with recently proven fertility, a subset of men can be identified who have sperm parameters well below WHO criteria [4]. It is interesting to note that WHO has repeatedly reclassified the semen analysis reference values over the last three decades. Semen analysis parameters of infertile men based initially on 1999 WHO reference criteria when reevaluated according to the most recent 2010 reference criteria resulted in some infertile men being reclassified as fertile [5].

The term "male factor infertility" is commonly used to describe infertility due to suboptimal sperm or semen parameters whereas "unexplained male infertility" refers to the inability of couples to conceive when the sperm parameters are within the normal range and the detailed evaluation of the female partner reveals no apparent cause of infertility. It is often difficult to assign the primary diagnosis of unexplained male infertility to a couple. The diagnosis of unexplained male infertility is further suspected in certain instances in men, who over time have been in more than one relationship, yet despite having normal semen parameters were unsuccessful in impregnating their reproductive age partner(s). As mentioned earlier, normal semen parameters reduce the probability of male infertility but do not completely eliminate the possibility of sperm dysfunction leading to failure of fertilization or poor embryonic development.

It is also important to make a distinction between two terms, namely, "unexplained male infertility" and "idiopathic

B. K. Gangrade (✉) · Z. Patel · S. D. Patel
Center for Reproductive Medicine, 3435 Pinehurst Ave, Orlando, FL 32804, USA
e-mail: Bhushan.gangrade@integramed.com, bkgangrade@hotmail.com

G. L. Schattman et al. (eds.), *Unexplained Infertility*, DOI 10.1007/978-1-4939-2140-9_31,

male infertility." In contrast to unexplained male infertility where sperm and semen values are within normal reference range, the term idiopathic male infertility refers to unexplained reduction in one or more semen parameters such as ejaculate volume, sperm concentration, total sperm count, sperm motility and progression, sperm viability, or sperm morphology. Idiopathic male infertility accounts for approximately one third of overall male infertility diagnoses [6]. In recent years, significant progress has been made toward understanding the regulation of spermatogenesis especially the role of microregions on the Y chromosome in men with defective spermatogenesis and poor sperm parameters. There is a need to develop tests that in conjunction with routine semen analyses may provide better identification of the underlying cause, and ultimately diagnosis and treatment of unexplained male infertility.

Unexplained Male Infertility: Possible Causes

As mentioned earlier, the obvious difficulties in assigning infertility diagnosis in couples with no abnormal finding prompts the healthcare providers to only suspect and infer the possible cause(s). In the following section, a brief description on possible causes and factors that may be associated with unexplained male infertility is presented since the matter is fully covered in a previous chapter: PART III: Pathophysiology: Male: "Potential Male Etiologies of Unexplained Male Infertility".

Chromosomal Abnormalities in Sperm

Despite normal diagnostic sperm parameters in some men, spermatozoa may exhibit high degree of structural or numerical chromosomal aberrations. The background numerical chromosome abnormalities in sperm of fertile men are between 1 and 2% whereas the background frequency of structural chromosomal abnormalities in these men ranges from 7 to 14%. In men heterozygous for different chromosomal translocations, the frequencies of sperm chromosomal abnormalities are elevated from 33 to 92% [7]. Infertile men despite having a normal somatic karyotype, exhibit an increased risk of chromosomally abnormal sperm and resulting embryo. Men with normal karyotype in somatic cells but abnormal cell lines in the testes (germinal or gonadal mosaics) often require infertility treatment in order to impregnate their partners. Infertile men show higher frequency of numerical chromosomal abnormalities especially disomy for chromosome 1 and XY as determined by FISH karyotyping [8]. In some men, increased incidence of sperm chromosome aneuploidy appears to play a key role in unexplained recurrent pregnancy loss [9].

In recent years, techniques, such as single sperm polymerase chain reaction (PCR) for sperm typing, have advanced our knowledge regarding meiotic recombination, errors of chromosome pairing, synapsis, and the production of aneuploid sperm. Interestingly, the frequency of morphologically abnormal sperm does not appear to correlate with abnormal chromosomal makeup [10–12]. It has been reported that no relationship exists between sperm chromosome abnormalities and sperm morphology in fertile men [13]. The dissociation between normal sperm morphology and chromosomal make up is further evident from the observation that the frequency of both structural and numerical chromosomal aberrations significantly increases in cancer patient following radiation therapy however, in such men no increase in morphologically abnormal sperm is noted [14–16]. It should be however noted that the abnormal sperm morphology in above studies largely refers to subtle morphological deviations in the sperm that prompt the classification of sperm as abnormal. Several distinct sperm abnormalities such as enlarged head or small (pin) head, on the other hand have been definitely linked to polyploidy and aneuploidy [17, 18].

Paternal Age

Unlike maternal age, the effect of paternal age on fertility potential in men is controversial. Even though men retain their fertility potential all through their life span, advanced paternal age may be associated with subtle decrease in male fertility as evidenced by lower success of IUI cycles [19–21]. Higher incidence of abnormal reproductive outcome such as pregnancy loss [22], developmental and morphological birth defects [23], nervous system disorders [24], and certain types of childhood cancers [25] are associated with advanced paternal age. Children of men over 50 years of age are approximately eight times more likely to be affected with achondroplasia as compared to those fathered by younger (25–29 years) males. Older men (>50 years) also have a 9.5-fold higher risk of having children diagnosed with Apert syndrome than younger men [26]. A significant increase in nondisjunction of sex chromosomes, frequency of chromosomal breaks and autosomal translocation in older men has been reported [27]. It seems plausible that high frequency of chromosomal aberrations in sperm in some men might be the underlying cause of unexplained infertility and recurrent pregnancy loss.

Sperm DNA Damage

The integrity of both the maternal and the paternal genome in gametes is of utmost importance for successful pregnancy and the birth of genetically normal progeny. The DNA is tightly packaged in sperm head in such a way that the volume occupied by sperm chromatin is less than 10% of a somatic cell. This compaction of sperm chromatin confers a high degree of protection to the genome from genotoxic factors and thus conserves the integrity of the paternal DNA. In order to attain this supercompaction of sperm chromatin, histones, the predominant protein component of chromatin in somatic cells, are largely replaced by protamines. The compaction of the sperm chromatin takes place during the postmeiotic phase of spermatogenesis. Despite the protection conferred to the sperm chromatin by compaction, several intrinsic and extrinsic factors are capable of damaging the sperm DNA.

It is well known that in women fertility declines when the oocytes exhibit high incidence of genetic abnormalities especially chromosomal aberrations with advancing age. In contrast to the decline in fertility in women, the effect of DNA damage in sperm and its role in fertility in the male has been less clear. Men with proven fertility have low levels of DNA damage in spermatozoa whereas infertile men especially with abnormal semen parameters exhibit increased DNA damage. Approximately 8% of infertile men with normal sperm parameters show high incidence of DNA damage in sperm [28–30]. Moreover, when approximately 30% of the sperm exhibit DNA damages; it may be the cause of infertility in the male [31, 32]. The fertilizing capability of spermatozoa with high degree of DNA damage does not appear to be compromised, however, poor embryonic development and high rate of miscarriage in such couples seem to reflect the importance of the integrity of sperm DNA [33, 34]. According to a recent report [35], the negative effect of sperm DNA damage on pregnancy and live birth rate is also evident in patients undergoing IVF. Men with <25% DNA fragmentation had a live birth rate of 33% as compared to couples with >50% DNA fragmentation (13% live birth rate). In contrast, in men undergoing IVF with intracytoplasmic sperm injection (ICSI) there was no difference in the live birth rate in high DNA fragmentation (>50%) group versus low DNA fragmentation group (<25%) [35]. It thus appears that sperm DNA damage may be less informative in couples undergoing ICSI since this technique of fertilization bypasses the natural selection barriers like sperm–zona binding, acrosome reaction, and fusion.

Based on evidence suggesting high incidence of sperm DNA damage in unexplained male infertility, diagnostic testing for sperm DNA integrity in addition to conventional semen analysis may provide a better measure of male fertility potential than semen analysis alone. There are several tests to evaluate DNA damage in spermatozoa. These include sperm chromatin structure assay (SCSA), single-cell gel electrophoresis assay (Comet assay), terminal deoxynucelotidyl transferase-mediated dUTP-nick end-labeling or "TUNEL" assay. Other assays to determine sperm chromatin integrity such as sperm nuclear maturity test, nuclear protein composition assay, and DNA oxidation assay are also available [30]. Despite differences in the principle and methodology in these assays, there is general consensus in the results achieved.

Oxidative Stress

Reactive oxygen species (ROS) are produced during normal cellular metabolism and play an important role in cell signaling and homeostasis. The production of free oxygen radicals in sperm bears immense physiological importance in terms of cAMP-mediated tyrosine phosphorylation associated with sperm capacitation. Supraphysiological concentrations of free oxygen radicals on the other hand cause irreversible damage to sperm DNA. Oxidative stress is defined as imbalance between the prooxidant and antioxidant ratio caused by limited availability of fewer antioxidants in relation to excessive amounts of oxidizing agents such as free oxygen radicals. Seminal plasma is rich in several antioxidant molecules (such as glutathione peroxidase, superoxide dismutase, ascorbic acid, alpha-tocopherol, and hypotaurine) secreted by the male reproductive tract [36, 37] that protect the sperm from the oxidative stress caused by ROS. Presence of high numbers of white blood cells in the semen results in excessive production of ROS which can cause damage to spermatozoa. High levels of ROS exert the detrimental effects on sperm at two levels viz. sperm membrane and sperm DNA. At the membrane level, ROS cause peroxidation of lipids in the acrosome membrane resulting in loss of fluidity [38]. Excessive production of ROS in semen can also reduce acrosin activity [39] and block sperm–oocyte interaction [40–42]. At the level of nuclear DNA, free radicals have the ability to attack nucleic acids and deoxyribose backbone causing structural damage. There is a large body of evidence suggesting a correlation between oxidative stress and sperm DNA damage [43–47].

Infections

There is evidence to implicate certain infections of the male reproductive tract (especially sexually transmitted diseases) as a cause of infertility, however, the relevance of subclinical infections in the etiology of male infertility is less clear [48]. There is some evidence that acute Chlamydia infections may be associated with low sperm counts and abnormal sperm morphology [49]. The incidence of leukocytospermia in otherwise normospermic men may indicate asymptomatic subclinical genital tract infection and may lead to excessive production of reactive oxygen species (ROS) by white blood cells. The link between leukocytopsermia, excessive generation of ROS and infertility is well documented [50–52] and deserves attention while treating couples with unexplained infertility.

The role of antibiotic treatment in resolution of leukocytospermia has been advocated [53] as well as refuted [54]. In couples with unexplained infertility where men with otherwise normal semen analyses exhibit leukocytospermia, antibiotic treatment of males has been shown to result in significant improvement in pregnancy rates [55]. Improvement in semen quality and fertility in men with clinically suspected bacterial infections [56] has been reported. Even though there is lack of direct evidence to associate mycoplasma infections with male infertility, it has been reported that 85 % of men with infertile marriages of unexplained cause had semen cultures positive for ureaplasma compared with 23 % of fertile controls [57]. Additional studies on empiric treatment of infertile men might shed more light on the efficacy of antibiotic therapy in unexplained male infertility.

Diseases

Certain diseases in men can also alter reproductive functions and indirectly impair or reduce fertility. Metabolic disorders have wide effects on various organ systems including the reproductive system. There is evidence that spermatogenesis is affected by diabetes and that the diabetic patients have reduced sperm motility and semen volume [58, 59]. Sexual dysfunctions such as erectile and ejaculatory problems arising due to vascular and neuropathic causes further add to fertility impairment. There is also evidence that suggests that diabetes impairs spermatogenesis by affecting hypothalamo–hypophyseal–gonadal axis [60, 61]. Studies involving sperm nuclear and mitochondria DNA in men with insulin-dependent diabetes mellitus revealed increased nuclear DNA fragmentation and mitochondrial DNA deletions in sperm from diabetic males [62]. In addition, the deletions in mitochondrial DNA of sperm as noted in diabetic men are associated with impaired sperm motility and male infertility [63–65].

Some men with celiac disease suffer from reversible androgen resistance and testicular dysfunction [66, 67]. Studies on married men with celiac disease reveal that high percentages (20 %) of couples have infertile marriages. It has been reported that semen analysis in men with Crohn's disease show significant abnormalities in sperm morphology and motility. Interestingly a marked improvement in sperm morphology in celiacs following removal of dietary gluten was observed [67]. It should be noted that a recent report however found no correlation between the fertility potential in men with celiac disease and their age matched controls [68].

Fertilization Failure

Standard semen analysis has a limited ability to predict normal fertilization in vivo or by in vitro insemination of oocytes in IVF setting. Introduction of strict sperm morphology criteria [69] was offered as a means to enhance the diagnostic value and predictability of fertilization, however its efficacy in such prediction has been both supported and refuted [70–73].

Calcium ions play an important role in the process of sperm–oocyte fusion. There is evidence to show that calcium channel blockers used as antihypertensive medication in men can cause failure of fertilization in IVF setting. The spermatozoa in normospermic men taking calcium antagonists do not express head-directed mannose-ligand receptors and also fail to undergo spontaneous acrosome loss [74]. The inhibition of sperm fertilizing potential appears to be mediated through insertion of lipophilic calcium channel blockers into the lipid bilayer of the sperm plasma membrane.

Failure of fertilization may occur in 5–10 % of IVF cycles and may result from abnormal sperm parameters or poor oocyte quality [75, 76]. In approximately 56 % of the fertilization failures, there is no obvious oocyte anomaly but sperm fail to bind to the zona pellucida [77]. In a study, sperm proteomic profiles of patients with complete failure of fertilization and no sperm binding to the zona pellucida was compared with controls who exhibited normal fertilization. Differential expression of at least 14 proteins was recorded of which two (Laminin receptor LR67 and L-xylulose reductase) may play a role in sperm–egg interaction [77]. Beta-defensin 126 is a glycosylated protein that is encoded by DEFB126 gene present on chromosome 20. The beta-defensin is secreted in the epididymis and adsorbed on the sperm surface. This polypeptide has been implicated in immunoprotection as well as penetration of sperm through cervical mucus. Sequence variation in DEFB126 gene involving a two-nucleotide deletion results in abnormal mRNA and ultimately defective polypeptide. In a prospective study including married couples where men were found to be homozygous for the variant sequence of DEFB126 gene, it took longer to achieve pregnancy and live birth than control population [78].

The clinical significance of antisperm antibodies in male infertility remains controversial [79–81]. The reason for a lack of consensus on the role of sperm antibodies in infertility appears to be largely due to a large number of variables and testing methods. Variables such as types of immunoglobulins (IgA, IgG, IgM), location (sperm head or tail), effect (agglutination, immobilization, cytotoxicity), and the lack of standard methods to quantify the antibodies make such assessment difficult. Most studies however, have demonstrated a direct association between sperm surface antibodies and the fertility potential of the male [82–84].

Immunologic infertility due to sperm surface antibodies can result from impaired sperm transport, destruction of pre- and postmeiotic germ cells and gametes, and acrosome reaction abnormalities by inhibiting sperm–oocyte interaction [85]. Undoubtedly, absolute failure of fertilization or suboptimum fertilization may be the primary cause of infertility in some couples with unexplained male infertility. This possibility should be explored especially in couples who had multiple inseminations and despite high normal semen reference values have failed to achieve pregnancy.

Behavioral and Environmental Factors

There is growing body of evidence that lifestyle behaviors as well as environmental factors are intricately involved with their direct or indirect effects on human sperm. Exposure to cigarette smoke, alcohol, caffeine, and environmental pollutants is known to negatively affect male fertility [86, 87]. It is well established that cigarette smoke is enriched with mutagens, carcinogens, and oxidants. Adverse effects of smoking as well as passive smoke inhalation on male fertility and semen quality have also been extensively studied [88, 89]. There is some evidence that sperm parameters such as concentration, motility, progression, and possibly morphology are also negatively affected in smokers [90, 91]. A significant and dose-dependent reduction in sperm motility averaging 22 % in smokers as compared with nonsmoking men strongly indicates the deleterious effect of smoking on semen quality [92]. Sperm from men who smoke nicotine possess higher levels of DNA strand breaks [93]. The alteration in sperm chromatin structure may not only affect fertility potential in the male but also predisposes the offspring to greater risk of malformations, cancers, and genetic diseases. Cigarette smoke contains high levels of oxidants. It also adversely affects plasma and tissue levels of antioxidants such as tocopherol and ascorbate. The reduced levels of protective antioxidants in tissues and plasma appear to induce further damage to sperm DNA [94]. Despite the strong correlation between smoking and semen quality, there is no evidence to warrant that sperm parameters in smokers fall significantly below normal reference range. It is however possible that, men in lower range of normal reference values for semen may be affected to induce enough DNA damage in spermatozoa to impair or reduce fertility.

There is an ample evidence to suggest that exposure to environmental pollutants introduced and spread by human activities contributes to reproductive problems often leading to decrease in fertility potential [95]. The detrimental effect of these chemicals on fertility may be more pronounced and apparent in men with borderline semen parameters. Pollutants often affect spermatogenesis by disturbing the endocrine pathways, namely, hypothalamo–hypophyseal–gonadal axis. However, there is some evidence suggesting direct effect of chemical pollutants on sperm cells. Men exposed to polychlorinated biphenyls and p,p'-dichlorodiphenyldichloroethylene (p,p'-DDE) exhibit increased rates of chromosomal aberrations especially sex–chromosome disomy [96] and this may result in reduced fertility. Polychlorinatedbiphenyls (PCBs) that were widely used (but have been banned now) in coolants, capacitors, transformers, and electrical motors adversely affect sperm motility while certain pesticides such as DDT and organophosphates affect sperm count. Exposure of men to phthalates which are ubiquitously present in plastics and many industrial and consumer products can occur by oral route or dermal absorption. It has been shown that phthalate esters impact sperm count and motility in men and this effect is linked to phthalate levels [97]. There also exists a relationship between urinary concentrations of certain phthalate metabolites (such as monoethyl phthalate and mono-(2-ethylhexyl) phthalate) and sperm DNA damage among men seeking infertility treatment [98]. Exposure to heavy metals has also been linked to male infertility due to sperm oxidative damage and testicular cell apoptosis [99]. A significant decrease in fertility associated with higher miscarriage rate has been observed in the partners of men working in lead battery factory suggesting the detrimental effects of heavy metals on reproductive success [100].

Urologic Workup and Treatment Options

As mentioned earlier, semen analysis is often used as the primary diagnostic test for the evaluation of the fertility potential of the male. Despite normal reference values for various semen parameters, 8–30 % of males may have male factor infertility [101]. Furthermore, what is considered "normal" with regards to semen parameters has changed significantly over time since the WHO put forth its first guidelines in 1987 [102].

Many couples with unexplained infertility may have subfertile variants that, once identified, may be then used to aid in reproductive outcomes. To understand the utility of searching for such variants, it is necessary to identify the difference between semen parameters and sperm parameters. Although the recent 5th edition of the WHO guidelines [103] is useful in determining norms among fertile men, it is important to realize that these guidelines identify trends among populations of spermatozoa rather than an individual sperm's ability to allow for fertilization or that individual sperm's DNA's ability to complement appropriately with the oocyte counterpart. In order to further elucidate the properties of the sperm–oocyte interface, a series of tests have been developed to aid in diagnosis and therapy for men that may have a defect in one or all of these interactions.

One of those interactions pertains to the integrity of sperm DNA to withstand the process of unwinding and undergoing recombination. DFI testing, as outlined earlier, is a diagnostic index to assess this process. Though standardizations of the various assays have made interpretation difficult [104] abnormal results may have clinical consequences [105]. Although the mechanism underlying increased nuclear DNA damage in sperm from normozoospermic infertile men is unclear, it has been proposed that inherent defects in sperm chromatin packaging may not be associated with other stages of sperm development or maturation, and thus normozoospermic men may have a fundamental defect allowing for early embryo loss [106]. In cases of recurrent early ICSI/IUI failures and high DFI values, testicular extraction combined with ICSI have yielded improved pregnancy success [107].

Another clinically useful evaluation in the workup of the normozoospermic infertile male is an evaluation of ROS [108]. High ROS may lead to only mild changes in semen parameters but may ultimately lead to loss of integrity within the sperm nucleus [43]. High ROS may be secondary to inherent defects in oxidative enzymes in the testicle or secondarily to increased insult from pyospermia or gonadotoxins [109].

Antioxidants may be helpful, though there is limited evidence supporting their clinical utility [110]. The most commonly implicated are L-carnitine, vitamin C, D3, E, folic acid, zinc, and selenium. However, the nutraceutical with perhaps most robust data supporting use is coenzyme Q10, which has been shown to reduce ROS and improve semen parameters as well [111, 112]. In men with persistently high ROS, testicular sperm extraction may be necessary.

Idiopathic asthenozoospermia may have a multitude of causes and likely reflects a wide range of disorders. At present due to lack of an alternative treatment approach, isolated genetic defects (e.g., glutathione s-transferase gene polymorphisms) or other sperm deficits can only be treated by assisted reproduction—most often ICSI [113, 114]. Although the spectrum of diseases that leads to a diagnosis of idiopathic asthenozoospermia has yet to be delineated, there is promise of more directed therapies addressing fundamental defects in sperm that may lead to spontaneous return of reproductive potential in the future [115].

In similar fashion, isolated idiopathic teratozoospermia may likewise be problematic to treat in a clinical arena. However, the clinical importance of teratozoospermia remains elusive, as the normal thresholds listed in the most recent WHO manual [103] suggest even traditionally very low strict morphologies may still be compatible with spontaneous pregnancy. In essence from urologist's point of view, at present there are limited treatment options for the management of unexplained male infertility. The referral of couples to reproductive endocrinologists and treatment by IVF with ICSI appears to be the most effective strategy.

Management of Infertile Couple with Suspicion of Unexplained Male Infertility: A Reproductive Endocrinologist's Approach

Management of a couple who presents with unexplained infertility typically is focused on an empiric approach that sequentially gets more aggressive until pregnancy is achieved. A diagnosis of unexplained infertility is assigned to a couple who has completed an infertility workup including hysterosalpingogram, documentation of ovulatory function, and ovarian reserve, and an assessment for other etiologies (i.e., endometriosis, PCOS) as clinically appropriate for the female patient [116] with no abnormal findings. The male partner should have undergone a semen analysis which shows semen and sperm parameters within normal reference values. The initial treatment approach involves discussion aimed at optimizing the couples' fertility through natural means (optimizing their BMI, cessation of tobacco, alcohol) [116].

Although estimates will vary, the percentage of couples with unexplained infertility is between 10–15% [117]. Couples with unexplained infertility are affected by both decreased and delayed fecundity. Average cycle fecundity in couples with a diagnosis of unexplained infertility is significantly low in nonrandomized studies [118]. Treatment is therefore designed to empirically improve low cycle fecundity and includes expectant management, controlled superovulation with IUI and in vitro fertilization.

Expectant Management

The likelihood of pregnancy without treatment among couples with unexplained infertility is suboptimal compared to the fertile population but cumulative data provides cautious optimism. Cumulative pregnancy rates range between 30 and 80% over 3 years [116]. This large variation is due to differences in female age and the duration of infertility. A cumulative pregnancy rate of 50–80% as a function of female age has been reported. When calculated as a function of the duration of infertility over 3 years, the cumulative pregnancy rate is between 30 and 80% [119].

Controlled Superovulation with Intrauterine Insemination

In an ovulatory female with a partner whose semen analysis is within the normal range, controlled superovulation with IUI is an effective therapeutic modality. Intrauterine insemination (IUI) using male partner's ejaculated sperm is one of the first lines of treatment for certain types of infertility including unexplained infertility. It is an inexpensive and minimally invasive technique that offers successful outcome in a fraction of couples seeking infertility treatment. The success of IUI depends on several variables including female age, etiology of infertility, and importantly sperm parameters.

Even though there appears to be some disagreement on the predictive value of normal sperm morphology on IUI success, majority of the reports are in favor of a strong correlation [120]. The number of motile sperm in insemination fraction is another important variable that is positively correlated with the pregnancy rate following IUI. The inseminating motile count (IMC) of less than 1×10^6 is highly predictive of IUI failure. [121].

For couples with normal seminal parameters and the diagnosis of unexplained infertility, pregnancy rates following artificial insemination (IUI) do not significantly improve when compared with traditional timed coitus [122]. There is a small benefit when using oral ovulation induction medication in addition to IUI [118]. This is further confirmed with the utilization of gonadotropin superovulation with IUI, in that IUI increases pregnancy rates (31 %) over gonadotropin stimulation alone (19%) [123]. Couples with unexplained infertility achieve most benefit in terms of pregnancy by undergoing three controlled superovulation cycles with IUIs [124]. IUI in couples with antisperm antibodies is not as effective since the intrauterine placement of prepared spermatozoa does not alter the distribution or the adverse action of antisperm antibodies [125].

In Vitro Fertilization

IVF is a treatment modality that is advocated by many clinicians based upon classical literature for the management of unexplained infertility. As compared to IUI, IVF enables a clinician to further diagnostically assess whether there is an anatomic factor preventing transport of the oocyte, an oocyte–sperm binding obstruction, or suboptimal functional embryo quality. It may even lend suspicion to unexplained male infertility in addition to providing a strong therapeutic benefit. According to the Society for Assisted Reproductive Technology (SART) in USA, in 2010 pregnancy rates from IVF were 47.8 % per embryo transfer in women under age 35 (www.sart.org).

In patients with unexplained infertility, IVF will enable a couple to shorten their time to pregnancy [126]. ICSI as discussed below will enable correction of fertilization impairment or occurrence of antisperm antibodies. The trend for the management of unexplained male infertility is toward the utilization of IVF with ICSI.

The Role of the Laboratory in the Management of Unexplained Male Infertility

The involvement of the reproductive laboratory in the diagnosis and treatment of male infertility starts with the standard semen analysis. The etiology of infertility and treatment options for couple, to a large extent depend on the semen analysis report and information provided by the laboratory to the physician. It is important to implement a good quality control and quality assurance (QC/QA) program in the andrology laboratory in order to have uniform high standard of accuracy and reproducibility. The periodic evaluation of intra- and intertechnician variability in semen analysis should be an integral part of QC/QA. Accurate semen analysis by the laboratory facilitates the physicians to counsel the couples on their treatment plan.

As mentioned earlier, when the semen values are within normal reference range on at least two occasions and female infertility has been ruled out by the reproductive endocrinologist, the diagnosis of unexplained infertility seems logical. A detailed history of male partner to rule out occupational, environmental, or behavioral exposures to substances or chemicals that may cause excessive damage to sperm DNA is essential. The treatment of unexplained infertility often involves IUI using partner's sperm. The ejaculated spermatozoa are washed to remove seminal plasma prior to insemination. The simple washing procedure involves centrifugation of culture medium-diluted liquefied semen. The resulting sperm pellet consists of the mixed population of motile, nonmotile, and dead sperm. In addition to round cells, epithelial cells, and leukocytes may also be present in varying numbers. Leucocytes are a potent source of free oxygen radicals which in the tight vicinity of spermatozoa in the washed pellet may cause oxidative damage in sperm DNA [127]. Simple washing of sperm is therefore not recommended especially if there is concern to avoid the ROS-induced DNA damage in sperm. Several other sperm preparation methods such as swim up, gradient separation, glass-wool filtration, etc. are also used to separate motile sperm population from other cellular and nonmotile sperm fraction. Swim up of spermatozoa directly from liquefied semen avoids the initial centrifugation of semen to form a tight sperm pellet and close contact of motile sperm with ROS-producing cells. Use of density gradients for isolating motile sperm has gained wide acceptance in reproductive laboratories largely due to high recovery and yield. Density gradient separation of sperm effectively removes the majority of white blood cells and other cellular debris and produces highly motile sperm fraction for IUI or IVF. The choice of sperm wash method by the laboratory is critical and various semen parameters in the prewash sample as well as the end use of washed sperm (IUI, IVF, or ICSI) are taken into consideration in choosing the method. As noted in the earlier section, IUI may provide a cost-effective first approach toward the treatment of unexplained infertility with pregnancy rates in the range of 12–15 %. Majority of the patients, who are unsuccessful in achieving pregnancy after 3–4 inseminations proceed to in vitro fertilization as the next step in treatment. In women with multiple failed IUIs, the possibility of fertilization failure and insemination of oocytes by ICSI should be discussed. In the event, a fair number of oocytes are retrieved, split insemination by IVF and ICSI can be offered. This strategy insures fertilization by ICSI in case oocytes inseminated by standard IVF fail to fertilize. Alternatively if the standard insemination results in fertilization, the couple will not require ICSI in future IVF attempts.

The development of the techniques of ICSI has revolutionized the management of male infertility and essentially rendered other modalities of male infertility treatment relatively inefficient and outdated. ICSI involves the injection of a single viable sperm into the ooplasm of the mature oocyte. Spermatozoa irrespective of the source (ejaculate, testis, and epididymis) are highly effective in fertilizing the eggs following ICSI. Sperm attributes such as morphology, motility, and progression exert little effect if any, on the rate of fertilization of sperm-injected oocytes. Broadly speaking, the viability of the sperm used for injection is the main determinant for successful fertilization. Even though ICSI was initially offered as a treatment modality for male factor patients, it has been successfully employed to treat couples with immunological infertility, unexplained infertility, and those with a history of failed fertilization. As mentioned earlier, presence of antisperm antibodies in either partner may adversely affect sperm motility, sperm transport through female reproductive tract and ultimately sperm–zona binding/fusion. Insemination using ICSI bypasses these initial obstacles, and results in high fertilization and pregnancy rates [128, 129]. In a study [130], patients with a history of failed fertilization were offered a repeat cycle with random splitting of oocytes for ICSI and IVF. Insemination by ICSI resulted in normal fertilization rate of approximately 63 %. None of the sibling MII oocytes which were inseminated by standard IVF with a higher concentration of sperm than in previous attempt showed normal zygote formation. In couples undergoing IVF for unexplained infertility, fertilization rate of oocytes by ICSI appears to be higher than standard insemination [131, 132].

It has been suspected that spermatozoa may carry structural defects that may not be detected at standard optical magnification (200–400×) commonly used for ICSI. Spermatozoa that appear normal at this magnification may in fact carry subtle ultrastructural alterations in the head, middle piece, or tail. Bartoov et al. [133] reported that it is possible to detect such defects in motile sperm at higher magnification (6600×). This technique, "motile sperm organellae morphology examination (MSOME)" was later used by Hazout et al. [134] to identify and select normal sperm for ICSI at 6000× magnification. This modified ICSI technique was called intracytoplasmic morphologically selected sperm injection (IMSI). These investigators reported significant improvement in pregnancy outcome in patients undergoing IMSI as compared with those with previous failed ICSI attempts. In another prospective randomized study [135] to compare the efficacy of ICSI with IMSI, 446 couples were divided into two groups. IMSI resulted in a significant higher clinical pregnancy rate (39.2 %) as compared with ICSI (26.5 %). Interestingly, approximately 30 % of the patients with multiple previous failed attempts undergoing IMSI had clinical pregnancy as compared with 13 % who had standard ICSI method for fertilization. Patients in the IMSI group also exhibited significantly decreased miscarriage rate (17.4 %) as compared to ICSI group (37.5 %). Additional studies to support the effectiveness of IMSI over ICSI are needed.

Due to superior fertilization rate and avoidance of the probability of total fertilization failure, some clinics offer ICSI as the only technique for fertilization of oocytes following oocyte retrieval. This approach however has not been embraced by the majority of the assisted reproductive clinics and ICSI is reserved for patients based on the clinical history and semen parameters.

Conclusion

Unexplained male infertility is a condition that is difficult to diagnose with certainty and often is the last resort in terms of assigning an etiology as the cause of infertility. Significant advances have been made in recent years that have helped to elucidate the mechanisms of sperm DNA damage and structural chromosomal aberrations leading to male infertility. The realm of unexplained male factor infertility dwindles with each molecular advance into the workings of sperm, and likewise does the clinical acumen in determining treatment modalities that may benefit patients in a more cost-effective and beneficial way than immediately shunting then to assisted reproduction. Even though there is no evidence to support the effectiveness of dietary supplements or vitamins on male fertility, supplements containing antioxidants like vitamin E and C, selenium, beta-carotene, and other micronutrients like zinc, amino acids such as L-carnitine, B-multivitamins, and coenzyme Q10 may be helpful in improving fertility potential in men. We are in our infancy in determining many of the causes of unexplained infertility, and so our options are limited in providing management options other than assisted reproduction. Advances in the field of male infertility testing and development of new diagnostic and therapeutic pathways in future may improve outcomes. At present for couples with unexplained infertility, IUIs and if not successful, in vitro fertilization seems to be the preferred approach. Patients with unexplained male infertility may benefit from IVF with ICSI if fertilization failure is suspected as the cause of infertility.

References

1. Boivin J, Bunting L, Collins JA, Nygren KG. International estimates of infertility prevalence and treatment seeking: potential need and demand for infertility medical care. Hum Reprod. 2007;22:1506–12.
2. Mallidis C, Howard EJ, Balur HW. Variation of semen quality in normal men. Int J Androl. 1991;14:99–107.

3. World Health Organization. WHO laboratory manual for examination of human semen and sperm-cervical mucus interaction, 2nd edition. Cambridge: Cambridge University Press; 1987.
4. Irvine DS. Epidemiology and aetiology of male infertility. Hum Reprod. 1998;13:33–44.
5. Murray KS, McGeady JA, Reed ML, Kuang WW, Nangia AK. The effect of the new 2010 World Health Organization criteria for semen analyses on male infertility. Fertil Steril. 2012;98:1428–31.
6. Lipschultz LI. Office evaluation of the subfertile male. In: Lipschults LI, Niederberger CS, editors. Infertility in the male, 4th edition. Cambridge: Cambridge University Press; 2009. p. 153–76.
7. Martin RH. Chrosomal abnormalities in human sperm. In: Robaire B, Hales BE, editors. Advances in male-mediated developmental toxicity. New York: Plenum Press; 2003. p. 181–8.
8. Moosani N, Pattinson HA, Carter MD, Rademaker AW, Martin RH. Chromosomal analysis of sperm from men with idiopathic infertility using sperm karyotyping and fluorescence in situ hybridization. Fert Steril. 1995;64:811–17.
9. Carrell DT, Wilcox AL, Lowy L, Peterson CM, Jones KP, Erickson L, Hatasaka HH. Elevated sperm chromosome aneuploidy and apoptosis in patients with unexplained recurrent pregnancy loss. Obstet Gynecol. 2003;101:1229–35.
10. Balkan W, Martin RH. Chromosome segregation into the spermatozoa of two men heterozygous for different reciprocal translocations. Hum Genet. 1983;63:345–48.
11. Balkan W, Martin RH. Segregation of chromosomes into the spermatozoa of a men heterozygous for a 14; 21 Robertsonian translocation. Am J Med Genet. 1983;16:169–72.
12. Martin RH. Analysis of human sperm chromosome complements from a male heterozygous for a reciprocal translocation t(11;22)(q23;q11). Clin Genet. 1984;25:357–61.
13. Martin RH, Rademaker A. The relationship between sperm chromosomal abnormalities and sperm morphology in humans. Mutat Res. 1988;207:159–64.
14. Martin RH, Rademaker A, Barnes M, Arthur K, Ringrose T, Douglas GA. A prospective serial study of the effects of radiotherapy on semen parameters, and hamster egg penetration rates. Clin Invest Med. 1985;8:239–43.
15. Martin RH, Hildebrand K, Yamamoto J, Rademaker A, Barnes M, Douglas G, Arthur K, Ringrose T, Brown IS. An increased frequency of human sperm chromosomal abnormalities after radiotherapy. Mutat Res. 1986;174:219–25.
16. Martin RH, Rademaker A, Hildebrand K, Barnes M, Arthur K, Ringrose T, Brown IS, Douglas G. A comparison of chrosomal aberrations induced by in vivo radiotherapy in human sperm and lymphocytes. Mutat Res. 1989;226:21–30.
17. Devillard F, Metzler-Guillemain C, Pelletier R, DeRobertis C, Bergues U, Hennebicq S, Guichaoua M, Sele B, Rousseaux S. Polyploidy in large-headed sperm: fish study of three cases. Hum Reprod. 2002;17:1292–8.
18. Bernardini L, Borini A, Preti S, Conte N, Flamigni C, Capitanio GL, et al. Study of aneuploidy in normal and abnormal germ cells from semen of fertile and infertile men. Hum Reprod. 1988;13:3406–13.
19. Mathieu C, Ecochard R, Bied V, Lornage J, Czyba JC. Andrology: cumulative conception rate following intrauterine artificial insemination with husband's spermatozoa: influence of husband's age. Hum Reprod. 1995;10:1090–97.
20. Bellver J, Garrido N, Remohí J, Pellicer A, Meseguer M. Influence of paternal age on assisted reproduction outcome. Reprod Biomed Online. 2008;17:595–604.
21. Demir B, Dilbaz B, Cinar O, Karadag B, Tasci Y, Kocak M, Goktolga U. Factors affecting pregnancy outcome of intrauterine insemination cycles in couples with favourable female characteristics. J Obstet Gynaecol. 2011;31:420–3.
22. Slama R, Bouyer J, Windha G, Fenste L, Werwatz A, Swan SH. Influence of paternal age on the risk of spontaneous abortion. Am J Epidem. 2005;161:816–23.
23. Green RF, Devine O, Crider KS, Olney RS, Archer N, Olshan AF, Shapira SK. Association of paternal age and risk for major congenital anomalies from the national birth defects prevention study, 1997–2004. Ann Epidemiol. 2010;20:241.
24. Saha S, Barnett AG, Foldi C, Burne TH, Eyles DW, Buka SL, McGrath JJ. Advanced paternal age is associated with impaired neurocognitive outcomes during infancy and childhood. PLoS Med. 2009;6.3:e1000040.
25. Hemminki K, Kyyrönen P. Parental age and risk of sporadic and familial cancer in offspring: implications for germ cell mutagenesis. Epidemiology. 1999;10:747–51.
26. Risch N, Reich EW, Wishnick MM, McCarthy JG. Spontaneous mutation and parental age in humans. Am J Hum Genet. 1987;41:218–48.
27. Sartorelli EMP, Mazzucatto LF, de Pina-Neto JM. Effect of paternal age on human sperm chromosomes. Fertil Steril. 2001;76:1119–23.
28. Kodama H, Yamaguchi R, Fukuda J, Kasai H, Tanaka T. Increased oxidative deoxyribonucleic acid damage in the spermatozoa of infertile male patient. Fertil Steril. 1997;68:519–24.
29. Spano H, Bonde JP, Hjollund HI, Kolstad HA, Cordelli E, Leter G. The Danish first pregnancy planner study team. Sperm chromatin damage impairs human fertility. Fertil Steril. 2000;73:43–50.
30. Zini A, Libman J. Sperm DNA damage: clinical significance in the era of assisted reproduction. Can Med Assoc J. 2006;175:495–500.
31. Evenson DP, Jost LK, Marshall D, Zinaman MJ, Clegg E, Purvis K, de Angelis P, Claussen OP. Utility of sperm chromatin structure assay as a diagnostic and prognostic tool in the human fertility clinics. Hum Reprod. 1999;14:1039–49.
32. Evenson DP, Larson KL, Jost LK. Sperm chromatin structure assay: its clinical use for detecting sperm DNA fragmentation in male infertility and comparisons with the other techniques. J Androl. 2002;23:25–43.
33. Carrell DT, Liu L, Peterson CM, Jones KP, Hatasaka HH, Erickson L, Campbell B. Sperm DNA fragmentation is increased in couples with unexplained recurrent pregnancy loss. Arch Androl. 2003;49:49–55.
34. Tesarik J, Greco E, Mendoza C. Late, but not early, paternal effect on human embryo development is related to sperm DNA fragmentation. Hum Reprod. 2004;19:611–15.
35. Simon L, Proutaski I, Stevenson M, Jennings D, McManus J, Lutton D, Lewis SEM. Sperm DNA damage has a negative association with live-birth rates after IVF. Reprod Biomed Online. 2013;26:68–78.
36. Twigg J, Irvine DS, Houston P, Fulton N, Michael L, Aitken RJ. Iatrogenic DNA damage induced in human spermatozoa during sperm preparation: protective significance of seminal plasma. Mol Hum Reprod. 1998;4:439–45.
37. van Overveld FW, Floris WPC, Rhemrev J, Vermeiden JPW, Bast A. Tyrosine as important contributor to the antioxidant capacity of seminal plasma. Chem Biol Interact. 2000;127:151–61.
38. Jones R, Mann T, Sherins R. Peroxidative breakdown of phospholipids in human spermatozoa, spermicidal properties of fatty acid peroxides, and protective action of seminal plasma. Fertil Steril. 1979;31:531.
39. Zalata AA, Ahmed AH, Allamanemi SS, Comhaire FH, Agarwal A. Relationship between acrosin activity of human spermatozoa and oxidative stress. Asian J Androl. 2004;6:313–18.
40. Aitken RJ, Clarkson JS, Fishel S. Generation of reactive oxygen species, lipid peroxidation, and human sperm function. Biol Reprod. 1989;41:183–97.
41. Ichikawa T, Oeda T, Ohmori H, Schill WB. Reactive oxygen species influence the acrosome reaction but not acrosin activity in human spermatozoa. Int J Androl. 1999;22:37–42.
42. Jedrzejczak P, Fraczek M, Szumala-Kakol A, Taszarek-Hauke G, Pawelczyk L, Kurpisz M. Consequences of semen inflammation and lipid peroxidation on fertilization capacity of spermatozoa in in vitro conditions. Int J Androl. 2005;28:275–83.

43. Saleh RA, Agarwal A. Oxidative stress and male infertility: from research bench to clinical practice. J Androl. 2002;23:737–52.
44. Oger I, Da Cruz C, Panteix G, Menezo Y. Evaluating human sperm DNA integrity: relationship between 8-hydroxydeoxyguanosine quantification and the sperm chromatin structure assay. Zygote. 2003;11:367–71.
45. Henkel R, Kierspel E, Stalf T, Mehnert C, Menkveld R, Tinneberg HR, Schill WB, Kruger TF. Effect of reactive oxygen species produced by spermatozoa and leukocytes on sperm functions in non-leukocytospermic patients. Fertil Steril. 2005;83:635–42.
46. Kao SH, Chao HT, Chen HW, Hwang TI, Liao TL, Wei YH. Increase of oxidative stress in human sperm with lower motility. Fertil Steril. 2008;89:1183–90.
47. Tremellen K. Oxidative stress and male infertility–a clinical perspective. Hum Reprod Update. 2008;14:243–58.
48. Fowler JE. Infections of the male reproductive tract and infertility: a selected review. J Androl. 1981;3:121–31.
49. Berger RE, Alexander ER, Harnisch JP, Paulson CA, Monda GD, Ansel J, Holmes KK. Etiology, manifestations and therapy of acute epididymitis: prospective study of 50 cases. J Urol. 1979;121:750–4.
50. Agarwal A, Ikemoto I, Loughlin KR. Relationship of sperm parameters with levels of reactive oxygen species in semen specimens. J Urol. 1994;152:107–10.
51. Wolff H, Politch JA, Martinez A, Haimovici F, Hill JA, Anderson DJ. Leukocytospermia is associated with poor semen quality. Fertil Steril. 1990;53:528–36.
52. Wolff H. The biologic significance of white blood cells in semen. Fertil Steril. 1995;63:1143–57.
53. Branigan EF, Muller CH. Efficiency of treatment abd recurrence rate of leukocytospermia in infertile men with prostatitis. Fertil Steril. 1994;62:580–4.
54. Yanushpolsky ET, Politch JA, Hill JA, Anderson DJ. Antibiotic therapy and leukocytospermia: a prospective randomized controlled study. Fertil Steril. 1995;63:142–7.
55. Branigan EF, Spadoni LR, Muller CH. Identification and treatment of leukocytospermia in couples with unexplained infertility. J Reprod Med. 1995;40:625–9.
56. Ulstein M, Capell P, Holmes KK, Paulsen CA. Nonsymptomatic genital tract infection and male infertility. In: Hafez ESE, editor. Human semen and fertility regulation in men. Mosby. St. Louis; 1976. p. 355–362.
57. Gnarpe H, Freiberg J. T mycoplasmas on spermatozoa and infertility. Nature. 1973;245:97–8.
58. Bartak V. Sperm quality in adult diabetic men. Int J Fertil. 1979;24:226–32.
59. Glenn DR, McClure N, Lewis SE. The hidden impact of diabetes on male sexual dysfunction and fertility. Hum Fertil. 2003;6:174–9.
60. Baccetti B, La Marca A, Piomboni P, Capitani S, Bruni E, Petraglia F, DeLeo V. Insulin-dependent diabetes in men is associated with hypothalamo-pituitary derangement and with impairment in semen quality. Hum Reprod. 2002;10:2673–77.
61. Ballester J, Munoz MC, Dominguez J, Rigau T, Guinovart JJ, Rodriguez-Gil JE. Insulin-dependent diabetes affects testicular function by FSH-and LH-linked mechanisms. J Androl. 2004;25:706–19.
62. Agbaje IM, Rogers DA, McVicar CM, McClure N, Atkinson AB, Malladis C, Lewis SEM. Insulin-dependent diabetes mellitus: implications for male reproductive function. Hum Reprod. 2007;22:1871–77.
63. Lestienne P, Reynier P, Chretien MF, Penisson-Besnier I, Malthiery Y, Rohmer V. Oligoasthenospermia associated with multiple mitochondrial DNA arrangements. Mol Hum Reprod. 1997;3:811–14.
64. Kao SH, Chao HT, Wei YH. Multiple deletions of mitochondrial DNA are associated with the decline of motility and fertility of human spermatozoa. Mol Hum Reprod. 1998;4:657–66.
65. Spiropoulos J, Turnbull DM, Chinnery PF. Can mitochondrial DNA mutations cause sperm dysfunction. Mol Hum Reprod. 2002;8:719–21.
66. Green JR, Goble HL, Edwards CR, Dawson AM. Reversible insensitivity to androgens in men with untreated gluten enteropathy. Lancet. 1977;1:1280–2.
67. Farthing MJ, Edwards CR, Rees LH, Dawson AM. Male gonadal function in celiac disease: 1. Sexual dysfunction, infertility, and semen quality. Gut. 1982;23:608–14.
68. Zugna D, Richiardi L, Akre O, Stephansson O, Ludvigsson JF. Celiac disease is not a risk factor for infertility in men. Fertil Steril. 2011;95:1709–11.
69. Kruger TF, Acosta AA, Simmons KF, Swanson RJ, Matta JF, Veeck LL, Morshedi M, Brugo S. New method of evaluating sperm morphology with predictive value for human in vitro fertilization. Urology. 1987;30:248–51.
70. Kruger TF, Acosta AA, Simmons KF, Swanson RJ, Matta JF, Oehninger S. Predictive values of abnormal sperm morphology in in vitro fertilization. Fertil Steril. 1998;49:112–17.
71. Check JH, Adelson HG, Schubert BR, Bollendorf A. Evaluation of sperm morphology using Kruger's strict criteria. Arch Androl. 1992;28:15–7.
72. Eggert-Kruse W, Schwarz H, Rohr G, Demirakca T, Tilgen W, Runnebaum B. Sperm morphology assessment using strict criteria and male fertility under in-vivo conditions of conception. Hum Reprod. 1996;11:139–46.
73. Ghirelli-Filio M, Mizrahi FE, Pompeo ACL, Glina S. Influence of strict morphology on the results of classic in vitro fertilization. Int Braz J Urol. 2012;38:519–28.
74. Benoff S, Cooper GW, Hurley I, Mandel FS, Rosenfeld DL, Scholl GM, Gilbert BR, Hershlag A. The effect of calcium ion channel blockers on sperm fertilization potential. Fertil Steril. 1994;62:606–17.
75. Hull MG, Williams JA, Ray B, McLaughlin EA, Akande VA, Ford WC. The contribution of subtle oocyte or sperm dysfunction affecting fertilization in endometriosis-associated or unexplained infertility: a controlled comparison with tubal infertility and use of donor spermatozoa. Hum Reprod. 1998;7:1825–30.
76. Wolf JP, Bulwa S, Ducot B, Rodrigues D, Jouannet P. Fertilizing ability of sperm with unexplained in vitro fertilization failures, as assessed by the zona-free hamster egg penetration assay: its prognostic value for sperm-oolema interaction. Fertil Steril. 1996;65:1196–201.
77. Frapsauce C, Pionneau C, Booley J, de Larouziere V, Berthaut I, Ravel C, Antoine JM, Soubrier F, Madelbaum J. Unexpected in vitro fertilization failure in patients with normal sperm: a proteomic analysis. Gynecol Obstet Fertil. 2009;37:796–802.
78. Tollner TL, Venners SA, Hollox EJ, Yudin AI, Liu X, Tang G, Xing H, Kays RJ, Lau T, Overstreet JW, Xu X, Bevins CL, Cherr GN. A common mutation in the defensin DEFB126 causes impaired sperm function and subfertility. Sci Trans Med. 2011;3:92.
79. Barratt CL, Dunphy BC, McLeod I, Cooke ID. The poor prognostic value of low to moderate levels of sperm surface-bound antibodies. Hum Reprod. 1992;7:95–8.
80. Jarow JP, Sanzone JJ. Risk factors for male partner antisperm antibodies. J Urol. 1992;148:1805–7.
81. Rajah SV, Parslow JM, Howell RJ, Hendry WF. The effects of in-vitro fertilization of autoandibodies to spermatozoa in subfertile men. Hum Reprod. 1993;8:1079–82.
82. Hjort T, Hansen KB. Seminal antigens in man with particular regard to possible immunological contraception. In: Shulman S, Dondero F, editors. Immunological factors in human contraception. Rome: Acta Medica; 1983. p. 47–56.
83. Hammitt DG, Muench MM, Williamson RA. Antibody binding to greater than 50 % of the tail tip does not impair male fertility. Fertil Steril. 1988;49:1.

84. Acosta AA, van der Merwe JP, Doncel G, Kruger TF, Sayilgan A, Franken DR, Kolm P. Fertilization efficiency of morphologically abnormal spermatozoa in assisted reproduction is further impaired by antisperm antibodies on the male partner's sperm. Fertil Steril. 1994;62:826–33.
85. Shushan A, Schenker JG. Immunological factors in infertility. Am J Reprod Immunol. 1992;28:285–7.
86. Robbins WA, Vine MF, Trung KY, Everson RB. Use of fluorescence in situ hybridization (FISH) to assess effects of smoking, caffeine and alcohol on aneuploidy load in sperm of healthy men. Environ Mol Mutagen. 1997;30:175–83.
87. Rubes J, Lowe X, Moore D, Perrault S, Slott V, Evenson D, Selevan SG, Wyrobek AJ. Smoking cigarettes is associated with increased sperm disomy in teenage men. Fertil Steril. 1998;70:715–23.
88. Hughes EG, Brennan BG. Does cigarette smoking impair natural or assisted fecundity? Fertil Steril. 1996;66:679–89.
89. Richthoff J, Elzanaty S, Rylander L, Hagmer L, Giwercman A. Association between tobacco exposure and reproductive parameters in adolescent males. Int J Androl. 2007;31:31–9.
90. Vine MF, Margolin BH, Morrison HI, Hulka BS. Cigarette smoking and sperm density: a meta-analysis. Fertil Steril. 1994;61:35–43.
91. Vine MF, Tse CK, Hu P, Truong KY. Cigarette smoking and semen quality. Fertil Steril. 1996;65:835–42.
92. Practice Committee of the American Society for Reproductive Medicine. Smoking and infertility: a committee opinion. Fertil Steril. 2012;98(6):1400–6.
93. Zenzes MT, Bielecki R, Reed TE. Detection of benzo(a)pyrene diol epoxide-DNA adducts in sperm of men exposed to cigarette smoke. Fertil Steril. 1999;72:330–35.
94. Fraga CG, Motchnik PA, Wyrobek AJ, Rempel DM, Ames BN. Smoking and low antioxidant levels increase oxidative damage to sperm DNA. Mutat Res. 1996;351:199–203.
95. Hauser R. The environment and male fertility: recent research on emerging chemicals and semen quality. Sem Reprod Med. 2006;24:156–67.
96. McAuliffe ME, Williams PL, Korrick SA, Altshul LM, Perry MJ. Environmental exposure to polychlorinated biphenyls and p, p′-DDE and sperm sex-chromosome disomy. Environ Health Persp. 2012;120:535–40.
97. Duty SM, Silva MJ, Barr DB, Brock JW, Ryan L, Chen Z, Herrick RF, Christani DL, Hauser R. Phthalate exposure and human semen parameters. Epidemiology. 2003;14:269–77.
98. Hauser R, Meeker JD, Singh NP, Silva MJ, Ryan L, Duty S, Calafat AM. DNA damage in human sperm is related to urinary levels of phthalate monoester and oxidative metabolites. Hum Reprod. 2007;22:688–95.
99. Xu DX, Shen HM, Zhu QX, Chua L, Wang QN, Chia SE, Ong CN. The association among semen quality, oxidative DNA damage in human spermatozoa and concentrations of cadmium, lead and selenium in seminal plasma. Mutat Res. 2003;534:155–63.
100. Gennart JP, Buchet JP, Roels H, Ghyselen P, Ceulemans E, Lauwerys R. Fertility of male workers exposed to cadmium, lead, or manganese. Am J Epidemiol. 1992;135:1208–19.
101. Thonneau P, Marchand S, Tallec A, ferial ML, Ducot B, Lansac J, Lopes P, Tabaste JM, Spira M. Incidence and main causes of infertility in a resident population (1,850,000) of three French regions (1988–1989). Hum Reprod. 1991;6:811–6.
102. Patel ZP, Niederberger CS. Male factor assessment in infertility. Med Clin North Am. 2011;95:223–34.
103. World Health Organization. WHO laboratory manual for examination and processing of semen, 5th ed., 2010.
104. Barratt CL, Aitken RJ, Bjorndahl DT, Carrell DT, de Boer U, Kvist SE, Perrault SD, Perry MJ, Ramos L, Robaire B, Ward S, Zini A. Sperm DNA: organisation, protection, and vulnerability: from basic science to clinical applications–a position report. Hum Reprod. 2010;25:824–38.
105. Larson KL, DeJonge CJ, Barnes AM, Jost LK, Evenson DP. Sperm chromatin structure assay parameters as predictors of failed pregnancy following assisted reproductive techniques. Hum Reprod. 2000;15:1717–22.
106. Saleh RA, Agarwal A, Nelson DR, Nada EA, El-Tonsy MH, Alvarez JG, Thomas AJ, Sharma RK. Increased sperm nuclear DNA damage in normozoospermic infertile men: a prospective study. Fertil Steril. 2002;78:313–18.
107. Practice Committee of the American Society for Reproductive Medicine. The clinical utility of sperm DNA integrity testing. Fertil Steril. 2008;90:S178–80.
108. Aktan G, Dogru-Abbasoglu S, Kucukgergin C, Kadioglu A, Ozdemirler-Erata G, Kocak-Toker N. Mystery of idiopathic male infertility: is oxidative stress an actual risk? Fertil Steril. 2013;99:1211–15.
109. Erenpreiss J, Hlevica S, Zalkalns J, Erenpreisa J. Effect of leukocytospermia on sperm DNA integrity: a negative effect in abnormal semen samples. J Androl. 2002;23:717–23.
110. Greco E, Romano S, Iacobelli M, Ferrero S, Baroni E, Minasi MG, Ubaldi F, Rienzi L, Tesarik J. ICSI in cases of sperm DNA damage: beneficial effect of oral antioxidant treatment. Hum Reprod. 2005;20:2590–4.
111. Safarinejad MR. Efficacy of coenzyme Q10 on semen parameters, sperm function, and reproductive hormones in infertile men. J Urol. 2009;182:237–48.
112. Safarinejad MR, Safarinejad S, Shafiei N, Safarinejad S. Effects of the reduced form of coenzyme Q10 (ubiquinol) on semen parameters in men with idiopathic infertility: a double-blind, placebo controlled, randomized study. J Urol. 2012;188:526–31.
113. Li X, Pan J, Liu Q, Xiong E, Chen Z, Zhou Z, Su Y, Lu G. Glutathione S-transferases gene polymorphisms and risk of male idiopathic infertility: a systematic review and meta-analysis. Mol Biol Rep. 2013;40:2431–8.
114. Salvolini E, Buldreghini E, Lucarini G, Vignini A, Lenzi A, Di Primio R, Balercia G. Involvement of sperm plasma membrane and cytoskeletal proteins in human male infertility. Fertil Steril. 2013;99:697–704.
115. Hamada A, Esteves SC, Agarwal A. Unexplained male infertility: potential causes and management. Hum Androl. 2011;1:2–16.
116. Practice Committee of the American Society for Reproductive Medicine. Effectiveness and treatment of unexplained infertility. Fertil Steril. 2006;86 (Suppl 4):S111–4.
117. Guzick DS, Grefenstette I, Baffone K, Berga SL, Krasnow JS, Stovall DW. Infertility evaluation in fertile women: a model for assessing the efficacy of infertility testing. Hum Reprod. 1994;9:2306–10.
118. Guzick DS, Sullivan MW, Adamson GD, Cedars MI, Falk RJ, Peterson EP, Steinkampf MP. Efficacy of treatment for unexplained infertility. Fertil Steril. 1998;70:207–13.
119. Hull MG, Glazener CM, Kelly NJ, Conway DI, Foster PA, Hinton RA Coulson C, Lambert PA, Watt EM, Desai KM. Population study of causes, treatment, and outcome of infertility. Br Med J. 1985;291:1693–7.
120. Van Waart J, Ktuger F, Lombard CJ, Ombelet W. Predictive value of normal sperm morphology in intrauterine insemination (IUI): a structured literature review. Hum Reprod Update. 2001;7:495–500.
121. Ombelet W, Vandeput H, Van de Potte G, Cox A, Janssen M, Jacobs P, Bosmans E, Steeno O, Kruger T. Intrauterine insemination after ovarian stimulation with clomiphene citrate: predictive potential of inseminating motile count and sperm morphology. Hum Reprod. 1997;12:1458–63.
122. Kirby CA, Flaherty SP, Godfrey BM, Warnes GM, Matthews CD. A prospective trial of intrauterine insemination of motile spermatozoa versus timed intercourse. Fertil Steril. 1991;56:102–7.
123. Guzick DS, Carson SA, Coutifaris C, Overstreet JW, Factor-Litvak P, Steinkampf MP, et al. Efficacy of superovulation and intrauterine insemination in the treatment of infertility. National

Cooperative Reproductive Medicine Network. N Engl J Med. 1999;340:177–83.
124. Aboulghar M, Mansour R, Serour G, Abdrazek A, Amin Y, Rhodes C. Controlled ovarian hyperstimulation and intrauterine insemination should be limited to three trials. Fertil Steril. 2001;75:88–91.
125. Horvath PM, Beck M, Bohrer MK, Shelden RM, Kemmann E. A prospective study on the lack of development of antisperm antibodies in women undergoing intrauterine insemination. Am J Obstet Gynecol. 1989;160:631–7.
126. Stanford J, Mikolajczyk R, Lynch C, Simonsen S. Cumulative pregnancy rate probability among couples with subfertility: effects of varying treatments. Fertil Steril. 2010;93:2175–81.
127. Saleh RA, Agarwal A, Kandirali E, Sharma RK, Thomas AJ, Nada EA, Evenson DP, Alvarez JG. Leukocytospermia is associated with increased reactive oxygen species production by human spermatozoa. Fertil Steril. 2002;78:1215–24.
128. Nagy ZP, Verheyen G, Liu J, Joris H, Janssenswillen C, Wisanto A, Van Steirteghem AC. Andrology: results of 55 intracytoplasmic sperm injection cycles in the treatment of male-immunological infertility. Hum Reprod. 1995;10:1775–80.
129. Check ML, Check JH, Katsoff D, Summers-Chase D. ICSI as an effective therapy for male factor with antisperm antibodies. Syst Biol Reprod Med. 2000;45:125–30.
130. Kastrop PMM, Weima SM, van Kooij RJ, Velde ER. Comparison between intracytoplasmic sperm injection and in vitro fertilization (IVF) with high insemination concentration after total fertilization failure in a previous IVF attempt. Hum Reprod. 1998;14:65–9.
131. Hershlag A, Paine T, Kupail G, Feng H, Napolitano B. In vitro fertilization- intracytoplasmic sperm injection split: an insemination method to prevent fertilization failure. Fertil Steril. 2002;77:229–32.
132. Jaroudi K, Al-Hassan S, Al-Sufayan H, Al-Mayman H, Qeba M, Coskun S. Intracytoplasmic sperm injection and conventional in vitro fertilization are complementary techniques for management of unexplained infertility. J Assist Reprod Genet. 2003;20:377–81.
133. Bartoov B, Berkovitz A, Eltes F, Kogosowski A, Menezo Y, Barak Y. Real time fine morphology of motile human sperm cells is associated with IVF-ICSI outcome. J Androl. 2002;23:1–8.
134. Hazout A, Dumont-Hassan M, Junca AM, Cohen BP, Tesarik J. High magnification ICSI overcomes paternal effect resistant to conventional ICSI. Reprod Biomed Online. 2006;12:19–25.
135. Antinori M, Licata E, Dani G, Cerusico F, Versaci C, d'Angelo D, Antinori S. Intracytoplasmic morphologically selected sperm injection: a prospective randomized trial. Reprod Biomed Online. 2008;6:835–41.

Future Perspectives in the Diagnosis and Management of Unexplained Male Infertility

32

Avinash Maganty, Ranjith Ramasamy and Peter N. Schlegel

Stem Cell Biology

During a man's reproductive life, a pool of spermatogonial stem cells (SSCs), or germ cells, undergo self-renewal and differentiation to produce sperm through spermatogenesis. Fetal spermatogonia transform into adult dark spermatognoia (A_{Dark}). These A_{Dark} cells are diploid SSCs which have the ability to undergo self-renewal and differentiation. Through the process of asymmetric division, they are able to replace themselves and produce a differentiated progenitor daughter cell. These progenitor daughter cells are known as adult pale (A_{pale}) spermatogonia. A_{pale} cells produce B spermatogonia, and these spermatogonia can proliferate and differentiate to form spermatocytes. Spermatocytes undergo meiosis to form haploid spermatids that eventually mature into spermatozoa. The progression from the initial diploid SSC to the haploid spermatid to the mature spermatozoa takes approximately 64 days [1].

The male germline stem cells are able to produce sperm through the lifetime of an adult. Additionally, these stem cells are capable of indefinite self-renewal, making them ideal for therapeutic use. Harvesting the power of these stem cells and using them to grow sperm using *in vitro* would provide significant therapeutic options for men with unexplained infertility. To further understand the processes behind spermatogenesis and stem cells, several *in vivo* and *in vitro* models have been designed to recreate the testis environment.

In Vivo Studies

The differentiation and sell-renewal capability of germ cells is regulated by gene expression and external signals from the microenvironment, often referred to as a niche, in which the stem cell resides. Within the testis, the niche consists of Sertoli, Leydig, and peritubular cells. Each cell type plays a role in maintaining and regulating stem cells. Sertoli cells form the blood–testis barrier and secrete numerous factors such as growth factors, steroids, androgen binding protein, and extracellular matrix components that help to regulate spermatogenesis [2]. Leydig cells, following stimulation by luteinizing hormone, produce androgens that are necessary for the regulation of spermatogenesis and the development of secondary sexual characteristics. Peritubular cells have contractile function and secrete substances that serve to modulate Sertoli cell function. *In vivo* models utilize this idea of a niche to promote germ cell maturation and spermatogenesis. Two such models include the SSC transplantation and the xenograft model.

Spermatogonial Stem Cell Transplantation

SSCs can maintain the stem cell population and produce progeny cells leading to mature spermatozoa. Transplantation of these cells occurred in 1994 in a breakthrough study conducted by Brinster and Zimmerman in which they devised a technique for transplanting SSCs and demonstrated their ability to undergo spermatogenesis. They transferred SSCs from donor mice into mice treated with chemotherapy, generating germ cell aplasia. However, the cells making up the testicular niche, such as the Sertoli cells, were resistant to the effects of the chemotherapy. When the SSCs were injected into the seminiferous tubules where it is believed they established themselves in the functional niche along the seminiferous epithelium, they were able to proliferate and differentiate, thereby restoring spermatogenesis in the recipient. They were able to successfully restore spermatogenesis following this transplantation using the both fresh and cryopreserved donor SSCs. Spermatogenesis in the recipient mice showed normal morphology and produced mature spermatozoa [3]. This initial model has paved the way for the potential use of SSCs in the restoration of fertility,

P. N. Schlegel (✉) · A. Maganty · R. Ramasamy
Department of Urology, New York—Presbyterian Hospital, Weill Cornell Medical College, 525 East 68th St, Starr 900, New York, NY 10065, USA
e-mail: pnschleg@med.cornell.edu

G. L. Schattman et al. (eds.), *Unexplained Infertility*, DOI 10.1007/978-1-4939-2140-9_32,

especially in males who have undergone chemotherapy and radiation for the treatment of cancer.

This model has been expanded to other animals, including rats [4], dogs [5], goats [6], and primates [7]. Additionally, this technique has been further studied in terms of its ability to produce functional sperm that result in the production of live offspring. Goossens et al. demonstrated that SSC transplanted mice can produce live offspring; however, the litter sizes following *in vivo* conception were smaller than those obtained by control mice with normal fertility [8]. Fertilization rates after *in vitro* fertilization (IVF) were also reduced. Goossens et al. sought to identify possible reasons for reduced fertility rates in SSC transplanted mice and demonstrated that post-transplantation mice had a lower concentration of spermatozoa with reduced motility compared to controls [9].

Further advances of this model offer the possibility of its use in humans as a means of restoring fertility. One potential clinical application could be the preservation of fertility in prepubertal cancer patients. While postpubertal cancer patients have the ability to cryopreserve sperm before receiving chemo or radiation therapy, prepubertal patients cannot. The use of SSC transplantation offers a method of preserving fertility by harvesting SSCs prior to therapy, and reintroducing them at the appropriate time after completion of therapy.

While this model has significant potential clinical benefits, there are still several barriers to its use in humans. One such barrier is that the number of SSC that can be harvested from prepubertal testis is low and be insufficient to restore fertility upon transplantation [2]. The work by Sadri-Ardekani et al. has demonstrated the ability to culture and propagate human postpubertal SSCs, allowing for the opportunity to expand an SSC population before transplantation [10]. However, it is not yet known whether prepubertal cells will behave the same way. Another risk to utilizing this model in humans is that autologous SSC transplantation back into a patient who has been treated for cancer may result in the transplantation of malignant cells. One possible method of surpassing this limitation is through the use of flow cytometry. Fujita and colleagues isolated SSCs from leukemic mice and used flow cytometry to enrich for germ cells positive for H-2Kb/H-Kd and negative for CD45 (leukemic surface marker). They transplanted germ cell enriched fractions into mice treated with alkylating agents. The SSCs colonized successfully and the recipient mice survived to produce progeny. Transplantation without flow cytometry enrichment resulted in all transplanted mice developing leukemia [11]. While this method is promising, it is still not considered safe enough to allow SSC injections for humans.

SSC transplantation offers a potential therapy to unexplained male infertility (UMI), however more work remains to be done. Future work to be done includes analysis of risks to offspring obtained from SSC transplantation, methods of safely isolating SSCs from malignant cells, and the role of *in vitro* expansion of SSC populations.

Xenograft Transplantation Model

A xenograft transplantation model involves the transplantation of immature testis tissue into immunodeficient mice. Xenografts can allow for spermatogenesis to occur and the sperm obtained from the graft can be used with assisted reproduction to potentially produce offspring. This model offers another means of preserving the male fertility through transplantation of the germ cells as well as the surrounding cells that compose the microenvironment. While SCC transplantation is a valuable tool to study spermatogensis, it can be expensive to study larger animals. Additionally, SCC transplantation of germ cells from more phylogenetically distant species does not result in complete spermatogenesis, possibly due to incompatible microenvironments. The xenograft models allow for the study of larger animals by experimentation in smaller rodents by transferring small pieces of testis tissue, and thereby transferring the microenvironment as well [12]. Honoarammooz and colleagues first demonstrated that grafting immature mammalian testis tissue from a different donor species onto an immunodeficient mouse can lead to successful spermatogenesis and steroidgenesis. They also demonstrated that tissue previously cryopreserved could also be grafted and maintain the ability to undergo complete spermatogenesis. This has been achieved for a variety of animals including mice [12], pigs [13], goats [6], cats [14], and nonhuman primates [15]. Additionally, fertile offspring can be obtained by using assisted reproductive technology and sperm obtained from the grafts [16].

While other mammalian xenograft studies have been done, models using immature human testis is limited due to the lack of donors. Schlatt and colleagues grafted adult testis tissue from patients with infertility into immunodeficient mice and found that the adult tissue undergoes regression of spermatogenesis. However, when spermatogenesis was suppressed in the donor either through chemotherapy or hormonal treatment, there was better graft survival [17]. These results are also reflected in studies done with mature animals which have also shown that testis tissue grafts from mature donors do not support germ cell differentiation, but rather show degeneration of the tubules or the grafts. The reason for poor survival of mature testis tissue xenografts is unknown. Possible theories include a lack of Sertoli cell proliferation in mature tissue, transient ischemia before and immediately after grafting, and diminished testosterone production from mature Leydig cells [18].

In contrast to the mature testis grafting, immature human testis tissue grafting has been shown to allow increased germ cell survival. Yu et al. demonstrated that fetal testis tissue grafts were able to survive in immunodeficient mice for more than 135 days. They measured the success of their grafts by demonstrating increased graft weight, Sertoli cell differentiation, and germ cell migration to the basal lamina over time [19]. Sato et al. demonstrated spermatogenesis in xenografts of infant testicular tissue derived from 3-month old patients with testicular cancer. They showed that spermatogenesis progressed from the SSCs to pachytene spermatocytes. They also showed Sertoli and Leydig cell differentiation that was comparable to normal testicular development [20]. Goossens et al. obtained prepubertal testicular tissue from sickle cell patients prior to bone marrow depletion (placing them at increased risk for sterility) and grafted them onto immunodeficient mice. Wyns et al. reported xenograft survival of tissue derived from prepubertal patients for more than 6 months. They demonstrated spermatogonial survival and production of premeiotic spermatocytes. However, they did not observe normal spermatogenesis with production of mature sperm cells [21]. Goossens et al. observed graft survival greater than 9 months, however, only Sertoli cells and a few spermatogonia were observed at the end of the 9 months. Spermatogenesis was never observed [22].

While human xenograft models offer a potential means of preserving fertility especially for patients undergoing treatment for childhood cancers, there are a number of limitations to the model. Although long-term survival of the graft, Sertoli cell maturation, and survival of germ cells has been observed, complete spermatogenesis has not yet been demonstrated. Future studies should evaluate relative survival of different fragment sizes to be grafted, impact of cryopreservation, and the role of gonadotropin supplementation. Further refinement of this model could also lead to its use for human reproductive toxicology studies. Rather than use healthy subjects, the xenograft model can be used to determine the reproductive impact of various chemicals and pharmacologic agents [2].

In Vitro Studies

In vitro models provide another future option for male fertility treatment by allowing the process of spermatogenesis to occur in a culture dish. *In vitro* models provide a means of producing male haploid gametes through the culturing and differentiation of SSCs. These gametes can then be used for ICSI as a way to circumvent male infertility.

Historical experiments of testicular tissue culture demonstrated that there was maintenance of specific architecture in which there was cell-to-cell communication between somatic and germ cells. However, these early studies did not demonstrate complete spermatogenesis, rather only showed arrest in meiosis [23–25]. Subsequent studies have provided refinements to the model and demonstrated that *in vitro* models require the presence of somatic and germ cells, incubation at a lower temperature compared to other cell types [26], and tissue should be derived from an immature donor [27].

A more current experimental approach involves using organ culture of testes fragments. This method allows for the maintenance of the testicular architecture, which is important for spermatogenesis. Sato and colleagues employed an organ culture technique in which they placed testis tissue fragments from neonatal mice on agarose gel half-soaked in medium lacking serum. They omitted the serum because they believed it may contain factors that inhibit spermatogenesis. Using this system, they were able to obtain sperm in 27–45 days that was reproductively competent as determined by microinsemination [28]. Through the preservation of the cytoarchitecture in this method, the endogenous factors were able to be released by the seminiferous epithelium to help in regulating the germ cells. With a multitude of signaling pathways involved in the germ cell differentiation process, researchers have also concentrated their efforts on identifying specific substances that may be associated with the differentiation pathway.

Newer culturing techniques have been developed that utilize a three-dimensional (3D) matrix of soft agar or methylcellulose in which germ and somatic cells are embedded. This system is based on the assumption that somatic cells provide both physical and paracrine support that enables germ cells to enter meiosis. This method employed by Stukenborg et al. was meant to reconstitute the 3D microenvironment of the seminiferous epithelium and allow for the maintenance of cell-to-cell contacts and signaling mechanisms necessary for germ cell differentiation [29]. Using this model, they were able to demonstrate the maturation of germ cells into normal spermatozoa. This 3D technique has not yet been attempted using human testicular tissue.

While there has been success in animal research, human studies are still needed. Coculturing techniques may be promising with regards to maturation of spermatocytes in humans. Cremades and colleagues have used a coculture system in which they were able to demonstrate *in vitro* maturation of round spermatids derived from azoospermic men to mature sperm when cocultured with Vero cells [30]. Vero cells are an immortalized kidney epithelial cell line from the green monkey and are embryological similar to the genital epithelial cells. They function by removing toxic compounds from the medium and provide important growth factors. Using similar techniques, Tanaka et al. obtained primary spermatocytes from azoospermic men and cocultured them with Vero cells. They demonstrated that the primary spermatocytes could mature into round spermatids, and confirmed their haploid status using Giemsa staining [31]. While coculture techniques with Vero cells may be promising, in order to apply them to a clinical setting, care must be taken with regards to infection transmission and tumorogenesis associated with Vero cell use.

In vitro models offer the capability of reproducing the biological processes occurring within the testes. In order to successfully do this, researchers are trying to imitate the *in vivo* processes. The hope is that this technology will eventually be able to reverse cases of incomplete spermatogenesis by producing gametes *in vitro* using culture techniques.

Pluripotent Stem Cells to Germ Cells *In Vitro*

Pluripotent stem cells as well as embryonic stem cells (ES cells) have the capability of self-renewal and differentiation. Differentiation of these stem cells into germ cells offers the possibility of generating sperm from pluripotent cells *in vitro*. This is essentially done by providing the ES cells with an environment (containing differentiating factors) within which they can differentiate *in vitro*. Of the multiple cell lineages produced by differentiation, germ cells can be specifically selected using germ cell specific cell surface markers and genetic profiles.

This methodology has been employed using mouse ES cells. Geijesen et al. were able to use this property to obtain primordial germ cells (PGCs) from mouse ES cells in culture. These germ cells were able to differentiate into gametes and using ICSI they demonstrated that these gametes were able to form embryos that reached the blastocyst stage [32]. Other groups took this idea further and generated male gametes from mouse ES cells *in vitro*. Using ICSI, these gametes were used to fertilize mouse oocytes to generate live offspring [33]. However, the efficiency of offspring production was low (7 out of 65 embryos) and many of the mice generated died prematurely.

While studies in mice have shown that PGCs can be obtained from mouse ES cells and can undergo further differentiation to produce mature gametes, studies in humans are not as advanced. There have been several recent developments in humans with regards to *in vitro* gamete development from ES cells. Tilgner and colleagues developed a protocol to differentiate two human ES cells lines into PGCs [34]. In addition to PGC production, Alfatoonian and colleagues were the first to produce postmeiotic spermatid cells *in vitro* [35]. Currently, the generation of mature sperm has not been demonstrated *in vitro* using human ES cells. While ES cells may offer a promising avenue for germ cell generation, ES cells are obtained from human embryo tissue and aborted fetus, making their use controversial.

Since much controversy and ethical issues surround the use of human ES cells, induced pluripotent stem cells have been developed from somatic cells through activation of specific genes [36]. Just like human ES cells, human induced pluripotent stem cells (iPSCs) have been used to produce not only PGCs, but haploid-like cells as well [37]. While iPSCs may provide a means to continue advancement while avoiding controversy, iPSC production may be associated with genetic instability [2]. High-resolution single-nucleotide polymorphism (SNP) analysis was performed on pluripotent samples and an increased frequency of copy number variations and mutations [38]. The results imply that there is a genetic instability in iPSCs and therefore their clinical use is limited until the implications of the instability can be deduced.

Male Infertility—Potential for Stem Cell Therapy

A substantial limitation of the application of stem cell therapy to male infertility is the likely genetic basis for most causes of severe spermatogenic dysfunction in the human. Where spermatogenic disruption is caused by a genetic factor, simply placing germ cells back into the genetically deficient host may not restore spermatogenesis, as the host is unable to efficiently support sperm development. In these cases, both stem cell therapy and management of the genetic defect may be needed.

Genetics and Gene Therapy in Male Infertility

Advances in stem cell therapy can help men with spermatogenic failure, especially those undergoing chemotherapy or radiation therapy. However, there is a predominant subset of men in whom genetic defects are responsible for infertility [39]. Gene therapy can be useful in these particular instances because it allows for the delivery of the missing genetic factors that are necessary for sperm production. Gene therapy is the introduction of a gene encoding a missing or mutated protein that is missing in a diseased cell. These genes could be introduced into the sperm or testes through the use of viral or nonviral vectors.

Gene Therapy Using Nonviral Vectors

Numerous methods utilizing nonviral vectors have been employed to introduce transgenes into sperm and testis. Nonviral vectors are advantageous in that they are cheap, have no DNA size limitations, and have a good safety profile [40]. However, expression of genes is short term and transfection efficiency is often low.

Sperm-mediated gene transfer (SMGT) emerged as means of generating transgenic animals through *in vitro* methods. SMGT is an *in vitro* method in which foreign DNA is introduced into sperm, which can then be used to fertilize an oocyte to create transgenic offspring. It has been demonstrated that sperm can spontaneously take up exogenous DNA through specific DNA binding and internalization [41]. Numerous studies have successful demonstrated the ability of sperm to take up exogenous DNA in a variety of species including mouse [42], chicken [43], pig [44], and the zebrafish [45]. Several studies have sought to improve the efficiency of gene transfer through the use of liposomes [46] and electroporation. Such methods have been used to successfully introduce transgenes into spermatozoa and fertilize oocytes with detection of the transgene in the offspring [47]. SMGT, however, is still not a reliable method for gene transfer because of its variability in transfer efficiency and gene expression.

Transgenes can also be introduced into testes by direct introduction of foreign DNA into the testes, a process known as testis-mediated gene transfer (TMGT). This is an *in vivo* method that allows for mass transfer of genes into the testes and subsequent natural mating. Similar to SMGT, various strategies of introduction have been explored. Mouse testis injected with plasmids encapsulated in liposomes resulted in transfer of DNA into testicular spermatozoa and subsequent detection of the transgenes in the offspring generated from mating with treated males [48]. *In vivo* electroporation is another technique that involves injecting a DNA construct into the testes with application of electric pulses that permeates cell membranes and allow DNA to enter the cells. Using *in vivo* electroporation, groups have demonstrated the ability to express transgenes in mature epididymal sperm in mice [49] and hamsters [50]. They also demonstrated that the use of electroporation *in vivo* does not lead to adverse effects on testicular integrity and sperm quality [49]. However, the expression of these transgenes is typically transient and may last as long as 60 days. Additionally, only 5–10% of sperm were found to carry the transgene indicating a low transfer rate [50].

Several groups were able to apply these techniques to assess the role of nonviral vector-based gene therapy in rescuing infertility. For example, Yomogida and colleagues were able to rescue spermatogenesis in mutant mice, that were rendered infertile by an alteration in stem cell factor in Sertoli cells, using gene transfer via electroporation [51]. Dobashi and colleagues used electroporation to introduce an erythropoietin gene into rat testes and found that it helped to reduce the risk of germ cell loss caused by cryptorchidism [52].

As previously mentioned, while there are a number of advantages to using nonviral vectors, the technique is not well controlled and lacks precision. Although the technique has utility in the production of transgenic animals, it is not currently appropriate for clinical applications.

Viral Vectors for Gene Therapy

Viral vectors offer a means of transfecting testicular cells *in vivo* and *in vitro*. They are more efficient in terms of transfection compared to nonviral vectors; however, they are limited by the size of DNA that can be inserted and immunogenicity of the vectors.

There are several types of viral vectors. Adenoviral vectors are most commonly used. They are able to infect dividing and differentiated cells and tend not to integrate into the host genome [40]. Using adenovirus vectors, transgenes were transferred to animal testes *in vivo*. When the viral vector was injected intratesticularly, expression of the transgene was strongest in the Leydig cells. Conversely, when the viral vector was injected intratubularly, the strongest expression was detected in Sertoli cells [53, 54]. No transgene expression was detected in germ cells using either of the injection methods [55]. Therefore, the transgene was not detected in offspring, suggesting germline transmission is very low.

Additional viral vectors include retroviral and lentiviral vectors. Retroviral vector is an established tool for gene transfer. Retroviruses only infect dividing cells and integrate transgenes into the genome [47]. Retroviral vectors were found to introduce transgenes into the germ line and spermatogonia *in vitro* [56] and *in vivo* [57]. Lentiviral vector use in basic science research has been increasing due to its capacity to efficiently transduce cells with long-term gene expression using large-sized DNA [40]. They can infect both dividing and nondividing cells.

Researchers have used viral vector-based gene therapy techniques in animals to study many diseases, including male infertility. Ikawa et al. demonstrated that mice Sertoli cells lacking expression of a transmembrane type c-kit ligand (involved in spermatogenesis) were able to achieve restoration of spermatogenesis using a lentiviral vector to transduce Sertoli cells [58]. The sperm generated was collected and able to generate offspring using ICSI. Additionally, none of the offspring carried the transgene which demonstrated that lentiviral vectors do not carry the risk of germline transmission, although other studies have shown transgene expression in the germ line when using lentivirus [59]. Using adenoviral-mediated gene transfer of hepatocyte growth factor (HGF) gene into the testis of cryptorchidism rats, HGF overexpression was induced in seminiferous epithelial cells and interstitial cells. This resulted in a decreased germ cell apoptosis and restoration of spermatogenesis [60]. An adenovirus with the HST-1/FGF-4 gene, previously shown to be important for spermatogenesis [61], was introduced into mouse testis. Its expression helped to ameliorate testicular toxicity induced using Adriamycin, an anticancer drug [62].

Future of Gene Therapy Techniques and the Treatment of Male Infertility

Spermatogenesis is a complex process involving differentiation of cells that occurs in a complicated microenvironment. Gene expression plays a significant role in the regulation of spermatogenic mechanisms. A potential cause of UMI may be gene defects. Therefore, understanding the genes involved in this process will aid in the developing treatment strategies for male infertility. Knockout mice studies have been invaluable in determining male fertility-associated genes [63].

While there is still no report regarding a clinical application of gene transfer to testes in humans, gene therapy techniques are continuing to advance and offer the potential for future clinical use. However, the administration of gene therapy on human germ cell line is prohibited. The prohibition is largely due to the potential adverse effects in subsequent generations as well as the ethical concerns associated with the therapy. Additionally, there are still significant risks associated with gene transfer, including toxicity and oncogenicity. While there are still ethical and technical barriers that must be overcome, gene therapy still offers an exciting tool to combat male infertility.

Since germ cell targeting is ethically questionable, targeting of Sertoli and Leydig cells is a potential future clinical application for treating male infertility using gene therapy techniques. Sertoli and Leydig cells are both important for spermatogenesis, and therefore are potential targets for transgene introduction. Since Sertoli and Leydig cell function is important for spermatogenesis, their dysfunction can lead to infertility. Rescue of their function by way of gene transfer is a potential future therapeutic option. There are a number of possible genes that are important for Sertoli cell function. Abnormalities in the maturation of Sertoli cells may lead to testicular dysfunction. Therefore, understanding expression patterns of genes that signify Sertoli cell maturity such as anti-Mullerian hormone, vimentin, aromatase, and inhibin alpha my provided a basis for gene therapy-based interventions [40]. Dysfunction of transcriptional regulation due to defective transcription factors (such as CREB, Sox3, PEM, and DAX1) may result in male infertility [40]. Leydig cells are also a potential gene therapy. Their dysfunction can lead to infertility, which is believed to be one of the mechanisms of infertility in Kleinfelter (47XXY) syndrome [40, 64]. Marker genes expressed involved in spermatogenesis that are expressed by Leydig cells have been identified [40, 65]. Additional information about these genes involved in Sertoli and Leydig cell function may make it more feasible to approach clinical treatment using gene therapy techniques in the future.

Conclusion

There has been significant advancement in therapeutic technology for the treatment of UMI. The *in vivo* animal studies offer hope of restoring spermatogenesis in germ cell deficient mice. While SCC transplantation and xenograft models have successfully restored spermatogenesis in animals, their remains limitations in humans. SCC transplantation is still not safe for human use. Xenograft models have yet to demonstrate complete spermatogenesis in humans. Much progress has been made with *in vitro* techniques in terms of replicating the testis microenvironment in rodents. However, more human studies are still needed. While the use of ES cells is interesting, there is significant ethical controversy that prevents its advancement. Induced pluripotent stem cells offer a means of circumventing the ethical concerns; however, their genetic stability is questionable and more work needs to be done to assess their safety. Gene therapy technology has become more sophisticated and offers a means of correcting infertility at the level of a single gene. However, both the risks and ethical concerns regarding the possibility of germline introduction of transgenes require additional studies to determine the clinical feasibility of this technique. Despite several developments, translational safety is required before any of these methods can be applied clinically.

References

1. Slobodan V, Čukuranović R, Bjelaković MD, Stefanović V. Possible therapeutic use of spermatogonial stem cells in the treatment of male infertility: a brief overview. The Sci World J. 2012;2012(Article ID 374151):8.
2. Lo KC, Domes T. Can we grow sperm? A translational perspective on the current animal and human spermatogenesis models. Asian J Androl. 2011;13:677–82.
3. Brinster RL, Zimmermann JW. Spermatogenesis following male germ-cell transplantation. Proc Natl Acad Sci U S A. 1994;91: 11298–302.
4. Zhang Z, Renfree MB, Short RV. Successful intra- and interspecific male germ cell transplantation in the rat. Biol Reprod. 2003;68: 961–7.
5. Kim Y, Turner D, Nelson J, Dobrinski I, McEntee M. Production of donor-derived sperm after spermatogonial stem cell transplantation in the dog. Reproduction. 2008;136:823–31.
6. Honaramooz A, Behboodi E, Blash S, Megee SO, Dobrinski I. Germ cell transplantation in goats. Mol Reprod Dev. 2003;64:422–8.
7. Schlatt S, Foppiani L, Rolf C, Weinbauer GF, Nieschlag E. Germ cell transplantation into X-irradiated monkey testes. Hum Reprod. 2002;17:55–62.
8. Goossens E, Frederickx V, De Block G, Van Steirteghem AC, Tournaye H. Reproductive capacity of sperm obtained after germ cell transplantation in a mouse model. Hum Reprod. 2003;18:1874–80.
9. Goossens E, De Block G, Tournaye H. Computer-assisted motility analysis of spermatozoa obtained after spermatogonial stem cell transplantation in the mouse. Fertil Steril. 2008;90(4):1411–6.

10. Sadri-Ardekani H, Mizrak SC, van Daalen SK, Korver CM, Roepers-Gajadien HL, et al. Propagation of human spermatogonial stem cells *in vitro*. JAMA. 2009;302:2127–34.
11. Fujita K, Hiroshi O, Tsujimura A, Takao T, Miyagawa Y, et al. Transplantation of spermatogonial stem cells isolated from leukemic mice restores fertility without inducing leukemia. J Clin Invest. 2005;115:1855–61.
12. Honaramooz A, Snedaker A, Boiani M, Schöler H, Dobrinskil I, Schlatt S. Sperm from neonatal mammalian testes grafted in mice. Nature. 2002;418:778–81.
13. Honaramooz A, Megee SO, Dobrinski I. Germ cell transplantation in pigs. Biol Reprod. 2002;66:21–8.
14. Snedaker AK, Honaramooz A, Dobrinski I. A game of cat and mouse: xenografting of testis tissue from domestic kittens results in complete cat spermatogenesis in a mouse host. J Androl. 2004;25:926–30.
15. Honaramooz A, Li MW, Penedo MC, Meyers S, Dobrinski I. Accelerated maturation of primate testis by xenografting into mice. Biol Reprod. 2004;70:1500–3.
16. Schlatt S, Honaramooz A, Boiani M, Schöler HR, Dobrinski I. Progeny from sperm obtained after ectopic grafting of neonatal mouse testes. Biol Reprod. 2003;68:2331–5.
17. Schlatt S, Honaramooz A, Ehmcke J, Goebell PJ, Rübben H, et al. Limited survival of adult human testicular tissue as ectopic xenograft. Hum Reprod. 2006;21:384–9.
18. Arregui L, Rathi R, Zeng W, Honaramooz A, Gomendio M, et al. Xenografting of adult mammalian testis tissue. Anim Reprod Sci. 2008;106:65–76.
19. Yu J, Cai ZM, Wan HJ, Zhang FT, Ye J, et al. Development of neonatal mouse and fetal human testicular tissue as ectopic grafts in immunodeficient mice. Asian J Androl. 2006;8:393–403.
20. Sato Y, Nozawa S, Yoshiike M, Arai M, Sasaki C, et al. Xenografting of testicular tissue from an infant human donor results in accelerated testicular maturation. Hum Reprod. 2010;25:1113–2.
21. Wyns C, Curaba M, Martinez-Madrid B, Van Langendonckt A, Francois-Xavier W, Donnez J. Spermatogonial survival after cryopreservation and short-term orthotopic immature human cryptorchid testicular tissue grafting to immunodeficient mice. Hum Reprod. 2007;22:1603–11.
22. Goossens E, Geens M, De Block G, Tournaye H. Spermatogonial survival in long-term human prepubertal xenografts. Fertil Steril. 2008;90:2019–22.
23. Champy C. Quelques résultats de la méthode de culture des tissus. Arch Zool Exp Gen. 1920;60:461–500.
24. Goldschmidt R. Some experiments on spermatogenesis *in vitro*. Proc Natl Acad Sci U S A. 1915;1:220–2.
25. Michailow M. Experimentell-histologische untersuchungen über die elemente der hodenkanälchen. Z Zellforsch. 1937;26:174–201.
26. Nakamura M, Romrell LJ, Hall PF. The effects of temperature and glucose on protein biosynthesis by immature (round) spermatids from rat testes. J Cell Biol. 1978;79:1–9.
27. Creemers LB, den Ouden K, van Pelt AM, de Rooij DG. Maintenance of adult mouse type A spermatogonia *in vitro* influence of serum and growth factors and comparison with prepubertal spermatogonial cell culture. Reproduction. 2002;124:791–9.
28. Sato T, Katagiri K, Gohbara A, Inoue K, Ogonuki N, et al. *In vitro* production of functional sperm in cultured neonatal mouse testes. Nature. 2011;471:504–7.
29. Stukenborg JB, Schlatt S, Simoni M, Yeung CH, Elhija MA, et al. New horizons for *in vitro* spermatogenesis? An update on novel three-dimensional culture systems as tools for meiotic and post-meiotic differentiation of testicular germ cells. Mol Hum Reprod. 2009;15:521–9.
30. Cremades N, Bernabeu R, Barros A, Sousa M. *In-vitro* maturation of round spermatids using co-culture on Vero cells. Human Reprod. 1999;14(5):1287–93.
31. Tanaka A, Nagayoshi M, Awata S, Mawatari Y, Tanaka I, et al. Completion of meiosis in human primary spermatocytes through *in vitro* coculture with Vero cells. Fertil Steril. 2003;79:795–801.
32. Geijsen N, Horoschak M, Kim K, Gribnau J, Eggan K, et al. Derivation of embryonic germ cells and male gametes from embryonic stem cells. Nature. 2004;427:148–54.
33. Nayernia K, Nolte J, Michelmann HW, Lee JH, Rathsack K, et al. *In vitro*-differentiated embryonic stem cells give rise to male gametes that can generate offspring mice. Dev Cell. 2006;11:125–32.
34. Tilgner K, Atkinson SP, Golebiewska A, Stojkovic M, Lako M, Armstrong L. Isolation of primordial germ cells from differentiating human embryonic stem cells. Stem Cells. 2008;26:3075–85.
35. Aflatoonian B, Ruban L, Jones M, Aflatoonian R, Fazeli A, Moore HD. *In vitro* post-meiotic germ cell development from human embryonic stem cells. Hum Reprod. 2009;24:3150–9.
36. Yamanaka S, Blau H. Nuclear reprogramming to a pluripotent state by three approaches. Nature. 2010;465:704–12.
37. Eguizabal C, Montserrat N, Vassena R, Barragan M, Garreta E, Garcia-Quevedo L, et al. Complete meiosis from human induced pluripotent stem cells. Stem Cells. 2011;29:1186–95.
38. Laurent LC, Ulitsky I, Slavin I, Tran H, Schork A, et al. Dynamic changes in the copy number of pluripotency and cell proliferation genes in human ESCs and iPSCs during reprogramming and time in culture. Cell Stem Cell. 2011;8:106–18.
39. Katherine LOFOB, Alex C, Varghese AC, Agarwal A. The genetic causes of male factor infertility: a review. Fertil Steril. 2010;93: 1–12.
40. Kojima YMK, Umemoto Y, Sasaki S, Hayashi Y, Kohri K. Therapeutic potential of gene transfer to testis; myth or reality? In: Kang C, editor. Gene therapy applications. Shanghai: InTech; 2011: 279–296.
41. Lavitrano M, French D, Zani M, Frati L, Spadafora C. The interaction between exogenous DNA and sperm cells. Mol Reprod Dev. 1992;31:161–9.
42. Maione B, Lavitrano M, Spadafora C, Kiessling AA. Sperm-mediated gene transfer in mice. Mol Reprod Dev. 1998;50:406–9.
43. Nakanishi A, Iritani A. Gene transfer in the chicken by sperm mediated methods. Mol Reprod Dev. 1993;36:258–61.
44. Lavitrano M, Bacci ML, Forni M, Lazzereschi D, Di Stefano C, Fioretti D. Efficient production by sperm-mediated gene transfer of human decay accelerating factor (hDAF) transgenic pigs for xenotransplantation. Proc Natl Acad Sci U S A. 2002;99:14230–5.
45. Khoo HW. Sperm-mediated gene transfer studies on zebrafish in Singapore. Mol Reprod Dev. 2000;56:278–80.
46. Bachiller D, Schellander K, Peli J, Ruther U. Liposome mediated DNA uptake by sperm cells. Mol Reprod Dev. 1991;30:194–200.
47. John Parrington KC, Joaquin G. Sperm and testis mediated DNA transfer as a means of gene therapy. Systems Biol Reprod Med. 2011;57:35–42.
48. Sato M, Gotoh K, Kimura M. Sperm-mediated gene transfer by direct injection of foreign DNA into mouse testis. Transgenics. 1999;2:357–69.
49. Coward K, Kubota H, Hibbit O, McIlhinney J, Kohri K, Parrington J. Expression of a fluorescent recombinant form of sperm protein phospholipase C zeta in mouse epididymal sperm by *in vivo* gene transfer into the testis. Fertil Steril. 2006;85:1281–9.
50. Hibbit O, Coward K, Kubota H, Prathalingham N, Holt W, Kohri K, Parrington J. *In vivo* gene transfer by electroporation allows expression of a fluorescent transgene in hamster testis and epididymal sperm and has no adverse effects upon testicular integrity or sperm quality. Biol Reprod. 2006;74:95–101.
51. Yomogida K, Yagura Y, Nishimune Y. Electroporated transgene-rescued spermatogenesis in infertile mutant mice with a sertoli cell defect. Biol Reprod. 2002;67:712–7.
52. Dobashi M, Goda K, Maruyama H, Fujisawa M. Erythropoietin gene transfer into rat testes by *in vivo* electropo-ration may reduce

the risk of germ cell loss caused by cryptorchidism. Asian J Androl. 2005;7:369–73.
53. Kojima Y, Sasaki S, Umemoto Y, Hashimoto Y, Hayashi Y, Kohri K. Effects of adenovirus mediated gene transfer to mouse testis *in vivo* on spermatogenesis and next generation. J Urol. 2003;170:2109–14.
54. Blanchard KT, Boekelheide K. Adenovirus-mediated gene transfer to rat testis *in vivo*. Biol Reprod. 1997;56:495–500.
55. Kojima Y, Hayashi Y, Kurokawa S, Mizuno K, Sasaki S, Kohri K. No evidence of germ-line transmission by adenovirus-mediated gene transfer to mouse testes. Fertil Steril. 2008;89:1448–54.
56. De Miguel MP, Donovan PJ. Determinants of retroviral-mediated gene delivery to mouse spermatogonia. Biol Reprod. 2003;68:860–6.
57. Kanatsu-Shinohara M, Toyokuni S, Shinohara T. Transgenic mice produced by retroviral transduction of male germ line stem cells *in vivo*. Biol Reprod. 2004;71:1202–7.
58. Ikawa M, Tergaonkar V, Ogura A, Ogonuki N, Inoue K, Verma IM. Restoration of spermatogenesis by lentiviral gene transfer: offspring from infertile mice. Proc Natl Acad Sci U S A. 2002;99:7524–9.
59. Coward K, Kubota H, Parrington J. *In vivo* gene transfer into testis and sperm: developments and future application. Arch Androl. 2007;53:187–97.
60. Goda K, Fujisawa M, Shirakawa T, Dobashi M, Shiota G, Zhang ZJ, Gotoh A, Kamidono S. Adenoviral-mediated HGF expression inhibits germ cell apoptosis in rats with cryptorchidism. J Gene Med. 2004;6:869–76.
61. Yamamoto H, Ochiya T, Takahama Y, Ishii Y, Osumi N, Sakamoto H, Terada M. Detection of spatial localization of Hst-1/Fgf-4 gene expression in brain and testis from adult mice. Oncogene. 2000;19:3805–10.
62. Yamamoto H, Ochiya T, Tamamushi S, Toriyama-Baba H, Takahama Y, Hirai K, Sasaki H, Sakamoto H, Saito I, Iwamoto T, Kakizoe T, Terada M. HST-1/FGF-4 gene activation induces spermatogenesis and prevents adriamycin-induced testicular toxicity. Oncogene. 2002;21:899–908.
63. Cram DS, O'Bryan MK, DE Kretser DM. Male infertility genetics–the future. J Androl. 2000;22(5):738–46.
64. Aksglaede L, Wikström AM, Rajpert-De Meyts E, Dunkel L, Skakkebaek NE, Juul A. Natural history of seminiferous tubule degeneration in Klinefelter syndrome. Hum Reprod Update. 2006;12:39–48.
65. Kojima Y, Sasaki S, Kohri K. Therapeutic options: current research and future prospects for gene therapy in andrology. In: Schill W-F, Comhaire FH, Hargreave TB, editors. Andrology for the clinician. Heidelberg:Springer; 2006. pp. 592–7.

Index

G. L. Schattman et al. (eds.), *Unexplained Infertility*, DOI 10.1007/978-1-4939-2140-9,

MIX
Papier aus verantwortungsvollen Quellen
Paper from responsible sources
FSC® C105338

If you have any concerns about our products,
you can contact us on
ProductSafety@springernature.com

In case Publisher is established outside the EU,
the EU authorized representative is:
Springer Nature Customer Service Center GmbH
Europaplatz 3, 69115 Heidelberg, Germany

Printed by Libri Plureos GmbH
in Hamburg, Germany